Practical Pharmaceutics

Practical Pharmaceutics

Edited by Mary Durrant

hayle medical

New York

Hayle Medical,
750 Third Avenue, 9th Floor,
New York, NY 10017, USA

Visit us on the World Wide Web at:
www.haylemedical.com

ISBN: 978-1-64647-109-6

Cataloging-in-Publication Data

Practical pharmaceutics / edited by Mary Durrant.
p. cm.
Includes bibliographical references and index.
ISBN: 978-1-64647-109-6
1. Pharmacy. 2. Drugs. 3. Pharmacology. 4. Materia medica. I. Durrant, Mary.
RS92 .P73 2022
615.1--dc23

Table of Contents

Preface

The purpose of the book is to provide a glimpse into the dynamics and to present opinions and studies of some of the scientists engaged in the development of new ideas in the field from very different standpoints. This book will prove useful to students and researchers owing to its high content quality.

The discipline within pharmacy which is involved in the process of turning a new chemical entity into medication which can be safely and effectively used by patients is known as pharmaceutics. It deals with the chemicals which have pharmacological properties and generally exist as white amorphous or crystalline powders. These chemicals need to be formulated into a dosage form. There are numerous branches of pharmaceutics such as pharmaceutical formulation, pharmaceutical manufacturing and dispensing pharmacy. Pharmaceutical formulation deals with the process through which different chemical substances are combined to produce a final medicinal product. Pharmaceutical manufacturing deals with the industrial scale synthesis of pharmaceutical drugs by pharmaceutical companies. This book provides significant information of this discipline to help develop a good understanding of pharmaceutics and related fields. The various studies that are constantly contributing towards advancing technologies and evolution of this field are examined in detail. This book includes contributions of experts and scientists which provide innovative insights into this field.

At the end, I would like to appreciate all the efforts made by the authors in completing their chapters professionally. I express my deepest gratitude to all of them for contributing to this book by sharing their valuable works. A special thanks to my family and friends for their constant support in this journey.

Editor

1

Stability Indicating Liquid Chromatographic Method for the Simultaneous Determination of Rosuvastatin and Ezetimibe in Pharmaceutical Formulations

Mathrusri Annapurna Mukthinuthalapati*, Venkatesh Bukkapatnam, Sai Pavan Kumar Bandaru

Department of Pharmaceutical Analysis & Quality Assurance, GITAM Institute of Pharmacy, GITAM University, Visakhapatnam-530045, India.

Article info

Keywords:
- RP-HPLC
- Rosuvastatin
- Ezetimibe
- Isocratic
- ICH guidelines

Abstract

Purpose: A simple stability indicating reverse phase liquid chromatographic method was developed for the simultaneous determination of rosuvastatin and ezetimibe in pharmaceutical formulations.

Methods: Best chromatographic response was achieved with C18 column (250 X 4.6 mm, 5μm) with photo diode array (PDA) detector. The mobile phase was composed of a mixture of sodium acetate buffer (pH 4.0) and acetonitrile (30:70, %v/v) with a flow rate of 1.2 mL/min. (UV detection at 254 nm). Rosuvastatin and ezetimibe were subjected to stress conditions of degradation and the method was validated as per ICH guidelines.

Results: The method shows linearity over a concentration range of 0.5–250 μg/ml for both rosuvastatin (r^2 = 0.9993) and ezetimibe (r^2 = 0.9996). Both the drugs are highly sensitive towards alkaline conditions in comparison to other stress conditions.

Conclusion: The proposed method can be successfully applied to perform long-term and accelerated stability studies for the simultaneous determination of rosuvastatin and ezetimibe in pharmaceutical formulations.

Introduction

Rosuvastatin (RST) is chemically designated as (3R, 5S, 6E) - 7 - [4 - (4 - fluorophenyl) - 2 - (N - methylmethanesulfonamido) - 6 - (propan - 2 - yl) pyrimidin - 5 - yl] - 3, 5 - dihydroxyhept - 6 - enoic acid (Figure 1A).[1] It is a member of the drug class of statins. It is used in the treatment of Hyperlipidemia. Rosuvastatin Calcium is a selective and competitive inhibitor of hydroxyl methyl glutaryl coenzyme A (HMG CoA) reductase (a precursor of cholesterol), the rate-limiting enzyme that converts 3-hydroxyl-3-methylglutaryl coenzyme A to mevalonate. It reduces levels of low-density lipoprotein, apolipoprotein B and triglycerides in the blood, while increasing levels of high-density lipoprotein in the management of hyper lipidaemias.[2] Ezetimibe (EZT) chemically designated as (3R, 4S) - 1 - (4 - fluorophenyl) - 3 - [(3S) - 3 - (4 - fluorophenyl) - 3 - hydroxypropyl] - 4 - (4 - hydroxyphenyl) azetidin - 2 - one (Figure 1B). [1] It is a selective cholesterol absorption inhibitor, used for the treatment of hyperlipidemia, which potentially inhibits the absorption of biliary and dietary cholesterol. Ezetimibe prevents intestinal absorption of cholesterol without affecting absorption of triglycerides, fatty acids and fat-soluble vitamins.[3-5]

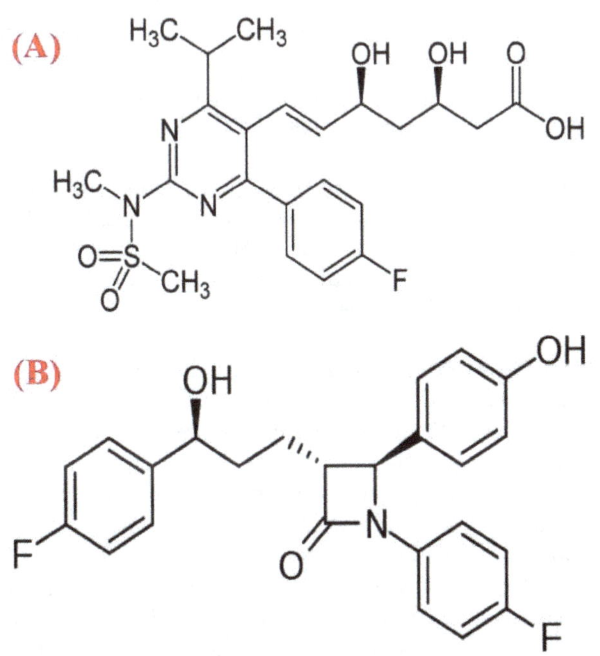

Figure 1. Chemical structures of rosuvastatin [A] and ezetimibe [B].

Various analytical techniques such as micellar liquid chromatography,[6] HPLC,[7-13] HPTLC,[14-15] densitometric

***Corresponding author:** Mathrusri Annapurna Mukthinuthalapati, Email: mathrusri2000@yahoo.com

TLC,[16] spectrophotometry[17-19] and spectrofluorimetry[20] have been developed for the simultaneous determination of rosuvastatin and ezetimibe in pharmaceutical formulations. In the present study an attempt has been made to develop a validated stability indicating RP-HPLC method for the simultaneous determination of rosuvastatin and ezetimibe in pharmaceutical formulations as per ICH guidelines.[21]

Materials and Methods

Chemicals

Reference standards of rosuvastatin (purity 99%) and ezetimibe (purity 99.5 %) were obtained from Glenmark Pharmaceuticals Ltd., India. The combination of rosuvastatin and ezetimibe is available as film-coated tablets (10 mg of rosuvastatin and 10 mg of ezetimibe) with brand names RAZEL-EZ® (Glenmark Pharmaceuticals Ltd., India) and ROSUVAS-EZ ® (Ranbaxy Laboratories Ltd., India) and were procured from the local pharmacy store. HPLC grade (Merck) solvents and chemicals were used for the entire study.

Instrumentation and chromatographic conditions

Chromatographic separation was attained by means of a Shimadzu Model CBM-20A/20 Alite HPLC system, equipped with SPD M20A prominence photodiode array detector and a Rheodyne injection valve with a 20 µL loop. The experimental conditions were optimized on a C18 (250 mm × 4.6 mm i.d., 5 µm particle size) column maintained at 25 °C. Isocratic elution was performed using sodium acetate buffer (pH 4.0) and acetonitrile (30:70, %v/v). The overall run time was 10 min. The flow rate was 1.2 ml/min. 20 µl of sample was injected into the HPLC system and all chromatographic conditions were performed at room temperature (25°C ± 2°C).

Preparation of sodium acetate buffer solution (pH 4.0)

The buffer solution was prepared by mixing 28.6 ml of glacial acetic acid with 10ml of 50% w/v NaOH in to a 1000 ml volumetric flask, dissolving and diluting to volume with HPLC grade water.

Preparation of rosuvastatin and ezetimibe stock solutions

Stock solutions of rosuvastatin (1000 µg/ml) and ezetimibe (1000 µg/ml) were prepared by accurately transferring 25 mg of rosuvastatin and ezetimibe separately in two 25 ml volumetric flasks and the volume was made up to volume with mobile phase. Working solutions for HPLC injections were prepared on a daily basis from the stock solution with mobile phase containing sodium acetate buffer and acetonitrile (30:70, % v/v). Solutions were filtered through a 0.45 µm membrane filter prior to injection.

Assay of marketed formulations

Twenty tablets from each marketed brands (RAZEL-EZ® and ROSUVAS-EZ®) were procured from pharmacy store and tablet powder equivalent to 25 mg of each of rosuvastatin and ezetimibe was accurately transferred to 25ml volumetric flask and extracted with acetonitrile. The solution was sonicated and filtered and the filtrate was further diluted with mobile phase as per the requirement. All the solutions were filtered through 0.45 mm nylon filter prior injecting in to HPLC system.

Method Validation

Linearity

A series of drug solutions were prepared containing both rosuvastatin and ezetimibe together from their stock solutions and 20 µL of each mixture was injected in to the HPLC system. The peak area of each drug in the chromatogram was recorded. A calibration curve was plotted by taking the concentration on the x-axis and the corresponding peak area on the y-axis for each drug separately.

Accuracy

The accuracy of the assay method was evaluated in triplicate at three concentration levels (50, 100 and 150%), and the percentage recoveries were calculated. Standard addition and recovery experiments were conducted to determine the accuracy of the method for the quantification of rosuvastatin and ezetimibe in the marketed product. The study was carried out in triplicate at 150, 200 and 250 µg/ml and the percentage recovery in each case was calculated.

Precision

The intra-day and inter-day precision of the method were evaluated at three different concentration levels (10, 50 and 100 µg/ml) (n=3) against a qualified reference standard. The intra-day precision study was conducted on the same day where as the inter-day precision study was conducted on three different days i.e. day 1, day 2 and day 3.

Robustness

The robustness of an analytical procedure refers to its ability to remain unaffected by small and deliberate variations in method parameters and provides an indication of its reliability for routine analysis.[21] The robustness of the method was evaluated by assaying the drug solution by deliberately changing the different analytical parameters such as the detection wavelength (252 and 256 nm i.e. ± 2 nm), the mobile phase composition (sodium acetate buffer: acetonitrile, 32:68 and 28:72 i.e. ± 2 %, v/v), the flow rate (1.1 and 1.3 ml/min i.e. ± 0.1 ml/min) etc. and the % RSD was calculated.

Sensitivity/ Limit of detection and limit of quantitation

The limit of quantification (LOQ) and limit of detection (LOD) were based on the standard deviation of the response and the slope of the constructed calibration curve (n=3), as described in International Conference on Harmonization guidelines Q2 (R1).[21] Sensitivity of the method was established with respect to limit of detection

(LOD) and LOQ for analytes. LOD and LOQ were established by slope method as mentioned below.

$$\text{LOD} = \frac{3.3 \times \text{standard deviation of calibration curve}}{\text{Slope of the calibration curve}}$$

$$\text{LOQ} = \frac{10 \times \text{standard deviation of calibration curve}}{\text{Slope of the calibration curve}}$$

Forced Degradation Studies

Stress studies were performed to evaluate the specificity of the method.[22] All samples were diluted with mobile phase to give a final concentration 100 µg/ml and filtered through 0.45 µm nylon filter before injection.

Acidic degradation

Acidic degradation was performed by treating the drug solution mixture (containing each of 1 mg/ml rosuvastatin and ezetimibe) with 0.1 N hydrochloric acid for 30 min in a thermostat maintained at 80 °C. The drug solution mixture was cooled, neutralized with 0.1 N sodium hydroxide and then diluted with mobile phase as per the requirement and 20 µL of the solution was injected in to the HPLC system.

Alkaline degradation

Alkaline degradation was performed by treating the drug solution mixture (containing each of 1 mg/ml rosuvastatin and ezetimibe) with 0.1 N sodium hydroxide for 30 min in a thermostat maintained at 80 °C. The drug solution mixture was cooled, neutralized with 0.1 N hydrochloric acid and then diluted with mobile phase as per the requirement and 20 µL of the solution was injected in to the HPLC system.

Oxidation degradation

Oxidation degradation was performed by treating the drug solution mixture (containing each of 1 mg/ml rosuvastatin and ezetimibe) with 30% H_2O_2 for 30 min in a thermostat maintained at 80 °C. The drug solution mixture was cooled and then diluted with mobile phase as per the requirement and 20 µL of the solution was injected in to the HPLC system.

Photolytic degradation

The drug solution mixture (containing each of 1 mg/ml rosuvastatin and ezetimibe) was exposed to UV light (365 nm) for 3 hours, diluted with mobile phase as per the requirement and 20 µL of the solution was injected in to the HPLC system.

Thermal degradation

The drug solution mixture (containing each of 1 mg/ml rosuvastatin and ezetimibe) was in a thermostat maintained at 80 °C for 10 hours, cooled and 20 µL of the solution was injected in to the HPLC system after necessary dilution with mobile phase.

Results and Discussion

HPLC method development and optimization

Initially the stressed samples were analyzed using a mobile phase consisting of sodium acetate: acetonitrile (60:40, % v/v) at a flow rate of 1.2 mL/min. Under these conditions, a broad peak was eluted for rosuvastatin at 9.775 min and therefore the mobile phase composition was changed to 55: 45, v/v) with the same flow rate under which a sharp peak was observed with slight tailing. Finally the mobile phase composition was changed as 30:70, % v/v where a sharp peak was eluted at 2.563 min for rosuvastatin. In similar conditions ezetimibe was also eluted at 3.629 min and therefore mobile phase consisting of sodium acetate: acetonitrile (30:70, % v/v) with a flow rate of 1.2 mL/min was chosen as the best chromatographic response for the simultaneous determination of rosuvastatin and ezetimibe. UV detection was carried out at 254 nm (PDA detector).

Method Validation

Linearity

The combination of rosuvastatin and ezetimibe shows linearity over a concentration range of 0.5 to 250 µg/ml and the linear regression equations were found to be y = 30291x + 53405 (r^2 = 0.9993) and y = 39595x + 53321 (r^2 = 0.9996) for rosuvastatin and ezetimibe respectively. The chromatogram of the mobile phase (blank) and that of the combination of rosuvastatin and ezetimibe was shown in Figure 2.

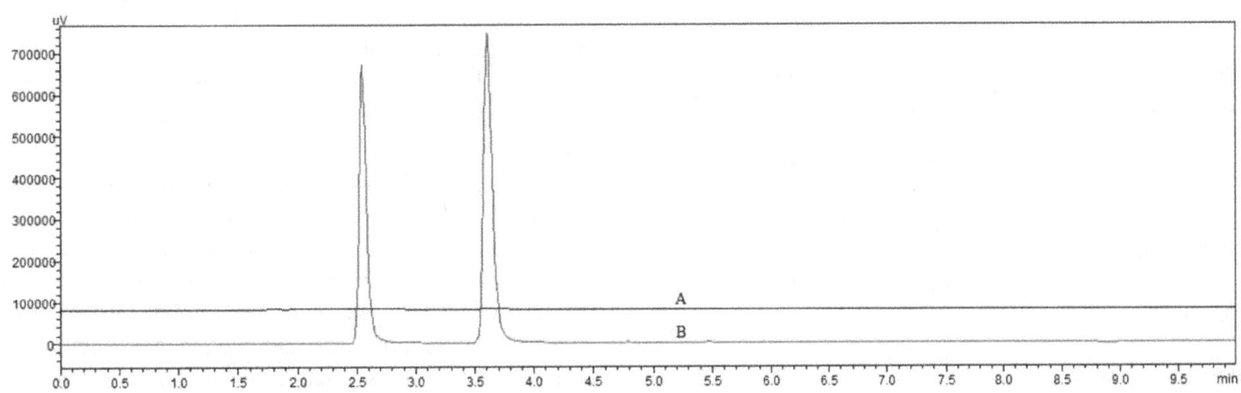

Figure 2. Typical chromatograms of blank [A], rosuvastatin and ezetimibe [B].

Accuracy

The method accuracy was proved by the recovery test. A known amount of rosuvastatin and ezetimibe standards (100 µg/ml) were added to aliquots of sample solutions and then diluted to yield the total concentrations of 150, 200 and 250 µg/ml as described in Table 1. The assay was repeated over three consecutive days and the resultant % RSD was found to be 0.21-0.41 and 0.50-0.73 with a recovery of 98.29-101.48 % and 99.41-99.81 % for rosuvastatin and ezetimibe respectively.

Table 1. Accuracy studies of rosuvastatin and ezetimibe

Drugs	Conc. (µg/mL)			*Mean peak area ± SD (%RSD)	Drug found (µg/mL)	% Recovery
	Formulation	Pure drug	Total			
Rosuvastatin	100	50	150	4602347.33±15847.32 (0.35)	150.21	100.14
	100	100	200	6202425.00±25385.87 (0.41)	202.95	101.48
	100	150	250	7500280.33±15623.15 (0.21)	245.73	98.29
Ezetimibe	100	50	150	5956160.67±35196.04 (0.60)	149.11	99.41
	100	100	200	7932586.67±57655.07 (0.73)	198.97	99.48
	100	150	250	9936336.33±49615.788 (0.50)	249.51	99.81

* Mean of three replicates

Precision

The intra-day precision of the method was determined by assaying three samples of each at three different concentration levels (10, 50 and 100 µg/ml) on the same day. The inter-day precision was calculated by assaying three samples of each at three different concentration levels (10, 50 and 100 µg/mL) on three different days. The % RSD for intra-day precision was found to be 0.41-0.94 and 0.31-0.59 for rosuvastatin and ezetimibe respectively whereas the inter-day precision was found to be 0.68-0.95 and 0.68-1.02 for rosuvastatin and ezetimibe respectively (Table 2).

Table 2. Precision studies of rosuvastatin and Ezetimibe

Drugs	Conc. (µg/mL)	Intra-day precision		Inter-day precision	
		Conc. (µg/mL) found	% RSD	Conc. (µg/mL) found	% RSD
Rosuvastatin	10	9.93	0.94	9.97	0.89
	50	50.05	0.74	49.91	0.76
	100	100.28	0.41	100.03	0.68
Ezetimibe	10	9.94	0.44	9.91	0.68
	50	49.98	0.59	50.06	0.89
	100	100.11	0.31	100.04	1.02

Sensitivity/ Limit of quantification (LOQ) and limit of detection (LOD)

The LOD and LOQ were found to be 0.1149 µg/ml and 0.3483 µg/ml for rosuvastatin and the LOD and LOQ for Ezetimibe were 0.1365 µg/ml and 0.4135 µg/ml respectively.

Robustness

The results of the robustness study were given in Table 3. The slight changes in flow rate, mobile phase composition etc. affects the chromatographic response such as retention time, tailing factor and theoretical plates etc. The % RSD obtained was 0.52-0.95 % and 0.71-1.38 % for rosuvastatin and ezetimibe respectively (< 2.0%) indicating that the proposed method is robust.

Analysis of commercial formulations

The proposed method was applied for the determination of rosuvastatin and ezetimibe in marketed formulations available (RAZEL-EZ® and ROSUVAS-EZ®). The % recovery was found to be 96.48 and 96.97 respectively.

Forced Degradation Studies

The specificity of the developed method can be determined from the stress studies and the percentage drug recovery was calculated from the peak area of the resultant chromatograms.

30.27 % of rosuvastatin has undergone alkaline degradation. The carboxylic acid group present in the rosuvastatin chemical structure is highly responsible for the alkaline degradation. Lactonization of the β-hydroxy acid and lactone ring formation can takes place at the same time and reports on such interconversion process have been seen in the literature for statins (Ex: Atorvastatin).[23] Ezetimibe also has undergone alkaline degradation (43.94 %) and the phenolic hydroxyl group present in the chemical structure may be responsible for it. During the oxidation an extra peak was observed at 1.915 min. During the acidic, oxidative, photolytic and thermal degradations the percentage of decomposition was found to be less than 20.0 %. The chromatograms obtained during the stress degradation conditions were shown in Figure 3A-3E.

Table 3. Robustness studies of rosuvastatin (100 μg/mL) and ezetimibe (100 μg/mL)

Parameter		Condition	Conc. (μg/mL) found	% RSD	% Assay
Rosuvastatin	Flow rate (mL/min)	1.1 1.2 1.3	99.84	0.52	99.84
	Detection wavelength (nm)	252 254 256	99.67	0.42	99.67
	Mobile phase composition (v/v)	32:68 30:70 28:72	100.17	0.76	100.17
	pH ± 0.1	3.9 4.0 4.1	99.28	0.95	99.28
Ezetimibe	Flow rate (mL/min)	1.1 1.2 1.3	99.40	0.71	99.40
	Detection wavelength (nm)	252 254 256	98.88	0.99	98.88
	Mobile phase composition (v/v)	32:68 30:70 28:72	100.21	1.38	100.21
	pH ± 0.1	3.9 4.0 4.1	99.60	0.93	99.60

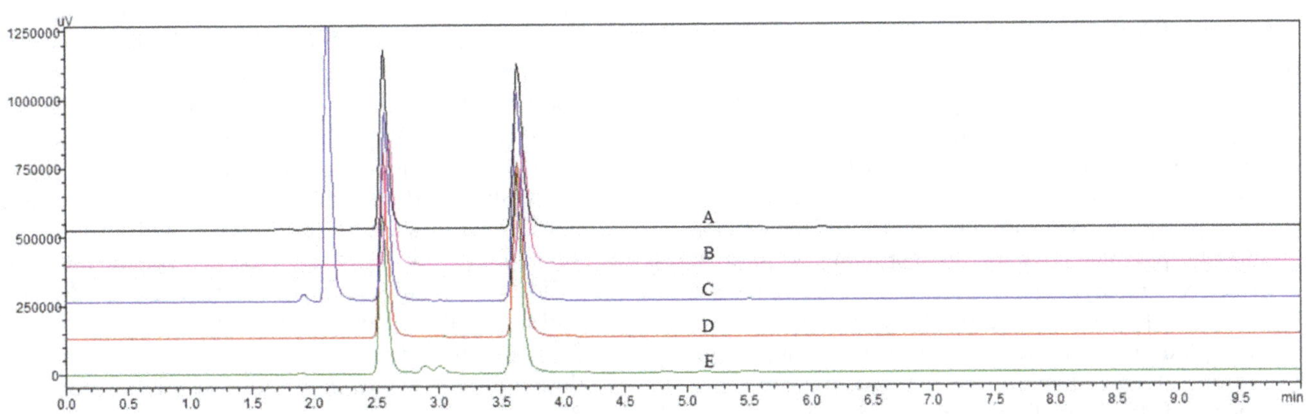

Figure 3. Typical Chromatograms of rosuvastatin and ezetimibe on acidic [A], alkali [B], oxidation [C], thermal [D] and photolytic [E] degradations.

The system suitability parameters for all the degradation studies were shown in Table 4. The number of theoretical plates (N) is used to determine the performance and effectiveness of the column. The efficiency of a column can be measured by the number of theoretical plates per meter. It is a measure of band spreading of a peak. Smaller the band spread, higher is the number of theoretical plates, indicating good column and system performance. Columns with N ranging from 5,000 to 100,000 plates / meter are ideal for a good system. Efficiency can be calculated by using the formula: $N = 5.54\ [R/W_{h/2}]^2$

Where 'W' is the peak width, 'h' is the height of the peak and 'R_t' is the retention time of the drug peak. The theoretical plates were found to be more than 2000 and the tailing factor was less than <1.5 –2 or <2 indicating that the method is more selective and specific.

Table 4. Forced degradation studies of rosuvastatin and ezetimibe

Stress conditions		% Drug recovered	% Drug decomposed	Theoretical plates	Tailing factor	% RSD
Rosuvastatin	Standard drug	100	0	6091.624	1.471	0.21
	Acidic degradation	98.92	1.08	6021.477	1.485	0.35
	Alkaline degradation	69.73	30.27	5923.741	1.495	0.23
	Oxidative degradation	97.61	2.39	6137.202	1.480	0.54
	Photolytic degradation	87.92	12.08	5546.035	1.450	0.48
	Thermal degradation	99.63	0.37	6017.274	1.488	0.57
Ezetimibe	Standard drug	100	0	8432.386	1.415	0.42
	Acidic degradation	80.95	19.05	8600.699	1.479	0.85
	Alkaline degradation	56.06	43.94	9001.826	1.432	0.74
	Oxidative degradation	99.43	0.57	8807.580	1.423	0.56
	Photolytic degradation	98.67	1.33	8528.807	1.414	0.23
	Thermal degradation	96.22	3.78	8385.751	1.436	0.62

* Mean of three replicates

Conclusion

The proposed method for the simultaneous determination of rosuvastatin and ezetimibe is simple, specific, precise, accurate, and robust and validated as per the ICH guidelines and can be applied for the long term stability studies as well as for the kinetic studies of the pharmaceutical formulations. The method was validated as per the ICH guidelines.

Acknowledgements

The authors are grateful to M/s GITAM University, Visakhapatnam for providing the research facilities and UGC, New Delhi for their financial support.

Conflict of interest

The authors report no conflicts of interest.

References

1. Budavari S. The Merck Index: an encyclopedia of chemicals, drugs, and biologicals. 13th ed. New Jersey: Merck and Company, Inc; 2001.
2. Mctaggart F, Buckett L, Davidson R, Holdgate G, Mccormick A, Schneck D, et al. Preclinical and clinical pharmacology of Rosuvastatin, a new 3-hydroxy-3-methylglutaryl coenzyme A reductase inhibitor. *Am J Cardiol* 2001;87(5A):28B-32B.
3. Kosoglou T, Statkevich P, Johnson-Levonas AO, Paolini JF, Bergman AJ, Alton KB. Ezetimibe: a review of its metabolism, pharmacokinetics and drug interactions. *Clin Pharmacokinet* 2005;44(5):467-94.
4. Van Heek M, France CF, Compton DS, Mcleod RL, Yumibe NP, Alton KB, et al. In vivo metabolism-based discovery of a potent cholesterol absorption inhibitor, SCH58235, in the rat and rhesus monkey through the identification of the active metabolites of SCH48461. *J Pharmacol Exp Ther* 1997;283(1):157-63.
5. Knopp RH, Bayes H, Manion CV, Lipka LJ, Melani L, LeBeaut AP, et al. Effect of ezetimibe on serum concentrations of lipid soluble vitamins. *Atherosclerosis* 2001;2(2):90.
6. Sharma S, Sharma MC, Kohli DV, Chaturvedi SC. Micellar liquid chromatographic method development for determination of rosuvastatin calcium and ezetimibe in pharmaceutical combination dosage form. *Der Pharma Chemica* 2010;2(1):371-7.
7. Mohammed IB, Vanitha Prakash K, Krishna Mohan G. RP-HPLC method for the simultaneous estimation of rosuvastatin and ezetimibe from their combination tablet dosage form. *Int J Chem Anal Sci* 2013;4(4):205-9.
8. Sree Janardhanan V, Manavalan R, Valliappan K. Chemometric technique for the optimization of chromatographic system: Simultaneous HPLC determination of rosuvastatin, telmisartan, ezetimibe and atorvastatin used in combined cardiovascular therapy. *Arab J Chem* 2012. Inpress.
9. Varma D PSRChNP, Lakshmana Rao A, Dinda SC. Development and validation of stability indicating RP-HPLC method for simultaneous estimation of rosuvastatin and ezetimibe in combined tablet dosage form. *Rasayan J Chem* 2012;5(3):269-79.
10. Anuradha KG, Vishal DS. Development and validation of a stability-indicating reversed-phase HPLC method for simultaneous estimation of rosuvastatin and ezetimibe from their combination dosage forms. *Eurasian J Anal Chem* 2010;5(3):265-83.
11. Eswarudu MM, Mounica P, Venkatesh D, Nagalakshmi B. Method development and validation for simultaneous estimation of rosuvastatin calcium and ezetimibe in pharmaceutical dosage form by RP-HPLC. *Int Res J Pharm App Sci* 2012;2(1):24-36.
12. Joshi H, Kumar S, Yadav YC, Seth AK. New analytical method development and validation of rosuvastatin and ezetimibe in tablet dosage form. *Int J Drug Discov Med Res* 2012;1(2):22-9.
13. Sharma S, Sharma MC, Kohli DV, Chaturvedi SC. Simultaneous estimation of rosuvastatin calcium and ezetimibe in tablet dosage form by reverse phase high

performance liquid chromatography. *Optoelectron Adv Mat Rapid Comm* 2010;4(2):238-41.

14. Varghese SJ, Ravi TK. Determination of rosuvastatin and ezetimibe in a combined tablet dosage form using high-performance column liquid chromatography and high-performance thin-layer chromatography. *J AOAC Int* 2010;93(4):1222-7.
15. Sharma MC, Sharma S, Kohli DV, Sharma AD. A validated HPTLC method for determination of simultaneous estimation rosuvastatin calcium and ezetimibe in pharmaceutical solid dosage form. *Arch Apll Sci Res* 2010;2(1):1-7.
16. Hiral JP, Bhanubhai NS. Method development and validation of LC and densitometric-TLC for simultaneous estimation of rosuvastatin calcium and ezetimibe in combined dosage forms. *Der Pharma Chemica* 2013;5(3):208-15.
17. Anuradha KG, Vishal DS. Simultaneous UV-spectrophotometric estimation of rosuvastatin and ezetimibe in their combined dosage forms. *Int J Pharm Sci* 2010;2(1):131-8.
18. Pandya CB, Channabasavaraj KP, Shridhara HS. Simultaneous estimation of rosuvastatin calcium and ezetimibe in bulk and tablet dosage form by simultaneous equation method. *Int J Chem Tech Res* 2010; 2(4):2140-4.
19. Anuradha GK, Vishal DS. Simultaneous estimation of rosuvastatin and ezetimibe by ratio spectra derivative spectrophotometry method in their fixed dosage forms. *Intl J Pharm Tech Res* 2010;2(1):404-10.
20. El-bagary RI, Elkady EF, Kadry AM. Spectrofluorometric determination of certain anti-hyperlipidemic agents in bulk and pharmaceutical preparations. *Spectrosc- Int J* 2012;27(2):83-92.
21. ICH, Validation of analytical procedures: Text and methodology, Q2 (R1). International Conference on Harmonization; IFPMA, Geneva, 2005.
22. ICH, Stability testing of new drug substances and products, Q1A(R2). International Conference on Harmonization; IFPMA, Geneva, 2003.
23. Mohammadi A, Rezanour N, Ansari Dogaheh M, Ghorbani Bidkorbeh F, Hashem M, Walker RB. A stability-indicating high performance liquid chromatographic (HPLC) assay for the simultaneous determination of atorvastatin and amlodipine in commercial tablets. *J Chromatogr B Analyt Technol Biomed Life Sci* 2007;846(1-2):215-21.

D-optimal Design for Preparation and Optimization of Fast Dissolving Bosentan Nanosuspension

Elham Ghasemian, Parisa Motaghian, Alireza Vatanara*

Pharmaceutics Department, Faculty of Pharmacy, Tehran University of Medical Sciences, Tehran, Iran.

Article info

Keywords:
· Bosentan
· Nanosuspension
· Optimization
· D-optimal
· Stabilizer

Abstract

Purpose: Bosentan is a drug currently taken orally for the treatment of pulmonary arterial hypertension. However, the water solubility of bosentan is very low, resulting in low bioavailability. The aim of this study was preparation and optimization of bosentan nanosuspension to improve solubility and dissolution rate.

Methods: The different formulations designed by Design Expert® software. Nanosuspensions were prepared using precipitation method and the effects of stabilizer type and content and drug content on the particle size, polydispersity (PDI) and yield of nanosuspensions were investigated.

Results: Particle size, PDI and yield of the optimal nanosuspension formulation were 200.9 nm, 0.24 and 99.6%, respectively. Scanning electron microscopy (SEM) results showed spherical morphology for bosentan nanoparticles. Thermal analysis indicated that there was a partial crystalline structure and change in the pholymorphism of bosentan in the nanoparticles. In addition, reduction of particle size, significantly increased *in vitro* dissolution rate of the drug.

Conclusion: Optimization by design expert software was shown to be a successful method for optimization and prediction of responses by less than 10% error and formulation with 15.8 mg span 85 as an internal stabilizer and 45 mg drug content were introduced as the optimum formulation. The solubility of bosentan in the optimal formulation was 6.9 times higher than coarse bosentan and could be suggested as promising drug delivery systems for improving the dissolution rate and possibly the pharmacokinetic of bosentan.

Introduction

Pulmonary arterial hypertension (PAH) is a devastating and progressive disease that usually characterized by remodeling of the pulmonary vasculature.[1] The progressive vasculopathy increases the pulmonary arterial pressure and pulmonary vascular resistance, eventually culminating in limited patients exercise capacity, right ventricular failure and death.[2] Endothelin plays a major role in the pathogenesis of pulmonary arterial hypertension and induction of vasoconstriction.[3] Additionally, endothelin 1 is a smooth-muscle mitogen, and can potentially raise the vascular tone and pulmonary vascular hypertrophy.[4]

Bosentan is an orally active, selective and competitive non-peptide dual endothelin receptor (both ET_A and ET_B) antagonist and usually used in cure of PAH.[5] Bosentan is also being considered for treatment of other conditions such as Eisenmenger syndrome,[6] persistent pulmonary hypertension of the newborn,[7] digital ulcer prevention in patients with systemic sclerosis,[8] adolescent and adult patients who have undergone Fontan operation,[9] vascular remodeling and dysfunctional angiogenesis in diabetes[10] and possibly even depression.[11]

For treatment of PAH, bosetan is currently administered at the daily dose of 125-250 mg.[12] The maximum plasma peak is seen within 3-5 h after oral intake and the half-life of drug is 5.4 h.[13] Moreover, the bioavailability of bosentan after oral administration is approximately low (50%)[14] and variability is seen in bosentan absorption which may get back to its poor water solubility.[13] The water solubility of bosentan is low (1 mg/100 ml)[15] and classified in class II of BCS.[16] So, increasing the solubility of bosentan can improve its pharmacokinetics and dose reduction and variability in drug exposure among individuals can be solved.[17]

One of the strategies in solubility enhancement is particle size reduction.[18] Nanoparticle are colloidal drug delivery systems usually between 10-1000 nm in size. Due to the high surface to volume ratio, nanoparticles can provide better solubility, adsorption and improve therapeutic outcomes.[19] Pharmaceutical nanosuspensions can be designed to be taken orally and topically or through parenteral or inhalation routes.

The aim of this study is preparation, characterization and optimization of bosentan nanosuspention by using of experimental design to enhance the solubility and dissolution rate.

***Corresponding author:** Alireza Vatanara, Email: vatanara@tums.ac.ir

Materials and Methods

Materials

Bosentan was provided by Pajouhesh Darou Arya, Iran. Sodium dodecyl sulfate (SDS) and HPβCD were purchased from Sigma Aldrich, USA. Tween 20, Tween 80, Span 85 and acetonitrile were from Merck. Acetone was from Applichem, Germany.

Preliminary study on nanosuspension formulation

Bosentan nanosuspensions were prepared by the antisolvent precipitation method in the presence of different types of surfactants in aqueous phase. First, the screening was done on the effect of some formulation parameters on the characterization of prepared nanoparticles as presented in Table 1. In summary, a combination of bosentan, 25 mg tween 80 (internal stabilizer) and 1 ml acetone were placed in a beaker and mixed (organic phase). In another beaker, the aqueous phase was prepared by dissolving of 2 mg/ml external stabilizer in distilled water. Subsequently, the organic phase was emulsified dropwise in aqueous phase. Emulsification was carried out using a homogenaizer (High Shear T25D, IKA, Germany) for 3 min in 18000 rpm. Then, the emulsion was treated with an ultrasonic probe (UP400S_Ultrasonic processor, Hielscher, Germany) at power input of 320W and a cycle of 0.7 per second for 3 min.

Next, acetone was eliminated by evaporation under reduced pressure using a rotary evaporator (Buchi, Switzerland). Nanoparticles were recovered by centrifugation (sigma, Germany) at 20000 rpm for 25 min at 25 °C.

Table 1. Screening formulation for evaluation effect of external stabilizer type, aqueous volume and drug content on the size and PDI of prepared nanosuspension formulation

Stabilizer type	Water amount	Drug content (mg)	Size (nm)	PDI
Tween80	25	25	2190	0.3
		15	Large	1.0
	40	25	3323	0.2
		15	2250	0.4
βCD	25	25	1426	0.6
		15	1561	0.9
	40	25	1216	0.6
		15	950	0.8
HPβCD	25	25	732	0.5
		15	440	0.8
	40	25	443	0.3
		15	400	0.4
SDS	25	25	2132	1.0
		15	601	0.9
	40	25	1652	0.3
		15	700	0.6

Experimental design

Experimental design is one of the most reliable methods for selection of the best formulation as optimized, when different factors and variables are involved. The information obtained from this mathematical method can yield the combination of variables that can make up the best formulation. In the current research, 17 formulations with 3 variables –two levels of qualitative variable and 3 levels of quantitative variable (low, medium and high) - were assessed using D-optimal design and Design Expert® V6 (DX6) software for design of experiments (DOE). Experimental factors and factor levels were determined in preliminary studies. The independent variables included the type and content of internal stabilizer as well as the drug concentration. The dependent outcomes were the size and yield of the formulations (Table 2). The relationships linking the main factors and their interactions to the responses were determined and presented as a general form in the following equation:

$$Y = \text{intercepts} + \sum \text{main effects} + \sum \text{interactions} \qquad \text{(Eq.1)}$$

Equation coefficients were calculated using coded values; hence the various terms were compared directly, regardless of magnitude. A positive parameter coefficient indicates that output increases at a higher level evaluation for a variable and vice versa. Values are given as mean±SD. Statistical significance of the results was determined using one-way analysis of variance (ANOVA), employing a confidence interval of 95%. The numerical output of ANOVA includes the F-value, stating magnitude of the impact of each factor and P-value as representative of the statistical significance with smaller figures signifying greater importance.

Table 2. Run parameters and responses for experimental design

Runs	Stabilizer type (C)	Stabilizer content (A)	Drug content (B)
R_1	Span 85	15	45
R_2	Tween 80	15	30
R_3	Span 85	15	45
R_4	Span 85	15	15
R_5	Span 85	30	45
R_6	Tween 80	30	30
R_7	Span 85	15	15
R_8	Tween 80	15	45
R_9	Tween 80	15	15
R_{10}	Span 85	22.5	30
R_{11}	Span 85	30	15
R_{12}	Tween 80	30	15
R_{13}	Tween 80	30	45
R_{14}	Tween 80	22.5	45
R_{15}	Span 85	30	45
R_{16}	Span 85	30	15
R_{17}	Tween 80	22.5	15

Physiochemical characterization of nanoparticles

Particle size analysis

The mean hydrodynamic size (z-average) of prepared nanoparticles was determined by photon correlation spectroscopy (Zetasizer®, Malvern Instruments, UK) at 25 °C. Particle sizes were analyzed immediately after preparation and without dilution. The experiments were performed in triplicates.

Yield

Bosentan nanosuspensions were centrifuged (Sigma, Germany) at 20000 rpm for 25 min. The concentration of drug in the supernatant was quantified using isocratic HPLC system (Waters 600E, USA) and C18 column (5 µm, 15 cm). The mobile phase consisted of potassium dihydrogen orthophosphate buffer (pH=4.7) and acetonitrile (45:55) at a flow rate of 1 ml/min with UV detection at 270 nm. All experiments were performed in triplicate. The yield was calculated by means of the equation below:

$$\text{Yield (\%)} = \frac{\text{Total drug} - \text{dissolved drug}}{\text{Total drug}} \times 100 \quad \text{(Eq. 2)}$$

Scanning electron microscopy (SEM)

The surface morphology of unprocessed bosentan and optimal nanoparticles (NPs) was evaluated using a scanning electron microscope (S-4160, Hitachi, Japan) at a voltage of 20 kV. Coarse bosentan and a few drops of the freshly prepared nanosuspensions were spread on stubs using double side carbon tape and then sputtered with gold using a sputter coater (BAL-TEC, Switzerland).

Differential scanning calorimetry (DSC)

A differential scanning calorimeter (Mettler Toledo, Switzerland) was employed to evaluate the thermal behavior of all materials used in the optimal nanoparticles. The equipment was calibrated using indium and zinc. Then, accurately weighed sample powders (8 mg) were heated in aluminum pans within the range of 20-330 °C at a scanning rate of 20 °C/min under nitrogen gas.

Dissolution study

The solubility of coarse bosentan and the freeze-dried optimized nanosuspension were studied in phosphate buffer (PBS) at a pH of 7.4 as dissolution medium. For this purpose, Amounts of powders equal to 20 mg of bosentan were dispersed in screw-capped glass vials, (100 ml) containing 50 ml of medium, by shaking at 50 rpm at 37 ± 0.5 °C in shaker incubator (LABOTEC, Germany). At predetermined time intervals (1, 5, 10 and 15 min) 1 ml of the dispersion were taken away and replaced with 1 ml of fresh PBS. The samples were filtered through 0.22 µ syringe filter and the amount of dissolved bosentan was determined using HPLC method that described previously. All tests were carried out in triplicate.

Results

Preliminary formulations

Bosentan nanosuspensions were successfully prepared using the antisolvent precipitation method. In the first step, the effect of various external stabilizer types, drug content and volume of aqueous phase were studied (Table 1) to achieve the most favorable particle size. As seen in Table 1, the smallest size of nanoparticles was seen when HPβCD was used as an external stabilizer. In addition, by increasing the drug content in formulation that HPβCD was as an external stabilizer, the size of particles increased. Furthermore, when a larger volume of aqueous phase applied in the formulation of nanoparticles, the size of formed particles was smaller. So, HPβCD was selected as an external stabilizer in next investigations.

In the next step, several formulations having Tween 20, Tween 80 and Span 85 as internal stabilizers were prepared. Particles that formed in presence of span 85 (220.3 nm) had smaller size as compare to tween 80 (550 nm) and tween 20 (1432 nm). Therefore, span 85 and tween 80 were selected for more investigation.

Experimental design

After determination of the type and levels of variables from the preliminary formulation studies, the Design Expert software was used to design of experiments.

Size measurements

The hydrodynamic size of prepared nanoparticles measured by nano zetasizer. The particle size of nanoparticles was in the range of 188.3-2816 nm and all formulations had a PDI of less than 0.7.

The quadratic model was the best fitted model on the data ($p< 0.001$). As presented in Table 3, the most effective parameter on the size of nanoparticle was stabilizer type with F-value 32.87 ($p<0.001$). The relation of parameters and size of particles presented in equation 3:

$$\text{Size} = +1104.19 +64.92*A +156.93*B +508.78*C +973.88*A2 -1152.47*B2 -92.87*A*B -96.23*A*C +124.38*B*C \quad \text{(Eq. 3)}$$

As shown in Figure 1, the produced particles in formulations with span 85 as an internal stabilizer had smaller size than formulations with tween 80. In addition, increase of drug content up to midpoint and stabilizer content in the lower and upper level increased the particle sizes.

PDI measurements

The PDI of nanoparticle formulations varied within ranges of 0.17-0.69. The reduced quadratic model is the best fitted model on PDI data with F value of 9.31 ($p<0.001$). As presented in Table 3, the only significant parameter affects the PDI was stabilizer content (F value = 4.83 and $p<0.05$). Increase in stabilizer content up to middle of studied range (22.5 mg), causes decrease in PDI. But more increase in stabilizer content results in the higher polydispersity index (Figure 2). This fact is in agreement with positive value of stabilizer content. The relation of parameters and PDI of formulation presented in equation 4:

$$PDI = +0.48 + 0.063*A - 0.042*B - 0.017*C + 0.18*A2 - 0.27*B2 \quad (Eq.4)$$

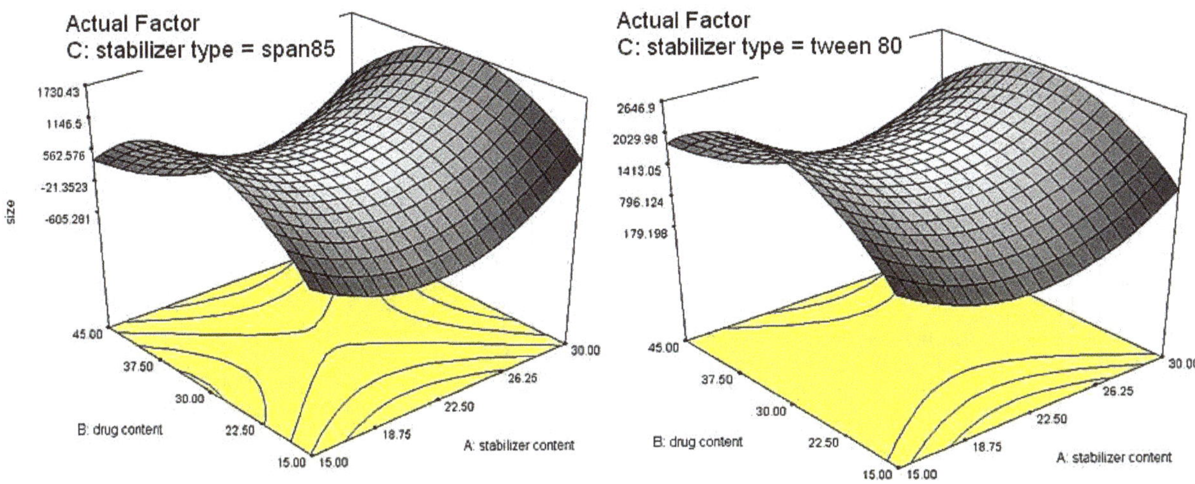

Figure 1. The effect of stabilizer content and drug content on the particle size

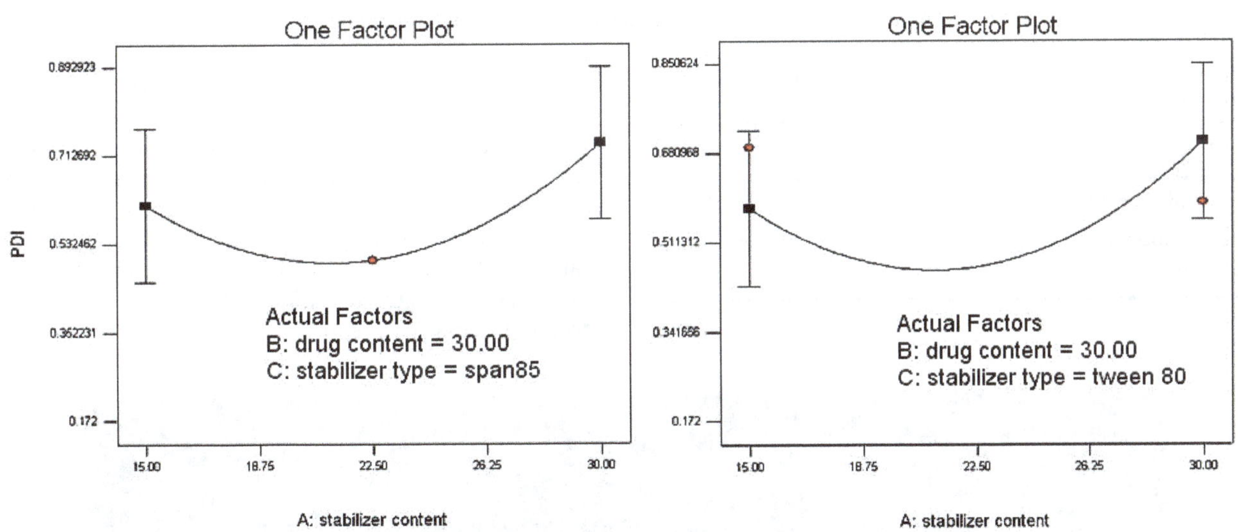

Figure 2. The effect of stabilizer content on the PDI

Table 3. The contribution and significance of different formulation parameters on different nanoparticle attributes

Parameters	F-value in size	F-value in yield	F-value in PDI
A	0.46	2.58	4.83*
B	2.68	24.11**	2.13
C	32.87**	1.31	0.42
A^2	17.50	-	6.16
B_2	24.51	-	15.19
AB	0.82	-	-
AC	1.01	-	-
BC	1.68	-	-

*: $P < 0.05$ and **: $P < 0.001$

Yield

The yield of fabricated nanoparticles was in the range of 80.79-96.97%. Furthermore, ANOVA analysis showed that the drug content is a factor significantly affects the yield (F value = 24.11, $p<0.001$). As shown in Figure 3, the increase in drug content leads to a relative increase in the yield of nanoparticles. The linear model that explains the relationship of parameters and yield of formulation presented in equation 5:

$$Yield = +92.28 + 1.52*A + 4.64*B - 0.98*C \quad (Eq.5)$$

Optimization

After confirming the polynomial equations relating the response and independent factors, the optimization model was constructed by combining the size, PDI and yield of formulations. Optimization was performed by using a desirability function to obtain the levels of drug content, stabilizer type and content which maximized yield, while minimizing PDI and size of particles less than 500 nm. Simultaneously, the formulation with 15.8 mg span 85 as an internal stabilizer and drug content of 45 mg suggested as an optimized formulation. This formulation prepared and evaluated. Predicted and actual amounts of responses are compared and shown in Table 4. As seen in Table 4, the amount of responses for optimized formulation have lower than 10% difference with the predicted amount of D-optimal design.

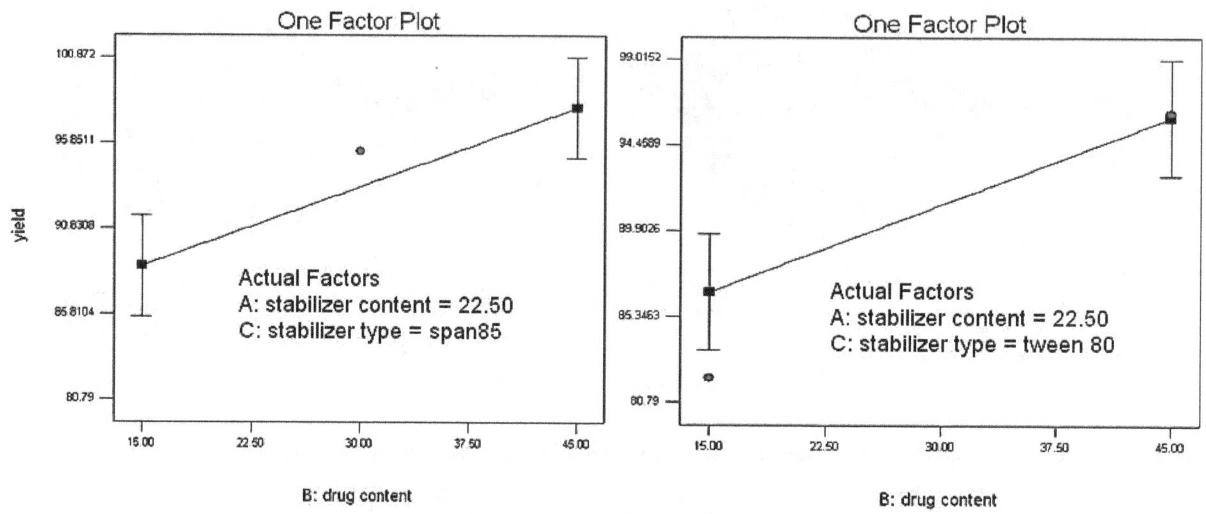

Figure 3. The effect of drug content on the yield of nanoparticles

Table 4. Comparison of actual and predicted responses for optimal formulation

	Size (nm)	PDI	Yield (%)
Predicted response	188.3	0.265	96.55
Actual response	200.7	0.285	99.54
Error (%)	6.6	7.7	3.1

Physiochemical properties of the nanoparticles

Morphology

The morphology of coarse bosentan and optimized nanoparticles were studied by SEM (Figure 4). Coarse bosentan particles were needle-shaped crystals or squama like with rough surfaces (Figure 4A); whereas, nanoparticles were relatively spherical in shape with some degree of agglomeration that could be related to the drying process (Figure 4B).

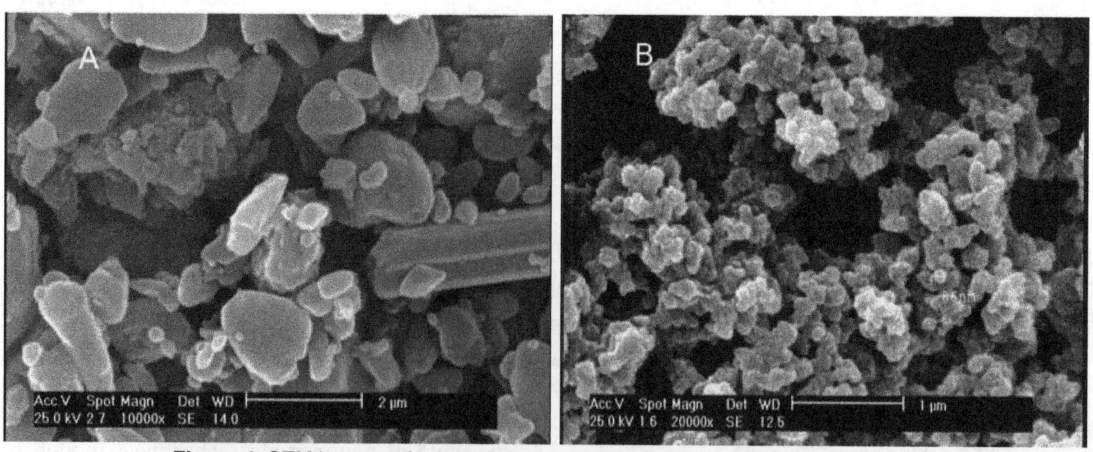

Figure 4. SEM images of coarse bosentan (A) and optimized nanoparticles (B)

Thermal analysis

Figure 5 shows the DSC thermograms of coarse bosentan, HPβCD and the lyophilized optimized formulation.

In Figure 5 was shown that coarse bosentan had 2 endothermic peaks in 130 °C and 80 °C. In the case of HPβCD, an extended endothermic feature is seen around 90 °C. In the optimized nanoparticles, the endothermic peak of bosentan in 80 °C and extended peak of HPβCD were disappeared and the endothermic peak of bosentan in 130 °C was seen by lower intensity.

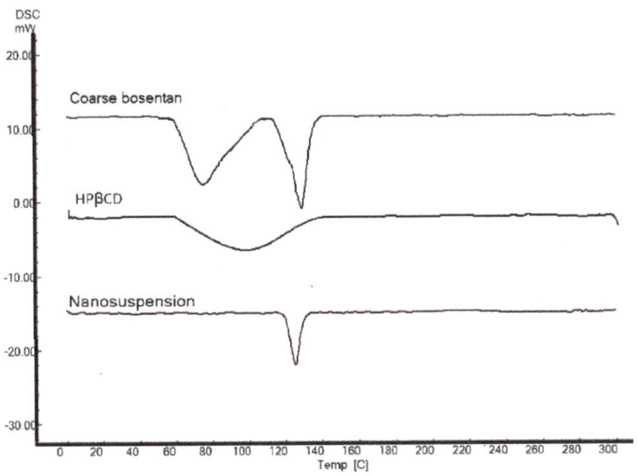

Figure 5. DSC thermograms of coarse bosentan, HPβCD and the lyophilized optimized nanosuspension

Dissolution study

The dissolution profiles of coarse bosentan and fabricated nanoparticles were studied and the results have been shown in Figure 6.

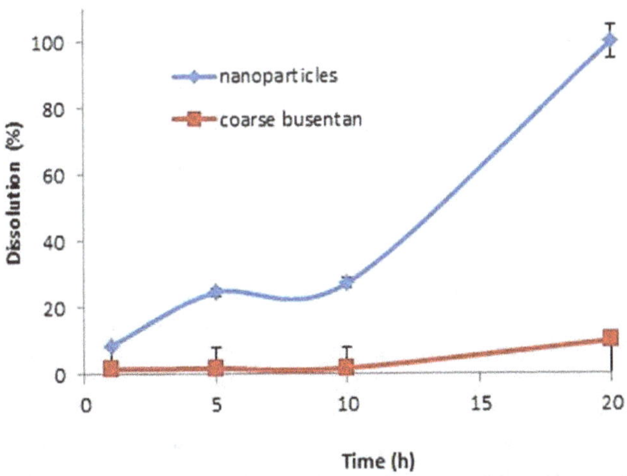

Figure 6. The dissolution profiles of coarse bosentan and fabricated nanoparticles

As seen in Figure 6, about 30% of drug content of nanoparticle formulation dissolved after 5 min and the drug content completely dissolved after 20 min. But, the maximum amount of dissolved coarse bosentan was 10% after 20 min.

The maximum solubility of optimized nanoparticles and coarse bosentan was measured in phosphate buffer (pH=7.4) after 24 h. The maximum solubility of lyophilized nanoparticles was 6.9 mg/100 ml, while coarse bosentan is was 1 mg/100ml. On the other words, the bosentan nanoparticles had around 7- fold higher solubility than unprocessed bosentan.

Discussion

Bosentan is a drug with low water solubility and belongs to class II of BCS.[20] Thus, increasing the solubility and dissolution rate can increase the absorption and efficacy of the drug.[21] Decreasing particle size and incorporating drugs in the structure of nanoparticles is a strategy widely used for increasing the solubility and dissolution rate of pharmaceuticals.[22]

In this study, nanosuspension formulations of bosentan were fabricated to improve its solubility by nanoprecipitation (antisolvent) method.

As indicated in the results section, formulations with Span 85 as an internal stabilizer had smaller size than Tween 80. This finding could be justified by focusing on the properties of these surfactants. Since Span85 has a higher tendency to organic phase compared to Tween 80 and drug was dissolved in organic phase, better coverage of drug particles in fabrication process was done by span 85 and result in smaller particles.

Increasing the stabilizer content initially lead to decreasing PDI; however, further increase results in increasing in PDI. The initial decrease in PDI can be attributed to favorable coverage of nanoparticles surface. However, further increase in stabilizer content can also lead to increase in viscosity of the solution and can lead to increase in nanoparticle aggregation and PDI.[23]

Increase in the drug content could directly increase the yield of formulation. One of the role of surfactants in formulations is solubility enhancing.[18] However, when the drug content increased and stabilizer amount was fixed, the ability of surfactant for dissolving is fixed and the amount of precipitated drug and as a result yiled was increased.

Subsequently, according to the predictions of experimental design software, the optimized formulation was suggested to be composed of 15.8 mg Span 85 and 45 mg of bosentan. The difference in experimental and predicted values was less than 10%, which refers to the ability of the software in prediction of parameters for optimized formulation.

In SEM images were shown that optimized nanoparticles have a spherical shape (compared to coarse bosentan which was crystal-like). This change in shape can influence the dissolution behavior of bosentan.

In DSC thermogram of coarse bosentan, 2 endothermic peaks were seen which are related to the polymorphism structures of bosentan.[24] In the case of bosentan nanoparticles, this endothermic peak of 80 °C was disappeared and it can be explain by changing this polymorph of bosentan to more stable of polymorph that be appear in 130 °C. On the other hand, the endothermic peak of nanoparticle had a lower intensity than coarse bosentan in this point. It can be a sign of partial crystallization of bosentan in nanoparticles which can be favorable in terms of drug dissolution.

As presented in Figure 6, the dissolution extent and rate of nanoparticles are higher than coarse bosentan. This phenomenon can be due to the increase in the effective surface area between drug and the solvent provided by size reduction in nanoparticles. Overall, nanoparticles increased the saturation solubility of bosentan to 6.9 mg/100ml which is 7 fold higher than the solubility of unprocessed bosentan (1 mg/100 ml) which can be due to increase in dissolution pressure.[25]

Conclusion

The data confirm that antisolvent-precipitation method is a feasible method for preparation of bosentan nanosuspension. Besides, the experimental design software successfully could determine the optimal conditions to achieve the desired responses. This optimum condition could be proposed as a beginning to scale up and industrialization of bosentan nanoparticle formation to utilize in the form of tablets or processed in the presence of inhalable sugars to form a dry powder for inhalation purposes. As compared to unprocessed bosentan, the formed nanocrystalline structures can significantly enhance solubility properties and dissolution rate of the drug.

Conflict of Interest

The authors declare that there are no conflicts of interests.

References

1. Schermuly RT, Ghofrani HA, Wilkins MR, Grimminger F. Mechanisms of disease: Pulmonary arterial hypertension. *Nat Rev Cardiol* 2011;8(8):443-55. doi: 10.1038/nrcardio.2011.87
2. Howard LS. Prognostic factors in pulmonary arterial hypertension: Assessing the course of the disease. *Eur Respir Rev* 2011;20(122):236-42. doi: 10.1183/09059180.00006711
3. Galié N, Manes A, Branzi A. The endothelin system in pulmonary arterial hypertension. *Cardiovasc Res* 2004;61(2):227-37. doi: 10.1016/j.cardiores.2003.11.026
4. Stewart DJ, Levy RD, Cernacek P, Langleben D. Increased plasma endothelin-1 in pulmonary hypertension: Marker or mediator of disease? *Ann Intern Med* 1991;114(6):464-9. doi: 10.7326/0003-4819-114-6-464
5. Rubin LJ, Badesch DB, Barst RJ, Galiè N, Black CM, Keogh A, et al. Bosentan therapy for pulmonary arterial hypertension. *N Engl J Med* 2002;346(12):896-903. doi: 10.1056/NEJMoa012212
6. Abd El Rahman MY, Rentzsch A, Scherber P, Mebus S, Miera O, Balling G, et al. Effect of bosentan therapy on ventricular and atrial function in adults with eisenmenger syndrome. A prospective, multicenter study using conventional and speckle tracking echocardiography. *Clin Res Cardiol* 2014;103(9):701-10. doi: 10.1007/s00392-014-0703-5
7. Sharma V, BerKelhamer S, Lakshminrusimha S. Persistent pulmonary hypertension of the newborn. *Matern Health Neonatol Perinatol* 2015;1:14. doi: 10.1186/s40748-015-0015-4
8. Romaniello A, Viola G, Salsano F, Rosato E. In systemic sclerosis patients, bosentan is safe and effective for digital ulcer prevention and it seems to attenuate the development of pulmonary arterial hypertension. *Rheumatology* 2014;53(3):570-1. doi: 10.1093/rheumatology/ket424
9. Hebert A, Mikkelsen UR, Thilen U, Idorn L, Jensen AS, Nagy E, et al. Bosentan improves exercise capacity in adolescents and adults after fontan operation: The tempo (treatment with endothelin receptor antagonist in fontan patients, a randomized, placebo-controlled, double-blind study measuring peak oxygen consumption) study. *Circulation* 2014;130(23):2021-30. doi: 10.1161/CIRCULATIONAHA.113.008441
10. Abdelsaid M, Kaczmarek J, Coucha M, Ergul A. Dual endothelin receptor antagonism with bosentan reverses established vascular remodeling and dysfunctional angiogenesis in diabetic rats: Relevance to glycemic control. *Life Sci* 2014;118(2):268-73. doi: 10.1016/j.lfs.2014.01.008
11. Pinho-Ribeiro FA, Borghi SM, Staurengo-Ferrari L, Filgueiras GB, Estanislau C, Verri WA Jr. Bosentan, a mixed endothelin receptor antagonist, induces antidepressant-like activity in mice. *Neurosci Lett* 2014;560:57-61. doi: 10.1016/j.neulet.2013.12.018
12. Channick RN, Simonneau G, Sitbon O, Robbins IM, Frost A, Tapson VF, et al. Effects of the dual endothelin-receptor antagonist bosentan in patients with pulmonary hypertension: A randomised placebo-controlled study. *Lancet* 2001;358(9288):1119-23. doi: 10.1016/S0140-6736(01)06250-X
13. Dingemanse J, van Giersbergen PL. Clinical pharmacology of bosentan, a dual endothelin receptor antagonist. *Clin Pharmacokinet* 2004;43(15):1089-115. doi: 10.2165/00003088-200443150-00003
14. J Meyer RB. In vitro binding of the endothelin receptor antagonist ro 47-0203 to plasma proteins in man and animals, and red blood cell/plasma partitioning. *Basel F: Hoffmann-La Roche Ltd;* 1996.
15. Roux S, Breu V, Ertel SI, Clozel M. Endothelin antagonism with bosentan: A review of potential applications. *J Mol Med (Berl)* 1999;77(4):364-76. doi: 10.1007/s001090050363
16. Maiya S, Hislop AA, Flynn Y, Haworth SG. Response to bosentan in children with pulmonary hypertension. *Heart* 2006;92(5):664-70. doi: 10.1136/hrt.2005.072314
17. Wong SM, Kellaway IW, Murdan S. Enhancement of the dissolution rate and oral absorption of a poorly water soluble drug by formation of surfactant-containing microparticles. *Int J Pharm* 2006;317(1):61-8. doi: 10.1016/j.ijpharm.2006.03.001
18. Savjani KT, Gajjar AK, Savjani JK. Drug solubility: Importance and enhancement techniques. *ISRN Pharm* 2012;2012:195727. doi: 10.5402/2012/195727

19. Uhrich KE, Cannizzaro SM, Langer RS, Shakesheff KM. Polymeric systems for controlled drug release. *Chem Rev* 1999;99(11):3181-98.
20. Zhu J. Bosentan salts. Google Patents; 2009. Pat No: US20090291974.
21. Amidon GL, Lennernas H, Shah VP, Crison JR. A theoretical basis for a biopharmaceutic drug classification: The correlation of in vitro drug product dissolution and in vivo bioavailability. *Pharm Res* 1995;12(3):413-20. doi: 10.1208/s12248-014-9620-9
22. Merisko-Liversidge E, Liversidge GG, Cooper ER. Nanosizing: A formulation approach for poorly-water-soluble compounds. *Eur J Pharm Sci* 2003;18(2):113-20. doi: 10.1016/S0928-0987(02)00251-8
23. Budhian A, Siegel SJ, Winey KI. Haloperidol-loaded plga nanoparticles: Systematic study of particle size and drug content. *Int J Pharm* 2007;336(2):367-75. doi: 10.1016/j.ijpharm.2006.11.061
24. Gaitonde A, Manojkumar B, Mekde S, Bansode P, Shinde D, Phadtare S. Crystalline forms of bosentan. Google Patents; 2013. Pat No: WO 2011058524 A2.
25. Hu J, Johnston KP, Williams RO 3rd. Nanoparticle engineering processes for enhancing the dissolution rates of poorly water soluble drugs. *Drug Dev Ind Pharm* 2004;30(3):233-45. doi: 10.1081/DDC-120030422

3

Optimized and Validated RP-UPLC Method for the Determination of Losartan Potassium and Chlorthalidone in Pharmaceutical Formulations

Tadiboyina Sirisha[1]*, Bannimath Gurupadayya[1], Sridhar Siddiraju[2]

[1] *Department of Pharmaceutical Chemistry, JSS College of Pharmacy, JSS University, Mysore, India.*
[2] *Department of Pharmaceutical Chemistry, Malla Reddy College of Pharmacy, Osmania University, Secunderabad, India.*

Article info

Keywords:
· Chromatography
· Losartan
· Chlorthalidone

Abstract
Purpose: A validated ultra performance liquid chromatography (UPLC) method has been developed and validated for the simultaneous determination of losartan potassium and chlorthalidone in pharmaceutical preparations.
Methods: Waters-Acquity UPLC system equipped with Auto Sampler, PDA detector and operated with Empower-2 software was used for the present study. Detection was done at wavelength of 230 nm, HSS C18, 100 mm x 2.1x 1.8 μm column with a reverse phase elution and mobile phase composed of A and B mixed in the ratio 56:44 v/v (Where mobile phase A consists of potassium dihydrogen phosphate buffer of pH 3.0 and Mobile phase B consists of acetonitrile and methanol mixed in the ratio of 90:10 v/v) used at a flow rate of 0.4ml per minute.
Results: The retention times for losartan potassium and chlorthalidone were observed at 0.72 and 1.89 minutes. The developed method was validated as per ICH guidelines. Linearity ranges were found to be 12.5-125 μg/ml and 3.125-31.25 μg/ml for losartan potassium and chlorthalidone, respectively.
Conclusion: This method is fast, accurate, precise and sensitive hence it can be employed for routine quality control of tablets containing both drugs in industries.

Introduction

Losartan potassium (LSP), an angiotensin II receptor antagonist used in the treatment of hypertension. Losartan potassium is given to delay progression of diabetic nephropathy and also to reduce renal disease progression in patients with type 2 diabetes. Chlorthalidone (CLD), a thiazide diuretic used in the treatment of hypertension. Chlortalidone increases the excretion of sodium, chloride, and water into the renal lumen by inhibiting sodium ion transport across the renal tubular epithelium. Losartan and Chlorthalidone combination therapy is prescribed because they have complementary mechanism of action which allows for synergistic lowering of blood pressure and more over this combination therapy allows lower dosage requirements of each individual agent which leads to decreased side effects and improved compliance. The chemical structure of LSP and CLD were presented in Figure 1.

A number of analytical and bioanaytical methods have been reported for the estimation of LSP by using UV,[1,2] HPLC,[3-7] LC/MS/MS[8-11] and voltammetry.[12] A few of analytical methods have been reported for the estimation of chlorthalidone by using Potentiometry,[13] UV,[14] HPLC,[15] Capillary electrophorosis[16,17] and also by LC/MS/MS.[18]

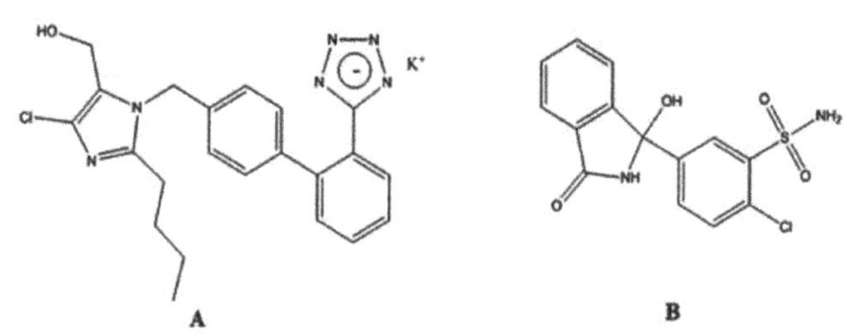

Figure 1. Chemical Structures of Losartan Potassium (A) and Chlorthalidone (B)

From the above literature, it was found that, there are no chromatographic methods available for the simultaneous estimation of losartan potassium and chlorthalidone in their combined dosage form, this work holds a challenge for developing a new method in ultra performance liquid chromatography. Moreover, among the existing liquid chromatographic methods, there exists no method in which LSP is eluted below 4 min. Hence UPLC was selected in order to reduce the elution time of both the drugs which in turn reduce the consumption of mobile phase and time of analysis.

***Corresponding author:** Tadiboyina Sirisha, Email: tadiboyina.sirisha@gmail.com

Materials and Methods

Instrumentation

Waters-Acquity UPLC system equipped with auto sampler, binary gradient pump, and PDA detector was used for the separation. An analytical column; HSS C18, (100 mm x 2.1x 1.8 μm) was used in the analysis. For data collection and processing Chromatographic software Empower -2 was used.

Chemicals and Reagents

Losartan potassium pure drug was obtained from Chemit laboratories, Hyderabad and chlorthalidone pure drug was obtained from Hetero Drugs, Hyderabad. The commercially available formulations of losartan potassium and chlorthalidone(ctd-L 25/6.25mg) were purchased from the local market. The HPLC grade water was obtained from Millipore. Acetonitrile and methanol of HPLC grade were obtained from E. Merck. (India) Ltd., Mumbai. Potassium dihydrogen phosphate and ortho phosphoric acid of analytical grade were purchased from Chempure pvt Ltd., India.

Preparation of standard solution

Stock solution (50μg/mL, 12.5 μg/mL) of losartan potassium and chlorthalidone was prepared by dissolving accurately weighed 25 mg of losartan potassium standard and 6.25mg of chlorthalidone standard into a 25ml volumetric flask, dissolved and made up to the volume. A series dilute solutions ranging from 12.5 to 125 μg/mL of losartan potassium and 3.125 to 31.25 μg/mL of chlorthalidone were prepared by taking different aliquots (0.125 to 1.25 mL) of the stock solution and diluted to 10ml with diluent in similar manner.

Preparation and sample solution

About 20 tablets of ctd-L were weighed and powdered and from that powder the amount of powder equivalent to 25mgof losartan potassium and 6.25mg of chlorthalidone was dissolved in 25 mL of diluent in a volumetric flask, sonicated and made up to the mark. Further working standard (50μg/mL ,12.5 μg/mL) of losartan potassium and chlorthalidone was prepared by transferring 0.5 mL of the stock solution into 10 mL volumetric flask and diluted up to the mark with diluent, sonicated and filter through 0.45 mm filter.

Results and Discussion

Optimisation of chromatographic method

The chromatographic separation was carried out under the isocratic conditions. The mobile phase was allowed to flow through the column at a flow rate of 0.4 mL/min for 3 min to equilibrate the column at ambient temperature. Chromatographic separation was achieved by injecting a volume of 0.5μl of standard into HSS C18, (100 mm x 2.1x 1.8 μm) column .The mobile phase of composition 560 mL of solution A (1.36g of potassium dihydrogen phosphate buffer of pH 3.0) and 440ml mL of solution B (acetonitrile and methanol in 9:1 ratio) was allowed to flow through the column at a flow rate of 0.4 ml per minute for a period of 3.0 min. Detection of the component was carried out at a wavelength of 230 nm. The retention time of the components were found to be 0.72 and 1.89min for losartan potassium and chlorthalidone respectively (Figure 2). The system suitability parameters such as tailing factor and theoretical plate count were found to 1.36, 1.25 and 11040, 8325, respectively.

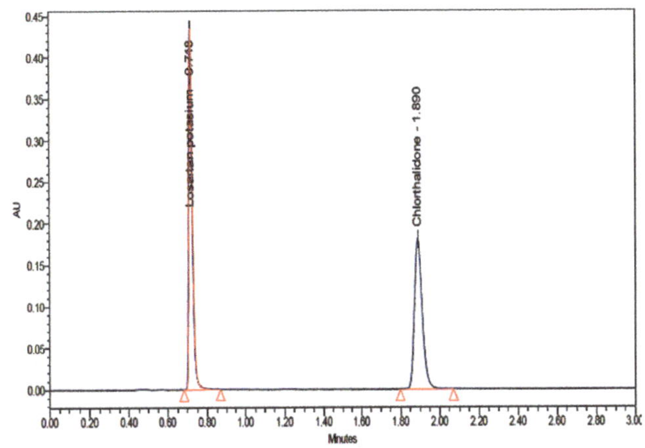

Figure 2. UPLC overlay chromatogram of Losartan Potassium and Chlorthalidone

Validation results of the method

Validation of the proposed method was done according to ICH[19] guidelines. In the repeatability study, the % relative standard deviation (%RSD) was 0.51 & 0.37 for the retention times of losartan potassium and chlorthalidone and 0.13 & 1.31 for the peak areas of both the drugs. In the intermediate precision which is the study of reproducibility of results in different days, the % relative standard deviation for the retention times and peak areas were 0.831, 0.523 and 0.522, 0.849 for both the drugs.

The limit of detection (LOD) and LOQ concentrations were estimated by using signal to noise ratio method.[20] At 3:10 S/N ratio the LOD and LOQ were found to be 497ng/mL and 1508 ng/mL for losartan potassium and 71 ng/ mL and 217 ng/ mL for chlorthalidone.

Good linearity was observed over the concentration range of 12.5 to 125 μg/ mL for losartan and 3.125 to 31.25 μg/ mL for chlorthalidone with correlation coefficient > 0.999 for both the drugs and data was presented in Table 1.

Table 1. Validation parameters of developed UPLC method for analysis of LSP and CLD

Parameters		LSP	CLD
Regression equation (y=mx+c)	Slope (m)	5919.3	2044.7
	Intercept (c)	8407.3	216.57
Correlation coefficient (r^2)		0.9994	0.9997
LOD (ng/mL)		497	71
LOQ(ng/mL)		1508	217
Precision (%RSD) (n=5)	Intra day	0.132	1.31
	Inter day	0.522	0.849

The standard addition and recovery experiments were conducted for both the drugs in triplicate at 50,100 and 150% of analyte concentration. The recovery was calculated from the slope and y-intercept of the calibration curve and the % recovery was ranged from 99.56% to 100.03% for losartan potassium and 98.73% to 100.34% for chlorthalidone (Table 2).

Table 2. Accuracy data

Drug name	%Concentration	Area	Amount added(μg/mL)	Amount found(μg/mL)	Mean %Recovery	%RSD
	50%	452060	25	24.95	99.81	1.44
LSP	100%	600403	50	50.01	100.03	1.10
	150%	746352	75	74.67	99.56	1.25
	50%	38595	6.25	6.27	100.34	1.21
CLD	100%	51002	12.5	12.34	98.73	0.41
	150%	89762	31.25	31.30	100.17	1.59

The chromatographic resolution of losartan potassium and chlorthalidone peaks was used to evaluate the method robustness under the modified conditions like change in flow rate, pH of the buffer and composition of organic phase. The resolution between both the peaks was greater than 2 under all the tested conditions; also both the drug peaks passed the system suitability parameters.

No significant change in the losartan potassium and chlorthalidone drug content was observed during solution stability and mobile phase stability experiments. Hence, standard solutions and mobile phase were stable for upto 48hr during assay determination.

Conclusion

The proposed RP-UPLC method was found to be simple, fast, precise, accurate and rugged. Both the drugs were eluted below 2min hence reduces the run time and the mobile phase composition, made the method economical. The drugs were found to be stable throughout the assay period. Therefore the developed method can be used as an alternative method for routine analysis in quality control.

Acknowledgments

The authors would like to thank Prinicipal, and administrative officer, JSS College of pharmacy, Mysore for providing us the laboratory facilities for research work.

Conflict of Interest

The authors declare no conflict of interest.

References

1. Lastra OC, Lemus IG, Sánchez HJ, Pérez RF. Development and validation of an UV derivative spectrophotometric determination of Losartan potassium in tablets. *J Pharm Biomed Anal* 2003;33(2):175-80.
2. Singh S, Patel K, Agrawal VK, Chaturvedi S. Simultaneous estimation of S(-) Amlodipine Besylate Hemipentahydrate and Losartan Potassium in Combined Dosage Form by Using UV-Spectroscopy. *Der Pharmacia Lettre* 2012;4(3):897-905.
3. Mhaske RA, Sahasrabudhe S, Mhaske AA. Rp-HPLC method for Simultataneous determination of irbesartan, losartan, hydro-chlorothiazide and chlorthalidone-application to commercially available drug products. *Int J Pharm Sci Res* 2012;3(4):1116-23.
4. Jalalizadeh H, Souri E, FARSAM H, Ansari M. A High-Performance Liquid Chromatographic Assay for the Determination of Losartan in Plasma. *Iran J Pharmacol Ther* 2003;2(1):18-21.
5. Dorado P, Machín E, De Andrés F, Naranjo ME, Peñas-Lledó EM, Llerena A, et al. Development of a HPLC method for the determination of losartan urinary metabolic ratio to be used for the determination of CYP2C9 hydroxylation phenotypes. *Drug Metabol Drug Interact* 2012;27(4):217-33.
6. Priyanka Patil R, Sachin Rakesh U, Dhabale PN, Burade KB. RP- HPLC Method for Simultaneous Estimation of Losartan potassium and Amlodipine besylate in Tablet Formulation. *Int J ChemTech Res* 2009;1:464-9.
7. Siddiqui MMA, Syed SQ, Abueida EY. Isocratic RP-HPLC method validation and verification of losartan potassium in pharmaceutical formulations with stress test stability for drug substance. *Der Pharmacia Lettre* 2011;3(5):160-7.
8. Karra VK, Pilli NR, Inamadugu JK, Rao JV. Simultaneous determination of losartan, losartan acid and amlodipine in human plasma by LC-MS/MS and its application to a human pharmacokinetic study. *Pharm Methods* 2012;3(1):18-25.
9. Prasad SVSGB, Shiva Kumar S, Sudhir T, Mital R, Devala Rao G. LC/MS/MS Method for the simultaneous estimation of losartan potassium and irbesartan in rat plasma. *Int J Pharm Pharm Sci* 2009;1(Suppl 1):206-15.
10. Salvadori MC, Moreira RF, Borges BC, Andraus MH, Azevedo CP, Moreno RA, et al. Simultaneous determination of losartan and hydrochlorothiazide in human plasma by LC/MS/MS with electrospray ionization and its application to pharmacokinetics. *Clin Exp Hypertens* 2009;31(5):415-27.

11. Shah HJ, Kundlik ML, Patel NK, Subbaiah G, Patel DM, Suhagia BN, et al. Rapid determination of losartan and losartan acid in human plasma by multiplexed LC-MS/MS. *J Sep Sci* 2009;32(20):3388-94.
12. Ensafi AA, Hajian R. Determination of losartan and triamterene in pharmaceutical compounds and urine using cathodic adsorptive stripping voltammetry. *Anal Sci* 2008;24(11):1449-54.
13. Fleuren HL, Van Ginneken CA, Van Rossum JM. Differential potentiometric method for determining dissociation constants of very slightly water-soluble drugs applied to the sulfonamide diuretic chlorthalidone. *J Pharm Sci* 1979;68(8):1056-8.
14. Parmar kreny E, Mehta RS. First order derivative spectrophotometric method for simultaneous estimation of telmisartan and chlorthalidone in bulk and pharmaceutical dosage form. *Int Res J Pharm* 2013;4(3):224-8.
15. Brijesh S, Patel DK, Ghosh SK. A reversed-phase high performance liquid chromatographic method for determination of chlorthalidone in pharmaceutical formulation. *Int J Pharma Pharmaceu Sci* 2009;1(2):24-9.
16. Balesteros MR, Faria AF, de Oliveira MAL. Determination of losartan associated with chlorthalidone or hydrochlorothiazide in capsules by capillary zone electrophoresis. *J Braz Chem Soc* 2007;18(3):554-8.
17. Al Azzam KM, Saad B, Aboul-Enein HY. Simultaneous determination of atenolol, chlorthalidone and amiloride in pharmaceutical preparations by capillary zone electrophoresis with ultraviolet detection. *Biomed Chromatogr* 2010;24(9):977-81.
18. Khuroo A, Mishra S, Singh O, Saxena S, Monif T. Simultaneous determination of Atenolol and Chlorthalidone by LC-MS-MS in human plasma. *Chromatographia* 2008;68(9-10):721-9.
19. International Conference on Harmonization. ICH Harmonised Tripartite Guideline, Validation of Analytical Procedures: Text and Methodology (Q2(R1)), Geneva. 2005.
20. Snyder LR, Kirkland JJ, Glajch JL. Practical HPLC method development. 2nd Ed. New York: Wiley-Interscience; 1997.

Triamcinolone Acetonide Oromucoadhesive Paste for Treatment of Aphthous Stomatitis

Hamed Hamishehkar[1], Ali Nokhodchi[2], Saeed Ghanbarzadeh[3], Maryam Kouhsoltani[4]*

[1] *Drug Applied Research Center, Tabriz University of Medical Sciences, Tabriz, Iran.*

[2] *Medway School of Pharmacy, Universities of Kent and Greenwich, Central Ave., Chatham Maritime, Kent ME4 4TB, United Kingdom.*

[3] *Biotechnology Research Center, Tabriz University of Medical Sciences, Tabriz, Iran.*

[4] *Dental and Periodontal Research Center and Faculty of Dentistry, Tabriz University of Medical Sciences, Tabriz, Iran.*

Article info

Keywords:
- Aphthous stomatitis
- Triamcinolone acetonide
- Plastibase
- Oral paste

Abstract

Purpose: The aim of this study was to prepare the optimized oral paste formulation of Triamcinolone acetonide intended to be used in aphtous stomatitis.

Methods: Plastibases were prepared using mineral oil and polyethylene (95:5). Oral paste formulations were prepared with different mixtures of three hydrocolloids solids, including gelatin, pectin and sodium carboxymethylcellulose, with different ratios, as well as Plastibase. Long-term and short-term stability of prepared formulations were studied in the case of color and consistency of pastes. Franz diffusion cell and dialysis membrane were employed for release study. Release data were fitted in the kinetic models to find out the mechanism of drug release.

Results: Formulation containing 60% plastibase, 3.3% pectin, 6.6% gelatin and 30% carboxymethylcellulose showed desired durability of adhesion, spreadability and rheology property in healthy volunteers and was compared with reference formulation (Adcortyl®) in the case of release profile. Although, optimized formulation and Adcortyl followed the Higuchi and first order release kinetics respectively, optimized formulation showed similar release profile to reference formulation.

Conclusion: Optimized oral paste formulation of Triamcinolone Acetonide showed similar characteristics with reference formulation and could be used as an effective drug delivery system for the treatment of recurrent aphthous stomatitis.

Introduction

The mucosa lining of the oral cavity is susceptible to many inflammatory, atrophic and ulcerative conditions, including aphthous stomatitis, lichen planus, erythema multiforme and Behcet's syndrome. Recurrent aphthous stomatitis (RAS), usually known as canker sores, is a disease of the oral mucosa involving the repeated development of one or more painful ulcers. The oral symptoms of RAS include pain, weakness and major alterations in oral functions, such as speech, chewing and swallowing. Despite multiple investigations about this disease, its etiology remains unknown.[1-3] The main treatment strategy of RAS and other inflammatory conditions of the mouth is the use of corticosteroids. These corticosteroids are normally formulated in ointments, pastes, lozenges and mouthwashes, and applied topically in order to avoid systemic side effects.[4-6] Triamcinolone Acetonide, a medium to high potency corticosteroid, is a fluorinated prednisolone derivative and considered an intermediate-acting glucocorticoid. It is effective in the treatment of dermatoses, asthma and allergic rhinitis and is used in the decreasing of the signs and symptoms of many oral inflammatory conditions, including RAS. Triamcinolone Acetonide dental paste was used for adjunctive treatment and temporary relief of symptoms associated with oral inflammation and gingival disorders.[7-9] For effective therapy in conditions of the oral mucosa, the concentration of corticosteroid in the buccal mucosa should be preserved with minimal systemic absorption which could be achieved by incorporation of drugs in special dosage forms, resulting in enhanced mucosal concentrations of drugs with reduced systemic absorption. The amount of drug absorption is dependent to the time of exposure of the drug to the buccal membrane.[10,11] Drug delivery systems for delivering drugs to the oral mucosa include mouthwashes, tinctures, buccal formulations and ointments. The contact time of mouthwash is very short as compared with the other dosage forms. However, addition of a mucoadhesive polymer in the formulations could provide longer contact time. Mucoadhesive polymers such as hydroxypropylcellulose, carbopol, sodium carboxymethylcellulose, gelatin and pectin have been employed in formulations used for the oral cavity.[9,12,13] Tinctures are easily applied to oral lesions but may be swallowed within a rather short time period after application. Buccal formulations retain in the oral

***Corresponding author:** Maryam Kouhsoltani, Email: mkoohsoltani@yahoo.com

cavity for longer periods than tinctures, however, they are usually larger in size and thus uncomfortable to keep in the oral cavity. Conventional ointment formulations may be readily applied, however, in many cases, they removed from the oral cavity during speaking, eating or by salivation, as well as tongue movement and swallowing. In addition, bleeding of active ingredients from ointments during storage or after application to oral lesions results inefficient drug contact to the lesions and/or migration by saliva to other locations in the oral cavity.[10,12,14-17] Therefore, a new formulation with suitable adhesion potential with capability for sustained drug release for a period of time is needed. The objective of the present study was to prepare an oromucoadhesive formulation of Triamcinolone Acetonide with desired release of Triamcinolone Acetonide.

Materials and Methods

Materials

Triamcinolone Acetonide was kindly donated from Jaber Ebne Hayyan Pharmaceutical Company (Iran). Gelatin was supplied from Fluka biochemika Company (Germany). Pectin (from citrus peel, Galacturonic acid ≥74.0 % (dried basis)) and high viscosity sodium carboxymethylcellulose (NaCMC) (average M_w ~700,000) were bought from Sigma-Aldrich (USA) and mineral oil was purchased from Merck Company (Germany). Low density and high density polyethylene were prepared from Tabriz Petrochemical Company (Iran). Adcortyl in Orabase (Triamcinolone Dental Paste) was provided from the market manufactured by Bristol-Myers Squibb Pharmaceuticals Ltd.

Preparation of Plastibase

Plastibases were prepared using mineral oil and polyethylene (95:5). Two types of polyethylene (PE), high density polyethylene (HDPE) and low density polyethylene (LDPE) were dissolved in mineral oil at 120-130 °C. After complete dissolving of polyethylene in mineral oil, the mixtures were cooled immediately by pouring the oil on a metal surface cold by ice. The rapid cooling process is crucial in an appropriate gel formation.

Preparation of oral paste

Oral drug delivery systems were provided by compositions which included three hydrocolloids solids, including gelatin, pectin and NaCMC, with different ratios, and base comprising of mineral oil containing polyethylene (Plastibase®). For prevention of formulations from hardening upon prolonged storage due to the presence of humidity, solid colloids were dried in an oven (60 °C) for at least 16 hrs. The first step (A) formulations (Table 1) were designed to find the most appropriate Plastibase® ratio. To obtain the best formulation with desired characteristics, different formulations with various ratios of gelatin, pectin and NaCMC were prepared at two pre-formulation stages, formulations B and C based on triangle phase diagram (Figure 1 and Table 2).

Table 1. Plastibase and colloid ratios of different formulation of pastes containing equivalent amount of gelatin, pectin and sodium carboxymethylcellulose

Formulation code	Plastibase: Colloids (w/w)
A1	30:70
A2	40:60
A3	50:50
A4	60:40
A5	70:30
A6	80:20

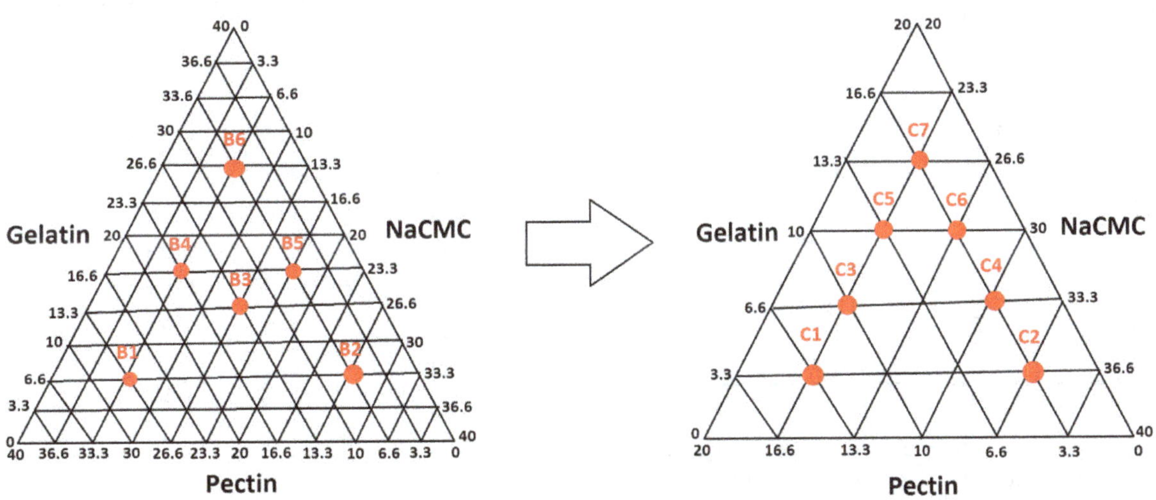

Figure 1. Formulation development of oromucoadhesive paste based on triangle phase diagram.

In vitro release study

Dialysis membrane was mounted between the donor and receptor chamber of Franz diffusion cells filled with 50% ethanol solution in receptor phase ensuring that there were no air bubbles between the formulation and donor surface to keep the sink condition for

Tramcinolone Acetonide. The surface area available for diffusion was 2.5 cm^2 and receptor volume was 25 cm^3. Accurately weighed of different formulations (0.5 g of Triamcinolone Acetonide paste, 0.1 % w:w) was applied to the surface of the dialysis membranes and spread by means of a spatula. The receptor fluid was maintained at 37 ± 0.5 °C and continuously stirred at 700 rpm using a transdermal tester (Erweka HDT6, Germany). Samples from receptor medium (2 mL) were withdrawn at specific time intervals over a 6 hrs period and immediately replaced with fresh prewarmed hydroethanolic solution. The samples were quantified spectrophotometrically at 240 nm using a calibration curve which was linear in the range of 1.25 - 20 µg/mL (r^2=0.9997). Each formulation was investigated in 3 cells. Based on release study, dissolution parameters indicating drug release behavior were calculated and reported as the following. The dissolution efficiency (DE) of a pharmaceutical dosage form is defined as the area under the dissolution curve up to the time t, expressed as the percentage of the area of the rectangle:

$$DE\% = \frac{\int_0^t y\,dt}{y_{100}\,t} \times 100$$

Where y is the percentage of Triamcinolone Acetonide dissolved at time t.

Table 2. Formulations with different composition of gelatin, pectin and sodium carboxymethylcellulose (NaCMC).

Formulation code	Pectin (%w/w)	Gelatin (%w/w)	NaCMC (%w/w)
B1	26.6	6.6	6.6
B2	6.6	6.6	26.6
B3	13.3	13.3	13.3
B4	16.6	16.6	6.6
B5	6.6	16.6	16.6
B6	6.6	26.6	6.6
C1	13.3	3.3	23.3
C2	3.3	3.3	33.3
C3	10	6.6	23.3
C4	3.3	6.6	30
C5	6.6	10	23.3
C6	3.3	10	26.6
C7	3.3	13.3	23.3

Another approach to achieve a parameter that explains the dissolution rate is the mean dissolution time (MDT). This parameter is the most likely time taken for a molecule to be dissolved from a solid dosage form. In other words, MDT is the mean time for the drug to dissolve under in vitro dissolution conditions. This is calculated using the following equation:

$$MDT = \frac{\sum_{j=1}^{n} t_j \Delta M_j}{\sum_{j=1}^{n} \Delta M_j}$$

Where j is the sample number, t_j is the midpoint of the jth time period (easily calculated with ((t+t−1)/2) and M_j is the additional amount of drug dissolved between t_j and t−1. The mean dissolution rate (MDR) can be calculated according to the following equation:

$$MDR = \frac{\sum_{j=1}^{n} \frac{\Delta M_j}{\Delta t}}{n}$$

Where n is the number of dissolution sample times, t is the time at the midpoint between t and t−1 (easily calculated with [t+(t−1)/2]).

Stability study

Long-term and short-term stability of prepared formulations were studied in the case of color and consistency of pastes. Long-term stability of prepared formulations was conducted for 6 months at three temperatures, 4 °C, 25 °C and 40 °C. Short-term stability test was performed as four 24 hr temperature cycles (4 °C and 40 °C).

Drug release kinetic study

The dissolution results have served as a means to evaluate different formulations (Table 3). The kinetic models have been used in interpretation of drug release data and dissolution data of formulations were fitted to the kinetic models. The equations of the kinetic models and coefficient of correlation of each formulation are presented in Table 4.

Table 3. Drug dissolution parameters

Formulation code	DE (%)[a]	MDR (%.h^{-1})[b]	MDT (h)[c]
A1	28.9	9.3	2.23
A2	48.4	15.7	2.22
A3	44.2	14.7	2.08
A4	41.7	13.3	1.76
A5	36.4	11.9	2.03
A6	13.9	4.6	1.87
B1	40.9	13.4	2.06
B2	34.5	11.3	2.17
B3	34.1	11.2	2.23
B4	23.2	7.5	2.08
B5	34.3	11.6	1.55
B6	34.3	11.6	1.55
C1	43.5	14.2	2.18
C4	34.6	11.5	2.24
Adcortyl®	30.0	11.15	2.24

[a]Dissolution efficiency
[b]Mean dissolution rate
[c]Mean dissolution time

Table 4. Kinetic models used for analysis of selected formulations release data

Formulation code	Zero order (F=kt)		First order (ln (1-F) = - $k_f t$)		Higuchi (F= k $t^{0.5}$)	
	MRSQ	K	MRSQ	K	MRSQ	K
A1	0.955	0.144	0.986	0.001	0.996	2.865
A2	0.960	0.192	0.998	0.004	0.996	4.811
A3	0.973	0.143	0.997	0.002	0.999	3.558
A4	0.915	0.001	0.958	0.002	0.979	0.031
A5	0.978	0.001	0.995	0.001	0.993	0.283
A6	0.979	0.003	0.982	0.004	0.983	0.008
B1	0.978	0.003	0.999	0.002	0.998	0.329
B2	0.990	0.001	0.999	0.002	0.990	0.282
B3	0.960	0.001	0.990	0.002	0.998	0.033
B4	0.957	0.001	0.976	0.001	0.998	0.205
B5	0.972	0.004	0.997	0.003	0.998	0.034
B6	0.954	0.001	0.974	0.001	0.994	0.184
C1	0.974	0.001	0.999	0.002	0.999	0.032
C4	0.977	0.001	0.977	0.002	0.999	0.032
Adcortyl®	0.985	0.001	0.998	0.002	0.996	0.349

F denotes fraction of drug released up to time t.

Statistical analysis

The data was demonstrated as mean ± SD. Analysis of variance (ANOVA) was performed for multiple comparisons (SPSS 15). A level of significance of $P < 0.05$ was set to determine any significant difference between the formulations.

Results and Discussion

The preparation of Plstibase with both LDPE and HDPE showed that LDPE provides better Plastibase based on the least paraffin oil leak during the storage for one month in different storage conditions. Preliminary studies revealed that formulations containing about 60% of Plastibase® and 40 % of solid colloids with equivalent amount of gelatin, pectin and NaCMC (A4), suitable characteristics (Table 1). In the next stage, B2 formulation was selected the most proper formulation in the point of mucoadhesion and consequently the next triangle phase diagram was designed based on B2 formulation. Finally, after further investigations on the formulations with different ratios of solid colloids, formulation C4 and C1 were chosen as a formulation with desired organoleptic properties durability of adhesion, spreadability and rheology property in healthy volunteers.

In vitro release study

Figure 2 illustrates the cumulative release of different formulations of Triamcinolone Acetonide over 6 hrs through the formulations with different base to colloids ratios. In formulations A2-A6, by increase in Plastibase® ratio drug release was decreased probably as a result of drug entrapment into PE network. The lower drug release rate observed in formulation A1 may be attributed to the high viscosity of paste caused by the presence of high amounts of hygroscopic colloids in the formulation composition. The lower DE and MDR values for formulations A1 and A6 than other formulations implies the sustained release pattern of these formulations (Table 3). Accordingly, in formulations B1-B6, by increasing concentration of gelatin and Sodium CMC concentrations a decrease in drug release were observed (Figure 3). The role of Sodium CMC in the control of drug release through the paste was much clear in the comparison of C1 and C4 in Figure 4. Both optimized formulations especially formulation C4 showed similar release profile to that of the reference product. The dissolution parameters (DE, MDT and MDR) corresponding to C4 were also similar to the reference commercial brand (Adcortyl®) (Table 3).

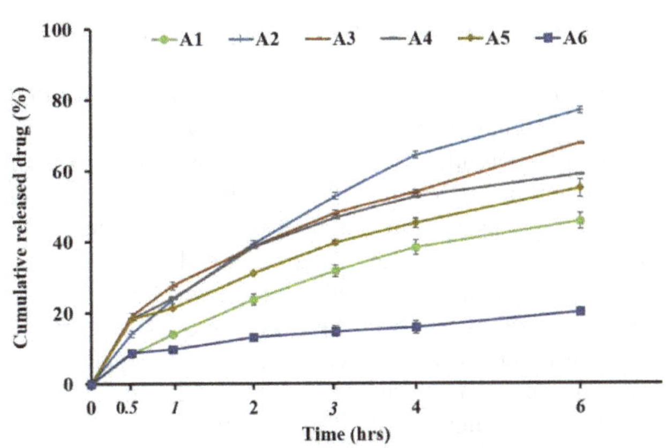

Figure 2. In vitro drug release patterns of different formulations vary in the base/mucoadhesive ingredients ratio.

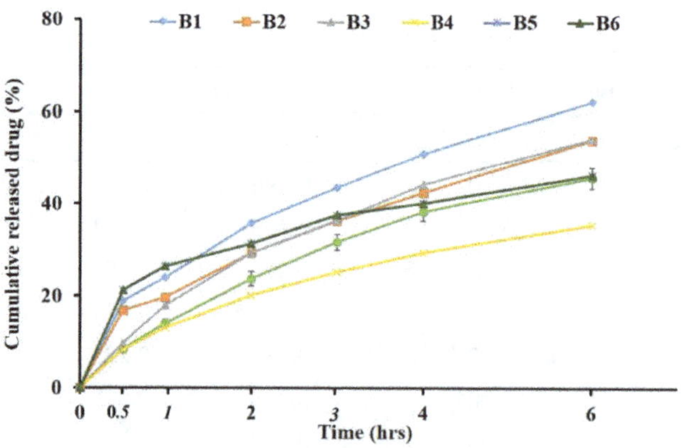

Figure 3. In vitro drug release patterns of different formulations vary in the ratios of mucoadhesive ingredients.

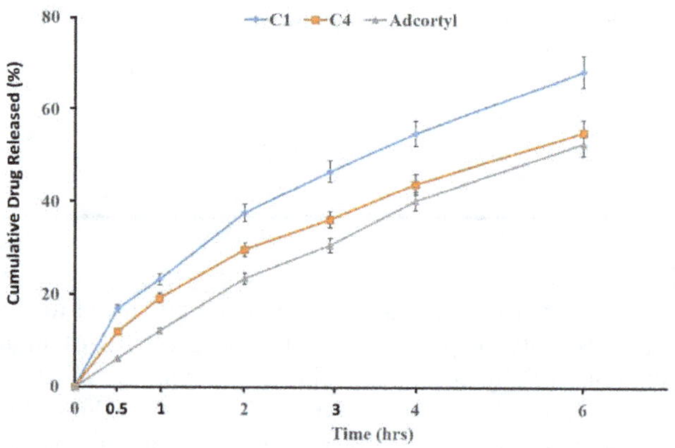

Figure 4. In vitro drug release patterns of the optimized formulations and Reference formulation (Adcortyl®).

Stability study

Short-term stability results of optimized formulation (C4) showed that the consistency and odor of formulations did not change significantly. Accordingly, long-term storage of formulations at 4 °C and 25 °C did not change consistency and odor of formulations. However, storage of formulation at 40 °C caused to the change in consistency without any effect on odor.

Drug release kinetic study

Kinetic study of drug release is often useful for comparative purposes and relating to the release parameters with bioavailability. To clarify the mechanism of release, the *in vitro* release data were fitted to different kinetic models. The accuracy and prediction ability of the models were compared by calculation of mean squared correlation coefficients (MRSQ) for all data sets (Table 4). Our finding revealed that, almost in all of the formulations the drug release data were fitted best to Higuchi models, even though some formulations also follow relatively from first order model. Therefore, diffusion could be considered as a major mechanism of drug release from the different formulations made from Plastibase®. Release of drug from Adcortyl® and formulation C4 followed from first order and Higuchi release kinetics, respectively.

Conclusion

Oral paste formulations of Triamcinolone Acetonide were prepared using plastibase as well as different ratios of pectin, gelatin and carboxymethylcellulose. Formulations were optimized after preliminary studies and formulation with desired durability of adhesion, spreadability and rheology property was compared with reference formulation in the case of release profile and kinetic. Release study and fitting release data in to kinetics models revealed that optimized formulation followed Higuchi release kinetics and had similar release pattern to the reference formulation.

Acknowledgments

The authors would like to thank Drug Applied Research Center, Tabriz University of Medical Sciences, Tabriz, Iran. This article is based on a thesis submitted for Pharm D degree (No. 3019) in Faculty of Pharmacy, Tabriz University of Medical Sciences, Tabriz, Iran.

Conflict of Interest

The authors report no conflicts of interest.

References

1. Albrektson M, Hedstrom L, Bergh H. Recurrent aphthous stomatitis and pain management with low-level laser therapy: a randomized controlled trial. *Oral Surg Oral Med Oral Pathol Oral Radiol* 2014;117(5):590-4. doi: 10.1016/j.oooo.2014.01.228
2. Porter SR, Hegarty A, Kaliakatsou F, Hodgson TA, Scully C. Recurrent aphthous stomatitis. *Clin Dermatol* 2000;18(5):569-78.
3. Ship JA. Recurrent aphthous stomatitis. An update. *Oral Surg Oral Med Oral Pathol Oral Radiol Endod* 1996;81(2):141-7.
4. Lee Y, Chien YW. Oral mucosa controlled delivery of LHRH by bilayer mucoadhesive polymer systems. *J Control Release* 1995;37(3):251-61. doi: 10.1016/0168-3659(95)00082-8
5. Miles DA, Bricker SL, Razmus TF, Potter RH. Triamcinolone acetonide versus chlorhexidine for treatment of recurrent stomatitis. *Oral Surg Oral Med Oral Pathol* 1993;75(3):397-402.
6. Scully C, Porter S. Oral mucosal disease: recurrent aphthous stomatitis. *Br J Oral Maxillofac Surg* 2008;46(3):198-206. doi: 10.1016/j.bjoms.2007.07.201
7. Browne RM, Fox EC, Anderson RJ. Topical triamcinolone acetonide in recurrent aphthous stomatitis. A clinical trial. *Lancet* 1968;1(7542):565-7. doi: 10.1016/s0140-6736(68)92833-x
8. Quijano D, Rodriguez M. Topical corticosteroids in recurrent aphthous stomatitis. Systematic review. *Acta Otorrinolaringol Esp* 2008;59(6):298-307. doi: 10.1016/s2173-5735(08)70242-4
9. Sveinsson SJ, Peter Holbrook W. Oral mucosal adhesive ointment containing liposomal

corticosteroid. *Intl J Pharm* 1993;95(1-3):105-9. doi: 10.1016/0378-5173(93)90396-w

10. Bernkop Schnurch A. Mucoadhesive systems in oral drug delivery. *Drug Discov Today Technol* 2005;2(1):83-7. doi: 10.1016/j.ddtec.2005.05.001
11. Rossi S, Sandri G, Caramella CM. Buccal drug delivery: A challenge already won? *Drug Discov Today Technol* 2005;2(1):59-65. doi: 10.1016/j.ddtec.2005.05.018
12. Salamat-Miller N, Chittchang M, Johnston TP. The use of mucoadhesive polymers in buccal drug delivery. *Adv Drug Deliv Rev* 2005;57(11):1666-91. doi: 10.1016/j.addr.2005.07.003
13. Smart JD. Drug delivery using buccal-adhesive systems. *Adv Drug Deliv Rev* 1993;11(3):253-70. doi: 10.1016/0169-409x(93)90012-s
14. Giunchedi P, Juliano C, Gavini E, Cossu M, Sorrenti M. Formulation and in vivo evaluation of chlorhexidine buccal tablets prepared using drug-loaded chitosan microspheres. *Eur J Pharm Biopharm* 2002;53(2):233-9. doi: 10.1016/s0939-6411(01)00237-5
15. Lee CH, Chien YW. Development and evaluation of a mucoadhesive drug delivery system for dual-controlled delivery of nonoxynol-9. *J Control Release* 1996;39(1):93-103. doi: 10.1016/0168-3659(95)00142-5
16. Sudhakar Y, Kuotsu K, Bandyopadhyay AK. Buccal bioadhesive drug delivery--a promising option for orally less efficient drugs. *J Control Release* 2006;114(1):15-40. doi: 10.1016/j.jconrel.2006.04.012
17. Wong CF, Yuen KH, Peh KK. Formulation and evaluation of controlled release Eudragit buccal patches. *Int J Pharm* 1999;178(1):11-22. doi: 10.1016/s0378-5173(98)00342-1

5

Preparation and Characterization of Nanosuspension of Aprepitant by H96 Process

Sunethra Kalvakuntla[1], Mangesh Deshpande[2], Zenab Attari[1], Koteshwara Kunnatur B[1]*

[1] Department of Pharmaceutics, Manipal College of Pharmaceutical Sciences, Manipal University, Manipal.
[2] Dr. Reddy's Laboratories Ltd., Hyderabad, India.

Article info

Keywords:
- Lyophilization
- Nanosuspension
- Particle size
- Second generation approach
- High pressure homogenization

Abstract

Purpose: Nanosuspension in drug delivery is known to improve solubility, dissolution and eventually bioavailability of the drugs. The purpose of the study was to compare particle size of nanosuspensions prepared by the first generation approach and H96 approach and to evaluate the effectiveness of H96 approach.
Methods: The nanosuspension of aprepitant was prepared by HPH and H96 approach. The prepared nanosuspensions were characterized for their particle size and zeta potential. The optimized nanosuspension was further evaluated for DSC, FT-IR, solubility and dissolution.
Results: The optimized nanosuspension (NCLH5) prepared using combination of tween 80 and poloxamer 188 as stabilizer, showed particle size of 35.82 nm and improved solubility and dissolution profile over pure drug. NCLH5 was chosen optimized formulation and further evaluated for other parameters after lyophilization. Lyophilization resulted in increase in particle size. The solubility and dissolution studies showed favorable increase in the performance. The FT-IR and DSC analysis showed change in the crystallinity after nanosizing.
Conclusion: The observations indicated that lyophilization prior to high pressure homogenization resulted in efficient particle size reduction yielding smaller particles than first generation preparation technique. H96 is a good and easy alternative to achieve efficient particle size reduction of drug in lesser time and increase its solubility and dissolution.

Introduction

Significant progress has been made in the area of supportive care in oncology over the last decade as chemotherapy-induced nausea and vomiting (CINV) has been a major problem leading to patients' refusal to continue chemotherapy. Aprepitant is an orally active NK 1 (neurokinin 1) receptor antagonist, used for the treatment of CINV.[1,2]

Aprepitant is given in combination with ondansetron and dexamethasone on day 1 and then continued on days 2 and 3 with dexamethasone which consequently improves acute, as well as delayed chemotherapy associated emesis. Aprepitant is a BCS class IV drug, having low solubility, low permeability). The bioavailability of aprepitant is dissolution rate limited following oral administration.[3,4]

Drug nanocrystals are a formulation approach to improve solubility of poorly soluble drugs and cosmetic actives. It has been first invented at the beginning of the 1990s and the first pharmaceutical product came in the year 2000. Arbitrarily, two generations of nanocrystals are proposed depending on the methods of preparation or technique used. The nanocrystal technology of the first generation comprises ball milling or high pressure homogenization (HPH) as a method of preparation.[5] SmartCrystals are the second generation nanocrystals prepared by the combination of methods. The production of smart crystals has been optimized by introducing modifications to the HPH process. This leads to faster production, smaller nanocrystals and an improved physical stability. This has also implications for improved *in vivo* performance after dermal application and oral or intravenous administration.[6]

In the previous study, we prepared nanosuspension of ibuprofen and aprepitant using combination of precipitation or ball milling with high pressure homogenization (HPH) and observed reduction in particle size with less processing time.[7] In present study two approaches i.e. HPH technique (first generation) and combination of lyophilization and HPH (second generation; H96 process) were evaluated for the production of aprepitant nanocrystals to enhance solubility and dissolution for enhancing bioavailability and reducing variability in systemic exposure.

Materials and Methods

The drug, aprepitant was provided as a kind gift by Dr. Reddy's Laboratories Ltd. All the chemicals and reagents used in the present study were of analytical grade. Tween 80 was procured from National Chemicals, Polyvinyl alcohol (PVA – Mw: 14000) from SD Fine-Chem. Ltd. and sodium lauryl sulfate (SLS) from Nice Chemicals Pvt. Ltd.

***Corresponding author:** Koteshwara KB, Email: kb.koteshwara@manipal.edu

Preparation of nanosuspensions

High pressure homogenization (HPH)

Aqueous solutions of stabilizers i.e. Tween 80, Poloxamer 188, PVA and SLS were prepared in various concentrations as shown in the Table 1 using purified water. Aprepitant (125 mg) was suspended in 10 ml of the stabilizer solution. The dispersion was homogenized using high speed homogenizer (Polytron PT 3100, Kinematica) at 10,000 rpm for 10 min to form homogeneous microsuspension. This was subjected to probe sonication (Vibracell VCX130; Sonis, USA) at amplitude of 80%, pulse 4 sec for 15 min to form presuspension. During this sonication, the temperature was maintained at 0°C using an ice bath. This presuspension was added dropwise to the remaining stabilizer solution and homogenized. Firstly, premilling step was conducted at 5000 psi for 5 cycles using high pressure homogenizer (Emulsiflex-C3, Avestin, USA). Then an HPH step was applied at 15000 psi for 10 cycles.

Table 1. Formulation batches by a) high pressure homogenization technique (First generation approach) and b) H96 process (Lyophilization + HPH)

Formulation code	Formulation Composition					
	Aprepitant (mg)	Tween 80 (%w/v)	Poloxamer 188 (%w/v)	PVA (%w/v)	SLS (%w/v)	Batch Size (ml)
a) Formulation batches by high pressure homogenization technique (First generation approach)						
NCH1	125	0.25	-	-	-	40
NCH2	125	0.5	-	-	-	40
NCH3	125	1	-	-	-	40
NCH4	125	2	-	-	-	40
NCH5	125	3	-	-	-	40
NCH6	125	-	0.25	-	-	40
NCH7	125	-	0.5	-	-	40
NCH8	125	-	1	-	-	40
NCH9	125	-	2	-	-	40
NCH10	125	-	3	-	-	40
NCH11	125	-	-	0.25	-	40
NCH12	125	-	-	0.5	-	40
NCH13	125	-	-	1	-	40
NCH14	125	-	-	2	-	40
NCH15	125	-	-	3	-	40
NCH16	125	-	-	-	0.25	40
NCH17	125	-	-	-	0.5	40
NCH18	125	-	-	-	1	40
NCH19	125	-	-	-	2	40
NCH20	125	-	-	-	3	40
NCH21	125	1	3	-	-	40
NCH22	125	1	-	0.25	-	40
NCH23	125	1	-	-	3	40
b) Formulation batches by H96 process (Lyophilization + HPH)						
NCLH1	125	1	-	-	-	40
NCLH2	125	-	3	-	-	40
NCLH3	125	-	-	0.25	-	40
NCLH4	125	-	-	-	3	40
NCLH5	125	1	3	-	-	40
NCLH6	125	1	-	0.25	-	40
NCLH7	125	1	-	-	3	40

H96 (lyophilization + HPH)

The H96 process is a combination of lyophilization and HPH techniques. The amount of drug and organic solvent are crucial factors to be considered for lyophilization in H96 process.[8] In the last step of drug (aprepitant) synthesis, no crystallization of the drug is performed but the drug solution was made using methanol as solvent. Methanol was solvent of choice as aprepitant was observed to be freely soluble in it. The prepared drug solution was then lyophilized. In the next step, the lyophilized product was dispersed in a various stabilizers solutions of concentrations (shown in the Table 1) using purified water, which was immediately passed through a homogenizer 15000 psi for 5 cycles. Four different stabilizers (Tween 80, Poloxamer 188, PVA and SLS) were screened in different concentrations, alone and in combinations (Table 1). The concentration of stabilizers was selected from the results obtained in HPH (first generation) process.

Shape and surface morphology: Scanning Electron Microscopy (SEM)

Immediately after freeze drying, the dry powder was examined for possible aggregation by visual inspection. Shape and surface morphology of the freeze dried nanocrystals was studied using SEM (JEOL, JSM 50A, Tokyo, Japan). An appropriate amount of freeze dried nanocrystals was mounted on metal (aluminium) stubs; the samples were mounted onto aluminium specimen stubs using double-sided adhesive tape and fractured with a razor blade. The samples were sputter-coated with gold/palladium for 120 sec at 14 mA under argon atmosphere for secondary electron emissive SEM and observed for morphology, at acceleration voltage of 20 KV.

Particle size and size distribution

The particle size and its distribution were determined using Zetasizer Nano ZS (Malvern instruments, U K) using a process called Dynamic Light Scattering (DLS). The zeta potential of a particle is the overall charge that the particle acquires in a particular medium. The particle size and zeta potential of nanosuspension samples were measured at 25°C. The nanosuspension by combination method showing the lowest particle size with acceptable zeta potential was selected for further studies. Though the zeta potential indicates the stability of the nanosuspension, however, the freeze drying is good for long term stability of colloidal nanoformulations and thus the optimized nanosuspensions were lyophilized using mannitol as cryoprotectant and subjected to various evaluation.[9]

Drug content

The drug content in the freeze dried product was analyzed by dissolving 10 mg of lyophilized nanocrystals in 10 ml of methanol. The sample was sonicated for 15 minutes and filtered using 0.22 μ membrane filter and after sufficient dilution, the amount of drug was determined spectrophotometrically at 210 nm (UV 1601PC, Shimadzu, Japan). The UV method was selected by scanning lower concentrations of the aprepitant in various media (methanol, pH 1.2 HCl buffer, pH 4.6 acetate buffer, pH 6.8 phosphate buffer, pH 7.4 phosphate buffer, distilled water, 2.2% SLS) to find out the maximum wavelength after nullifying the interference of the media.[10]

Saturation solubility

An excess amount of the freeze dried product was added separately to 4 ml each of distilled water, pH 1.2 HCl buffer + 2.2% w/v SLS, pH 4.6 acetate buffer + 2.2% w/v SLS, pH 6.8 phosphate buffer, pH 7.4 phosphate buffer, 2.2% w/v SLS solution. Then the mixtures were mounted on rotospin apparatus for 48 hrs at room temperature. The solution was filtered through a 0.22 μ membrane filter and the amount of the drug dissolved was analyzed using spectrophotometer at 210 nm.

Fourier-transform infra red spectroscopy (FT-IR) and differential scanning calorimetry (DSC)

The optimized formulation was subjected to FT-IR (Shimadzu FT-IR 8300 spectrophotometer) and DSC (DSC-60, Shimadzu, Japan) analysis and compared with that of pure drug to assess drug-excipient interaction and crystallinity of the drug in the formulation.

In vitro release studies

The *in vitro* dissolution study of nanocrystals and pure drug was carried out in 900 ml of different discriminating media such as 2.2% w/v SLS solution, pH 1.2 HCl buffer + 2.2% w/v SLS, pH 4.6 acetate buffer + 2.2% w/v SLS, pH 6.8 phosphate buffer + 2.2% w/v SLS, pH 7.4 phosphate buffer + 2.2% w/v SLS using USP type I dissolution apparatus at 75 rpm (US FDA dissolution methods).[11] The temperature of the dissolution medium was maintained at 37±0.5°C by a thermostatically controlled water bath. Five ml of sample was withdrawn at the time intervals of 10, 15, 20, 30 and 45 minutes and replaced with 5 ml of fresh buffer. The collected sample was filtered and analyzed spectrophotometrically at 210 nm. The dissolution profile of nanocrystal was compared with that of pure drug. The results were analyzed using student's t-test.

Results

Preparation and characterization of nanosuspension

The particle size of various batches of nanosuspension prepared by HPH perse and H96 process is depicted in Table 2. The stabilizers, Tween 80 and Poloxamer 188 resulted in smaller particle size compared to PVA and SLS. The combination of Tween 80 and Poloxamer 188 was observed to be effective in stabilization of prepared napsuspension. H96 process, i.e. combination of lyophilization and HPH resulted in smaller particle size than HPH perse. The particle size of NCH21 prepared by HPH perse using Tween 80 and Poloxamer 188 was found to be 320.4 nm whereas, NCLH5 prepared by H96 process using same stabilizers was observed to be 35.78 nm. The particle size of NCLH5 is smaller and thus chosen as optimized formulation, however, lyophilization resulted in increase in particle size. The particle size and zeta potential of the NCLH5 before and after lyophilization was depicted in the Table 3.

Shape and surface morphology: Scanning Electron Microscopy (SEM)

The freeze dried optimized nanocrystals (NCLH5) was observed for the shape and surface morphology by SEM. The SEM images of pure drug showed agglomerates (a) and that of the optimized formulation showed the particles are discrete without agglomeration (b) which could be attributed to the presence of stabilizer (Figure 1).

The SEM images confirmed that though an increase in particle size was observed after freeze drying, it was still in the submicron level and smaller in size in comparison with pure drug, but not below 100 nm (smart crystal).

Table 2. Particle size and zeta potential of nanosuspensions prepared by a) HPH process (First generation approach) and b) H96 process (Lyophilization + HPH)

Formulation	Particle size (nm)	PDI	ZP (mV)
a) Particle size and zeta potential of nanosuspensions prepared by HPH process (First generation approach)			
NCH1	516.2	0.293	-18.60
NCH2	443.2	0.218	-22.93
NCH3	433.1	0.288	-36.79
NCH4	373.9	0.306	-23.26
NCH5	351.0	0.278	-29.26
NCH6	840.9	0.331	-13.90
NCH7	815.8	0.294	-25.10
NCH8	890.7	0.298	-25.80
NCH9	784.6	0.269	-21.80
NCH10	840.0	0.256	-22.80
NCH11	960.2	0.227	-2.20
NCH12	1011.9	0.594	-6.61
NCH13	1169.4	0.369	-1.92
NCH14	1339.3	0.321	-2.37
NCH15	1502.9	0.341	-8.21
NCH16	1132.6	0.243	-8.41
NCH17	870.5	0.252	-6.21
NCH18	763.8	0.215	-4.08
NCH19	698.2	0.189	-13.64
NCH20	678.2	0.165	-10.22
NCH21	320.4	0.266	-28.80
NCH22	526.2	0.293	-15.10
NCH23	510.5	0.272	-16.92
b) Particle size and zeta potential of nanosuspensions prepared by H96 process (second generation approach)			
NCLH1	89.1	0.288	-20.60
NCLH2	125.1	0.141	-16.93
NCLH3	260.6	0.274	-5.79
NCLH4	178.7	0.255	-6.26
NCLH5	**35.78**	**0.257**	**-23.2**
NCLH6	126.5	0.181	-13.90
NCLH7	110.8	0.159	-18.10

Table 3. Particle size and zeta potential of optimized formulation before and after lyophilization

Optimized formulation (NCLH5)	Before lyophilization	After lyophilization
Particle size (nm)	35.78	119.9
Zeta potential (mV)	-23.2	-32.4

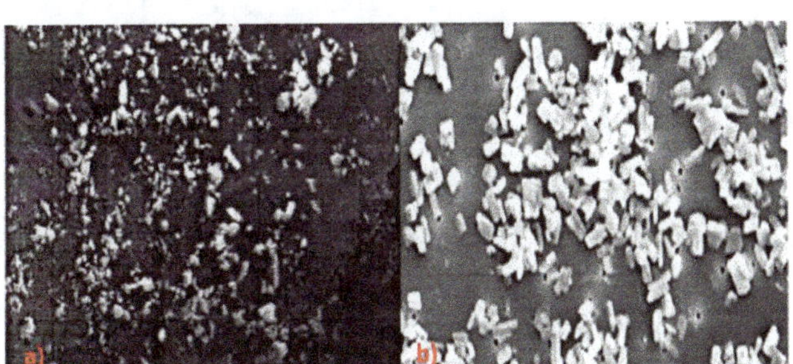

Figure 1. SEM images of a) pure drug and b) aprepitant nanocrystals

Drug content

The drug content of the freeze dried formulation (NCLH5) was found to be around 90%. The loss of drug can be attributed to the loss occurring during the preparation and lyophilization.[12] However, there was no change in color or aggregation observed.

Saturation Solubility

Saturation solubility study was carried out for both pure drug and nanocrystals in distilled water, pH 1.2 HCl buffer + 2.2% w/v SLS, pH 4.6 acetate buffer + 2.2% w/v SLS, phosphate buffer pH 6.8, phosphate buffer pH 7.4, 2.2% w/v SLS solution (as per FDA guidelines, pH 1 to 7.4).[13] However, it was found that drug was getting precipitated in HCl buffer pH 1.2 and acetate buffer pH 4.6, therefore, 2.2% w/v SLS was added to both the buffers. The saturation solubility of aprepitant was observed to increase over pure drug in all the vehicles used. This is due to the decrease in particle size when compared to pure dug according to Ostwald-Freundlich equation. Another possible explanation for the increase in saturation solubility can be given by Kelvin equation which states that the dissolution pressure increases with increasing curvature, which means decreasing particle size.[14] The curvature is enormous when the particle size is in the nanometer range. The fold increase in the solubility of nanocrystal over pure drug is depicted in Table 4.

Table 4. Saturation Solubility of pure drug and aprepitant nanocrystals

Medium	Pure drug Concentration (µg/ml) (Mean ± SD)	Nanocrystals Concentration (µg/ml) (Mean ± SD)	Fold increase in saturation solubility
Distilled water	2.90 ± 0.53	43.1 ± 5.10	14.86
pH 1.2 buffer + 2.2%w/v SLS	2736 ± 30.38	3314 ± 10.99	1.21
pH 4.6 buffer + 2.2%w/v SLS	3364 ± 12.59	3854 ± 8.17	1.15
Phosphate buffer pH6.8	3.4 ± 2.38	38.6 ± 3.94	11.35
Phosphate buffer pH7.4	3.52 ± 1.22	40.2 ± 5.10	11.42
2.2%w/v SLS in water	3910 ± 31.40	4610 ± 7.21	1.18

FT-IR and DSC

In the case of formulation NCLH5, disappearance of two peaks in the FT-IR spectrum was observed along with the attenuation of other peaks when compared to that of pure drug which may be due to the reduction in crystallinity of the drug (Figure 2).[15]

The assessment crystalline state helps in understanding the polymorphic changes that the drug might have undergone when subjected to nanosizing. So it is necessary to investigate the extent of amorphous state generated during the production of nanosuspensions. In DSC thermograms, pure drug showed an intense peak at 253.71°C whereas the drug peak in nanoformulation was observed at 244.70°C. The heat of melting was observed to be -17.94 J/g for pure drug and -1.13 J/g for nanoformulation. The shift in the peak and reduction in the peak intensity indicated a change in the crystallinity of the drug (Figure 2). The other reason could be presence of large amount of excipient, mannitol.[16]

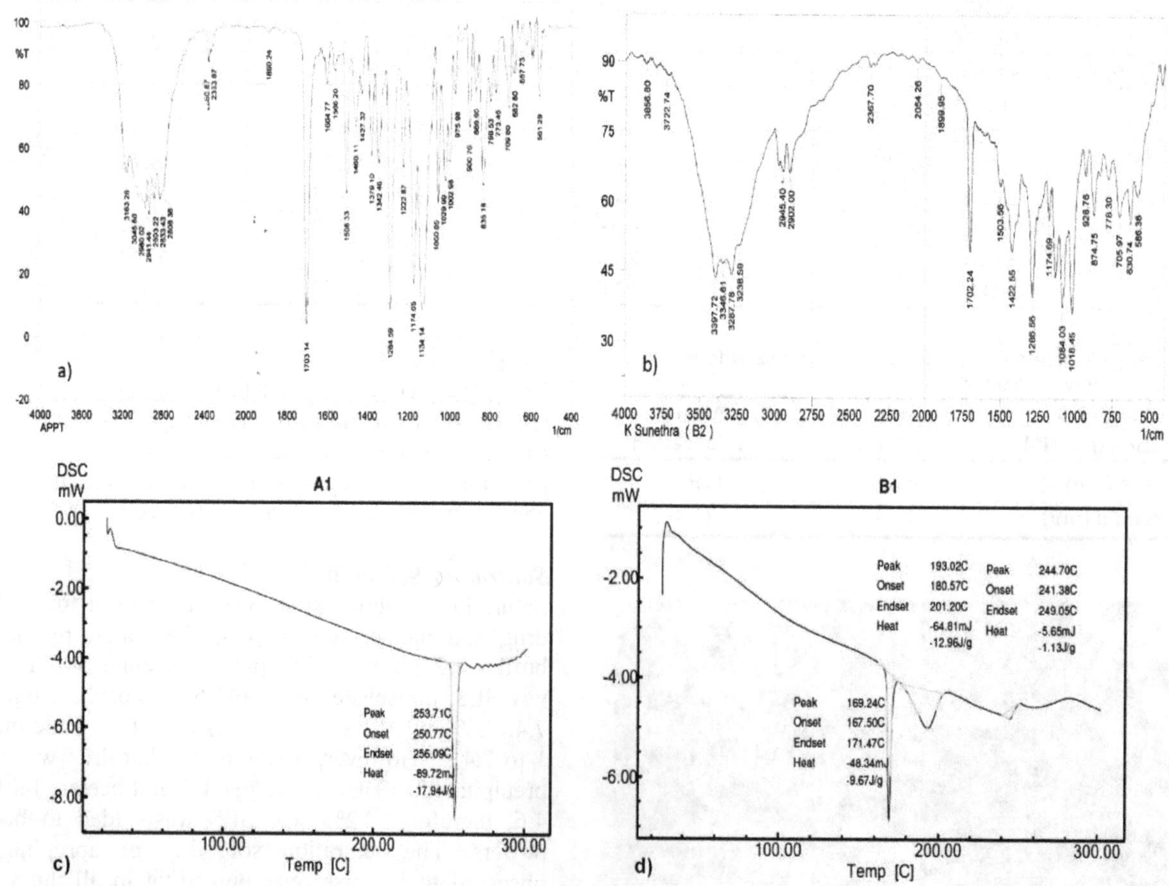

Figure 2. FT-IR spectra of a) aprepitant (pure drug) and b) aprepitant nanocrystal and DSC thermograms of c) aprepitant (pure drug) and d) aprepitant nanocrystal

In vitro dissolution studies

The *in vitro* dissolution studies were carried out in different media. 2.2% SLS was added in all the buffers to improve solubility of drug and avoid precipitation of drug. It was observed that dissolution of aprepitant crystal was significantly higher than the pure drug irrespective of the medium used. The two times fold increase in dissolution of the nanocrystals as compared to pure drug was observed at 45 minutes (see Table 5) and the dissolution profile of pure drug and nanocrystal are depicted in Figure 3.

Table 5. Percentage enhancement of dissolution of aprepitant nanocrystals as compared to pure drug at 45 minutes

Dissolution medium	%CDR at 45 minutes (Mean±SD)		Fold enhancement of dissolution of nanocrystal
	Pure drug	Nanocrystals	
2.2%w/v SLS	50.52 ± 1.05	100.05 ± 0.53	1.98
pH 1.2 HCl buffer + 2.2% w/v SLS	29.52 ± 0.55	85.05 ± 0.75	2.88
pH 4.6 acetate buffer + 2.2% w/v SLS	43.59 ± 0.55	88.05 ± 1.75	2.01
pH 6.8 phosphate buffer + 2.2% w/v SLS	49.18 ± 2.55	99.03 ± 1.83	2.01
pH 7.4 phosphate buffer + 2.2% w/v SLS	48.11 ± 1.13	100.93 ± 0.65	2.09

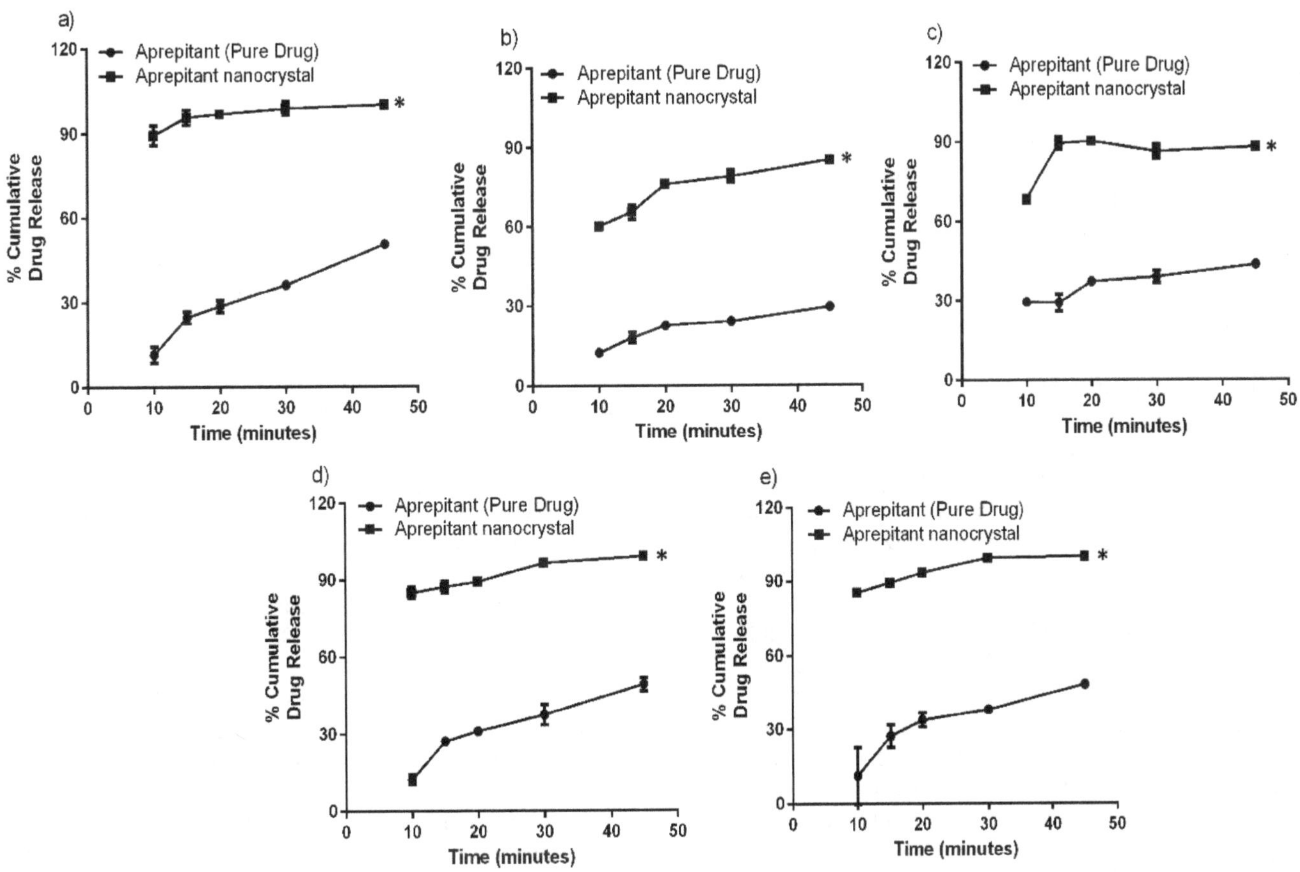

Figure 3. Dissolution profile of pure drug and aprepitant nanocrystal in various media a) 2.2% SLS, b) pH 1.2 HCl buffer + 2.2% SLS, c) pH 4.6 acetate buffer + 2.2% SLS, d) pH 6.8 phosphate buffer + 2.2% SLS and e) pH 7.4 phosphate buffer + 2.2% SLS
(* indicates significant difference between two groups at $p<0.05$ using student's t-test.)

Discussion

In first generation approach i.e. HPH, the stabilizers and its concentration were observed to greatly influence the particle size of the nanosuspensions. In case of PVA, it was observed that the particle size increased as the amount of stabilizer increased. While in case of Poloxamer 188 there was no significant change in particle size occurred with increase in the stabilizer concentration. In presence of Tween 80, particle size decreased with increase in concentration. Various reports suggest that combination of two stabilizers, particularly one surfactant stabilizer and one polymeric stabilizer gives more thermodynamically stable nanosuspensions.[17] Therefore, Tween 80 (surfactant stabilizer) was coupled with different polymeric stabilizers viz. PVA, SLS and Poloxamer 188 to achieve desired stability. The concentration of Tween 80 was fixed to 1%w/v as it was found that zeta potential of NCH3 was -36.79 mV which is expected to be a stable formulation according to the literature.[18]

The selected batches from first generation approach using specific concentration of stabilizers, which showed optimum particle size, were subjected to second generation process (H96 process). The particle size, PDI and zeta potential of nanosuspensions prepared by H96 process were summarized in Table 4. The particle size of the nanosuspension batch, NCLH1 using Tween 80 as stabilizer was found to be 89 nm (lower than 100 nm) a PDI of 0.288. The zeta potential was observed to be -20.60 indicating its stability however; sedimentation was seen after 24 hours. The particle size of nanosuspension with Poloxamer 188 was observed to be 125.1 nm (slightly above 100 nm) with a low PDI of 0.141. However, the zeta potential of -16.93 mV did not indicate its stability. In addition the sedimentation was also seen. The particle size of nanosuspensions with PVA (NCLH3) and SLS (NCLH4) was not even near to 100 nm and the nanosuspension was not stable. Thus, combination strategy using one surfactant stabilizer and one polymeric stabilizer was attempted here to improve the stability of the nanosuspensions. Tween 80 (surfactant stabilizer) was coupled with different polymeric stabilizers viz. PVA, SLS and Poloxamer 188 to achieve desired stability. Concentration of Tween 80 was fixed to 1%w/v as it showed highest stability in HPH process.

The use of Poloxamer 188 and Tween 80 (NCLH5), gave a particle size of 35.78 nm (Smart Crystals) with a PDI of 0.257 and an acceptable zeta potential of -23.2 mV (Figure 1). Earlier, Moschwitzer (2006) filed a patent for amphotericin B nanosuspension with 62 nm particle size prepared by H96 process.[19] Moschwitzer lyophilized the drug using liquid nitrogen, however, in the present case; the drug was lyophilized by storing at -80°C followed by freeze drying. The use of Tween 80 with PVA (NCLH6) and SLS (NCLH7) resulted in particle size near to 100 nm. These batches had a low PDI compared to NCLH5 but, their zeta potential was not indicating any stability. Hence, NCLH5 was chosen as optimized formulation and lyophilized for further studies. Although lyophilized powder was free flowing, there was significant increase in particle size which needs attention to overcome this (Table 5 and Figure 2).

H96 process led to efficient size reduction, eventually resulting in smaller particles of drug (aprepitant in our case) in nanosuspension than conventional approach (as reported by Salazar 2011).[20] It has been reported that lyophilization of drug dispersed in organic solvent lead to physical modification of drug particle which possess advantage of uniformly dispersed coarse drug in stabilizer solution and reduction in particle with less processing time and wear-tear effect.[21] We also observed that smaller particle size (35.78 nm) was obtained in 5 cycles of homogenization (lesser time than first generation approach - 10 cycles) and the PDI of 0.257 indicated uniform particle size distribution in nanosuspension.

The selected nanoformulation, NCLH 5 showed acceptable nanosized particles in SEM and by zetasizer and exhibited improved solubility and dissolution profile over pure drug in different media. These observations suggested that combination of size reduction methods, lyophilization with HPH in the present case, can be successfully employed to improve solubility of drugs or active compounds in lesser time. Furthermore, it needs to be evaluated for its application in large scale production of different dosage forms.

Acknowledgments

The authors are thankful to Manipal university for providing the facilities to carry out the present work and also would like to thank Dr. Reddy's Laboratories Ltd. for providing us the drug.

Conflict of Interest

The authors declare no conflict of interest.

Abbreviations

CINV – chemotherapy induced nausea and vomiting; NK 1 – neurokinin 1; BCS – biopharmaceutics classification system; HPH – high pressure homogenization; SEM – scanning electron microscopy; DLS – dynamic light scattering; FT-IR – fourier-transform infra red; DSC – differential scanning calorimetry

References

1. Chawla SP, Grunberg SM, Gralla RJ, Hesketh PJ, Rittenberg C, Elmer ME, et al. Establishing the dose of the oral nk1 antagonist aprepitant for the prevention of chemotherapy-induced nausea and vomiting. *Cancer* 2003;97(9):2290-300. doi: 10.1002/cncr.11320
2. Hesketh PJ, Grunberg SM, Gralla RJ, Warr DG, Roila F, de Wit R, et al. The oral neurokinin-1 antagonist aprepitant for the prevention of chemotherapy-induced nausea and vomiting: A multinational, randomized, double-blind, placebo-controlled trial in patients receiving high-dose cisplatin--the aprepitant protocol 052 study group. *J Clin Oncol* 2003;21(22):4112-9. doi: 10.1200/JCO.2003.01.095
3. Majumdar AK, Howard L, Goldberg MR, Hickey L, Constanzer M, Rothenberg PL, et al. Pharmacokinetics of aprepitant after single and multiple oral doses in healthy volunteers. *J Clin Pharmacol* 2006;46(3):291-300. doi: 10.1177/0091270005283467
4. Bergstrom M, Hargreaves RJ, Burns HD, Goldberg MR, Sciberras D, Reines SA, et al. Human positron emission tomography studies of brain neurokinin 1 receptor occupancy by aprepitant. *Biol Psychiatry*

2004;55(10):1007-12. doi: 10.1016/j.biopsych.2004.02.007

5. Muller RH, Peters K. Nanosuspensions for the formulation of poorly soluble drugs: I. Preparation by a size reduction technique. *Int J Pharm* 1998;160(2):229-37. doi:10.1016/S0378-5173(97)00311-6
6. Keck C, Kobierski S, Mauludin R, Muller RH. Second generation of drug nanocrystals for delivery of poorly soluble drugs: Smartcrystal technology. *Dosis* 2008;24(2):124-8.
7. Attari Z, Kalvakuntla S, Reddy MS, Deshpande M, Rao CM, Koteshwara KB. Formulation and characterisation of nanosuspensions of BCS class II and IV drugs by combinative method. *J Exp Nano* 2016;11(4):276-88.
8. Salazar J, Ghanem A, Muller RH, Moschwitzer JP. Nanocrystals: Comparison of the size reduction effectiveness of a novel combinative method with conventional top-down approaches. *Eur J Pharm Biopharm* 2012;81(1):82-90. doi: 10.1016/j.ejpb.2011.12.015
9. Abdelwahed W, Degobert G, Stainmesse S, Fessi H. Freeze-drying of nanoparticles: Formulation, process and storage considerations. *Adv Drug Deliv Rev* 2006;58(15):1688-713. doi: 10.1016/j.addr.2006.09.017
10. Benjamin T, Rajyalakshmi Ch, Rambabu C. Derivative spectrophotometric methods for determination of aprepitant in bulk and pharmaceutical formulation. *Der Pharma Chem* 2013;5(1):156-60.
11. Dissolution methods. U.S. Food and Drug Administration, U.S. Department of Health and Human Services. Available from: http://www.accessdata.fda.gov/scripts/cder/dissolution/dsp_SearchResults_Dissolutions.cfm
12. Katteboinaa S, Chandrasekhar VSRP, Balaji S. Drug nanocrystals: A novel formulation approach for poorly soluble drugs. *Int J Pharmtech Res* 2009;1(3):682-94.
13. Shah VP, Lesko LJ, Fan J, Fleischer N, Handerson J, Malinowski H, et al. FDA Guidance for Industry: Dissolution Testing of Immediate Release Solid Oral Dosage forms. *Dissolut Technol* 1997;4(4):15-22.
14. Junyaprasert VB, Morakul B. Nanocrystals for enhancement of oral bioavailability of poorly-water soluble drugs. *Asian J Pharm Sci* 2015;10(1):13-23. doi:10.1016/j.ajps.2014.08.005
15. Liu J, Zou M, Piao H, Liu Y, Tang B, Gao Y, et al. Characterization and pharmacokinetic study of aprepitant solid dispersions with soluplus(r). *Molecules* 2015;20(6):11345-56. doi: 10.3390/molecules200611345
16. Surolia R, Pachauri M, Ghosh PC. Preparation and characterization of monensin loaded plga nanoparticles: In vitro anti-malarial activity against plasmodium falciparum. *J Biomed Nanotechnol* 2012;8(1):172-81. doi:10.1166/jbn.2012.1366
17. Wu L, Zhang J, Watanabe W. Physical and chemical stability of drug nanoparticles. *Adv Drug Deliv Rev* 2011;63(6):456-69. doi: 10.1016/j.addr.2011.02.001
18. Gao L, Zhang D, Chen M. Drug nanocrystals for the formulation of poorly soluble drugs and its application as a potential drug delivery system. *J Nanopart Res* 2008;10(5):845-62. doi: 10.1007/s11051-008-9357-4
19. Möschwitzer J, Lemke A. Method for carefully producing ultrafine particle suspensions and ultrafine particles and use thereof. *WO/2006/108637*. Unitied states patent US; 2006.
20. Salazar J, Heinzerling O, Muller RH, Moschwitzer JP. Process optimization of a novel production method for nanosuspensions using design of experiments (doe). *Int J Pharm* 2011;420(2):395-403. doi: 10.1016/j.ijpharm.2011.09.003
21. Hu X, Chen X, Zhang L, Lin X, Zhang Y, Tang X, et al. A combined bottom-up/top-down approach to prepare a sterile injectable nanosuspension. *Int J Pharm* 2014;472(1-2):130-9. doi: 10.1016/j.ijpharm.2014.06.018

Development and Characterization of Solid Dispersion for Dissolution Improvement of Furosemide by Cogrinding Method

Mohammad Reza Siahi-Shadbad[1,2], **Saeed Ghanbarzadeh**[2,3,4], **Mohammad Barzegar-Jalali**[1,2]*, **Hadi Valizadeh**[2], **Alireza Taherpoor**[2], **Ghobad Mohammadi**[5], **Azim Barzegar-Jalali**[6], **Khosro Adibkia**[1,2,4]

[1] *Drug Applied Research Center, Tabriz University of Medical Science, Tabriz, Iran.*
[2] *Faculty of Pharmacy, Tabriz University of Medical Science, Tabriz, Iran.*
[3] *Student Research Committee, Tabriz University of Medical Sciences, Tabriz, Iran.*
[4] *Research Center for Pharmaceutical Nanotechnology, Tabriz University of Medical Sciences, Tabriz, Iran.*
[5] *School of Pharmacy, Kermanshah University of Medical Science, Kermanshah, Iran.*
[6] *Faculty of Medicine, Islamic Azad University, Ardabil Branch, Ardabil, Iran.*

Article info

Keywords:
- Furosemide
- Solid dispersion
- Dissolution rate
- Release kinetic

Abstract

Purpose: The purpose of this study was to prepare and characterize solid dispersion formulation of furosemide to enhance dissolution rate.
Methods: Solid dispersions with different drug: carrier ratios were prepared by cogrinding method using crospovidone and microcrystalline cellulose as carrier. The physical state and interactions between the drug and carrier were characterized by Fourier transform infrared spectroscopic (FT-IR) and X ray diffraction (XRD).
Results: Solid dispersions (especially with drug: Carrier ratio of 1:2) showed a higher dissolution rate than their respective physical mixture and pure furosemide. Dissolution rate in pH 5.8 was also higher than pH 1.2. The XRD analysis showed that crystalline form was changed to the amorphous state in the solid dispersions. FT-IR analysis did not show any physicochemical interactions in the solid dispersion formulations. Release kinetic of formulations were fitted best to the Weibull and Wagner log probability (linear kinetic) as well as suggested 2 and Gompertz (non-linear kinetic) models.
Conclusion: The dissolution properties of furosemide were improved with the use of hydrophilic carriers in solid dispersions due to change in the crystalline form of the drug and more intimate contact between drug and carriers which was dependent on the type and ratio of carrier as well as dissolution medium pH.

Introduction

Oral drug delivery is the simplest and easiest way of drugs administering, because of the greater stability, smaller bulk, and easy production. Nearly 40% of new discovered chemical are poorly water soluble. Dissolution is the rate limiting step for the poorly water soluble drugs. Poor solubility results in low bioavailability, increase in the dose, large inter and intra subject variation and large variations in blood drug concentrations depending on fed and fasted conditions. Enhancement of solubility and dissolution rate is an important step in drug development. For better absorption and quick onset of action, dissolution rate enhancement is critical.[1-4] To improve the dissolution and bioavailability of poorly water-soluble drugs, researchers have employed various techniques such as micronization, solubilization, salt formation, use of surfactant, use of cosolvent, complexation with polymers, use of prodrug and drug derivatization, pH alteration and others.[5-10] Among various approaches, the solid dispersion (SD) technique is a promising and most successful method in improving the dissolution and bioavailability of poorly soluble drugs because it is simple, economical and advantageous. A solid dispersion can be defined as the dispersion of one or more active ingredients in an inert carrier matrix in solid-state prepared by a melting (fusion), solvent, or melting-solvent method. The increased dissolution rates from solid dispersions are mostly attributed to the reduction of particle size of the drug within the dispersions and increased wettability.[11-14] Solid dispersion has advantages like, increase in the dissolution with absorption enhancement and therapeutic efficacy of dosage form, obtaining a homogeneous distribution of a small quantity of drug in a solid state, stabilization of unstable drugs, formulation of sustained release product of soluble drugs by using poorly soluble and insoluble carriers and increase in the rate and extent of the absorption of the drug. Higher drug dissolution rates from a solid dispersion can be facilitated by optimizing the wetting characteristics of the compound surface, as well as particle size reduction and increasing the interfacial area available for drug dissolution.[15-20] Various hydrophilic carriers such as polyethylene glycols, polyvinylpyrrolidone, gelucires, poloxamers, sugars, urea,

***Corresponding author:** Mohammad Barzegar-Jalali, Email: mahbarja@gmail.com

HPMC and gums have been investigated for improving the dissolution rate and bioavailability of poorly water soluble drugs.[21-27]

Furosemide is practically insoluble in water (Class-II of Biopharmaceutical classification system, BCS). The solid dispersion approach has been widely and successfully applied to improve the solubility, dissolution rate and consequently the bioavailability of poorly soluble drugs.[28-30] The objective of the present investigation was to formulate FUR solid dispersion to enhance its dissolution rate.

Materials and Methods

Materials

Furosemide was purchased from Jinaram Mandel Factory (India). Microcrystalline cellulose (Avicel PH-101) was obtained from Blanver Company (Korea). Crospovidone was supplied by BASF Company (Germany). HCl, NaOH and KH_2PO_4 were obtained from Merck Company (Germany).

Preparation of physical mixture

The physical mixtures were prepared by weighing the calculated amounts of FUR and carriers and then mixing them in a glass mortar by trituration. The resultant physical mixtures were passed through 40-mesh sieve and stored in desiccator until used for further studies.

Preparation of solid dispersions

Solid dispersions of FUR with crospovidone and microcrystalline cellulose were prepared by the cogrinding method. Accurately weighed quantities (10 g) of FUR and the respective dispersion carrier were transferred into a Ball Mill (Fritsch, Germany). The mixtures were then rotate (rpm=360) at room temperature for 3 hrs.

Characterization of formulations

Fourier Transform Infrared (FT-IR) spectroscopic analysis

FT-IR spectra of moisture free powdered samples of FUR and its physical mixtures and solid dispersion with crospovidone and Avicel (1:2 drug: carrier) were obtained using a spectrophotometer (Bomem, USA) by potassium bromide (KBr, 150 bar) pellet method. The scanning range was 450–4000 cm^{-1}, and the resolution was 1 cm^{-1}.

X-Ray diffraction (XRD) studies

The X-ray diffraction patterns were determined for pure drug, carriers, physical mixtures and solid dispersions. X-ray diffractograms were obtained using the X-ray diffractometer (Siemens, Germany) and Cu-kα radiation (λ=1.54). Diffractograms were run at scanning speed of 2°/min and a chart speed of 0.6°/min.

Particle size analyzing

The particle size and size distribution of the prepared solid dispersions were determined using the laser diffraction particle size analyzer (Shimadzu, Japan) equipped with the Wing software (version 2101). The mean diameter and size distribution of the resulted homogeneous suspension were assessed. Each value resulted from triplicate determinations.

In vitro release study

In vitro dissolution study was performed in a paddle type dissolution apparatus (USP Type II). A fixed amount of each batch of formulation and pure FUR powder, containing 20 mg equivalent of FUR were used for dissolution study purpose. Simulated Gastric Fluid (SGF) without pepsin and Phosphate buffered saline (PBS), pH 5.8, was used as dissolution media, where 900 mL of it was taken in each dissolution vessel at a temperature of 37±0.5 °C and a paddle speed of 100 rpm. The dissolution test was carried out for 60 min and 5 ml sample was withdrawn at predetermined intervals of 5, 10, 15, 20, 30, 45 and 60 min. The dissolution samples were then analyzed spectrophotometrically by UV-VIS spectrophotometer (SHIMADZU, Japan) at 234 nm in pH 1.2 (linear in the range of 1-5 µg/mL, R^2= 0.9997) and at 272 nm in pH 5.8 (linear in the range of 2.5-20 µg/mL, R^2= 0.9997).

Release kinetic analysis

The release data obtained from *in vitro* dissolution studies were fitted to ten linear and seven non-linear kinetic equations to find out the mechanism of drug release (Table 1).[31,32] The precision and prediction power of the modes were evaluated by calculation of mean percent error (MPE) for each set as well as overall mean percent error (OMPE) for all set using following equations.[33]

$$MPE = \frac{100 \times \sum \frac{|Fcal - Fobs|}{Fobs}}{N}$$

$$OMPE = \frac{\sum_{1}^{14} MPE}{14}$$

Where, 14 is the number of formulations.

Where Fobs and Fcal are the measured and calculated fraction of the drug released in each sampling time, and N is the number of sampling times.[5,34]

Dissolution profile of different formulations were compared using calculation of mean percent dissolution (MPD) and time needed to release 30% of incorporated drug (t30%) in pH 1.2 and 5.8.

MPD was calculated according to following equation.[35]

$$MPD = \frac{\sum_{i=1}^{n} D\%}{n}$$

Where D is the percent of drug dissolved at different sampling times.

Table 1. Mean squared correlation coefficients (MRSQ), mean percent error (MPE) and percent of total number of error (NE) of the kinetic models used for analysis of drug release data.

Models	Equation	MRSQ	MPE	NE<5	NE<10	NE<12
Zero	$F = K_0 t$	0.898	18.333	16.667	14.286	46.429
First	$\ln(1-F) = -k_f t$	0.962	51.415	25.000	25.000	36.905
Higuchi	$F = k_H \sqrt{t}$	0.943	12.346	29.762	29.762	64.286
Pepas	$\ln F = \ln k_p + p \ln t$	0.959	15.325	16.667	16.667	42.857
Hixon–Crowell	$1-\sqrt[3]{1-F} = k_{\frac{1}{3}} t$	0.960	49.488	1.190	1.190	13.095
Square root of mass	$1-\sqrt{1-F} = k_{\frac{1}{2}} t$	0.947	14.459	23.810	23.810	52.381
Three seconds root of mass	$1-\sqrt[3]{(1-F)^2} = k_{\frac{2}{3}} t$	0.931	16.271	19.048	19.048	50.000
Weibull	$\ln[-\ln(1-F)] = \beta \ln t_d + \beta \ln t$	0.970	5.308	64.286	64.286	88.095
Wagner Linear	$Z = Z_0 + qt$	0.919	15.432	25.000	25.000	63.095
Wagner Log probability	$Z = Z_0' + q' \ln t$	0.962	7.638	41.667	41.667	85.714
Gompertz	$F = e^{\left(-a \times e^{-b \log t}\right)}$	0.971	8.028	42.857	42.857	71.429
Skrdla (homogen)	$F = 1 - e^{\left(ate^{-bt^2} - 1\right)}$	0.925	10.447	33.333	33.333	63.095
Skrdla (hetrogen)	$F = 1 - e^{\left(\frac{-a}{t\left(e^{bt^2} - 1\right)}\right)}$	0.869	25.368	13.095	13.095	42.857
Logistic	$F = e^{\left(\frac{a + b \log t}{1 + e^{(a + b \log t)}}\right)}$	0.979	9.657	45.238	45.238	73.810
Reciprocal powered time (suggested 1)*	$\left(\frac{1}{F} - 1\right) = \frac{m}{t^b}$	0.939	17.076	16.667	16.667	51.190
Suggested 2*	$n < 1 \quad 1-(1-F)^{1-n} = kt$	0.979	8.411	52.381	67.857	71.429
Suggested 3*	$n > 1 \quad \frac{1}{(1-F)^{n'-1}} - 1 = (n'-1) k_{n'-1} t$	0.968	22.406	53.571	66.667	67.857

F denotes fraction of drug released up to time t. k_0, k_f, k_H, p, k_p, $k_{1/3}$, $k_{1/2}$, $k_{2/3}$, t_d, β, Z_0, Z_0', q, q', a and b are parameters of the models. Z and Z' are probits of fraction of drug released at any time. Z_0 and Z_0' are the values of Z and Z' when t=0 and t=1 respectively.
*See reference 31

Results and Discussion

Characterization of the solid dispersions

Particle size analysis

The particle size analysis results showed that mean particle size of ground powders were decreased significantly ($p<0.05$) compared to the pure drug (Figure 1).

The ground powders had a reduced geometric diameter and as a result higher surface area than that of pure FUR. According to the Noyes–Whitney equation, the amount of solute dissolved per unit time, dM/dt, is related to the surface area of the solute.

$$\frac{dM}{dt} = \frac{DS}{h}(C_S - C)$$

Where D is the diffusion coefficient of the solute in solution, h stands for the thickness of the diffusion layer, C_s and C are the solubility and the concentration of the solute in the solution, respectively.[20,36]

Therefore, one of the reasons of higher dissolution rate of the solid dispersions comparing to pure FUR maybe be explained by particle size reduction during solid dispersion process.

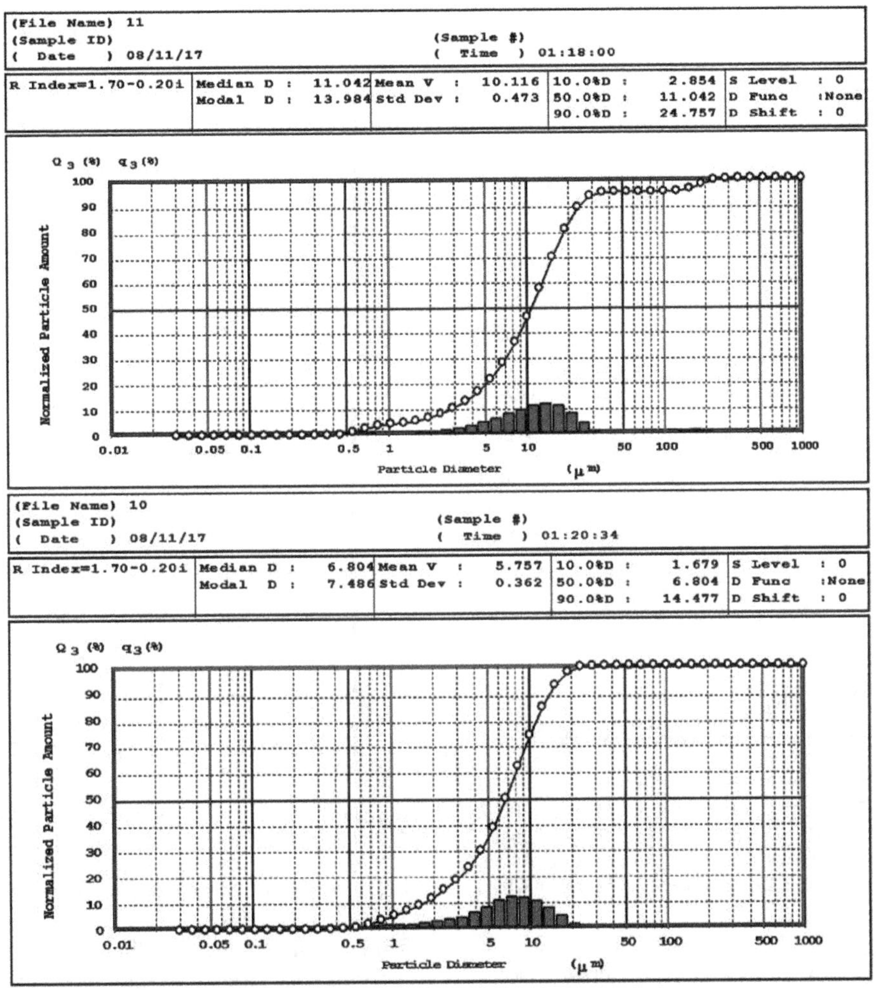

Figure 1. Particle size distribution of pure (Top) and treated powder (Below) of Furosemide

X-Ray diffraction studies

XRD diffractograms revealed that pure FUR showed distinctive peaks in 2θ=18, 18.9, 24.7 and 28.6 which indicate the crystalline nature of pure FUR. However, in treated FUR powder, the height and number of peaks were decreased, indicating the reduced crystallinity of the treated FUR powder. Comparing height of the peaks in the physical mixtures of both carriers demonstrated the reduction in magnitude of peaks due to the dilution effect of the carriers. Reduction in the height of the peaks and absence of some major peaks were seen in XRD patterns of the solid dispersions represented a decrease in FUR crystallinity in these preparations (Figure 2). The results confirmed the transformation of crystalline polymorph of FUR into its amorphous polymorph in the form of solid dispersion.

Fourier Transform Infrared Spectroscopy

In order to find out the possible intermolecular interactions between the FUR and carriers, FTIR studies were conducted. The FT-IR peaks of pure and treated FUR as well as carriers, physical mixture (drug: carrier 1:2) and solid dispersion (drug: carrier 1:2) are presented in Figure 3. There are three absorption peaks in 3340, 3260 and 16650 cm^{-1} which are related to the amino group, as well as 1560 and 1318 cm^{-1} which belong to carboxyl and sulphonyl groups, respectively. Lack of any new peaks in the solid dispersions and also no differences in the positions of the absorption bands, indicate the absence of significant interactions between FUR and carriers during cogrinding.

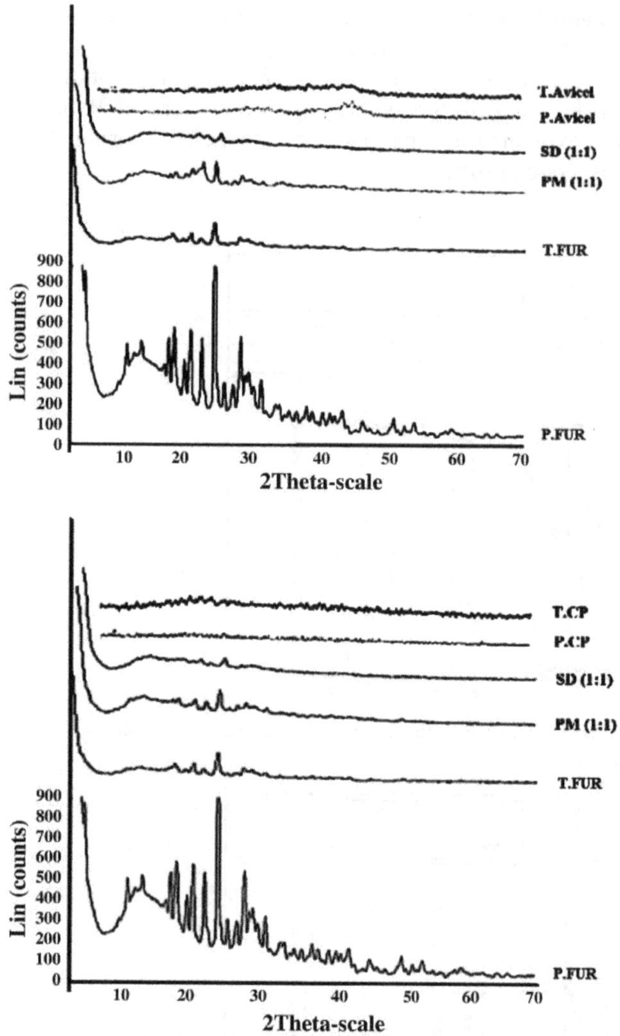

Figure 2. Powder X-Ray Diffraction patterns of pure FUR (P.FUR), treated FUR (T.FUR), physical mixtures (PM) 1:2, solid dispersions (SD) 1:2, pure Avicel (P.Avicel) and treated Avicel (T.Avicel), pure Crospovidone (P.CP) and treated Avicel (T.CP).

In vitro drug release

Dissolution profiles of physical mixtures, solid dispersions, pure and treated FUR powders prepared with various drug: carrier ratios of both carriers at pH 1.2 and 5.8 are presented in Figure 4 and 5. Dissolution rate of all formulations in pH 5.8 is considerably faster than pH 1.2 in the presence or absence of carriers. This could be due to the better solubility of the FUR, a weak acid, because of a greater ionization at higher pH values. In addition, as a result of lower particle size in treated powder compared with pure FUR (10.12 μm and 5.76 μm respectively), dissolution rate was also higher than pure FUR powder in both pHs. On the other hand, the physical mixtures of both carriers exhibited noticeably faster dissolution rates than the pure and treated FUR, which may be is due to high hydrophilicity of the carriers. Hydrophilic polymers caused aggregation reduction, wettability improvement and local solubilization in the diffusion layer and thereby increasing in the dissolution rate. Although, a direct relationship between the amount of carrier and FUR dissolution rate could not be established from the dissolution profiles of the different physical mixtures, but dissolution rate of all physical mixtures were much higher than the pure FUR. The solid dispersions of FUR and both carriers with different drug to polymer ratios showed the higher drug release rate when compared to the respective physical mixtures and pure drug.

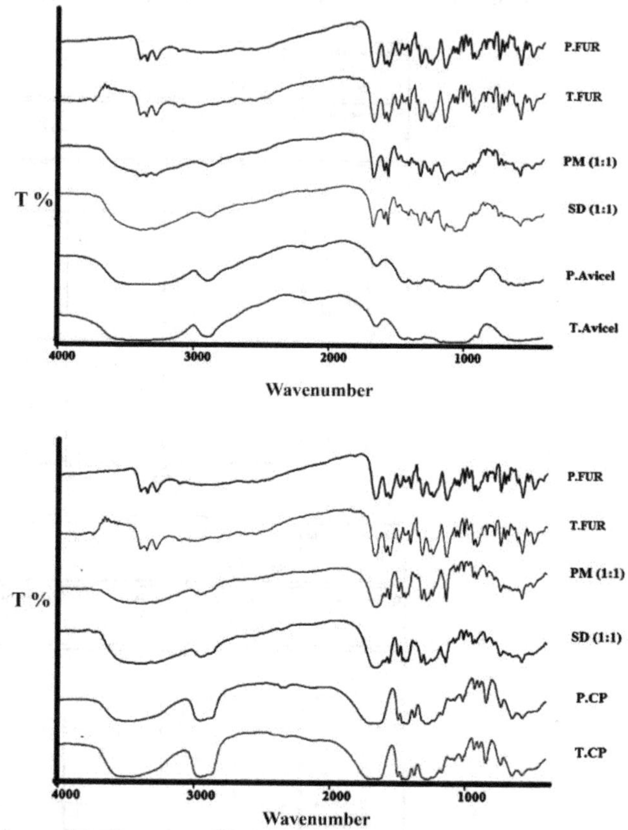

Figure 3. Powder FT-IR patterns of pure FUR (P.FUR), treated FUR (T.FUR), physical mixtures (PM) 1:2, solid dispersions (SD) 1:2, pure Avicel (P.Avicel) and treated Avicel (T.Avicel), pure Crospovidone (P.CP) and treated Avicel (T.CP).

Table 2 illustrates the time needed to release 30% of incorporated drug and the mean percent dissolution of pure FUR, treated FUR, physical mixtures and solid dispersions. Dissolution rate is considered faster, if the value of $t_{30\%}$ is lower and MPD value is higher. Similarly, these model independent parameters also verified that the drug is released faster from the solid dispersions. The improved drug release rate could be attributed to the drug crystallinity reduction in the FUR loaded solid dispersions prepared by Avicel and Crospovidone. It is generally well known that a drug in a solid dispersions system every so often exists in an amorphous form. The amorphous form of a drug has a higher thermodynamic activity than its crystalline form, leading to rapid dissolution of the drug. Furthermore, the reduced particle size and accordingly elevated surface area could enhance the dissolution rate of FUR in the solid dispersions. In addition to latter evidences, increasing drug wettability and solubility as well as deaggregation of the drug particles brought about by the polymers could be the reasons for enhanced drug release rate from the solid dispersions.[5,20,37]

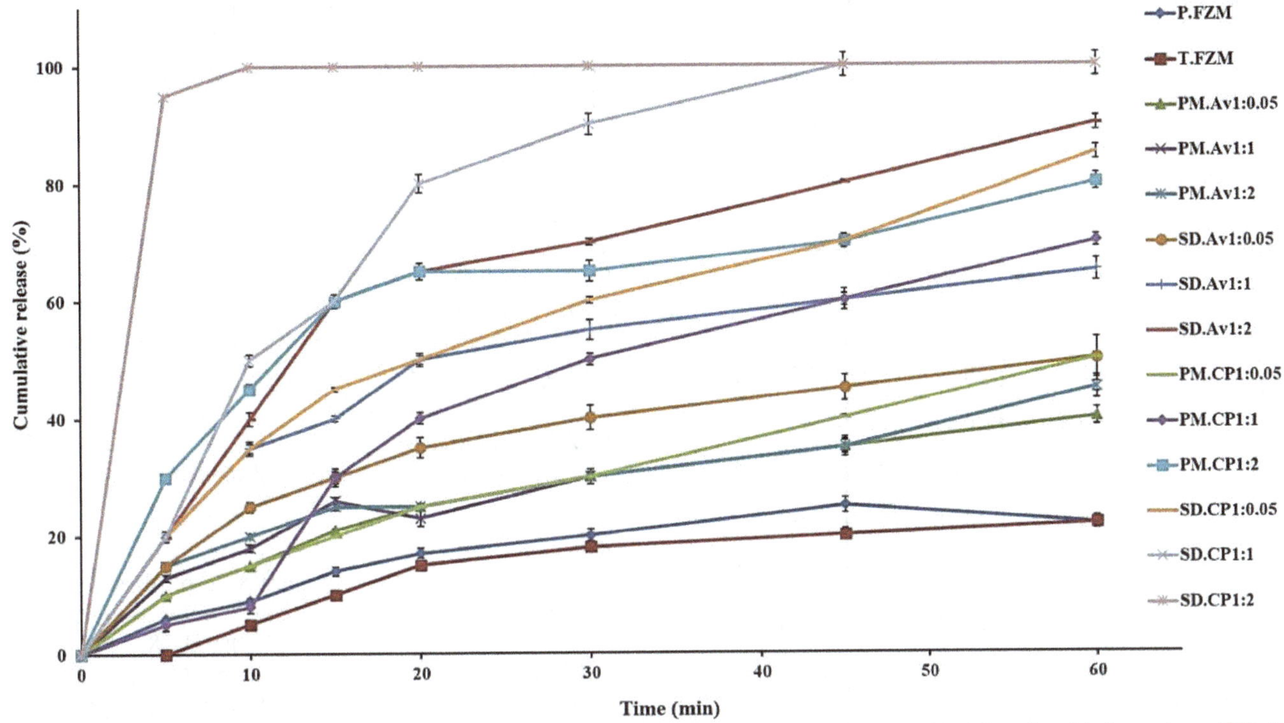

Figure 4. Dissolution profiles of pure FUR (P.FUR), treated FUR (T.FUR) physical mixtures (PM) 1:2 and solid dispersions (SD) 1:1 containing Avicel (AV) and Crospovidone (CP) in pH 1.2. (mean ± SD, n=3)

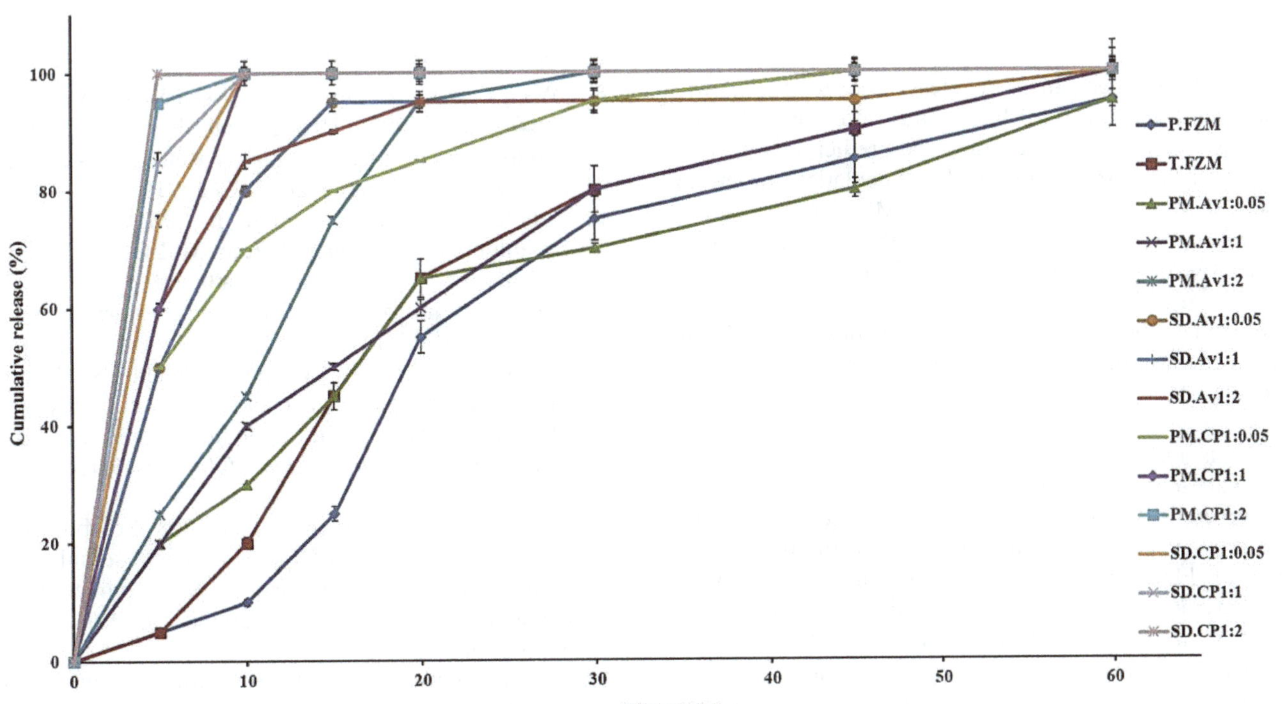

Figure 5. Dissolution profiles of pure FUR (P.FUR), treated FUR (TFUR) physical mixtures (PM) and solid dispersions (SD) containing Avicel (AV) and Crospovidone (CP) in pH 5.8. (mean ± SD, n=3).

Drug release rate was enhanced as a consequence of increasing carrier concentration, while solid dispersions showed the maximum release rate at the drug: carrier ratio of 1:1 and 1:2 (Table 2 as well as Figure 4 and 5). However, solid dispersions with drug: carrier ratio of 1:1 are economically the best formulation to enhance dissolution rate of FUR.

Table 2. Mean percent dissolution (MPD) and time needed to release 30% of incorporated drug (t30%) of Furosemide formulations in pH 1.2 and 5.8

Formulation		pH 1.2		pH 5.8	
		MPD	$t_{30\%}$	MPD	$t_{30\%}$
Pure Furosemide		12.27	84.5	50.33	10.8
Treated Furosemide		16.49	62.2	60.52	7
Avicel	PM 1:0.5	17.02	44.8	54.19	9.6
	PM 1:1	20.78	39	56.52	6.8
	PM 1:2	26.52	26.6	63.67	5.4
	SD 1:0.5	30.90	21.2	-	4.2
	SD 1:1	44.81	6	-	3
	SD 1:2	68.18	3	53.65	2
Crospovidone	PM 1:0.5	24.97	27.4	59.39	6.2
	PM 1:1	39.75	17.2	63.73	2.2
	PM 1:2	67.24	3.2	98.48	1
	SD 1:0.5	48.43	13.8	73.94	2
	SD 1:1	78.43	2.2	85.11	1.2
	SD 1:2	89.95	1.8	98.88	0.8

Release kinetics

To clarify the mechanism of release, the *in vitro* release data were fitted in to 10 linear and 7 non-linear kinetic models (Table 1). The accuracy and prediction ability of the models were compared by calculation of mean squared correlation coefficients (MRSQ) and mean percent error (MPR). Considering the RSQ and mean percent error values, release data of the all formulations were fitted best to the Weibull and Wagner log probability models from linear kinetics as well as Gompertz and suggested 2 models from nonlinear kinetic models.

Conclusion

Bioavailability of poorly water soluble drugs could be improved as a result of release rate enhancement. Thus, the present study was aimed to enhance the dissolution rate of FUR by means of cogrinding method using Crospovidone and microcrystalline cellulose as hydrophilic carriers. The results showed that both carriers enhanced dissolution rate in solid dispersion formulations in all three ratios and also physical mixture of Crospovidone in drug: carrier ratio of 1:2 compared with drug powder at both dissolution medium (pH 1.2 and 5.8). Drug: carrier ratio, type of polymer and pH can carry out a major role to control the dissolution rate from the solid dispersion. The best economical drug: carrier ratio of both carriers was 1:1. The solid state studies confirmed that solid dispersion of FUR with both carriers can decrease crystallinity or increase amorphousness of the drug. In conclusion, solid dispersion can be beneficially applied to enhance the dissolution rate of the poorly water-soluble drugs. Overall, the increased dissolution rate of solid dispersions can be described by the several factors including the increased surface area and creation of amorphous polymorph of the drug.

Acknowledgments

The authors would like to thank Biotechnology Research Center, Tabriz University of Medical Sciences, Tabriz, Iran. This article is based on a thesis submitted for PharmD degree (No. 3504) in Faculty of Pharmacy, Tabriz University of Medical Sciences, Tabriz, Iran.

Conflict of Interest

The authors report no conflicts of interest.

References

1. Humberstone AJ, Charman WN. Lipid-based vehicles for the oral delivery of poorly water soluble drugs. *Adv Drug Deliv Rev* 1997;25(1):103-28.
2. Merisko-Liversidge E, Liversidge GG. Nanosizing for oral and parenteral drug delivery: A perspective on formulating poorly-water soluble compounds using wet media milling technology. *Adv Drug Deliv Rev* 2011;63(6):427-40.
3. Sprunk A, Strachan CJ, Graf A. Rational formulation development and in vitro assessment of SMEDDS for oral delivery of poorly water soluble drugs. *Eur J Pharm Sci* 2012;46(5):508-15.
4. Wang XQ, Zhang Q. pH-sensitive polymeric nanoparticles to improve oral bioavailability of peptide/protein drugs and poorly water-soluble drugs. *Eur J Pharm Biopharm* 2012;82(2):219-29.
5. Adibkia K, Barzegar-Jalali M, Mohammadi G, Ebrahimnejhad H, Alaei-Beirami M. Effect of sodium alginate chain length and Ca2+and Al 3+on the release of diltiazem from matrices. *Pharmaceutical Sciences* 2011;16(4):221-8.
6. Cirri M, Maestrelli F, Corti G, Furlanetto S, Mura P. Simultaneous effect of cyclodextrin complexation, pH, and hydrophilic polymers on naproxen solubilization. *J Pharm Biomed Anal* 2006;42(1):126-31.
7. Dong Y, Ng WK, Surana U, Tan RB. Solubilization and preformulation of poorly water soluble and hydrolysis susceptible N-epoxymethyl-1,8-naphthalimide (ENA) compound. *Int J Pharm* 2008;356(1–2):130-6.
8. Jain P, Yalkowsky SH. Solubilization of poorly soluble compounds using 2-pyrrolidone. *Int J Pharm* 2007;342(1–2):1-5.
9. Linares M, De Bertorello MaM, Longhi M. Solubilization of naphthoquinones by complexation with hydroxypropyl-β-cyclodextrin. *Int J Pharm* 1997;159(1):13-8.
10. Rao VM, Nerurkar M, Pinnamaneni S, Rinaldi F, Raghavan K. Co-solubilization of poorly soluble

drugs by micellization and complexation. *Int J Pharm* 2006;319(1–2):98-106.

11. Barmpalexis P, Koutsidis I, Karavas E, Louka D, Papadimitriou SA, Bikiaris DN. Development of PVP/PEG mixtures as appropriate carriers for the preparation of drug solid dispersions by melt mixing technique and optimization of dissolution using artificial neural networks. *Eur J Pharm Biopharm* 2013;85(3 Pt B):1219-31.
12. Dinunzio JC, Brough C, Hughey JR, Miller DA, Williams RO 3rd, Mcginity JW. Fusion production of solid dispersions containing a heat-sensitive active ingredient by hot melt extrusion and Kinetisol® dispersing. *Eur J Pharm Biopharm* 2010;74(2):340-51.
13. Giri TK, Kumar K, Alexander A, Ajazuddin, Badwaik H, Tripathi DK. A novel and alternative approach to controlled release drug delivery system based on solid dispersion technique. *Bulletin of Faculty of Pharmacy, Cairo University* 2012;50(2):147-59.
14. Li S, Liu Y, Liu T, Zhao L, Zhao J, Feng N. Development and in-vivo assessment of the bioavailability of oridonin solid dispersions by the gas anti-solvent technique. *Int J Pharm* 2011;411(1–2):172-7.
15. Hussain MD, Saxena V, Brausch JF, Talukder RM. Ibuprofen–phospholipid solid dispersions: Improved dissolution and gastric tolerance. *Int J Pharm* 2012;422(1–2):290-4.
16. Konno H, Handa T, Alonzo DE, Taylor LS. Effect of polymer type on the dissolution profile of amorphous solid dispersions containing felodipine. *Eur J Pharm Biopharm* 2008;70(2):493-9.
17. Lust A, Laidmäe I, Palo M, Meos A, Aaltonen J, Veski P, et al. Solid-state dependent dissolution and oral bioavailability of piroxicam in rats. *Eur J Pharm Sci* 2013;48(1–2):47-54.
18. Nepal PR, Han H-K, Choi HK. Enhancement of solubility and dissolution of Coenzyme Q10 using solid dispersion formulation. *Int J Pharm* 2010;383(1–2):147-53.
19. Vo CL, Park C, Lee BJ. Current trends and future perspectives of solid dispersions containing poorly water-soluble drugs. *Eur J Pharm Biopharm* 2013;85(3 Pt B):799-813.
20. Adibkia K, Barzegar-Jalali M, Maheri-Esfanjani H, Ghanbarzadeh S, Shokri J, Sabzevari A, et al. Physicochemical characterization of naproxen solid dispersions prepared via spray drying technology. *Powder Technol* 2013;246:448-55.
21. Al-Hamidi H, Edwards AA, Mohammad MA, Nokhodchi A. To enhance dissolution rate of poorly water-soluble drugs: Glucosamine hydrochloride as a potential carrier in solid dispersion formulations. *Colloids Surf B Biointerfaces* 2010;76(1):170-8.
22. Goddeeris C, Willems T, Houthoofd K, Martens JA, Van Den Mooter G. Dissolution enhancement of the anti-HIV drug UC 781 by formulation in a ternary solid dispersion with TPGS 1000 and Eudragit E100. *Eur J Pharm Biopharm* 2008;70(3):861-8.
23. Karavas E, Georgarakis E, Sigalas MP, Avgoustakis K, Bikiaris D. Investigation of the release mechanism of a sparingly water-soluble drug from solid dispersions in hydrophilic carriers based on physical state of drug, particle size distribution and drug–polymer interactions. *Eur J Pharm Biopharm* 2007;66(3):334-47.
24. Papadimitriou SA, Barmpalexis P, Karavas E, Bikiaris DN. Optimizing the ability of PVP/PEG mixtures to be used as appropriate carriers for the preparation of drug solid dispersions by melt mixing technique using artificial neural networks: I. *Eur J Pharm Biopharm* 2012;82(1):175-86.
25. Sjökvist E, Nyström C. Physicochemical aspects of drug release. VI. Drug dissolution rate from solid particulate dispersions and the importance of carrier and drug particle properties. *Int J Pharm* 1988;47(1–3):51-66.
26. Sjökvist E, Nyström C. Physicochemical aspects of drug release. XI. Tableting properties of solid dispersions, using xylitol as carrier material. *Int J Pharm* 1991;67(2):139-53.
27. Van Den Mooter G, Weuts I, De Ridder T, Blaton N. Evaluation of Inutec SP1 as a new carrier in the formulation of solid dispersions for poorly soluble drugs. *Int J Pharm* 2006;316(1–2):1-6.
28. De Zordi N, Moneghini M, Kikic I, Grassi M, Del Rio Castillo AE, Solinas D, et al. Applications of supercritical fluids to enhance the dissolution behaviors of Furosemide by generation of microparticles and solid dispersions. *Eur J Pharm Biopharm* 2012;81(1):131-41.
29. Perioli L, D'alba G, Pagano C. New oral solid dosage form for furosemide oral administration. *Eur J Pharm Biopharm* 2012;80(3):621-9.
30. Shin SC, Kim J. Physicochemical characterization of solid dispersion of furosemide with TPGS. *Int J Pharm* 2003;251(1–2):79-84.
31. Barzegar-Jalali M. A model for linearizing drug dissolution data. *Int J Pharm* 1990;63(2):9-11.
32. Mohammadi G, Barzegar-Jalali M, Valizadeh H, Nazemiyeh H, Barzegar-Jalali A, Siahi Shadbad MR, et al. Reciprocal powered time model for release kinetic analysis of ibuprofen solid dispersions in oleaster powder, microcrystalline cellulose and crospovidone. *J Pharm Pharm Sci* 2010;13(2):152-61.
33. Barzegar-Jalali M, Adibkia K, Valizadeh H, Shadbad MR, Nokhodchi A, Omidi Y, et al. Kinetic analysis of drug release from nanoparticles. *J Pharm Pharm Sci* 2008;11(1):167-77.
34. Adibkia K, Javadzadeh Y, Dastmalchi S, Mohammadi G, Niri FK, Alaei-Beirami M. Naproxen-eudragit RS100 nanoparticles: Preparation and physicochemical characterization. *Colloids Surf B Biointerfaces* 2011;83(1):155-9.

35. Barzegar-Jalali M, Dastmalchi S. Kinetic Analysis of Chlorpropamide Dissolution from Solid Dispersions. *Drug Dev Ind Pharm* 2007;33:63-70.
36. Adibkia K, Barzegar-Jalali M, Nokhodchi A, Siahi Shadbad MR, Omidi Y, Javadzadeh Y, et al. A review on the methods of preparation of pharmaceutical nanoparticles. *Pharmaceutical Sciences* 2009;15(4):303-14.
37. Adibkia K, Barzegar-Jalali M, Javadzadeh Y, Maheri-Esfanjani H. A review on the methods and applications of spray drying technology. *Pharmaceutical Sciences* 2012;18(2):119-32.

7

Prediction of Optimum Combination of Eudragit RS/Eudragit RL/Ethyl Cellulose Polymeric Free Films Based on Experimental Design for Using as a Coating System for Sustained Release Theophylline Pellets

Abbas Akhgari[1]*, Ali Tavakol[2]

[1] *Targeted Drug Delivery Research Center, School of Pharmacy, Mashhad University of Medical Sciences, Mashhad, Iran.*
[2] *Nanotechnology Research Center and School of Pharmacy, Ahvaz Jundishapur University of Medical Sciences, Ahvaz, Iran.*

Article info

Keywords:
- Sustained release
- Permeability
- Swelling
- Theophylline
- Ethylcellulose
- Eudragit

Abstract

Purpose: The physicochemical properties of free films made from different mixtures of sustained release polymers were investigated, and an optimum formulation coating on drug containing pellets, based on the study of free film was evaluated.

Methods: In order to determine the effect of different variables on the permeability and swelling of films and procedure optimization, the experimental design was fulfilled based on the statistical method of a 3^3 full factorial design, and according to this method 27 formulations were prepared. The films were prepared using casting-solvent evaporation method. Water vapor permeability, the swelling and permeability of free films in both acidic and buffer media, were carried out. Then, the pellets containing theophylline were coated with the optimum formulation.

Results: The results of this study demonstrated that an increase in the free film thickness and Eurdragit RS ratio in films lowered the water vapor transmission (WVT), the swelling and the permeability of all formulations, while an increase in the quantity of ethylcellulose, up to a specific ratio (approximately 40%), decreased the permeability and swelling. The most optimum free film formulation was made up of 60% Eudragit RS and 40% ethylcellulose.

Conclusion: Pellets coated with a 10% coating level of ethylcellulose and Eudragit RS (4:6) showed suitable release properties and could serve as a favorable sustained release system for theophylline.

Introduction

Controlled release technology, which is used in the formulation of pharmaceutical product, has become increasingly important due to its significant role in recent pharmaceutical technology. A controlled release system has the advantages, including more constant or prolonged therapeutic effects, improved patient compliance, decreased side effects, and decreased costs. Film coating, based on polymeric substances, are widely used in oral dosage forms, with the aim of obtaining a sustained[1,2] and targeted drug delivery,[3,4] moisture barriers[5] and masking of the bitter taste of active ingredients in some drugs.[6] Several natural and synthetic polymers have proven to be suitable coating agents by providing different drug release kinetics.[7] However, it is often difficult to obtain the desired efficacy from each polymer alone, thus there is the need to combine the physicochemical characteristics of different macromolecules in order to achieve optimum response.

Ethyl cellulose (EC) is one of the most widely used hydrophobic polymers as a matrix former or coating material in sustained release dosage forms.[8,9] It offers moderate film forming properties, enabling suitable coatings to be produced. On the other hand, Eudragit RL (ERL) and Eudragit RS (ERS) are acrylic and methacrylic acid esters, respectively, having some hydrophilic properties due to the presence of quaternary ammonium groups; where ERL possesses higher amount (50 mEq/100 g polymer) of such groups than ERS (25 mEq/100 g polymer).[10] They are mainly used as film coatings in tablets, granules and other small particles, The release characteristics of film coated controlled release formulations are strongly dependent on the swelling ability and permeability of the film. From another point of view, the study on drug permeation through free films of polymeric materials could be useful in understanding and predicting the properties of coatings on the surface of a dosage form. A few number of studies focused on both permeation and release of drug from coated dosage forms. In a study, Ye et al. prepared mixed films of EC/hydroxypropyl methylcellulose and investigated the permeability of metoprolol tartrate through the films. Also, the drug release from pellets coated with the same formulation of polymer blends was evaluated. The authors included that the diffusion of drug through isolated plasticized

***Corresponding author:** Abbas Akhgari, Email: akhgaria@mums.ac.ir

polymer films was predictive for the release of film coated dosage forms.[11]

An experimental design approach allows for a reduction in the number of experiments, with a complete exploration of the experimental domain to be studied; where all the variables are studied at the same time. On the other hand, response surface methodology has been reported as an effective tool for optimizing a process when the independent variables have a combined effect on the desired response.[12]

Therefore, the objective of this study was to evaluate the properties of free films made from blends of three water insoluble polymers, Eudragit RS, Eudragit RL and ethylcellulose in different ratios, for the control of drug release, for the purpose of investigating the effect of each polymer on the swelling and permeation characteristics of the other polymers, and finally to predict the suitable formulation for coating of pellets in order to achieve the optimum controlled release dosage form. Theophylline was chosen as a model drug. This drug has long been used as a treatment for diseases, including bronchial asthma. However, due to its narrow therapeutic concentration range and meal dependent absorption, managing the dose of this drug has been rather difficult. The absorption of drug from a conventional matrix tablet is strongly influenced by its transition rate in the gastrointestinal tract. Also, the bioavailability of conventional matrix tablets varies widely[13] but a multiple-unit dosage form can overcome this problem. On the other hand, theophylline has been widely used as a model drug due to its ready availability, relatively low cost, ease of assay and chemical stability.[14]

Materials and Methods

Materials

Eudragit RS (ERS) (Rohm Pharma, Germany), Eudragit RL (ERL) (Rohm Pharma, Germany), ethylcellulose (EC) (Darusazi Arya, Iran), tributyl citrate (Merck, Germany), theophylline monohydrate (Cooper Rhone, France), talc (Merck, Germany), magnesium nitrate hexahydrate ($Mg(NO_3)_2.6H_2O$) (Merck, Germany), polyvinyl pyrrolidone (PVP K30) (Fluka, Switzerland), and non-pareil seeds (NP Pharm, France) were obtained from indicated sources. The other materials used were of analytical grade.

Methods

Experimental design

For the purpose of this study, a 3^3 full factorial design was used to investigate the effect of independent variables on the responses. The independent variables included film thickness (X_1), the ratio of EC to total polymer content (X_2), and the ratio of ERS: ERL in free films (X_3). The levels of independent factors and dependent variables are listed in Table 1.

Table 1. The levels of independent variables and responses

Independent variables	Levels			Responses
	-1	0	1	
				Y_1: Water Vapor Transmission of free films (mg/hm^{2}KPa)
X_1: film thickness (µ)	60	130	200	Y_2: swelling index in acidic media (%)
				Y_3: swelling index in buffer media (%)
X_2: the ratio of EC to total polymer content	0	40	80	Y_4: permeability in acidic media (cm/s)
X_3: the ratio of ERS: ERL	50	75	100	Y_5: permeability in buffer media (cm/s)
-	-	-	-	Y_6: ratio of permeability in acid:permeability in buffer

Preparation of free films

Free films comprising different amounts of polymers were prepared using casting-solvent evaporation method. Briefly, A 10% (w/v) solution of Eudragit RS 100, Eudragit RL 100 and/or ethylcellulose was prepared by dissolving granules or powders of these polymers in given ratios of isopropyl alcohol:distilled water (9:1; 4.5:1, and 3.5:1 ratio for films containing 0, 40, and 80% EC, respectively). Then, a fixed amount of triethyl citrate (1:6 ratio related to total polymer content) was added as a plasticizer. The resultant solution with a suspension volume of volume of 25 mL in each plate was transferred on to Teflon plates. The plates were then placed in an oven at a temperature of 50°C for 24 h until drying was completed. After keeping the plates in a desiccator of 100% relative humidity (RH) for 24 h, the films were cut into different special pieces with a scalpel for various experiments. The thickness of the films was measured at five different places using a micrometer. The free films were finally stored in a desiccator of 50% RH made from a saturated solution of magnesium nitrate hexahydrate at room temperature, until use. Different free films were prepared based on the experimental design. Table 2 summarizes the resultant formulations.

Water vapor transmission study

Water vapor transmission (WVT) of films was performed gravimetrically at a temperature of 25°C. Free films, with appropriate dimensions, were sealed in WVT cups containing 10 mL of distilled water. The cups were accurately weighed and placed in a desiccator containing silica gel and appropriate amounts of calcium chloride in order to create a climate of low relative humidity (approximately 0%). Then, reweighing of the cups was done again at designated intervals (24, 48, 72, 96 and 120 h), and the profile of mass change versus time was plotted for each free film. WVT was calculated using the following equation:

$$WVT = w/tAP_0(RH_1 - RH_2) \qquad \text{Equation 1}$$

Where w/t is the change in mass (flux, mg/h) resulting from the slope of profile of the mass change versus time, A is the area of the film surface exposed to the permeant (m^2), P_0 is the vapor pressure of pure water (kPa), and (RH_1-RH_2) is the relative humidity gradient. At a temperature of 25°C, the obtained $P0$ was 3.159 kPa.[15]

Table 2. Characteristics of investigated free films

Run	X_1 (μ)	X_2 (%)	X_3 (%)
F1	60	0	50
F2	60	0	75
F3	60	0	100
F4	60	40	50
F5	60	40	75
F6	60	40	100
F7	60	80	50
F8	60	80	75
F9	60	80	100
F10	130	0	5
F11	130	0	75
F12	130	0	100
F13	130	40	50
F14	130	40	75
F15	130	40	100
F16	130	80	50
F17	130	80	75
F18	130	80	100
F19	200	0	50
F20	200	0	75
F21	200	0	100
F22	200	40	50
F23	200	40	75
F24	200	40	100
F25	200	80	50
F26	200	80	75
F27	200	80	100

Water uptake experiments

Water uptake tests of free films were conducted in the media with a pH of 1.2 and 6.8 for acidic and buffer media, respectively. 1 cm^2 area of each free film was dried at 50°C for 24 h, and after accurate weighing it was immersed in a dissolution flask containing 250 ml of different media at 37°C. The swollen sample was withdrawn at specific intervals, with its surface water wiped off using a filter paper, and finally accurately reweighed. The swelling index, I_s, was calculated using the following expression:[16]

$$I_s(\%)=[(W_s-W_d)/W_d]\times 100 \quad \text{Equation 2}$$

Where W_d and W_s are the weights of the dried and swollen free films, respectively. All experiments on water uptake were applied in triplicate.

Permeability experiments

Samples of free films were retained between compartments of a side-by-side diffusion cell with a diffusion area of 3.46 cm^2. Each cell was continuously stirred and the temperature was maintained at 37°C. Permeability experiments were conducted in the acidic and buffer media, respectively for 3 h. The donor compartment was also composed of theophyllineas with an initial concentration of 3 g/L. Samples of 10 ml were taken from the acceptor cells at predetermined intervals and replaced together with the fresh medium. Then, the samples were assayed for theophylline spectrophotometrically at 272 nm. The permeability was calculated using the following equation:[17]

$$P=d_M/d_tSC_d \quad \text{Equation 3}$$

Where M is the amount of drug diffused (mg) through free films at time t, S is the effective diffusion area (cm^2), C_d is the concentration of drug in the donor cell and P is the permeability of free film (cm/s).

Preparation of drug containing pellets

Drug containing pellets were prepared by coating the theophylline onto the non-pareil beads (850 to 1180 μm) using fluidized bed coater (Wurster insert, Werner Glatt, Germany). A 30% w/v aqueous suspension of theophylline (<90 μm) was prepared by dispersing theophylline in a 9% w/v PVP K30 solution, and finally passing it through a 140 mesh sieve. The final suspension was coated onto non-pareils using fluidized bed coater. Table 3 presents a list of the coating conditions. The coating process continued until pellets having about 20% w/w drug load were produced. After coating, the pellets were extra fluidized for about 5 min, followed by storage in an oven at 40°C, for 2 h.

Content uniformity

Two hundred milligrams of theophylline pellets were ground and transferred into 250 ml volumetric flasks containing phosphate buffer at a pH of 6.8. The flasks were shaken in a shaking water bath at 25°C for 3 h. The concentration of the drug was determined spectrophotometrically in filtered solutions at 272 nm. All assays were carried out in triplicate.

Polymer coating

The two most optimum free film formulations (ERS-EC in the ratio of 60:40 and ERS) were chosen according to the contour plots and optimization of formulations. Then, 10% (w/w) solutions of the optimum formulations were prepared in isopropyl alcohol:water in ratios of 4.5:1 and 9:1, respectively. The solution was plasticized with triethyl citrate (in the ratio of 1:6 related to dry polymer) with talc added as a glidant (5% w/w, related to dry polymer). The final dispersion was coated onto 100 g of drug loaded pellets with a fluidized bed coating apparatus (Wurster insert, Werner Glatt). The process conditions were as follows: spray rate of 10 g min^{-1}, atomization pressure of 2 bars, nozzle diameter of 1 mm, inlet temperature between 40 and 45°C and outlet temperature between 30 and 35°C. Samples of coated pellets were removed from the apparatus upon reaching the coating loads of 5, 10, 15 and 20% (w/w), respectively.

Dissolution studies

Dissolution studies were conducted on a 900 ml medium at 37°C using a USP dissolution apparatus I (Pharmatest, PTWS, Germany) at a rotation speed of 50 rpm. Accurately weighed (100 mg) pellets were transferred into the dissolution medium and at predetermined intervals, the samples were taken from the vessel and ultra violetly (UV) assayed spectrophotometrically at 272 nm. Dissolution test was performed for 1 h in the medium with pH 1.2 (HCl 0.1 N), followed by 7 h in the medium with pH 6.8 (phosphate buffer). All experiments on dissolution were applied in triplicate.

Scanning electron microscopy

The surface characteristics of the powder samples were observed using scanning electron microscopy (SEM) (LEO 1450 VP, UK). The samples were sputter coated with silver for 1 min in a sputter coater (Polaron E5400, UK).

Statistical analysis of data

The effects of the independent variables on the responses were modelled using a second order polynomial equation:

$$Y=c+b_1X_1+b_2X_2+b_3X_3+b_4X_1^2+b_5X_2^2+b_6X_3^2+b_7X_1X_2+b_8X_1X_3+b_9X_2X_3+b_{10}X_1X_2X_3 \qquad \text{Equation 4}$$

The modeling was performed using SPSS (Version 16.0), with a backward, stepwise linear regression technique, and significant terms ($P < 0.05$) were chosen for the final equations. The resultant response surface plots and contour plots from the equations were obtained using Statgraphics 5.

Table 3. WVT, swelling and theophylline permeability of the formulations

Run	WVT index (mg/hm^2KPa)(mean±SD)	Swelling index in acid (%)(mean±SEM)	Swelling index in buffer (%)(mean±SEM)	Permeability in acid (cm/sec) (mean±SEM)*10^{-5}	Permeability in buffer (cm/sec) (mean±SEM)*10^{-5}	Ratio of permeability in acid:permeability in buffer (mean±SEM)
F1	43.545±0.500	39.81±2.06	48.77±4.72	4.433±0.031	5.363±0.015	0.827±0.005
F2	31.589±0.572	14.66±4.16	33.44±4.00	2.303±0.023	2.567±0.006	0.897±0.011
F3	21.279±0.687	12.93±2.36	19.92±3.21	0.125±0.007	0.133±0.008	0.947±0.020
F4	41.790±0.658	16.45±4.73	18.56±0.28	0.674±0.005	0.910±0.005	0.741±0.005
F5	38.280±0.762	15.63±4.68	27.27±2.60	0.529±0.007	0.705±0.003	0.751±0.188
F6	33.738±0.381	13.96±4.42	18.23±2.18	0.213±0.003	0.237±0.005	0.912±0.299
F7	43.106±1.432	14.07±3.54	21.46±2.60	0.504±0.008	0.467±0.023	1.081±0.179
F8	44.532±0.830	16.80±2.36	27.00±5.88	0.540±0.009	0.400±0.007	1.348±0.057
F9	43.213±0.681	13.49±2.44	20.72±3.26	0.417±0.007	0.331±0.006	1.259±0.051
F10	38.607±1.154	33.85±5.26	47.13±6.84	2.450±0.010	3.310±0.006	0.739±0.002
F11	26.980±0.660	17.85±1.26	27.79±6.98	1.220±0.006	1.920±0.010	0.634±0.004
F12	18.097±0.985	14.28±0.14	16.22±2.39	0.044±0	0.058±0	0.762±0
F13	33.233±1.138	10.46±2.25	19.43±4.72	0.376±0	0.480±0.007	0.783±0.11
F14	31.920±0.873	13.59±1.01	18.66±3.88	0.386±0.005	0.414±0.003	0.932±0.017
F15	29.947±0.980	9.62±4.22	15.85±7.81	0.112±0.002	0.116±0.002	0.966±0.034
F16	38.060±0.687	17.29±4.65	14.43±3.20	0.242±0.002	0.116±0.002	2.087±0.035
F17	39.606±0.832	18.41±1.28	22.09±2.19	0.233±0.002	0.254±0.002	0.918±0.009
F18	36.747±1.244	12.26±3.59	17.68±1.15	0.218±0.009	0.186±0.008	1.187±0.087
F19	29.387±0.685	28.02±4.45	37.87±3.24	1.456±0.006	1.970±0.010	0.739±0.019
F20	23.253±0.504	18.71±4.45	25.71±5.16	0.735±0.011	1.067±0.006	0.689±0.011
F21	13.382±0.687	6.78±2.43	13.74±8.21	0.018±0	0.013±0	1.353±0
F22	30.283±0.560	11.49±5.21	18.16±0.63	0.270±0.009	0.293±0.005	0.921±0.044
F23	27.202±0.687	15.35±2.70	20.22±9.09	0.193±0.003	0.233±0.002	0.831±0.018
F24	24.017±1.184	12.40±3.69	15.16±4.59	0.059±0.003	0.062±0.004	0.957±0.107
F25	34.770±1.159	10.41±1.72	18.94±10.26	0.159±0.005	0.188±0.003	0.848±0.038
F26	33.013±1.154	13.46±6.72	19.98±5.31	0.154±0.005	0.131±0.003	1.177±0.068
F27	31.370±1.008	8.13±2.59	19.36±5.44	0.146±0.034	0.117±0.006	1.261±0.342

Results and Discussion

The results of WVT experiments are shown in Table 3. From the results there was a decrease in WVT with increasing film thickness, and this could have resulted from the prolonged pathway of water vapor molecules through the films. The addition of ERS to the free films lowered the WVT index. From the comparison of the structure of ERS and ERL, it is obvious that ERS is more hydrophobic than ERL due to the less amounts of quaternary ammonium groups in its structure[18] and therefore gives rise to the less tendency of water vapor permeation through the free films.

The results of WVT were consistent with the data of another investigation in which WVT index of free films containing ERS was 13 mg/m^2hKPa, and the addition of EC increased the water vapor permeability of the films.[19]

In the present study, the WVT indices for free films compromising 100% ERS, with thicknesses of 60, 130 and 200 µ, were 21.729, 18.097 and 13.382 mg/m^2hKPa, respectively, which were the lowest amounts among all the given formulations. On the other hand, an increase in the ratio of EC to the other polymers in the formulations enhanced WVT, such that in a ratio of 80% EC, the WVT lowering effect of ERS was not significant. This outcome could have resulted from the less integration of free films, as illustrated in the scanning electron microscopy (SEM) (Figure 1) due to the presence of three different polymers, followed by a decrease in the resistance to water vapor transmission of the free films.

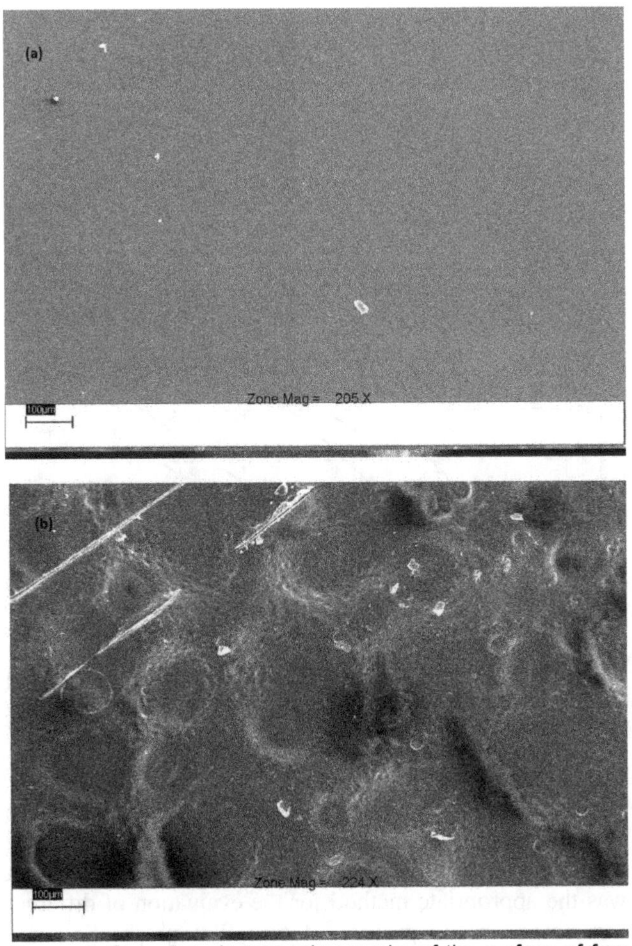

Figure 1. Scanning electron micrographs of the surface of free films; (a) ERS:ERL (50:50) (F10) and (b) ERS:ERL:EC (10:10:80) (F16) (magnification 200×).

The swelling index of formulations is presented in Table 3. As shown, formulations F15, F21 and F27 had the lowest swelling index in the acidic media. None of the three mentioned formulations had ERL in their compositions. It has been demonstrated in other studies that the swelling of ERS is partially restricted in the presence of chloride ion[18,20] which explains the small amounts of swelling of free films containing ERS. On the other hand, maximum amount of swelling in acidic and buffer media occurred in formulations containing ERS-ERL, with the ratio of 1:1 (F1, F10 and F19). A major decrease in swelling was observed when the film thickness increased in the presence of ERS. This effect diminished when ERS was partially substituted with ERL in free films. As a matter of fact, less amounts of ionizable quaternary ammonium groups in the structure of ERS restricted the accessibility of the functional groups, and swelling could be more influenced by variation in thickness compared with free films containing ERL. The presence of EC in the formulations compartment, in amounts up to 40%, lowered the swelling index in SGF and SIF. The larger amounts of EC showed no significant swelling controlling effect, especially in the presence of higher ratios of ERS, and this demonstrated that ERS was the most restrictive polymer on the swelling of free films.

The results of the permeability of theophylline for all formulations are shown in Table 3. Accordingly, formulations F1, F10 and F19, containing high elements of ERL in their compositions, exhibited minimum resistances to drug permeation in both acidic and buffer media. On the contrary, minimum amounts of permeability was attributed to formulations F12, F21, F24 ($p<0.01$) in which ERL was not present and the film thicknesses were either 130 or 200 µ. The latter formulation was made up of 40% EC, and could be assumed as a suitable ratio of EC to Eudragit for sustaining drug release.

The selection of accurate independent variables and dependent factors is a key parameter in an experimental design for optimization of process. The aim of the current study was to achieve an appropriate ratio of different time dependent polymers and to predict a suitable coating system for controlling the drug release from thepohylline pellets. Therefore, the ratios of ERS:ERL and EC:total polymer contents were assumed as the independent variables. With regards to the important effect of coating thickness on drug release, film thickness was selected as the third variable. Water vapor permeation of free films was selected as a response due to the importance of the protective effect of coating films against moisture permeation.[21] Also, according to the close relationship between drug release and the permeability of free films, the latter characteristic was the second candidate as a response for optimization. On the other hand, due to the need to predict a suitable formulation for controlled release product, the similar permeability in two simulated media, could be assumed as the sustained and uniform drug release in the gastro intestinal (GI) tract. Thus, the ratio of permeability in acidic: buffer media ($P_a:P_b$) was chosen as the other response for optimization (Table 3).

Mathematical equations were obtained for each response using the statistical program SPSS based on the relationship between the independent and dependent factors. The equations are listed as follows:

$$Y_1=72.663 - 0.142X_1 - 0.367X_2 - 0.479X_3+0.001X_1X_2 + 0.001X_1X_3+0.007X_2X_3-0.00001X_1X_2X_3 \quad \text{Equation 5}$$

$$Y_2=52.122-0.026X_1-0.664X_2-0.373X_3+0.003X_2X_2+0.005X_2X_3 \quad \text{Equation 6}$$

$$Y_3=54.676-0.037X_1-0.994X_2+0.004X_2X_2+0.008X_2X_3-0.003X_3X_3 \quad \text{Equation 7}$$

$$Y_4=99.998-0.429X_1-1.542X_2-0.930X_3+0.005X_1X_2+0.004X_1X_3+0.003X_2X_2+0.013X_2X_3-0.00005X_1X_2X_3 \quad \text{Equation 8}$$

$$Y_5=117.498-0.413X_1-1.890X_2-1.139X_3+0.006X_1X_2+0.004X_1X_3+0.004X_2X_2+0.016X_2X_3-0.000057X_1X_2X_3 \quad \text{Equation 9}$$

$$Y_6=1.487-0.025X_3+0.000016X_1X_3+0.0001X_2X_2+0.00018X_3X_3 \quad \text{Equation 10}$$

Analysis of variance (ANOVA) confirmed the significance of the assumed regression models for the responses. To prove the validity of the equations, values of X_1, X_2 and X_3 were substituted in the equations in order to obtain the predicted values of responses. Accordingly, the similarity between the results of the observed and predicted responses could be indicative of the accurate selection of the factorial design, variables and levels.

The selection of appropriate constraints for the responses was required for the optimization of the process and also to determine the optimum formulation(s). As the WVT of free films was indicative of the protection against moisture permeation, amounts less than 30 mg/m^2hKPa were assumed as the optimum Y_1 response. Also, the constraint used for Y_6 ranged from 0.95 to 1.05, levels in which the drug release from the formulations could be equal in both the acidic and buffer media. Contour plots were drawn for Y_1 and Y_6 (Figure 2). The best area for formulations was selected according to the contour plots and constraints. It was discovered that formulations F12, F15, F21 and F24 exhibited theoretical optimum responses. Of these, F15 and F24 (containing 40% EC and 60% ERS), which only differed in the film thickness also resulted in practical optimum responses. The two other formulations had only ERS in their compositions. Therefore, the coating systems containing ERS:EC (6:4) or ERS were selected as the optimum formulations for coating of theopylline pellets.

The drug release from the pellets was examined after preparation of the pellet. Figure 3 shows the drug release from the pellets containing optimum coating formulations with different coating thicknesses. As shown in the Figure, an increase in the coating thickness managed a slower release from the pellets, which was in direct relation with the higher tortuosity and path of drug molecules.[22] On the other hand, the addition of 40% EC to the coating formulations resulted in more sustained and controlled drug release, and the data were compatible with the data of permeability. Pellets coated with ERS:EC (6:4), and having coating thickness of 10%, met the suitable sustained drug release condition from a sustained release dosage form of theophylline defined by USP,[23] and such pellets could be selected as the optimum pellets.

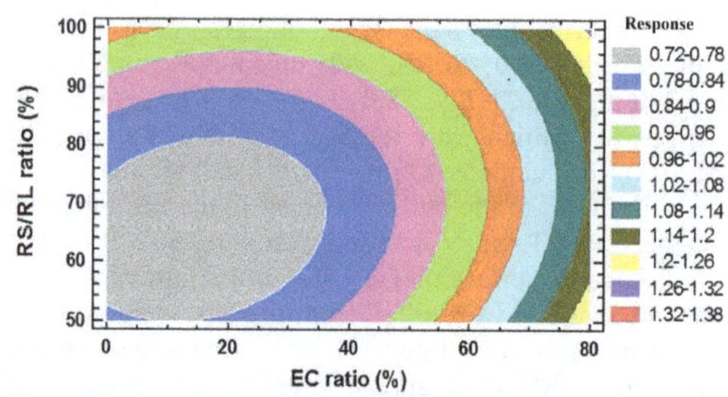

Figure 2. Contour plot for Y_6 response (ratio of permeability in acid:permeability in buffer).

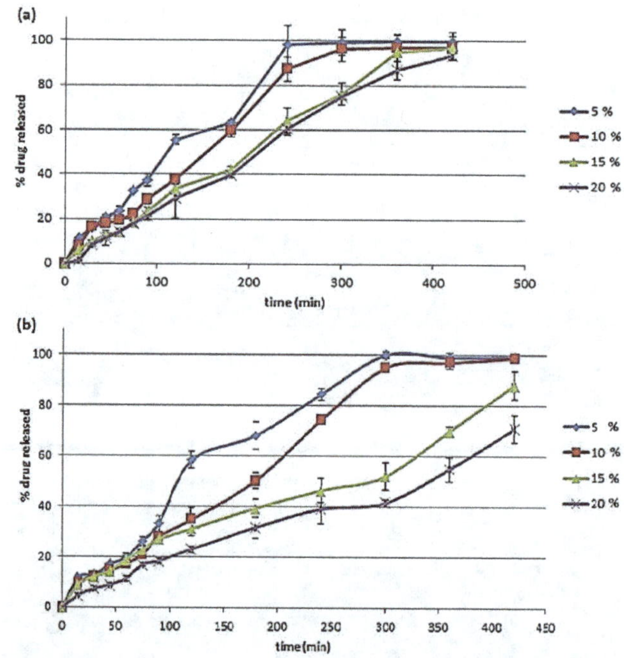

Figure 3. Drug release from theophylline pellets with coating thickness of 5, 10, 15 and 20% and coated with (a) ERS and (b) ERS:EC(6:4).

Conclusion

The results of this investigation demonstrated that the primary studies on free films could be valuable for the prediction of drug release from pellets. Factorial design was the appropriate method for the evaluation of different parameters in the process of free film preparation and optimization of the coating system.

According to the data, the formulation containing Eudragit RS:Ethylcellulose (in the ratio of 6:4) exhibited suitable conditions necessary for controlling drug release, and the pellets coated with this formulation could be selected as a theophylline controlled release dosage form.

Acknowledgments

This work is the Pharm. D thesis of Mr. A. Tavakol which is supported by a grant from research chancellor of Ahvaz Jundishapur University of Medical Sciences. The authors would like to thank Arya and NP Pharm for their collaboration and providing samples used in this paper.

Conflict of Interest

Authors declare no conflict of interest in this study.

References

1. Alnaief M, Antonyuk S, Hentzschel CM, Leopold CS, Heinrich S, Smirnova I. A novel process for coating of silica aerogel microspheres for controlled drug release applications. *Micropor Mesopor Mat* 2012;160:167-73. doi:10.1016/j.micromeso.2012.02.009
2. Haaser M, Karrout Y, Velghe C, Cuppok Y, Gordon KC, Pepper M, et al. Application of terahertz pulsed imaging to analyse film coating characteristics of sustained-release coated pellets. *Int J Pharm* 2013;457(2):521-6. doi: 10.1016/j.ijpharm.2013.05.039
3. Maroni A, Del Curto MD, Zema L, Foppoli A, Gazzaniga A. Film coating for oral colon delivery. *Int J Pharm* 2013;457(2):372-94. doi:10.1016/j.ijpharm.2013.05.043
4. Yadav D, Survase S, Kumar N. Dual coating of swellable and rupturable polymers on glipizide loaded mcc pellets for pulsatile delivery: Formulation design and in vitro evaluation. *Int J Pharm* 2011;419(1-2):121-30. doi: 10.1016/j.ijpharm.2011.07.026
5. Kugge C, Vanderhoek N, Bousfield DW. Oscillatory shear response of moisture barrier coatings containing clay of different shape factor. *J Colloid Interface Sci* 2011;358(1):25-31. doi: 10.1016/j.jcis.2011.02.051
6. Miyadai N, Higashi K, Moribe K, Yamamoto K. Optimization and characterization of direct coating for ibuprofen particles using a composite fluidized bed. *Adv Powder Technol* 2012;23(1):40-5. doi:10.1016/j.apt.2010.12.004
7. Van Savage G, Rhodes CT. The sustained release coating of solid dosage forms: a historical review. *Drug Dev Ind Pharm* 1995;21(1):93-118. doi: 10.3109/03639049509048098
8. Desai J, Alexander K, Riga A. Characterization of polymeric dispersions of dimenhydrinate in ethyl cellulose for controlled release. *Int J Pharm* 2006;308(1-2):115-23. doi: 10.1016/j.ijpharm.2005.10.034
9. Lokhande AB, Mishra S, Kulkarni RD, Naik JB. Influence of different viscosity grade ethylcellulose polymers on encapsulation and in vitro release study of drug loaded nanoparticles. *J Pharm Res* 2013;7(5):414-20. doi:10.1016/j.jopr.2013.04.050
10. Lehmann K. Chemistry and application properties of polymethacrylate coating systems. In: Mc Ginity GW, editors. Aqueous polymeric coating for pharmaceutical dosage form. USA: Marcel Dekker; 1997.
11. Ye ZW, Rombout P, Remon JP, Vervaet C, Van den Mooter G. Correlation between the permeability of metoprolol tartrate through plasticized isolated ethylcellulose/hydroxypropyl methylcellulose films and drug release from reservoir pellets. *Eur J Pharm Biopharm* 2007;67(2):485-90. doi: 10.1016/j.ejpb.2007.02.010
12. Srinivasa PC, Ravi R, Tharanathan RN. Effect of storage conditions on the tensile properties of eco-friendly chitosan films by response surface methodology. *J Food Eng* 2007;80:184-9. doi:10.1016/j.jfoodeng.2006.05.007
13. Abrahamsson B, Alpsten M, Bake B, Jonsson UE, Eriksson-Lepkowska M, Larsson A. Drug absorption from nifedipine hydrophilic matrix extended-release (er) tablet-comparison with an osmotic pump tablet and effect of food. *J Control Release* 1998;52(3):301-10.
14. Sriamornsak P, Thirawong N, Weerapol Y, Nunthanid J, Sungthongjeen S. Swelling and erosion of pectin matrix tablets and their impact on drug release behavior. *Eur J Pharm Biopharm* 2007;67(1):211-9. doi: 10.1016/j.ejpb.2006.12.014
15. Akhgari A, Farahmand F, Afrasiabi Garekani H, Sadeghi F, Vandamme TF. Permeability and swelling studies on free films containing inulin in combination with different polymethacrylates aimed for colonic drug delivery. *Eur J Pharm Sci* 2006;28(4):307-14. doi: 10.1016/j.ejps.2006.03.005
16. Blanchon S, Couarraze G, Rieg-Falson F, Cohen G, Puisieux F. Permeability of progesterone and a synthetic progestin through methacrylic films. *Int J Pharm* 1991;72(1):1–10. doi:10.1016/0378-5173(91)90374-W
17. Lin WJ, Lu CH. Characterization and permeation of microporous poly (ε-caprolactone) films. *J Membrane Sci* 2002;198(1):109-18. doi:10.1016/S0376-7388(01)00652-4
18. Bodmeier R, Guo X, Sarabia RE, Skultety PF. The influence of buffer species and strength on diltiazem hcl release from beads coated with the aqueous cationic polymer dispersions, eudragit rs, rl 30d. *Pharm Res* 1996;13(1):52-6.
19. Zheng W, Sauer D, McGinity JW. Influence of hydroxyethylcellulose on the drug release properties of theophylline pellets coated with eudragit rs 30 d. *Eur J Pharm Biopharm* 2005;59(1):147-54. doi: 10.1016/j.ejpb.2004.06.002
20. Wagner K, McGinity J. Influence of chloride ion exchange on the permeability and drug release of eudragit rs 30 d films. *J Control Release* 2002;82(2-3):385-97.
21. Elsabee MZ, Abdou ES. Chitosan based edible films and coatings: A review. *Mater Sci Eng C Mater Biol Appl* 2013;33(4):1819-41. doi: 10.1016/j.msec.2013.01.010
22. Fan TY, Wei SL, Yan WW, Chen DB, Li J. An investigation of pulsatile release tablets with ethylcellulose and eudragit l as film coating materials and cross-linked polyvinylpyrrolidone in the core tablets. *J Control Release* 2001;77(3):245-51.
23. United States Pharmacopeia 34/National Formulary 29. Rockville, MD, USA: United States Pharmacopeial Convention; 2011.

8

Aggregated Nanotransfersomal Dry Powder Inhalation of Itraconazole for Pulmonary Drug Delivery

Mehdi Hassanpour Aghdam[1], Saeed Ghanbarzadeh[2,3], Yousef Javadzadeh[4], Hamed Hamishehkar[3]*

[1] *Research Center for Pharmaceutical Nanotechnology, and Students' Research Committee, Tabriz University of Medical Sciences, Tabriz, Iran.*

[2] *Zanjan Pharmaceutical Nanotechnology Research Center, and Department of Pharmaceutics, Faculty of Pharmacy, Zanjan University of Medical Sciences, Zanjan, Iran.*

[3] *Drug Applied Research Center, Tabriz University of Medical Sciences, Tabriz, Iran.*

[4] *Biotechnology Research Center and Department of Pharmaceutics, Faculty of Pharmacy, Tabriz University of Medical Sciences, Tabriz, Iran.*

Article info

Keywords:
- Pulmonary drug delivery
- Dry powder inhaler
- Transfersome
- Itraconazole
- DPI

Abstract

Purpose: Local therapy is a valuable and strategic approach in the treatment of lung associated diseases and dry powder inhalation (DPI) formulations play the key role in this plan. Transfersome has been introduced as a novel biocompatible vesicular system with potential for administration in pulmonary drug delivery. The present study was designed to prepare Itraconazole-loaded nanotrantransfersomal DPI formulation.

Methods: Itraconazole-loaded nanotransfersomes with three different types of surfactant in varying concentrations were prepared and characterized in the point of particle size distribution and morphology by laser light scattering and scanning electron microscopy (SEM) methods. The optimized transferosomal formulations were co-spray dried with mannitol and the aerosolization efficiency and aerodynamic properties of dry powders were determined by next generation impactor using a validated HPLC technique.

Results: The volume mean diameter of optimized nanotransfersomal formulation with lecithin:Span® 60 in the ratio of 90:10 was 171 nm with narrow size distribution pattern which increased up to 518 nm after drug loading. Different types of surfactant did not influence the particle size significantly. SEM images confirmed the formation of aggregated nanoparticles in the suitable range (1-5 μm) for the pulmonary drug delivery. Aerosolization evaluation of co-spray dried formulations with different amounts of mannitol indicated that 2:1 ratio of mannitol:transfersome (w:w) showed the best aerosolization efficiency (fine particle fraction (FPF)=37%). Increasing of mannitol significantly decreased the FPF of the optimized formulations.

Conclusion: The results of this study was introduced the potential application of nanotransfersomes in the formulation of DPIs for lung delivery of various drugs.

Introduction

Itraconazole is a broad-spectrum synthetic triazole antifungal agent which is active against a broad spectrum of fungal species including *Cryptococcus, Candida, Aspergillus, Blastomyces* and *Histoplasma capsulatum.*[1] The lungs are suitable for both local and systemic drug delivery due to the presence of a large alveolar surface area with high permeability owing to their thin epithelial layer.[2] Development of drug delivery systems for pulmonary application had received considerable attention and high patient compliance in the last three decades due to be a noninvasive method of drug administration. Furthermore, the possibility to locally and more site-specific drug delivery at high concentrations into the diseased lung by avoiding the first-pass metabolism and reduced systemic doses would lead to maximum therapeutic efficiency and minimum side effects, respectively.[3-6] The use of liposomes as drug carriers for pulmonary delivery has been reported for different kinds of therapeutics.[7,8] The utilization of lipidic vesicular systems for pulmonary drug delivery has many potential advantages over aerosol delivery of the corresponding non-encapsulated drug, including carrier suitability for most lipophilic drugs, compatibility and reducing local irritation of lung tissue, prolonging local and systemic therapeutic drug levels and finally facilitating intracellular drug delivery especially to alveolar macrophages, tumor cells or epithelial cells.[9] Intensive research over the past 25 years led to the introduction and development of a new class of highly deformable liposomes resembling the natural cell vesicle, named transferosomes.[10-12] Transfersomes are composed of phospholipids like phosphatidylcholine and edge

***Corresponding author:** Hamed Hamishehkar, Email: Hamishehkarh@tbzmed.ac.ir

activators which self assembles into lipid bilayer in aqueous environment and closes to form a vesicle.[13,14] An edge activator is often a single-chain surfactant with a high radius of curvature that destabilizes the lipid bilayers of the vesicles and increases the deformability of the bilayers.[15] Spray drying has been considered as a simple one-step process for producing small particles for pulmonary administration, that can be easily scaled up.[16-18] Pressurized metered-dose inhalers (MDI), nebulizers, and dry powder inhalers (DPI) are the three main delivery systems used for aerosol inhalation in humans. Among these, DPI appears to be the most promising for future use. They are propellant-free, portable, easy to operate and low-cost devices with improved stability of the formulation as a result of the dry state.[19,20] According to our literature review, there is no report about the application of nanotransfersomes in pulmonary drug delivery. Therefore, the primary aim of this study was to introduce transfersomes as a carrier for pulmonary delivery in the form of dry powder inhalation formulation.

Materials and Methods

Materials

Acetonitrile, Tween® 80, Ursodiol, Chloroform and Ortho-phosphoric acid were purchased from Merck Chemicals Co. (Germany). Soybean phosphatidylcholine (SPC, purity >99%) was purchased from Lipoid GmbH (Ludwigshafen, Germany). Itraconazole was supplied from Cipla Company (India). Span® 60 and Span® 80 were supplied from Sigma Company (USA) and BDH laboratory (UK), respectively. D-Mannitol and ethyl alcohol were obtained from Fluka (Germany) and JATA (Iran) Companies, respectively.

Methods

Preparation of nanotransfersomes

Transfersomes were prepared by the thin film hydration method. Briefly, desired amounts of SPC (100 mg), Itraconazole (5 mg) and surfactant (5, 10, and 15 mg) were dissolved in an appropriate volume of organic solvent (Table 1). The container tightly closed, protected from light and maintained at room temperature for one day to make sure of formation of complete and homogeneous solution. The mixture was transformed to a round-bottomed flask for solvent removal using a rotary evaporator (Heidolph, Germany) at reduced pressure and above phase transition temperature of lecithin (60 °C). The dried film was hydrated for one hour at 60 °C and then sonicated using a prob sonicator (Sonix, Vibracell), with 0.5 sec on and 0.5 sec off intervals, for a total period of 15 min.[12,21]

Table 1. Composition of various nanotransfersome formulations. Data was presented as mean ± standard deviation (n=3).

Formulation code	Type of Surfactant	Surfactant (mg)	Itraconazole (mg)	VMD[a] (nm)	Span
T1	Span® 80	10	0	360 ± 21	1.18 ± 0.03
T2	Span® 80	5	5	556 ± 29	1.44 ± 0.04
T3	Span® 80	10	5	526 ± 31	1.74 ± 0.03
T4	Span® 80	15	5	598 ± 34	1.70 ± 0.06
T5	Span® 60	10	0	171 ± 28	1.03 ± 0.03
T6	Span® 60	5	5	535 ± 22	1.33 ± 0.03
T7	Span® 60	10	5	518 ± 23	1.07 ± 0.03
T8	Span® 60	15	5	534 ± 30	2.16 ± 0.14
T9	Ursodiol	5	5	545 ± 22	1.17 ± 0.04
T10	Ursodiol	10	5	522 ± 27	1.04 ± 0.04
T11	Ursodiol	15	5	594 ± 41	1.66 ± 0.04

[a] Volume median diameter

Spray drying process

For producing DPI formulations, different amounts of mannitol powder (100, 200, 300 and 600 mg named as F1, F2, F3 and F4, respectively) was co-spray dried with the nanotransfersomal dispersion (100 mg) with desired characteristics using a mini spray dryer at an inlet temperature of 100 ± 5 °C, outlet temperature of 60 ± 5 °C, aspiration setting of 90% and spray flow of 400 NL/h. Immediately after powder collection from the cyclone of spray dryer, spray-dried particles were packed into the tightly closed container wrapped in aluminum foil and desiccated over silica gel at room temperature until further studies.

Particle size analysis

The particle size and particle size distribution of prepared nanotransfersomal dispersions were determined by particle size analyzer (Wing SALD 2101, Japan). The size distribution was expressed by the volume median diameter (VMD) and span value. The smaller span values correspond to narrower size distribution. Span value calculated using following equation:

$$\text{Span}=\frac{D(v90\%)-D(v10\%)}{D(v50\%)}$$

Where D(v,90), D(v,10) and D(v,50) are the equivalent volume diameters at 90, 10 and 50% cumulative volume, respectively.[22,23]

Scanning electron microscopy (SEM)

The shape and surface morphology of the particles were studied by the scanning electron microscope (LEO 1430 VP, UK & Germany). Prior to scanning, the samples were coated with a thin layer of gold, using a direct current sputter technique (Emitechk450X, England).

In vitro aerosolization assessment

The *in vitro* aerodynamic parameters including aerodynamic diameter, aerosolization efficiency, dispersion and deposition characteristics of optimized Itraconazole-loaded nanotransfersomal dry powders were assessed by an aerolizer connected to the next generation impactor (NGI) with pre-separator and USP induction port (Copley Scientific, Nottingham, UK).[24] The NGI was assembled and operated in accordance with USP General Chapter 601 to assess the drug delivered. An appropriate number of hard gelatin capsules (N = 3) were filled with 10 mg of spray dried powder. To ensure efficient particle capture and prevent inter-stage losses due to particle bounce, the particle collection surface of each stage was coated with Tween® 80. For this purpose, every eight collection cups of the NGI were soaked into Tween® 80 ethanolic solution (1%) and placed under the fume hood until the complete evaporation of ethanol. The cups were placed into the apertures in the cup tray and the cup tray was located into the bottom frame and lowered into place. The impactor lid was closed with the sealed body attached and the handle was operated to lock the impactor together. Capsules were gathered after actuation for the study of remained powder. The content uniformity test was carried out for 10 mg of each formulation in 5 repetitions. The coefficient variation percentage (CV%) were less than 6% for all spray-dried powders. The batches that showed CV% above 6% were excluded from the study. The induction port was connected to the first stage of the NGI. The flow rate was calibrated using a flow meter (DFM 2000, Copley Scientific, Nottingham, UK) and fixed at 60 L/min. Fine particle fraction (FPF), mass median aerodynamic diameter (MMAD), and geometric standard deviation (GSD) indexes were calculated using the Copley Inhaler Testing Data Analysis Software (CITDAS, version 3.10). The MMAD is defined as the diameter at which 50% of the particles by mass are larger and 50% are smaller. FPF represents the percentage of emitted particles with an MMAD of 5 μm or less estimating the fraction of particles expected to deposit deep within the lungs. The emission was defined as the mass of drug delivered from the inhaler (i.e., total amount excluding the inhaler device and capsule), expressed as a percentage of the total amount of Itraconazole collected. Dispersibility was defined as the ratio of FPF per emission. Each value was expressed as the mean ± standard deviation.[25]

Chloroform as a solvent that can dissolve both SPC and Itraconazole was used as the washing solvent to rupture the transfersomes and extract Itraconazole. The whole process of washing was performed under the fume hood. The capsule shells, pre-separator, USP induction port and NGI stages were washed with suitable amount of chloroform. Chloroform containing extracted drug was moved into the test tubes. The test tubes were kept under nitrogen flow for complete removal of organic solvent. The tubes were filled with certain amount of acetonitrile, vortexed and sonicated for a few minutes to dissolve the extracted Itraconazole completely. 500 μl of acetonitrile was moved into the micro tubes and centrifuged at 13000 rpm for 10 minutes to separate the undissolved transfersome compositions and capsule residuals to yield a particle free solution suitable for HPLC analysis. After deposition onto the stages of the NGI, the mass deposited on each of the impactor pieces was collected and the total mass of drug was quantified by a validated HPLC system.

High performance liquid chromatography analysis

The Itraconazole content of each NGI stage was analyzed using a Knauer apparatus HPLC system (Germany) consisted of a model 1000 HPLC pump and a model 2600 tunable absorbance detector, with the following condition: Column: C-18 (150 × 4.6mm, 10 μm, 125 A°) (Germany) protected by a C-18 guard column, mobile phase: acetonitrile: water (90:10), flow rate: 1 mL/min, wave length: 263 nm and injection volume: 20 μl. The run time for Itraconazole appearance following the sample injection was approximately 3 min. The area under the curve (AUC) that demonstrates the Itraconazole concentration was calculated through the machine software (Chromgate® V3.3.1). An excess amount of sample was injected into the injector to make sure that the loop has been completely filled with the sample. Calibration curve was leaner in the range of 1.25 to 25 μg/mL (r^2=0.997).

Statistical analysis

Data are expressed as a mean value ± standard deviation (SD). Statistical analysis was performed using a one-way analysis of variance (ANOVA) with multiple comparisons between deposition data using a Tukey-Kramer HSD test by SPSS software (version 13.0, Chicago, IL, USA). A P value <0.05 was considered statistically significant.

Results

Preparation of Itraconazole-loaded nanotransfersomes

The effect of different kinds of surfactants and their concentration on the size of transfersomes are shown in Table 1. The size of blank transfersomes (T1 and T5) were smaller than drug-loaded transfersomes (T3 and T7) with the same compositions. Both drug free and drug-loaded transfersomes showed relatively narrow size distribution pattern (Figure 1). Although there are no statistically difference among the formulations composed of different type and amount of surfactants, formulations containing 10 mg of Span® 60 (T7) was selected for further experiments due to its lowest size and narrowest size distribution (Table 1). Results also showed that preparation of nanotransfersomal formulations with 10 mg of all types of surfactants resulted in the lowest size compared to using 5 and 15 mg of surfactant.

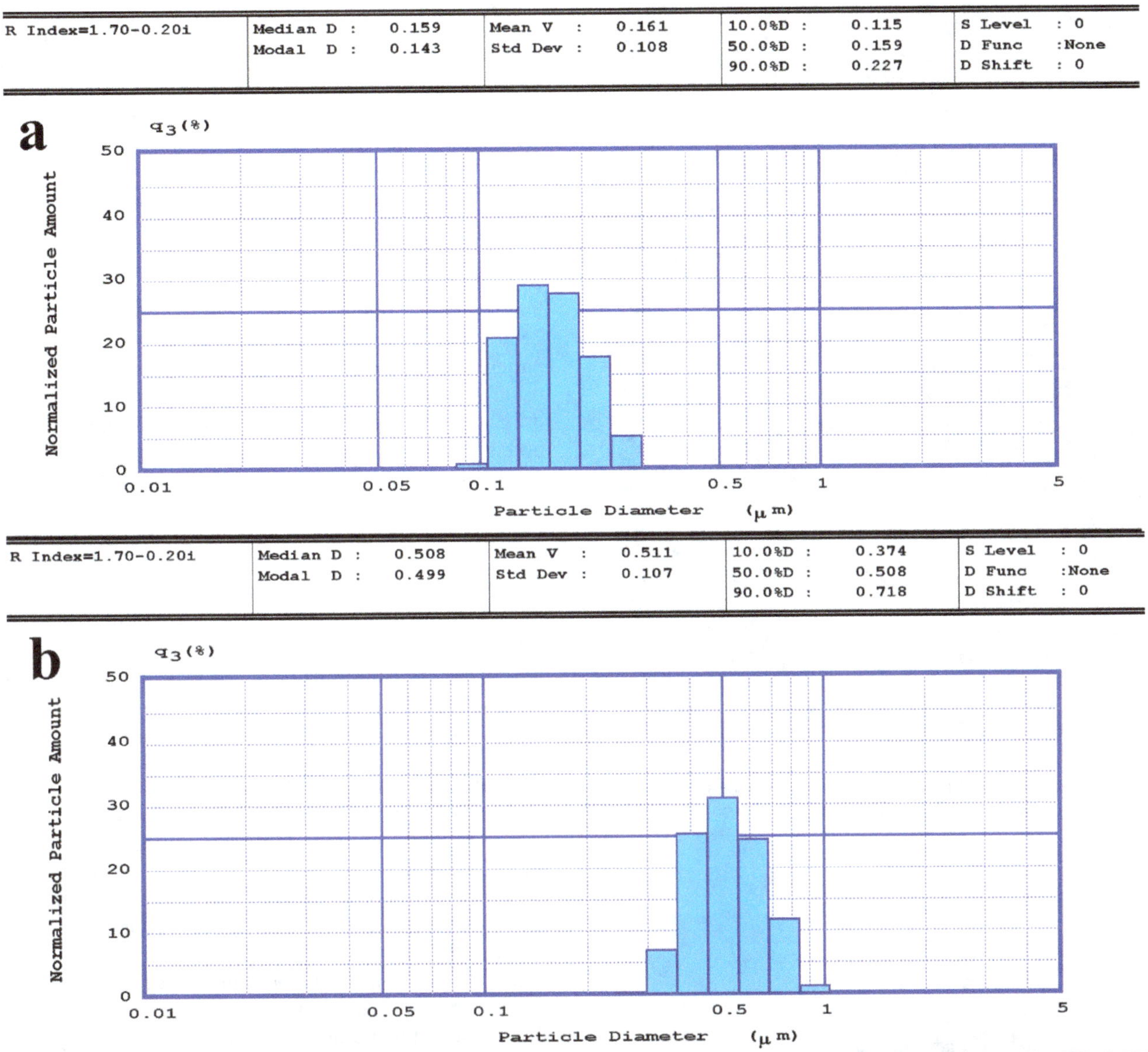

Figure 1. The size distribution pattern of a) drug free nanotransfersomes (T2) and b) drug loaded nanotransfersome (T7) formulations.

Preparation of DPI formulation

DPI formulations containing aggregated Itraconazol-loaded nanotransfersomes were prepared by various ratios of transfersomes to mannitol. The formulation F1 was not collected from the cyclone of the spray dryer and mostly adhered to the inner wall of heating chamber. It was reported that lecithin forms a viscous isotropic phase from 88 to 109 °C (the inlet temperature of spray dryer in our experiment) which may be responsible for the formulation adhesion to the spray dryer's chamber. The rest of the formulations with higher amounts of mannitol provided the suitable amounts of powder which were collected from the cyclone (yield value around 50 %) and assessed by NGI for determination of their aerosolization efficacy. Figures 2a and 2b show SEM images of the spray- dried particles (F2), confirmed the formation of aggregated nanoparticles in the suitable range for pulmonary drug delivery.

In vitro deposition

The amount of Itraconazole in each stage of NGI device was analyzed by HPLC method and illustrated in Figure 3. The in vitro parameters which were calculated according to the results of Figure 3 including FPF, MMAD and GSD are shown in Table 2. F2 showed the highest FPF and dispersibility, therefore, was selected as the optimized formulation. Although F4 had the best emission and GSD indicating its suitable flowability and aerodynamic size distribution, respectively, the main aerosolization indexes (FPF and dispersibility) are lower than other formulations.

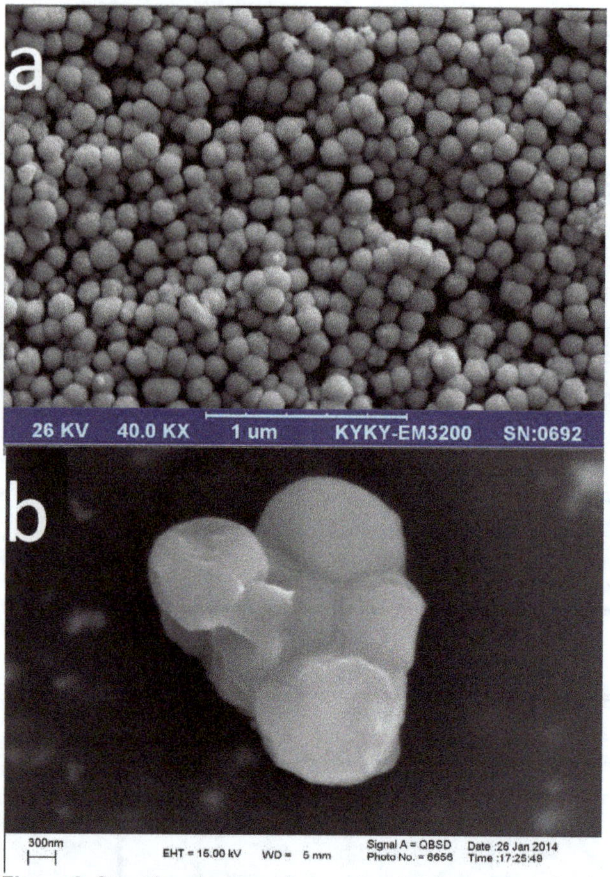

Figure 2. Scanning electron micrographs of a) Itraconazole-loaded nanotransfersomes (formulation T7) and b) those co-spray dried with mannitol (formulation F2).

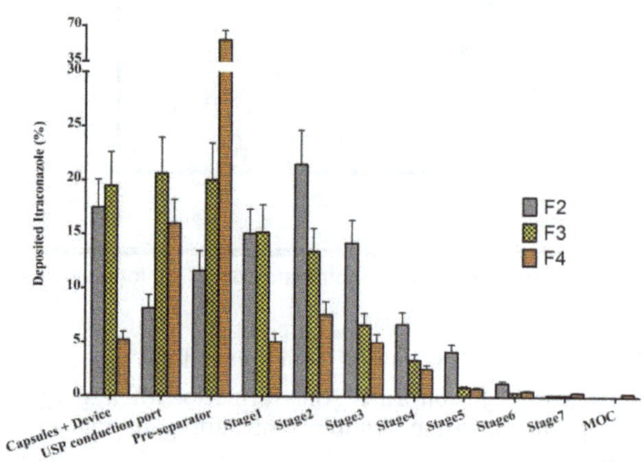

Figure 3. The percentage of Itraconazole from formulations F2, F3 and F4, deposited in various stages of NGI. Data was presented as mean ± standard deviation (n=3).

Table 2. Aerosolization efficiency indexes of selected Itraconazole-loaded nanotransfersomal dry powders measured by the NGI (mean ± SD, n= 3).

Parameters	[d]F2	F3	F4
[a]FPF (%)	37.3 ± 3.1	17.8 ± 2.9	10.4 ± 1.4
[b]MMAD (µm)	5.1 ± 0.7	6.5 ± 1	5.2 ± 0.9
[c]GSD	2.1 ± 0.2	2.1 ± 0.1	1.9 ± 0.1
Emission (%)	82.7 ± 2.6	80.5 ± 3.1	94.8 ± 0.8
Dispersibility	45.23 ± 2.9	22.11 ± 3.0	10.9 ± 1.1

[a] Fine Particle Fraction, [b] Mass Median Aerodynamic Diameter, [c] Geometric Standard Deviation, [d] F2, F3 and F4 were prepared by co-spray drying of 100 mg nanotransfersome and 200, 300 and 600 mg of mannitol, respectively

Discussion

Itraconazole is a poorly soluble drug that has displayed a low and variable oral absorption following oral administration. Absolute bioavailability of the oral Itraconazole capsule is 40% lower in the non-fed state compared to the fed state. To obtain a therapeutic level of drug at the site of lung infections, a high oral or intravenous dose must be administered which consequently increases the incidence of unwanted side effects associated with a high drug serum concentration.[26] In addition, gastrointestinal side effects have been reported in recipients of the oral solution up to 25% in a randomized trial and are the major reason for patient incompliance.[27] Local targeting of the drug at the usual site of infection (the lungs) means that less total drug may be required for dosing and therefore, the potential for side effects may be minimized due to a much reduced systemic concentration.[28] It has been reported that pulmonary delivery of nanoparticulate Itraconazole can achieve a significantly higher (more than 10-fold) lung tissue concentrations compared to conventional oral administration of Itraconazole. Effective and sustained lung tissue concentrations were achieved via inhalation of a nanoparticulate Itraconazole formulation.[29] Additionally, a targeted therapy may also initiate a quicker therapeutic onset and ultimately reduce the duration of treatment.[28] The utilization of lipidic vesicular systems for pulmonary drug delivery has many potential advantages over aerosol delivery of the corresponding nonencapsulated drug, including universal carrier suitability for most lipophilic drugs, compatibility and preventing local irritation of lung tissue, providing a pulmonary sustained release reservoir prolonging local and systemic therapeutic drug levels and facilitating intracellular drug delivery especially to alveolar macrophages, tumor cells or epithelial cells.[9] The present study explored a new idea for nanoparticle delivery to the lower respiratory regions of the lung using micrometer-sized carrier particles. In this investigation Itraconazole-loaded nanotransfersomes were incorporated as model drug delivery system by the lipid film hydration technique followed by sonication for size reduction. For the formulation of DPI, prepared nanotransfersomes should have a mean size below 5µm[30] to form inhalable carrier particles. This requirement was satisfied well when nanotransfersomes were co-spray dried with mannitol, a regularly used inert excipient in pulmonary drug delivery. The administered excipients (lecithin, mannitol, ursodiol, Span® 60 and Span® 80) were used because of their biocompatibility and pharmaceutical acceptability. The particle size of the transfersomes with different types of surfactant did not show a significant difference. These results indicate that the particle size of the vesicles was not significantly affected by the type of surfactant.[31] Spray drying is a low-cost, one-step pharmaceutical process that is widely used in the development of novel dry powder formulations.[3] Spray drying technique offers a number of potential advantages over lyophilization technique. Spray drying technique was utilized for stabilization of nanoliposomes and development of uniform sized particles with desired aerosolization properties for pulmonary administration to overcome constraints associated with lyophilization technique, such as formation of hard cake, need of micronization, addition of coarse carriers for aersolization, and heterogeneous size distribution pattern.[32] Once the nanotransfersome aggregates, with their large surface area, in the dry powder formulation is deposited in the aqueous lining fluid in the lung, the mannitol may quickly dissolve, resulting in the dispersion of nanotransfersomes in the respiratory tract fluids.[33] Carriers form the backbone structure of the solid particles during the spray drying process and facilitate pulmonary delivery.[32] The carrier of choice for DPI products is currently lactose monohydrate and almost all DPI products already in market are using lactose as a carrier. The advantages of lactose monohydrate are its well-investigated toxicity profile, its broad availability and its relatively low price.[19] However, it has some disadvantages that should be considered in its usage as carrier for DPIs. Lactose is incompatible with some drugs and compounds with a primary amine group. Lactose may develop a yellow brown color with browning aging that is accelerated by the process of spray drying. Lactose monohydrate is produced from bovine or with bovine-driven additives so that the Transmissible Spongiform Encephalopathy (TSE) discussion is still an issue for this compound. In addition, Lactose intolerance is a situation that requires a solution. For overcoming the above mentioned drawbacks of lactose, mannitol is a suitable substitute carrier that possesses further positive aspects.[20] For these reasons, mannitol was chosen as an excipient for co-spray drying with nanotransfersomes. Once the nanotransfersomes aggregate, with their large surface area, in the dry powder formulation is deposited in the aqueous lining fluid in the lung, the mannitol may quickly dissolve, resulting in the dispersion of nanotransfersomes in the respiratory tract fluids.[33] Due to the flexibility in use and high productivity, NGIs (a new impactor type specifically designed for testing pharmaceutical inhalers using the very newest and modern designed theory in 1997) have been used as the most popular testing machine within many inhaler research laboratories. NGI was launched in 2000 and was subsequently accepted into the European Pharmacopeia as Apparatus E and into the United States Pharmacopeia as Apparatus 5 and 6 in 2005. The ideal size for a therapeutic particle is not known exactly but it may be assumed that the MMAD should be not more than 5 µm to pass into the tracheobronchial tree and smaller airways if peripheral deposition is required.[34] Formulation F2 exhibited an MMAD of 5.1 ± 0.7 µm, and a higher FPF in comparison to the other formulations. In this study, it was shown that increase in mannitol ratio in the spray dried formulations caused a decrease in aerosolization efficiency (Table 2). Maximum FPF of 37.35 ± 3.1% was observed in formulation F2 containing 200 mg of mannitol as compared with F3 (300 mg of mannitol) of 17.8 ± 2.9% and F4 (600 mg of mannitol) of 10.4 ± 1.4%. Previous studies have indicated that increasing the lipid concentration in the spray drying feeds can decrease the residual water content in the powder[35] which consequently may improve the aerodynamic properties of the DPI formulation. Higher ratios of mannitol improved emission of formulation F4 which may be attributed to the powder flowability improvement by addition of carrier. The findings of this investigation showed that dry powder inhalation formulation of Itraconazole-loaded nanotransfersomes prepared by co-spray drying with mannitol possessed suitable aerosolization performance. Therefore, this formulation may have a potential to deliver Itraconazole to the site of infection in the lungs in the pulmonary aspergillosis. The results highlight the need to examine the enhanced *in vivo* therapeutic effects of pulmonary drug delivery via nanotransfersomal DPI formulations. The results of this study was introduced the potential application of nanotransfersomes in the formulation of DPIs for lung delivery of various drugs.

Acknowledgments

This paper was extracted from Pharm.D. thesis No. 3662 that was submitted to the Faculty of Pharmacy of Tabriz University of Medical Sciences and financially supported by grant No. 90/92 from the Drug Applied Research Center of the same university.

Conflict of Interest

The authors report no conflicts of interest.

References

1. Hong JY, Kim JK, Song YK, Park JS, Kim CK. A new self-emulsifying formulation of itraconazole with improved dissolution and oral absorption. *J Control Release* 2006;110(2):332-8. doi: 10.1016/j.jconrel.2005.10.002
2. Lu D, Hickey AJ. Liposomal dry powders as aerosols for pulmonary delivery of proteins. *AAPS PharmSciTech* 2005;6(4):E641-8. doi: 10.1208/pt060480
3. Sung JC, Pulliam BL, Edwards DA. Nanoparticles for drug delivery to the lungs. *Trends Biotechnol* 2007;25(12):563-70. doi: 10.1016/j.tibtech.2007.09.005
4. Ugwoke MI, Vereyken IJ, Luessen H. Microparticles and liposomes as pulmonary drug delivery systems: What are the recent trends? *Chapter VI* 2007:308-77.
5. Emami J, Hamishehkar H, Najafabadi AR, Gilani K, Minaiyan M, Mahdavi H, et al. Particle size design of plga microspheres for potential pulmonary drug delivery using response surface methodology. *J Microencapsul* 2009;26(1):1-8. doi: 10.1080/02652040802083900

6. Emami J, Hamishehkar H, Najafabadi AR, Gilani K, Minaiyan M, Mahdavi H, et al. A novel approach to prepare insulin-loaded poly(lactic-co-glycolic acid) microcapsules and the protein stability study. *J Pharm Sci* 2009;98(5):1712-31. doi: 10.1002/jps.21544
7. Gaspar MM, Bakowsky U, Ehrhardt C. Inhaled liposomes–current strategies and future challenges. *J Biomed Nanotechnol* 2008;4(3):245-57. doi: 10.1166/jbn.2008.334
8. Kaur IP, Agrawal R. Nanotechnology: A new paradigm in cosmeceuticals. *Recent Pat Drug Deliv Formul* 2007;1(2):171-82.
9. Chougule M, Padhi B, Misra A. Development of spray dried liposomal dry powder inhaler of dapsone. *AAPS PharmSciTech* 2008;9(1):47-53. doi: 10.1208/s12249-007-9024-6
10. Elsayed MM, Abdallah OY, Naggar VF, Khalafallah NM. Lipid vesicles for skin delivery of drugs: Reviewing three decades of research. *Int J Pharm* 2007;332(1-2):1-16. doi: 10.1016/j.ijpharm.2006.12.005
11. Singh D. Ultradeformable system: A carrier for transdermal drug delivery. *Int J Pharm Sci Res* 2013;4(11):98-104.
12. Ghanbarzadeh S, Arami S. Formulation and evaluation of piroxicam transferosomal gel: An approach for penetration enhancement. *J Drug Deliv Sci Technol* 2013;23(6):587-90. doi: 10.1016/S1773-2247(13)50089-X
13. Gharsallaoui A, Roudaut G, Chambin O, Voilley A, Saurel R. Applications of spray-drying in microencapsulation of food ingredients: An overview. *Food Res Int* 2007;40(9):1107-21. doi: 10.1016/j.foodres.2007.07.004
14. Ghanbarzadeh S, Valizadeh H, Zakeri-Milani P. Sirolimus nano liposomes. *Pharm Ind* 2013;75(8).
15. Ghanbarzadeh S, Khorrami A, Arami S. Nonionic surfactant-based vesicular system for transdermal drug delivery. *Drug Deliv* 2015;22(8):1071-7. doi: 10.3109/10717544.2013.873837
16. Faramarzi P, Haririan I, Ghanbarzadeh S, Yaqoubi S, Hamishehkar H. Development of carrier free montelukast dry powder inhalation formulation. *Pharm Ind* 2015;77(10):1535-42.
17. Rojanarat W, Changsan N, Tawithong E, Pinsuwan S, Chan HK, Srichana T. Isoniazid proliposome powders for inhalation-preparation, characterization and cell culture studies. *Int J Mol Sci* 2011;12(7):4414-34. doi: 10.3390/ijms12074414
18. Rahimpour Y, Hamishehkar H. Lactose engineering for better performance in dry powder inhalers. *Adv Pharm Bull* 2012;2(2):183-7. doi: 10.5681/apb.2012.028
19. Hamishehkar H, Emami J, Najafabadi AR, Gilani K, Minaiyan M, Mahdavi H, et al. Influence of carrier particle size, carrier ratio and addition of fine ternary particles on the dry powder inhalation performance of insulin-loaded plga microcapsules. *Powder Technol* 2010;201(3):289-95. doi:10.1016/j.powtec.2010.04.017
20. Hamishehkar H, Emami J, Najafabadi AR, Gilani K, Minaiyan M, Mahdavi H, et al. Effect of carrier morphology and surface characteristics on the development of respirable plga microcapsules for sustained-release pulmonary delivery of insulin. *Int J Pharm* 2010;389(1-2):74-85. doi: 10.1016/j.ijpharm.2010.01.021
21. Ghanbarzadeh S, Valizadeh H, Zakeri-Milani P. The effects of lyophilization on the physico-chemical stability of sirolimus liposomes. *Adv Pharm Bull* 2013;3(1):25-9. doi: 10.5681/apb.2013.005
22. Ghaderi S, Ghanbarzadeh S, Mohammadhassani Z, Hamishehkar H. Formulation of gammaoryzanol-loaded nanoparticles for potential application in fortifying food products. *Adv Pharm Bull* 2014;4(Suppl 2):549-54. doi: 10.5681/apb.2014.081
23. Hamishehkar H, Shokri J, Fallahi S, Jahangiri A, Ghanbarzadeh S, Kouhsoltani M. Histopathological evaluation of caffeine-loaded solid lipid nanoparticles in efficient treatment of cellulite. *Drug Dev Ind Pharm* 2015;41(10):1640-6. doi: 10.3109/03639045.2014.980426
24. United States Pharmacopeia 35/National Formulary 30. Rockville, MD, USA: United States Pharmacopeial Convention; 2015.
25. Yazdani A, Normandie M, Yousefi M, Saidi MS, Ahmadi G. Transport and deposition of pharmaceutical particles in three commercial spacer-mdi combinations. *Comput Biol Med* 2014;54:145-55. doi: 10.1016/j.compbiomed.2014.08.001
26. De Beule K. Itraconazole: Pharmacology, clinical experience and future development. *Int J Antimicrob Agents* 1996;6(3):175-81.
27. Alvarez CA, Wiederhold NP, McConville JT, Peters JI, Najvar LK, Graybill JR, et al. Aerosolized nanostructured itraconazole as prophylaxis against invasive pulmonary aspergillosis. *J Infect* 2007;55(1):68-74. doi: 10.1016/j.jinf.2007.01.014
28. McConville JT, Overhoff KA, Sinswat P, Vaughn JM, Frei BL, Burgess DS, et al. Targeted high lung concentrations of itraconazole using nebulized dispersions in a murine model. *Pharm Res* 2006;23(5):901-11. doi: 10.1007/s11095-006-9904-6
29. Vaughn JM, McConville JT, Burgess D, Peters JI, Johnston KP, Talbert RL, et al. Single dose and multiple dose studies of itraconazole nanoparticles. *Eur J Pharm Biopharm* 2006;63(2):95-102. doi: 10.1016/j.ejpb.2006.01.006
30. Joshi M, Misra A. Dry powder inhalation of liposomal ketotifen fumarate: Formulation and characterization. *Int J Pharm* 2001;223(1-2):15-27.
31. Duangjit S, Opanasopit P, Rojanarata T, Ngawhirunpat T. Characterization and in vitro skin permeation of meloxicam-loaded liposomes versus transfersomes. *J Drug Deliv* 2011;2011:418316. doi: 10.1155/2011/418316

32. Chougule M, Padhi B, Misra A. Nano-liposomal dry powder inhaler of tacrolimus: Preparation, characterization, and pulmonary pharmacokinetics. *Int J Nanomedicine* 2007;2(4):675-88.
33. Yang W, Tam J, Miller DA, Zhou J, McConville JT, Johnston KP, et al. High bioavailability from nebulized itraconazole nanoparticle dispersions with biocompatible stabilizers. *Int J Pharm* 2008;361(1-2):177-88. doi: 10.1016/j.ijpharm.2008.05.003
34. Newman SP, Clarke SW. Therapeutic aerosols 1--physical and practical considerations. *Thorax* 1983;38(12):881-6.
35. Rowe RC, Sheskey PJ, Owen SC, editors. Pharmaceutical Press and American Pharmacists Association. Handbook of pharmaceutical excipients. 4th ed. London: Pharmaceutical Press; 2006.

9

Formulation and Physicochemical Characterization of Lycopene-Loaded Solid Lipid Nanoparticles

Elham Nazemiyeh[1], **Morteza Eskandani**[2], **Hossein Sheikhloie**[1], **Hossein Nazemiyeh**[2,3]*

[1] *Department of Food Engineering, Maragheh Branch, Islamic Azad University, Maragheh, Iran.*
[2] *Research Center for Pharmaceutical Nanotechnology, Tabriz University of Medical Sciences, Tabriz, Iran.*
[3] *Faculty of Pharmacy, Tabriz University of Medical Sciences, Tabriz, Iran.*

Article info

Keywords:
· Lycopene
· Solid Lipid Nanoparticles (SLNs)
· Myristic acid
· Hot homogenization method
· Physicochemical characterization

Abstract
Purpose: Lycopene belongs to the carotenoids that shows good pharmacological properties including antioxidant, anti-inflammatory and anticancer. However, as a result of very low aqueous solubility, it has a limited systemic absorption, following oral administration.
Methods: Here, we prepared a stable lycopene-loaded solid lipid nanoparticles using Precirol® ATO5, Compritol 888 ATO and myristic acid by hot homogenization method with some modification. The size and morphological characteristics of nanoparticles were evaluated using Scanning Electron Microscopy (SEM). Moreover, zeta potential and dispersity index (DI) were measured using zeta sizer. In addition, encapsulation efficiency (EE%), drug loading (DL) and cumulative drug release were quantified.
Results: The results showed that the size and DI of particles was generally smaller in the case of SLNs prepared with precirol when compared to SLNs prepared with compritol. Scanning electron microscopy (SEM) and particle size analyses showed spherical SLNs (125 ± 3.89 nm), monodispersed distribution, and zeta potential of −10.06 ± 0.08 mV. High EE (98.4 ± 0.5 %) and DL (44.8 ± 0.46 mg/g) were achieved in the case of nanoparticles prepared by precirol. The stability study of the lycopene-SLNs in aqueous medium (4 °C) was showed that after 2 months there is no significant differences seen in size and DI compared with the fresh formulation.
Conclusion: Conclusively, in this investigation we prepared a stable lycopene-SLNs with good physicochemical characteristic which candidate it for the future *in vivo* trials in nutraceutical industries.

Introduction

With the increase of different incurable diseases, the nutraceutical scientist should pay more attention to man's feeding system. Lifestyle and nutrition can help preventing cancer. Carotenoids are common natural compounds in food booklet that play a significant role in the prevention of cancers. However, their low bioavailability due to their inadequate intestinal absorption and low solubility in the aqueous medium, and moreover chemical instability are important limiting factors in the food industry. Hence, there is urgent needs to develop new methods to increase their productivity and absorption as well. Carotenoids are fat-soluble pigments mostly appear in plants and microorganisms (algae and some bacteria) which have an essential role in photosynthesis.[1] In addition, the carotenoids play important pharmacological effects in animals including cells protection from free radicals,[2] coping with cancer cells and inhibition of the lipoxygenase activities,[3] and protection of fats against spontaneous oxidation.[4] In the food industry carotenoids are used widely in manufacturing of food products and soft/energy drinks as antioxidant, color and flavor modifier (especially bitter).[5] Due to the unsaturated structure of carotenoids, the compounds are susceptible to oxidative changes. Factors such as temperature, light and pH can also cause different changes in their color and nutritional value.[1] Recently, with the development of nanotechnology in food sciences and technology, investigators try to encapsulate these valuable resources in different nanoparticles to save their nutritional values, bioactivities and antioxidant properties as well as their stability and sustainability. The sparingly solubility of carotenoids hamper good intestinal absorption, thus reduce their bio-efficiency.

In the recent decade many attempts have been directed to overcome the solubility issues of carotenoids using their formulation in the lipid based nanoparticles e.g. liposomes,[6-9] micelle,[10-12] solid lipid nanoparticles[13] and nanostructured lipid carriers.[14,15] Solid lipid nanoparticles (SINs) are colloidal drug carrier with nanometer-sized, which contains the solid lipid matrix. SLNs consistent high biodegradability and biocompatibility and are good candidates as carriers for both hydrophilic and lipophilic compounds.[16] SLNs construction comprise a simple

***Corresponding author:** Hossein Nazemiye, Emails: nazemiyehh@tbzmed.ac.ir, nazemiyehh@yahoo.com

homogenization and solidification process that would allow successful scale up for industry.[17] In addition, compared with nanostructured lipid carriers (NLCs), SLNs display more controlled drug release effectiveness.[18] Altogether, SLNs possess different advantages in nutraceutical developments including high stability, protection of incorporated compound against chemical degradation,[19] biocompatibility of the carrier,[20] and avoidance of organic solvent during formulation.[21] Bioactive compounds in the solid core of SLNs have mobility limitation and speed of their distribution to the particle surface are lower than other nano-emulsions.[22] These features of SLNs make them suitable for the decrease of decomposition reactions such as oxidation of bioactive compounds e.g carotenoids. Different procedures are used for the preparation of SLNs including hot/cold homogenization, high pressure homogenization (HPH), ultrasonification, and emulsification and solvent evaporation method. Almost in all methods, emulsions are prepared in the first step, and then by mechanical means large droplets are break down into smaller particles.

In this investigation we tried to develop an enhanced lycopene loaded solid lipid nanoparticles (lycopene-SLNs) using simple hot homogenization method with some modification. Although in 2012 Riangjanapatee et al formulated lycopene-NLC and evaluated the surfactant type effects on the stability of the formulation,[23] to the best of our knowledge this investigation is a pioneering attempt in the formulation of lycopene in solid lipid nanoparticles composed of Precirol ® ATO 5 and Compritol 888 ATO as a lipid matrix to improve the pharmacokinetic behavior. Moreover, to enhance zeta potential of the formulated nanoparticles, to obtain a stable formulation, myristic acid was used during all formulation. Anionic lycopene-SLNs were physicochemically and morphologically characterized by means of zetaseizer and scanning electron microscopy (SEM). Moreover, we evaluated different physicochemical characterization including encapsulation efficiency (EE%), drug loading (DL) and stability.

Materials and Methods

Chemicals and reagents

All Chemical substances and compounds used in this investigation were pharmaceutical grade. Precirol® ATO5 and Compritol 888 ATO was gifted from Gattefosse (Nanterre, France). Tween 80, poloxamer 407 and myristic acid were purchased from Sigma-Aldrich (Poole, UK). All solvents used in this study were extra pure and purchased from Merck Co (Darmstadt, Germany).

Lycopene resources and extraction

Tomatoes needed to extract lycopene were purchased from a local market and after washing were air dried under the shade. Dried and ground tomatoes were extracted using petroleum ether aiding laboratory mixers for at least 30 minutes. After then the extract was filtrate using paper filter and solvent was removed *in vacuo* by rotary evaporator at maximum temperature of 40°C. The lycopene content of the extract was isolated using antisolvent precipitation method. For this, the crude extract was dissolved in ethyl acetate. Then methanol was added dropwise to the extract solution to completely precipitate lycopene. The sediment was dissolved in ethyl acetate and precipitation was repeated once again. Finally, the tartar was filtrate and remaining solvent was evaporated by a flow of nitrogen gas. Eventually dried red sediments were used for the production of solid lipid nanoparticles.

Preparation of Lycopene loaded solid lipid nanoparticles

Lycopene-SLNs were prepared by the hot homogenization method according to our previous work with some modification.[20] Briefly, lipid phase including lycopene and solid lipid (glyceryl palmitostearate (Precirol® ATO 5) or glyceryl behenate (Compritol® 888 ATO) was simply dispersed by unintended heating at ~10 °C above the lipids melting point. Moreover, myristic acid (< 0.5 % w/w) was added to the lipid phase as zeta enhancer. To prepared aqueous phase, an appropriate concentration of stabilizers (Poloxamer 407) was heated to the same temperature of the oil phase in distilled water. Then the hot aqueous phase was dropped to the oil phase during 30 minutes and homogenization (12 000 rpm and 70 °C). In the next step, the obtained emulsion was further homogenized (at 19 000 rpm) for additional 10 min. Lycopene-SLNs were finally obtained by allowing the hot nanoemulsion to cool down at room temperature, and then were stored at 4 °C. Blank SLNs also were prepared by the same method except instead of lycopene, an equal amount of precirol or compritol was used.

Size, zeta potential, and morphological characteristics of nanoparticles

Getting an appropriate system for lycopene nanoparticles (NPs) preparation, the size of the prepared NPs was measured immediately after fabrication by laser diffraction immediately after preparation (SALD-MS30, Schimadzu, USA). In this context, SLNs was diluted by distilled water to reach appropriate concentration. Moreover, particle size distribution [mean diameter and dispersity index (DI)] and zeta potential of suitable formulation system was determined in pH 8.3 using Malvern zetasizer (3000HS, Malvern Instruments, UK) in the final concentration which recommended by the manufacturer of the instrument. The morphology of the fabricated NPs was observed with Scanning Electron Microscopy (SEM) based on our previous published method.[16,21]

Encapsulation efficiency (%) and drug loading

The entrapment efficiency (EE) of the NPs were determined as the percentage of lycopene entrapped in the carriers compared to the total dug which was used for the formulation. For the measurement of the (EE), original suspension containing lycopene-SLNs and 0.3% tween 80 was placed in Ultra free tube with a cutoff of 10,000 Da (Ultrafree, MC Millipore, Bedford, USA) and centrifuged for 8 min at 14,000g (3K30, SIGMA Labrorzentrifugen GmbH, Germany). The filtrate was mixed by hexane (1:1) and hanged for at least 10 min and then the hydrophobe phase was separated by a separatory funnel and the quantity of free lycopene was determined using spectrophotometric method (λ max: 471 nm in hexane). To gain a calibration curve, working standard solutions were prepared by serially dilution with hexane. The stock solutions were prepared by dissolving pure lycopene in hexane at the concentrations of 6000 µg/mL. Each calibration curve consisted of 6 calibration points (600, 300, 100, 80, 40 and 20 µg/mL). Calibration curve was plotted by least square linear regression analysis. The drug EE in the SLNs was calculated from Eq. (1) and drug loading (DL) was obtained from Eq. (2).

$$\% \text{ Entrapment efficiency} = \frac{(total\ amount\ of\ lycopen\ taken) - (un-entraped\ lycopen)}{concentration\ of\ drug\ initially\ taken} \times 100 \qquad \text{Eq. (1)}$$

$$\text{Drug loading (mg/g)} = \frac{W_{LL}}{W_{Np}} \qquad \text{Eq. (2)}$$

where W_{LL} is the weight of lycopene loaded in nanoparticles and W_{NP} is the weight of nanoparticles solid mass.

In vitro release studies

Cumulative *in vitro* release of lycopene-SLNs was carried out based on dialysis method. Regarding to this, 1 mL of lycopene-SLNs was charged into dialysis bag (molecular weight cutoff: 12 kDa). The bag was then inserted in a glass holder containing 10 mL of dialysis buffer (0.3% W/V tween 80 in DW).[20] Moreover, intact lycopene also was dialyzed similarly to evaluate the permeability of lycopene to the membrane. During dialysis the media was continuously stirred at RT and 100 rpm and at the fixed time periods, 1 mL of medium was removed and 1 mL of fresh media was added to the receptacle. Drug concentration was determined by the spectrophotometric method mentioned earlier.

Physical stability studies

To evaluate the stability of the formulated SLNs, samples were stored for 2 months at a glass tube at refrigerator (4 °C). Then mean diameter, DI and EE were measured and compared with the fresh ones.[20]

Statistical analyses

All data represent the mean of at least three repeated experiments (error bars represent mean ± standard deviation). Independent Student's *t-test* was utilized to compare mean differences between two independent groups and one-way ANOVA was used to multiple comparisons. Post hoc pairwise comparisons were carried out using Tukey multiple comparison tests for those that showed significant mean differences (SPSS; version 13.0). We used Shapiro–Wilk test to compare the shape of sample distribution with the shape of a normal curve. The statistical significance was defined as $p<0.05$.

Results and Discussion

Preparation and physicochemical characterization of Lycopene-SLNs

SLNs of lycopene was developed by hot homogenization method without using of organic solvents by means of different solid lipids including Precirol® ATO 5 and Compritol® 888 ATO. The SLNs were stabilized using a surfactant, i.e. Tween 80 and Poloxamer 407. Moreover, myristic acid was used to enhance the zeta quantity of the particles surface. It is well known that the carbonyl carbon of the organic acid such as myristic acid is directly linked to, and in conjugation with, a second electronegative oxygen atom bearing a hydrogen atom. This electronic arrangement allows for loss of a proton and ionization because electron density is "pulled" from the hydroxyl hydrogen through the conjugated carboxyl group, and the negative charge formed upon ionization (in the conjugate base) is stabilized by resonance delocalization.[24]

The method and composition of the SLNs were optimized, and they were further considered in terms of total DL, EE, particle size, zeta potential, morphology, and stability studies. The characteristics of some formulated lycopene-SLNs and blank SLNs in this investigation are listed in Table 1. Our results showed that the size and DI was generally smaller in the case of SLNs prepared with precirol when compared to SLNs prepared with compritol (Table 1).

Particle size and morphology

The average size of the particles and their shapes may affect the drug release pattern, entrapment efficiency, cytotoxicity and pharmacokinetic behavior.[25] The results here showed that the size of the nanoparticles was generally in direct relation with the oil phase surfactant concentration. Clearly seen that nanoparticle size is reduced by increasing the amount of oil phase surfactant. However, our previous results showed that with the increase of tween 80 the cytotoxicity of NPs will increase.[16] Moreover, there is an obvious decrease of nanoparticle size with an increase of homogenizing duration time and speed (data not shown). Of the different formulation, F2 (blank SLNs) and F7 (lycopene-SLNs) at 25 °C exhibited mono dispersed characteristics with a mean diameter of 124 ± 5.24 nm and 125 ± 3.89 nm. Besides, F2 and F7 showed acceptable DI of 0.382 ± 0.142 and 0.253 ± 0.105, respectively. The DI values indicated a narrow particle size distribution. These results were approved more by Scanning Electron Microscopy (SEM) images (Figure 1). Moreover, SEM showed spherical and uniform SLNs. Zeta potential as important criteria can predict the particles long-term stability.

Table 1. Composition, particle size, and encapsulation efficiency (EE) of lycopene-loaded SLNs and blank SLNs formulation.

Formulation No	Lipid type and concentration (g)	Lycopene concentration (g)	Oil phase surfactant concentration[a] (g)	Aqueous phase surfactant concentration [b] (g)	Particle size(nm)	Dispersity index (DI)	Encapsulation Efficiency (EE%)	Drug Loading (DL,mg/g)
Blank SLNs	-	-	-	-	-	-	-	-
F1	Precirol (0.55)	-	0.01	0.52	153 ± 6.13	0.658 ± 0.131	-	-
F2	**Precirol (0.75)**	-	**0.05**	**0.65**	**124 ± 5.24**	**0.382 ± 0.142**	-	-
F3	Compritol (0.55)	-	0.07	0.55	162 ± 4.24	0.832 ± 0.121	-	-
F4	Compritol (0.75)	-	0.10	0.62	139 ± 3.13	0.927 ± 0.128	-	-
Lycopene-SLNs	-	-	-	-	-	-	-	-
F5	Precirol (0.59)	0.053	0.01	0.48	162 ± 7.01	0.444 ± 0.109	94 ± 0.2	51.8 ± 0.45
F6	Precirol (0.62)	0.049	0.06	0.55	155 ± 5.34	0.502 ± 0.151	96.7 ± 0.4	46.7 ± 0.39
F7	**Precirol (0.65)**	**0.052**	**0.09**	**0.69**	**125 ± 3.89**	**0.159 ± 0.105**	**98.4 ± 0.5**	**44.8 ± 0.46**
F8	Compritol (0.60)	0.048	0.01	0.44	166 ± 1.83	0.177 ± 0.221	86.6 ± 0.6	49.5 ± 0.63
F9	Compritol (0.67)	0.049	0.06	0.53	143 ± 3.89	0.253 ± 0.105	89.5 ± 0.3	47.6 ± 0.29
F10	Compritol (0.73)	0.054	0.09	0.71	129 ± 1.83	0.177 ± 0.221	93.1 ± 0.6	44.4 ± 0.33

Data are expressed as mean ± SD (n=3).
a: Tween 80 and *b:* Poloxamer 407 was used as the oil phase and aqueous phase surfactant in all formulations, respectively. 0.3% (w/w) myristic acid also was used in all formulation.

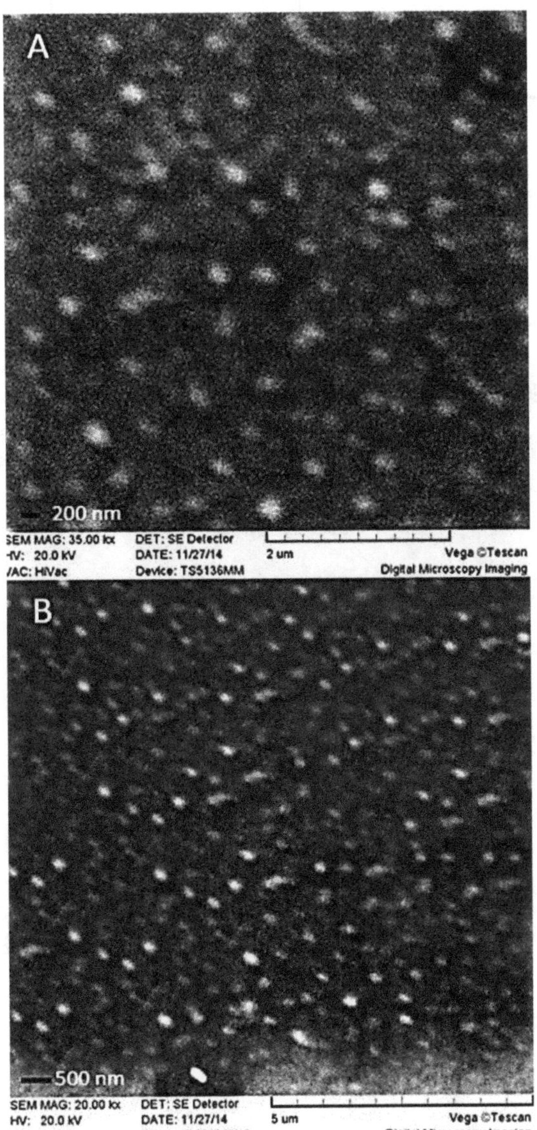

Figure 1. (A) SEM images of blank-SLNs (F2) and (B) lycopene-loaded SLNs (F7)

The zeta potential of higher than −60 mV for a colloidal dispersion forecast physically stable condition for the particles of the dispersion.[26] In this investigation, at pH of distilled water (8.3), zeta potential of the selected formulation, F2 and F7, were -14.21 ± 1.14 and -10.08 ± 2.06, respectively (Figure 2).

In vitro release studies

In this study the cumulative drug release was assessed using dialysis method. Figure 3 shows the release profile of lycopene-SLNs in DW containing 0.05% (W/V) tween 80 as co-solubilizer. The release profile showed that lycopene-SLNs exhibited no burst drug release and less than 30% of lycopene was released after 72 h. This type of sustained release profile of sparingly water soluble drug was also reported by others.[20, 27] It is may be mainly referring to the low diffusion of the drug from the lipid matrix of SLNs into aqueous media. However, as seen in Figure 3 approximately 23% of lycopene drug release was occurred in the first 24 h. This release may be attributed to those drugs which is located around the surface of the SLNs. Thought, all intact lycopene (>95%) was released to the media in the first 24 h which gives us confidence that lycopene could penetrate into the cellulose pores.

Physical stability studies

Of different formulations, the most suitable one – the formulation composed of 3.5% (w/w) lycopene, a surfactant consisting of 6.07% tween 80 and 46.55% poloxamer 407 in a solid lipid matrix of 43.85% precirol – was placed on long-term stability at 4 °C for 3 months. After three months, the NPs was checked for any potential aggregation, and SLNs were evaluated in terms of size, DI, and EE. Stability studies showed that in the usual dispersed aqueous medium (distilled water), coacervation and precipitation of lipid did not occur. The result of the stability studies showed that after three months storage of formulation at 4 °C, the mean diameter, entrapment efficiency and DI of lycopene-SLNs displayed no significant differences, as compared with the fresh preparation ($p > 0.05$) (Table 2).

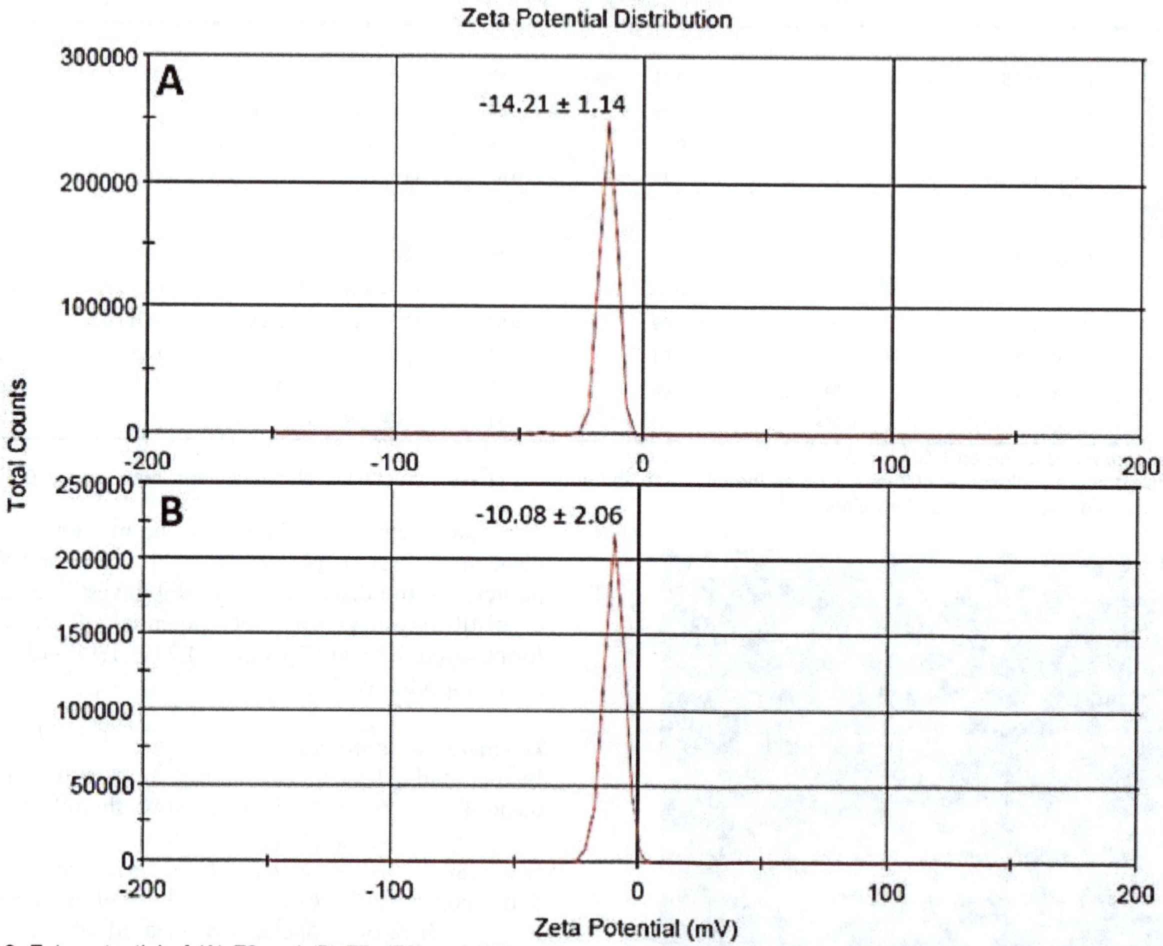

Figure 2. Zeta potential of (A) F2 and (B) F7. (F2) and (F7) represent the formulation code of 2 and 7 for blank SLNs and lycopene-SLNs, respectively.

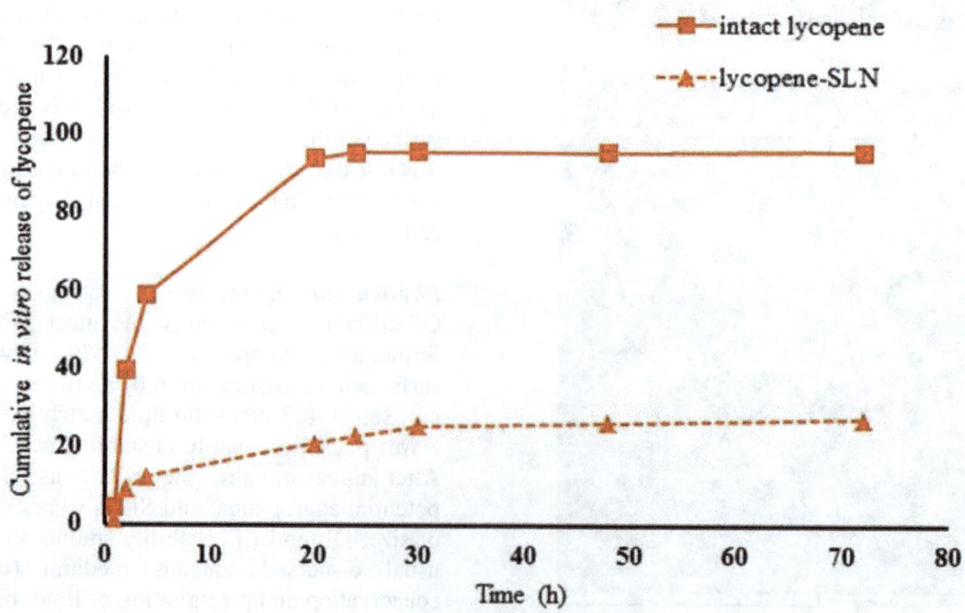

Figure 3. Cumulative release of lycopene. The release of intact lycopene was assessed in a same condition to evaluate the perme ability of the plain drug through the membrane

Table 2. Stability study of lycopene-SLNs. Data are presented here as mean ± SD (n=3).

Formulation	Mean diameter (nm)	Dispersity index	Entrapment efficiency (EE%)	Drug leakage
Blank SLNs	133 ± 3.78	0.146 ± 0.04	-	-
Fresh lycopene-SLNs (F7)	125 ± 3.89	0.159 ± 0.105	98.4±0.5	-
Lycopene-SLNs (F7) in 4 °C after 3 months	128 ± 7.52	0.173 ± 0.05	88.7 ± 0.19	9.7%

Conclusion

Here solid lipid nanoparticle containing lycopene successfully fabricated using simple hot homogenization procedure. Lycopene nanoparticles showed good physicochemical characterization in terms of good stability during storage times. The obtained small size of nanoparticles (110 to 130 nm) is hopeful characteristic to candidate lycopene-SLNs formulation to orally usage. There is enough observation revealed that the intestinal absorption of lycopene-SLNs formulated here will be good. Encapsulation efficiency of lycopene-SLNs stored for at least three months showed that an ignorable leakage is occurred in 4 °C. Finally, this investigation could be a pioneer study to propose that using of these types of carotenoid-SLNs (nano-nutraceutical) in the manufacturing of different beverages and dairy products as food supplementary materials.

Acknowledgments

The authors wish to thank Research Center for Pharmaceutical Nanotechnology (RCPN) for their technical and financial support.

Conflict of Interest

Authors declare no conflict of interest in this study.

References

1. Rao AV, Rao LG. Carotenoids and human health. *Pharmacol Res* 2007;55(3):207-16. doi: 10.1016/j.phrs.2007.01.012
2. Su Q, Rowley KG, Balazs ND. Carotenoids: Separation methods applicable to biological samples. *J Chromatogr B Analyt Technol Biomed Life Sci* 2002;781(1-2):393-418.
3. Nishino H, Tokuda H, Murakoshi M, Satomi Y, Masuda M, Onozuka M, et al. Cancer prevention by natural carotenoids. *BioFactors* 2000;13(1-4):89-94.
4. Timmons JS, Weiss WP, Palmquist DL, Harper WJ. Relationships among dietary roasted soybeans, milk components, and spontaneous oxidized flavor of milk. *J Dairy Sci* 2001;84(11):2440-9. doi: 10.3168/jds.S0022-0302(01)74694-2
5. Jaswir I, Noviendri D, Hasrini RF, Octavianti F. Carotenoids: Sources, medicinal properties and their application in food and nutraceutical industry. *J Med Plants Res* 2011; 5(33): 7119-31. doi: 10.5897/JMPRX11.011
6. Jiang J, Yu Z, Qiu Q, Wu Y. protective effects of beta-carotene liposome against rat neutrophile membrane damage caused by intra- or extra-cellular reactive oxygen species. *Zhongguo Yi Xue Ke Xue Yuan Xue Bao* 1996;18(5):387-91.
7. Tan C, Feng B, Zhang X, Xia W, Xia S. Biopolymer-coated liposomes by electrostatic adsorption of chitosan (chitosomes) as novel delivery systems for carotenoids. *Food Hydrocolloid* 2016;52:774-84. doi:10.1016/j.foodhyd.2015.08.016
8. Tan C, Zhang Y, Abbas S, Feng B, Zhang X, Xia S. Modulation of the carotenoid bioaccessibility through liposomal encapsulation. *Colloids Surf B Biointerfaces* 2014;123:692-700. doi: 10.1016/j.colsurfb.2014.10.011
9. Toniazzo T, Berbel IF, Cho S, Fávaro-Trindade CS, Moraes ICF, Pinho SC. β-carotene-loaded liposome dispersions stabilized with xanthan and guar gums: Physico-chemical stability and feasibility of application in yogurt. *LWT Food Sci Technol* 2014;59(2):1265-73. doi:10.1016/j.lwt.2014.05.021
10. Kotake-Nara E, Nagao A. Effects of mixed micellar lipids on carotenoid uptake by human intestinal caco-2 cells. *Biosci Biotechnol Biochem* 2012;76(5):875-82. doi: 10.1271/bbb.110777
11. White DA, Ornsrud R, Davies SJ. Determination of carotenoid and vitamin a concentrations in everted salmonid intestine following exposure to solutions of carotenoid in vitro. *Comp Biochem Physiol A Mol Integr Physiol* 2003;136(3):683-92.
12. Chen YJ, Inbaraj BS, Pu YS, Chen BH. Development of lycopene micelle and lycopene chylomicron and a comparison of bioavailability. *Nanotechnology* 2014;25(15):155102. doi: 10.1088/0957-4484/25/15/155102
13. Gomes GVdL, Borrin TR, Cardoso LP, Souto E, Pinho SCd. Characterization and shelf life of ²-carotene loaded solid lipid microparticles produced with stearic acid and sunflower oil. *Braz Arch Biol Techn* 2013;56(4):663-71.
14. Hejri A, Khosravi A, Gharanjig K, Hejazi M. Optimisation of the formulation of beta-carotene loaded nanostructured lipid carriers prepared by solvent diffusion method. *Food Chem* 2013;141(1):117-23. doi: 10.1016/j.foodchem.2013.02.080
15. Riangjanapatee P, Muller RH, Keck CM, Okonogi S. Development of lycopene-loaded nanostructured lipid

carriers: Effect of rice oil and cholesterol. *Pharmazie* 2013;68(9):723-31.

16. Eskandani M, Barar J, Dolatabadi JE, Hamishehkar H, Nazemiyeh H. Formulation, characterization, and geno/cytotoxicity studies of galbanic acid-loaded solid lipid nanoparticles. *Pharm Biol* 2015;53(10):1525-38. doi: 10.3109/13880209.2014.991836
17. Muller RH, Shegokar R, Keck CM. 20 years of lipid nanoparticles (sln and nlc): Present state of development and industrial applications. *Curr Drug Discov Technol* 2011;8(3):207-27.
18. Das S, Ng WK, Tan RB. Are nanostructured lipid carriers (nlcs) better than solid lipid nanoparticles (slns): Development, characterizations and comparative evaluations of clotrimazole-loaded slns and nlcs? *Eur J Pharm Sci* 2012;47(1):139-51. doi: 10.1016/j.ejps.2012.05.010
19. Fathi M, Mozafari MR, Mohebbi M. Nanoencapsulation of food ingredients using lipid based delivery systems. *Trends Food Sci Tech* 2012;23(1):13-27.
20. Eskandani M, Nazemiyeh H. Self-reporter shikonin-act-loaded solid lipid nanoparticle: Formulation, physicochemical characterization and geno/cytotoxicity evaluation. *Eur J Pharm Sci* 2014;59:49-57. doi: 10.1016/j.ejps.2014.04.009
21. Ezzati Nazhad Dolatabadi J, Hamishehkar H, Eskandani M, Valizadeh H. Formulation, characterization and cytotoxicity studies of alendronate sodium-loaded solid lipid nanoparticles. *Colloids Surf B Biointerfaces* 2014;117:21-8. doi: 10.1016/j.colsurfb.2014.01.055
22. Rao J, McClements DJ. Optimization of lipid nanoparticle formation for beverage applications: Influence of oil type, cosolvents, and cosurfactants on nanoemulsion properties. *J Food Eng* 2013;118(2):198-204. doi:10.1016/j.jfoodeng.2013.04.010
23. Riangjanapatee P, Okonogi S. Effect of surfactant on lycopene-loaded nanostructured lipid carriers. *Drug Discov Ther* 2012;6(3):163-8.
24. B. Pratt W, Taylor P. Principles of Drug Action: The Basis of Pharmacology. 3, illustrated ed. Michigan: Churchill Livingstone; 1990.
25. Muller RH, Mader K, Gohla S. Solid lipid nanoparticles (sln) for controlled drug delivery - a review of the state of the art. *Eur J Pharm Biopharm* 2000;50(1):161-77.
26. Freitas C, Müller RH. Effect of light and temperature on zeta potential and physical stability in solid lipid nanoparticle (SLN™) dispersions. *Int J Pharmaceut* 1998;168(2):221-9. doi:10.1016/S0378-5173(98)00092-1
27. Das S, Ng WK, Kanaujia P, Kim S, Tan RB. Formulation design, preparation and physicochemical characterizations of solid lipid nanoparticles containing a hydrophobic drug: Effects of process variables. *Colloids Surf B Biointerfaces* 2011;88(1):483-9. doi: 10.1016/j.colsurfb.2011.07.036

The Relation Between Thermodynamic and Structural Properties and Cellular Uptake of Peptides Containing Tryptophan and Arginine

Ali Shirani[1], Javid Shahbazi Mojarrad[2], Samad Mussa Farkhani[1], Ahmad Yari Khosroshahi[2], Parvin Zakeri-Milani[3], Naser Samadi[4], Simin Sharifi[5], Samaneh Mohammadi[1], Hadi Valizadeh[5]*

[1] *Research Center for Pharmaceutical Nanotechnology and Department of Medical Nanotechnology, Faculty of Advanced Medical Sciences, Tabriz University of Medical Sciences, Tabriz, Iran.*
[2] *Biotechnology Research Center and Faculty of Pharmacy, Tabriz University of Medical Sciences, Tabriz, Iran.*
[3] *Liver and Gastrointestinal Diseases Research Center and Faculty of Pharmacy, Tabriz University of Medical Sciences, Tabriz, Iran.*
[4] *Faculty of Advanced Medical Sciences, Tabriz University of Medical Sciences, Tabriz, Iran.*
[5] *Drug Applied Research Center and Faculty of Pharmacy, Tabriz University of Medical Sciences, Tabriz, Iran.*

Article info

Keywords:
- Cell-penetrating peptides (CPPs)
- Wimley-White scale
- GOR (Garnier-Osguthorpe-Robson) V method
- Model amphipathic peptide (MAP)

Abstract

Purpose: Cell-penetrating peptides (CPPs) are used for delivering drugs and other macromolecular cargo into living cells. In this paper, we investigated the relationship between the structural/physicochemical properties of four new synthetic peptides containing arginine-tryptophan in terms of their cell membrane penetration efficiency.
Methods: The peptides were prepared using solid phase synthesis procedure using FMOC protected amino acids. Fluorescence-activated cell sorting and fluorescence imaging were used to evaluate uptake efficiency. Prediction of the peptide secondary structure and estimation of physicochemical properties was performed using the GOR V method and MPEx 3.2 software (Wimley-White scale, helical wheel projection and total hydrophobic moment).
Results: Our data showed that the uptake efficiency of peptides with two tryptophans at the C- and N-terminus were significantly higher (about 4-fold) than that of peptides containing three tryptophans at both ends. The distribution of arginine at both ends also increased the uptake efficiency 2.52- and 7.18-fold, compared with arginine distribution at the middle of peptides.
Conclusion: According to the obtained results the value of transfer free energies of peptides from the aqueous phase to membrane bilayer could be a good predictor for the cellular uptake efficiency of CPPs.

Introduction

Transfer of cargos across cellular membranes is a major issue in cell biology and medicine. During the past few decades, significant progress has been made in focusing on the manufacture of new carriers for cargo delivery into cells. Cell-penetrating peptides or protein transduction domains (PTDs)[1] are new carriers that have been widely used to promote the uptake of various macromolecules. CPPs have been shown to efficiently improve transportation of PMO (phosphorodiamidate morpholinos),[2] PNA (peptide nucleic acids),[3] DNA,[4] siRNA (short interfering RNA),[5] drug,[6] and nanoparticles[7] across biological membranes. Recently several classes of CPPs have been introduced. Model amphipathic peptides (MAP) are one of the most common classes of CPPs that have been used in scientific research.[8] Amphipathic peptides contain hydrophobic and cationic residues in the backbone, this class of peptides have the ability to enter cells and can have antimicrobial properties.[9]

A group of amphipathic peptides containing tryptophan and arginine residue have been widely used as CPP for delivery of various drug and biological compounds.[10-12] Tryptophan has an aromatic side chain[13] and can participate in hydrophobic interactions to the lipid hydrocarbon chains of the cell membrane.[14] Arginine is a hydrophilic and basic amino acid;[15] the guanidino groups of arginine tend to bind with phosphate in the cell membrane lipids.[16] In this study, four amphipathic peptides containing tryptophan and arginine (RRWWWWRR, RRRWWWWRRR, WWRRRRWW and WWWRRRRWWW) were designed and synthesized in order to explore the relationships between the structural/physicochemical properties and penetration into the MCF-7 cells.

Materials and Methods

Materials

Fmoc–Trp (Boc) -OH, Rink amid AM and Fmoc-Arg (Pbf) -OH were purchased from AAPPTec (Louisville, KY, USA). N,N-Diisopropylethylamine (DIPEA) was obtained from Fluka (Buchs, Switzerland). O-(benzotriazol-1-yl)-N,N,N′,N′-tetramethyluronium tetrafluoroborate (TBTU) and triisopropylsilane (TIS) purchased from Sigma–Aldrich

***Corresponding author:** Hadi Valizadeh, Email: valizadeh@tbzmed.ac.ir

(St. Louis, MO, USA). 1,2-ethanedithiol (EDT), Trifluoroacetic acid (TFA) and other reagents were purchased from Merck (Darmstadt, Germany).

Peptide synthesis

The synthesis of peptides was carried out manually with Rink amide resin using the solid-phase synthesis method. O-(benzotriazol-1-yl)-N,N,N′,N′-tetramethyluronium tetrafluoroborate (TBTU) and N,N-diisopropylethylamine (DIPEA) in dimethylformamide (DMF) were used as coupling and activating reagents, respectively. Fmoc protecting group was removed from the resin and amino acids by addition of a solution of 20% (v/v) Piperidine/DMF. The Kaiser test was performed to monitor deprotection of peptides in solid phase peptide synthesis. A cleavage cocktail (TFA/H_2O/TIS/EDT: 94 /2.5 /2.5 /1) was used for side-chain deprotection and the final cleavage of the peptide from the Rink amide resin. Crude peptides were precipitated by cold diethyl ether under vigorous stirring. The peptides containing the cleavage cocktail and Et_2O were centrifuged at 4000 rpm for three minutes, followed by decantation in order to obtain the solid peptide precipitate.[17,18]

FITC Labeling of Peptides

A solution of 1.1 equivalent of FITC in pyridine/DMF/DCM (12:7:5) was prepared and incubated with the deprotected peptide for 12 h under gentle mixing conditions.[19] The completion of the reaction was confirmed by the Kaiser test. The obtained FITC-peptide was cleaved from resin with the cleavage cocktail and was precipitated by diethyl ether.

Cell Culture

The human breast cancer cell line MCF-7 was purchased from the Pasteur Institute (Tehran, Iran). The cells were grown on 25 cm^2 cell culture flasks with RPMI-1640 medium with 10% fetal bovine serum (Invitrogen, Carlsbad, CA, USA), sodium pyruvate (1 mM), penicillinG100 U/ml and streptomycin 100 μg/ml (AppliChem, Darmstadt, Germany) in a humidified atmosphere of 5% CO_2, 95% air at 37 °C.

Cytotoxicity analysis

The Mcf-7 cells were seeded in 200 μL of medium per well in 96-well plates 24 h prior to the experiment. The old medium was replaced by different concentrations of peptides synthesized in serum containing medium and plates incubated for 24–72 h at 37°C in a humidified atmosphere of 5% CO2. Cell viability was then determined by measuring the color intensity of the formazan solution at 570nm using an ELISA reader (Bioteck Instruments, Wmooski, VT, USA).

The percentage of inhibition of proliferation was calculated as follows:

$$\text{Inhibition of proliferation \%} = 100 \times \frac{\text{OD570(cells treated with peptide)} - \text{OD570(medium control)}}{\text{OD570(cells control)} - \text{OD570(medium control)}}$$

Fluorescent microscopy

The human breast cancer cell line MCF-7 was cultured in 6-well plates (200×10^3 cells/well) for 24 h in an incubator at 37°C in a 5% CO_2 environment. The Cells were treated with 15 μM concentration of R2W4R2-FITC, $W_2R_4W_2$- FITC, $W_3R_4W_3$-FITC and $R_3W_4R_3$-FITC. After 1 h incubation at 37 °C, the medium containing the peptide was removed. The cells were washed with PBS and examined with an emission filter of 530 nm BP (green emission) using an Olympus IX81 fluorescence microscope (Olympus Optical Co., Ltd., Tokyo, Japan).

Flow cytometry assay

Flow cytometry was used to determine the percentage of labelled cells and compared with control cells. MCF-7 cells were treated with 5 μM, 15 μM and 25 μM concentration of peptides in separate experiments for 1 h at 37°C and the cells were washed twice with phosphate buffered saline. However, because flow cytometry does not discriminate between cell membrane-bound and internalized FITC-peptides, the cells were treated with trypsin/EDTA (0.25% trypsin and 0.02% EDTA for 5 min) to minimize any contribution of peptides attached to the outer surface of the cell membrane.[20] Mean fluorescence ratios were determined for 10,000 cells sampled after the addition of peptides. Fluorescence ratios were calculated in arbitrary units set to a value of 100 for MCF-7 cells. The results were expressed as a percentage of gated populations and data were analysed using control cells. Flow cytometry was carried out using FACSCalibur (Becton Dickinson, San Jose, CA, USA) applying an argon laser. Excitation occurred at 488 nm for FITC.

***Peptide* secondary structure**

Structure prediction of synthesized peptides was performed to determine their secondary structure. We applied the GOR V algorithm in order to explain the different levels of uptake by MCF-7 cells. This method has high accuracy (Q3=73.5%) with a wide range of amino acid residues for predicting the secondary structures of peptides.[21] It is based on the use of information theory and Bayesian statistics for predicting the secondary structure of peptides and proteins,[22] by analysis and comparison of an input sequence with 513 proteins, to calculate the helix, sheet and coil probabilities at each residue position.[23] The GOR V server uses the FASTA sequence format and calculates the probability helix (α-helix), extended (β-sheet) and coil structures. The probabilities are then normalized to 0 and 1 using the following equation:[23,24]

$$P_H+P_E+P_C=1$$

The GOR V server is available online at http://gor.bb.iastate.edu (the Plant Sciences Institute at Iowa State University).

Helical wheel projection and thermodynamic parameters

Helical wheel projection illustrates the correct angular displacement from one amino acid to another amino acid in a cylindrical plot of the α-helix structure.[25] The Wimley-White is one of the most common scales that can be used for free energy calculation of peptides. This value is provided by the free-energy contributions of the side chains and backbone of peptides.[26] The free energy of peptides may be used to ascertain the feasibility of peptide transport across the cell membrane. Helical wheel projection, estimation of the transfer free energy and the total hydrophobic moment of peptides were performed by Membrane Protein Explorer (MPEx 3.2), free software provided by the Stephen White Laboratory at the University of California (Irvine, CA).

Results and Discussion

Cytotoxicity in cell culture

The cell viability of the human breast cancer cell line MCF-7 are summarized in Figure 1. Compared to control, the cells underwent reduced proliferation following treatment with $R_2W_4R_2$. All of the peptides had cytotoxic effects at concentrations of 25μM and 50 μM, following a 72- hour incubation period. The cell toxicity was dose and time dependent.

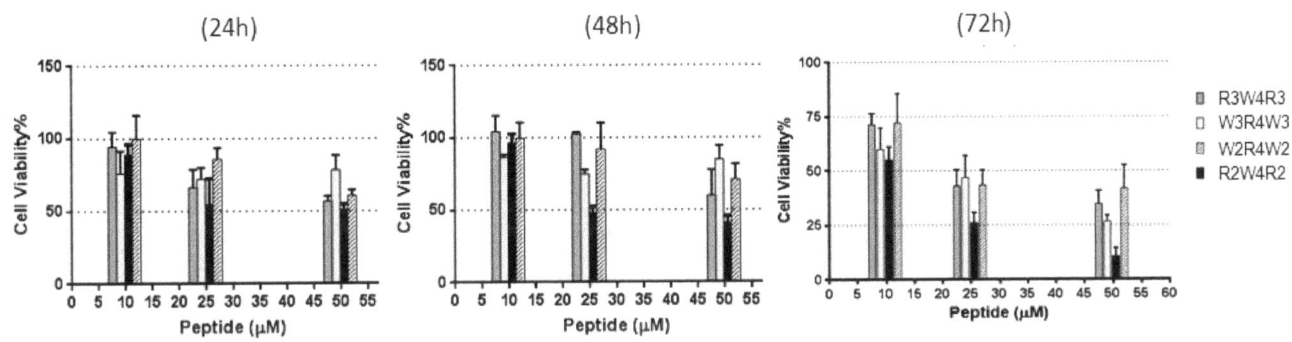

Figure 1. Cytotoxic effects of $R_3W_4R_3$, $R_2W_4R_2$, $W_3R_4W_3$, $W_2R_4W_2$. The peptides were incubated with 10^4 cells in 5, 25, and 50 μM concentrations for 24 h, 48h, and 72h. Each value is the mean ± SD of three separate determinations

Cellular Uptake and labeling

Increasing the concentration of all peptides resulted in an increased population of FITC-labelled cells (Figure 2). This effect was relatively linear in the concentration range of 5, 15 and 25μM of the peptides. The major difference was observed when comparing the two peptides containing four and six tryptophans at both ends. Accumulation of both $R_2W_4R_2$ and $R_3W_4R_3$ in MCF-7 was suitable. However the mean cellular uptake of $W_2R_4W_2$ and $W_3R_4W_3$ in 15μM concentrations of peptides was 2.52 and 7.18-fold less than that of $R_3W_4R_3$ respectively. According to the results, there was no significant difference between penetration of $R_2W_4R_2$ and $R_3W_4R_3$ sequences. It therefore appears that the location of tryptophan and arginine residues have a dramatic effect on cellular uptake. It seems that the number of tryptophan residues in $W_2R_4W_2$ and $W_3R_4W_3$ sequences affects the cellular uptake (Figure 2 and 3).

Secondary structure prediction

The results of prediction of secondary structure and the graphical model are shown in Table 1. According to the results, for $W_2R_4W_2$ sequence, coil structure is dominant with no α-helix structure. However, in other sequences, a high probability of α-helix formation was indicated. The amphipathic α-helical is important for the effective transportation of peptides across bilayer lipid membranes. It has been suggested that this structure leads to pore formation followed by peptide insertion into the cell membrane.[27] No relevance between the α-helix structure and cellular uptake of $W_2R_4W_2$ and $W_3R_4W_3$ sequences was observed.

Helical wheel* projection and *total hydrophobic moment

It has been suggested that the cellular uptake efficiency of peptide is dependent on the regular arrangement of hydrophobic and hydrophilic amino acid residues in one side of the helical wheel projection.[11,28] The helical wheel projection for $R_2W_4R_2$, $R_3W_4R_3$ and $W_3R_4W_3$ sequences are shown in (Figure 4). According to this projection, these peptides do not show any regular structure. Therefore, it cannot be used to explain differences in cellular uptake of the peptides.

The hydrophobic moment was performed to explain the high permeability of some irregular hydrophobic and hydrophilic residues in the α-helix structure, such as the amphiphilic peptide melittin.[29] The results of the total hydrophobic moment (μH) are shown in Table 2. Despite the fact that these peptides had the same value for the total hydrophobic moment, $W_3R_4W_3$ had much lower cellular uptake activity than the other peptides studied in this study.

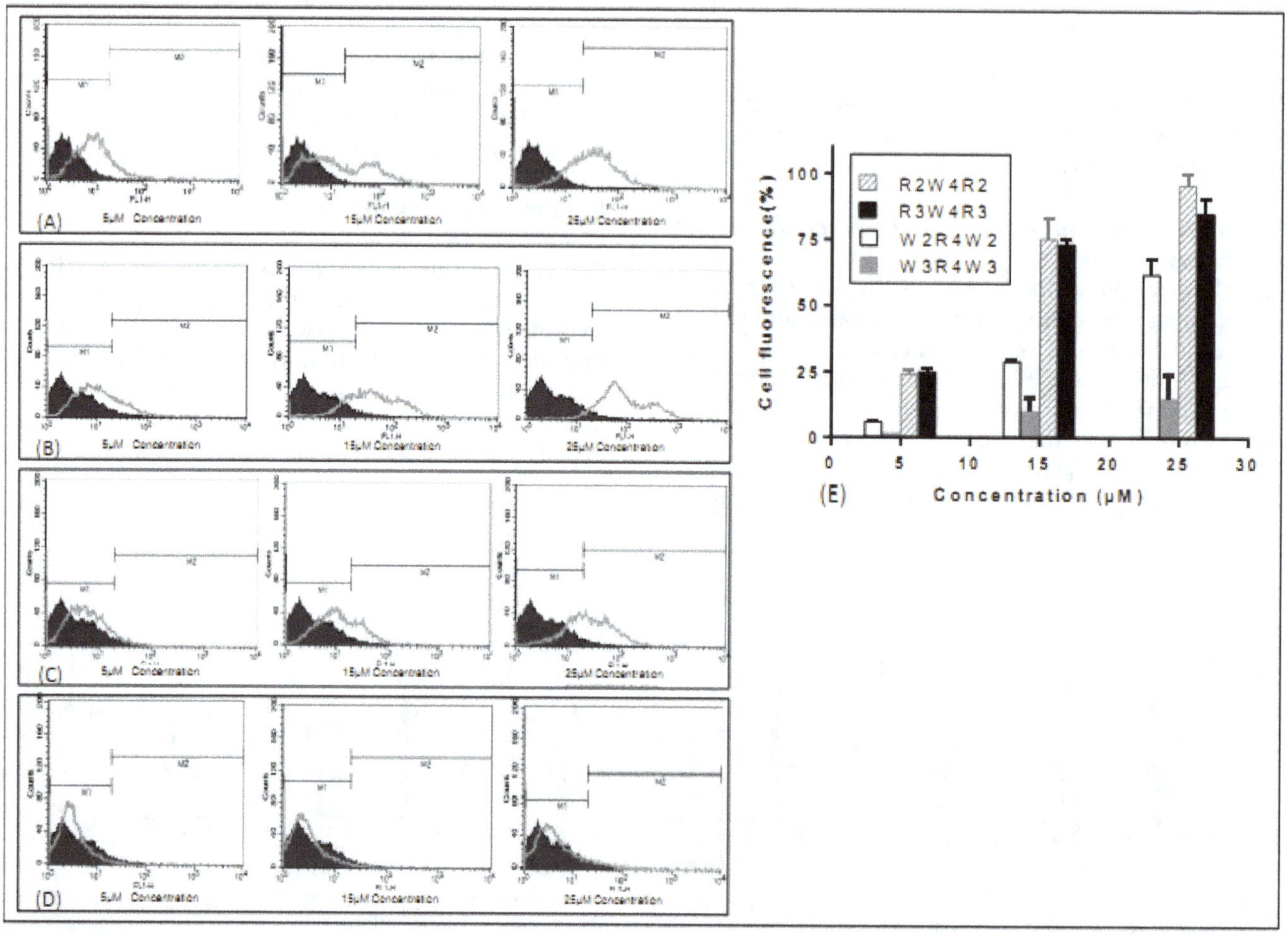

Figure 2. Cellular uptake of FITC-labeled peptides in live MCF-7 cells after incubation for 1 h at 37 °C. The uptake values of intensity are seen for $R_2W_4R_2$ (A) and $R_3W_4R_3$ (B), followed by, in order of decreasing intensity, $W_2R_4W_2$ (C), $W_3R_4W_3$ (D). (E) A comparison of the cellular uptake of peptides in 5, 15, and 25μM concentrations. The results are expressed as a percentage of gated populations. Each value is the mean ± SD of two separate determinations.

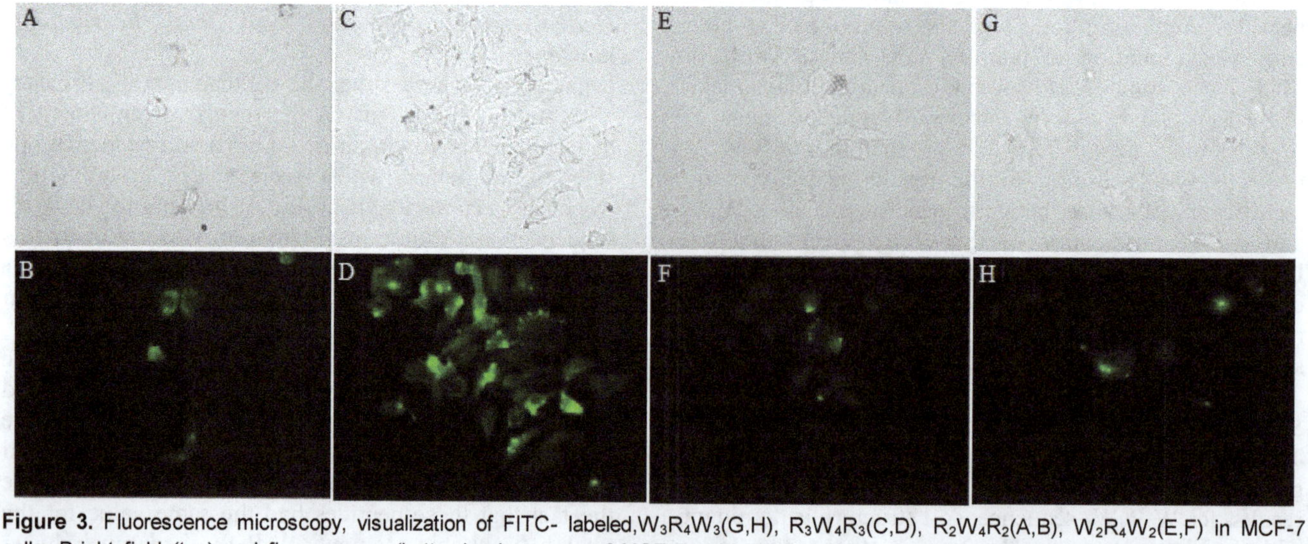

Figure 3. Fluorescence microscopy, visualization of FITC- labeled,$W_3R_4W_3$(G,H), $R_3W_4R_3$(C,D), $R_2W_4R_2$(A,B), $W_2R_4W_2$(E,F) in MCF-7 cells. Bright field (top) and fluorescence (bottom) microscopy of MCF-7 cells. Live cells were treated with 15 μM of peptides for 1h at 37°C.

Table 1. Prediction of secondary structural parameters of peptides, and graphical model

Sequence	Sequence index	Helix probability	Sheet probability	Coil probability	GOR V prediction	Graphical model
	1 W	0.114	0.129	0.758	C*	
	2 W	0.257	0.168	0.575	C	
	3 R	0.438	0.237	0.324	C	
WWRRRRWW	4 R	0.655	0.172	0.173	C	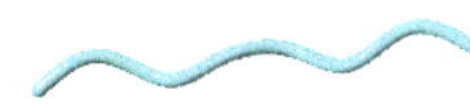
	5 R	0.632	0.178	0.190	C	
	6 R	0.427	0.221	0.352	C	
	7 W	0.310	0.162	0.528	C	
	8 W	0.113	0.127	0.760	C	
	1 W	0.175	0.135	0.689	C	
	2 W	0.312	0.151	0.537	C	
	3 W	0.488	0.217	0.296	H**	
	4 R	0.655	0.200	0.145	H	
WWWRRRRWWW	5 R	0.655	0.172	0.173	H	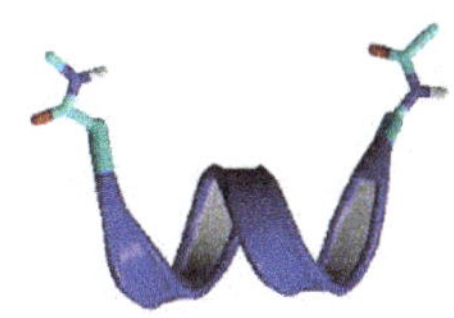
	6 R	0.632	0.178	0.190	H	
	7 R	0.549	0.253	0.197	H	
	8 W	0.421	0.245	0.334	H	
	9 W	0.247	0.166	0.586	C	
	10 W	0.123	0.133	0.743	C	
	1 R	0.102	0.170	0.728	C	
	2 R	0.246	0.241	0.513	C	
	3 W	0.399	0.267	0.334	H	
RRWWWWRR	4 W	0.543	0.286	0.171	H	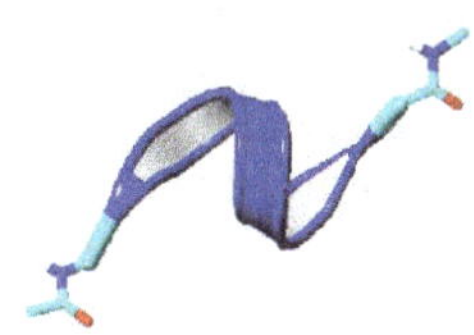
	5 W	0.595	0.255	0.150	H	
	6 W	0.512	0.265	0.222	H	
	7 R	0.387	0.213	0.400	C	
	8 R	0.234	0.150	0.616	C	
	1 R	0.074	0.146	0.779	C	
	2 R	0.179	0.268	0.553	C	
	3 R	0.393	0.267	0.340	H	
	4 W	0.531	0.291	0.178	H	
RRRWWWWRRR	5 W	0.543	0.286	0.171	H	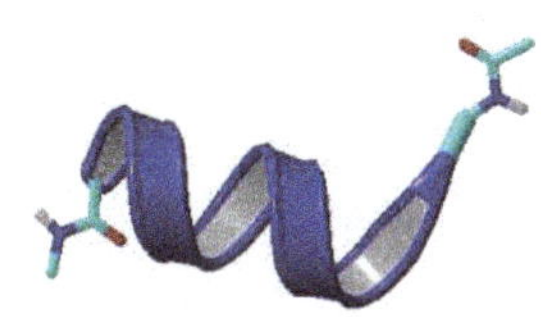
	6 W	0.595	0.255	0.150	H	
	7 W	0.648	0.224	0.128	H	
	8 R	0.542	0.229	0.229	H	
	9 R	0.435	0.204	0.360	H	
	10 R	0.213	0.137	0.649	C	

**α-helix (H),* coil (C).

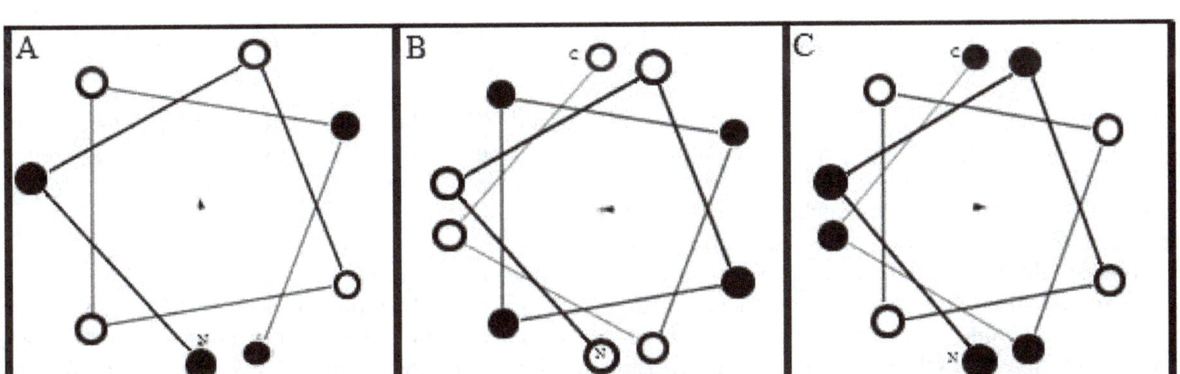

Figure 4. Illustration of sequences in helical wheel projection of $W_3R_4W_3$ (B), $R_2W_4R_2$ (A), and $R_3W_4R_3$ (C) generated using the program MPEx 3.2. Black symbols represent basics and hydrophilic residues (Arg), white, aromatics and hydrophobic residues (Trp).

Wimley-White **scales**

It is believed that difference between octanol hydrophobicity scale and interfacial hydrophobicity scale can be an effective parameter to predict behavior of peptides to penetrate the cell membrane. According to the research conducted in this field, peptides with $\Delta G°_{Oct\text{-}w} \leq 20$ kcal/mol^{-1} would be good candidates for penetrating the cell membrane.[30] Based on the values obtained from the W.W scale (Table 2) and flow cytometry data, $\Delta G°_{Oct\text{-}w}$ does not appear to be a suitable parameter for predicting cell penetrating peptides, since $\Delta G°_{Oct\text{-}w}$ of all peptides were less than 20 kcal/mol^{-1}.

Table 2. Hydrophobicity scales and the total hydrophobic moment

Sequence	NH2-R2W4R2-CONH2	NH2-R3W4R3-CONH2	NH2-W3R4W3-CONH2	NH2-W2R4W2-CONH2
Total. Hyd. Moment (μH)*	3.26	3.26	3.49	3.49
Wimley-White Scale(Oct-If)** (kcal mol^{-1})	9.51	11.51	9.03	9.51
Wimley-White Scale (Oct)*** (kcal mol^{-1})	3.18	6.8	-1	3.18

*Total. Hyd. Moment= the total hydrophobic moment

**Wimley–White Scale (Oct-If) ==difference between the Wimley–White whole-residue octanol hydrophobicity scale and interfacial hydrophobicity scale.

***Wimley–White Scale (Oct) = Wimley–White whole-residue octanol hydrophobicity scale

Another parameter used to predict the penetration efficiency of peptides is the transfer free energy values of peptide from water to membrane. The amount of energy required for transferring a random-coil and α-helix insertion into the hydrophobic core of the cell membrane is +1.15 kcal mol^{-1} ($\Delta G_{Oct} \geq +1.15$ kcal mol^{-1}).[31] According to the data in Table 2, $R_2W_4R_2$, $R_3W_4R_3$ and $W_2R_4W_2$ have enough energy for penetration from water to membrane. The data also shows that $W_3R_4W_3$ with lowest cellular uptake has not sufficient free energy value. It seems that uptake efficiency and transfer free energy values correlate with each other and this parameter may be used to explain differences in uptake of the peptides into the MCF-7 cells (Figure 5).

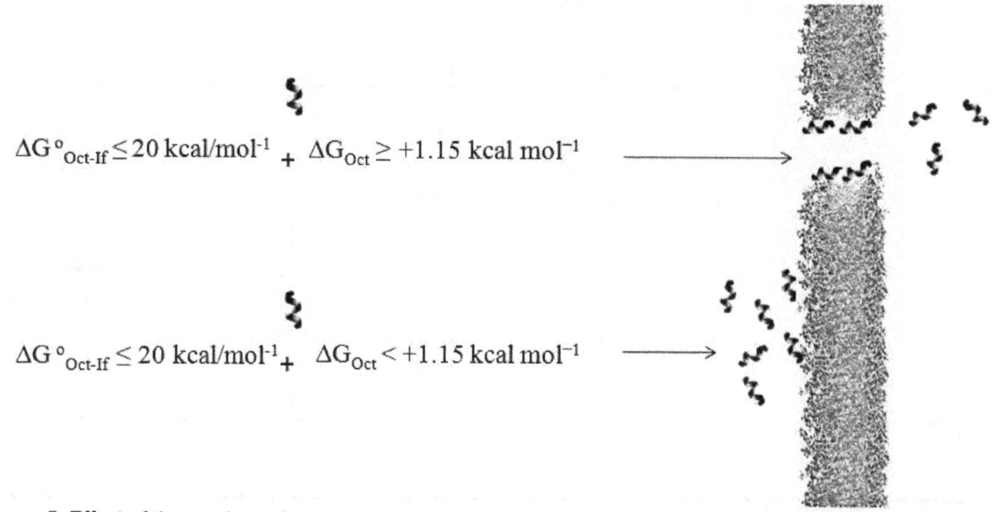

Figure 5. Effect of thermodynamic parameters for the transfer of peptide from water to the intracellular space.

Conclusion

In this study, four amphipathic peptides containing tryptophan and arginine amino acid residues were synthesized to assess the importance of different parameters in their cell uptake. The flow cytometry results showed different cellular uptake efficiency. Various thermodynamic and structural parameters that might influence peptide transport through the cell membrane were investigated. The secondary structure and the helical wheel projection failed to describe the differences in cellular uptake of the peptides. On the other hand it seems that the uptake efficiency correlates well with the transfer free energy values and this parameter may be used to describe the different uptake efficiency of the cell penetrating peptides into MCF-7 cells.

Acknowledgments

The financial support from the "Drug Applied Research Center" and "Research Center for Pharmaceutical Nanotechnology" of Tabriz University of Medical Sciences is greatly acknowledged. This paper is based on an MSc thesis submitted by A. Shirani in Faculty of

Advanced Medical Sciences, Tabriz University of Medical Sciences (Grant No. 5/79/1709).

Conflict of Interest

The authors report no conflicts of interest.

References

1. Vives E, Schmidt J, Pelegrin A. Cell-penetrating and cell-targeting peptides in drug delivery. *Biochim Biophys Acta* 2008;1786(2):126-38. doi: 10.1016/j.bbcan.2008.03.001
2. Yin H, Moulton HM, Betts C, Merritt T, Seow Y, Ashraf S, et al. Functional rescue of dystrophin-deficient mdx mice by a chimeric peptide-PMO. *Mol Ther* 2010;18(10):1822-9. doi: 10.1038/mt.2010.151
3. Siwkowski AM, Malik L, Esau CC, Maier MA, Wancewicz EV, Albertshofer K, et al. Identification and functional validation of PNAs that inhibit murine CD40 expression by redirection of splicing. *Nucleic Acids Res* 2004;32(9):2695-706. doi: 10.1093/nar/gkh584
4. Gottschalk S, Sparrow JT, Hauer J, Mims MP, Leland FE, Woo SL, et al. A novel DNA-peptide complex for efficient gene transfer and expression in mammalian cells. *Gene Ther* 1996;3(5):448-57.
5. Muratovska A, Eccles MR. Conjugate for efficient delivery of short interfering RNA (siRNA) into mammalian cells. *FEBS Lett* 2004;558(1-3):63-8. doi: 10.1016/s0014-5793(03)01505-9
6. Fernandez-Carneado J, Kogan MJ, Pujals S, Giralt E. Amphipathic peptides and drug delivery. *Biopolymers* 2004;76(2):196-203. doi: 10.1002/bip.10585
7. Sawant R, Torchilin V. Intracellular delivery of nanoparticles with CPPs. *Methods Mol Biol* 2011;683:431-51. doi: 10.1007/978-1-60761-919-2_31
8. Kilk K, Mahlapuu R, Soomets U, Langel U. Analysis of in vitro toxicity of five cell-penetrating peptides by metabolic profiling. *Toxicology* 2009;265(3):87-95. doi: 10.1016/j.tox.2009.09.016
9. Yamashita H, Demizu Y, Shoda T, Sato Y, Oba M, Tanaka M, et al. Amphipathic short helix-stabilized peptides with cell-membrane penetrating ability. *Bioorg Med Chem* 2014;22(8):2403-8. doi: 10.1016/j.bmc.2014.03.005
10. Yau WM, Wimley WC, Gawrisch K, White SH. The preference of tryptophan for membrane interfaces. *Biochemistry* 1998;37(42):14713-8. doi: 10.1021/bi980809c
11. Rydberg HA, Matson M, Amand HL, Esbjorner EK, Norden B. Effects of tryptophan content and backbone spacing on the uptake efficiency of cell-penetrating peptides. *Biochemistry* 2012;51(27):5531-9. doi: 10.1021/bi300454k
12. Sharma R, Shivpuri S, Anand A, Kulshreshtha A, Ganguli M. Insight into the role of physicochemical parameters in a novel series of amphipathic peptides for efficient DNA delivery. *Mol Pharm* 2013;10(7):2588-600. doi: 10.1021/mp400032q
13. Abidi F, Jacquot S, Lassiter C, Trivier E, Hanauer A, Schwartz CE. Novel mutations in Rsk-2, the gene for Coffin-Lowry syndrome (CLS). *Eur J Hum Genet* 1999;7(1):20-6. doi: 10.1038/sj.ejhg.5200231
14. Killian JA, Von Heijne G. How proteins adapt to a membrane-water interface. *Trends Biochem Sci* 2000;25(9):429-34. doi: 10.1016/s0968-0004(00)01626-1
15. Futaki S. Membrane-permeable arginine-rich peptides and the translocation mechanisms. *Adv Drug Deliv Rev* 2005;57(4):547-58. doi: 10.1016/j.addr.2004.10.009
16. Schug KA, Lindner W. Noncovalent binding between guanidinium and anionic groups: focus on biological- and synthetic-based arginine/guanidinium interactions with phosph[on]ate and sulf[on]ate residues. *Chem Rev* 2005;105(1):67-114. doi: 10.1021/cr040603j
17. Amblard M, Fehrentz JA, Martinez J, Subra G. Methods and protocols of modern solid phase Peptide synthesis. *Mol Biotechnol* 2006;33(3):239-54. doi: 10.1385/mb:33:3:239
18. Reichert J, Grasnick D, Afonin S, Buerck J, Wadhwani P, Ulrich AS. A critical evaluation of the conformational requirements of fusogenic peptides in membranes. *Eur Biophys J* 2007;36(4-5):405-13. doi: 10.1007/s00249-006-0106-2
19. Maurya IK, Thota CK, Sharma J, Tupe SG, Chaudhary P, Singh MK, et al. Mechanism of action of novel synthetic dodecapeptides against Candida albicans. *Biochim Biophys Acta* 2013;1830(11):5193-203. doi: 10.1016/j.bbagen.2013.07.016
20. Richard JP, Melikov K, Vives E, Ramos C, Verbeure B, Gait MJ, et al. Cell-penetrating peptides. A reevaluation of the mechanism of cellular uptake. *J Biol Chem* 2003;278(1):585-90. doi: 10.1074/jbc.m209548200
21. Kloczkowski A, Ting KL, Jernigan RL, Garnier J. Combining the GOR V algorithm with evolutionary information for protein secondary structure prediction from amino acid sequence. *Proteins* 2002;49(2):154-66. doi: 10.1002/prot.10181
22. Garnier J, Osguthorpe DJ, Robson B. Analysis of the accuracy and implications of simple methods for predicting the secondary structure of globular proteins. *J Mol Biol* 1978;120(1):97-120. doi: 10.1016/0022-2836(78)90297-8
23. Cheng H, Sen TZ, Kloczkowski A, Margaritis D, Jernigan RL. Prediction of protein secondary structure by mining structural fragment database. *Polymer (Guildf)* 2005;46(12):4314-21. doi: 10.1016/j.polymer.2005.02.040
24. Sen TZ, Jernigan RL, Garnier J, Kloczkowski A. GOR V server for protein secondary structure

prediction. *Bioinformatics* 2005;21(11):2787-8. doi: 10.1093/bioinformatics/bti408

25. Vance VB, Huang AH. The major protein from lipid bodies of maize. Characterization and structure based on cDNA cloning. *J Biol Chem* 1987;262(23):11275-9.
26. Wimley WC, White SH. Experimentally determined hydrophobicity scale for proteins at membrane interfaces. *Nat Struct Biol* 1996;3(10):842-8. doi: 10.1038/nsb1096-842
27. Oren Z, Shai Y. Mode of action of linear amphipathic alpha-helical antimicrobial peptides. *Biopolymers* 1998;47(6):451-63. doi: 10.1002/(SICI)1097-0282(1998)47:6<451::AID-BIP4>3.0.CO;2-F
28. Yandek LE, Pokorny A, Floren A, Knoelke K, Langel U, Almeida PF. Mechanism of the cell-penetrating peptide transportan 10 permeation of lipid bilayers. *Biophys J* 2007;92(7):2434-44. doi: 10.1529/biophysj.106.100198
29. Dathe M, Wieprecht T. Structural features of helical antimicrobial peptides: their potential to modulate activity on model membranes and biological cells. *Biochim Biophys Acta* 1999;1462(1-2):71-87. doi: 10.1016/s0005-2736(99)00201-1
30. Almeida PF, Pokorny A. Mechanisms of antimicrobial, cytolytic, and cell-penetrating peptides: from kinetics to thermodynamics. *Biochemistry* 2009;48(34):8083-93. doi: 10.1021/bi900914g
31. Wimley WC, White SH. Designing transmembrane alpha-helices that insert spontaneously. *Biochemistry* 2000;39(15):4432-42. doi: 10.1021/bi992746j

Formulation and Characterization of Cetylpyridinium Chloride Bioadhesive Tablets

Jafar Akbari[1]*, Majid Saeedi[1], Katayoun Morteza-Semnani[2], Hamidreza Kelidari[3], Maryam Lashkari[1]

[1] *Department of Pharmaceutics, Faculty of Pharmacy, Mazandaran University of Medical Sciences, Sari, Iran.*
[2] *Department of Medicinal Chemistry, Faculty of Pharmacy, Mazandaran University of Medical Sciences, Sari, Iran.*
[3] *Pharmaceutical Sciences Research Center, Mazandaran University of Medical Sciences, Sari, Iran.*

Article info

Keywords:
- Cetylpyridinium Chloride
- HPMC K100M
- Carbopol 974P
- Polycarbophill
- Bioadhesive

Abstract

Purpose: Bioadhesive polymers play an important role in biomedical and drug delivery applications. The aim of this study is to develop a sustained- release tablet for local application of Cetylpyridinium Chloride (CPC). This delivery system would supply the drug at an effective level for a long period of time, and thereby overcome the problem of the short retention time of CPC and could be used for buccal delivery as a topical anti-infective agent.

Methods: CPC bioadhesive tablets were directly prepared using 7 mm flat-faced punches on a hydraulic press. The materials for each tablet were weighted, introduced into the die and compacted at constant compression pressure. The dissolution tests were performed to the rotation paddle method and the bioadhesive strength of the tablets were measured.

Results: The results showed that as the concentration of polymer increased, the drug release rate was decreased. Also the type and ratio of polymers altered the release kinetic of Cetylpyridinium Chloride from investigated tablets. The bioadhesion strength increased with increasing the concentration of polymer and maximum bioadhesion strength was observed with HPMC K100M.

Conclusion: The selected formulation of CPC bioadhesive tablet can be used as a suitable preparation for continuous release of CPC with appropriate bioadhesion strength.

Introduction

Bioadhesive polymers play an important role in biomedical and drug delivery applications. Good adhesion and intimate contact between polymer carrier and tissue are desirable for use in these applications. Mucoadhesive systems are advantageous over conventional drug delivery systems due to their ability to increase the contact time of drug with the biological substrate, thus increasing drug absorption. Various bioadhesive mucosal dosage forms have been developed, which included adhesive tablets, gels, ointments, patches, and more recently films.[1] Mucoadhesion is provided by the formation of non-covalent bonds such as hydrogen bonds and ionic interactions or physical entanglements between the mucus gel layer and polymers. Mediated by mucoadhesive polymers, the residence time of dosage forms on the GI- mucosa should be prolonged, which allows a sustained drug release at a given target site to maximize the therapeutic effect.[2]

A major difficulty for the successful eradication of infections of oral cavity is the dilution and rapid elimination of topically applied drugs due to the flushing action of saliva. The delivery system in which the drug is incorporated is therefore an important consideration and should be formulated to prolong retention of the drug in the oral cavity. Efficient local delivery of actives such as dental bleaches and antimicrobials to the oral cavity is compromised by a number of factors that dramatically reduce residence time, most notably the shear forces associated with speaking, swallowing and mastication, as well as dilution and washout caused by continuous saliva production.[3]

Typical polymers that have been used as mucoadhesive drug carriers are poly (acrylic acid), poly (methacrylate acid), cellulose derivatives, poly (ethylene oxide), lectin and chitosan.[4] The PAA and its cross-linked commercial forms, Carbopol and polycarbophil exhibit strong mucoadhesive properties.[5] Many attempts have been undertaken to improve the mucoadhesive properties of polymers by preparing copolymers, polymer conjugates or interpolymer complexes.[6,7]

CPC, an amphiphilic quaternary compound, has been used extensively in oral hygiene formulations.[8] Valuable properties of CPC include solubility in water and alcohol, as well as its ability to reduce surface tension. A number of laboratory studies are available in the literature that report the broad spectrum activity of CPC on a range of organisms, including bacteria and yeast found in dental plaque.[9-11] Bonesvoll and Gjermo have shown that a moderate plaque inhibition was obtained

***Corresponding author:** Jafar Akbari, Email: JAkbari@mazums.ac.ir

when CPC was applied twice daily as a mouthwash. Only when the frequency was increased to 4 times daily did the plaque inhibitory effect approach that of chlorhexidine. The differences in clinical effect could be explained from the retention time of the drug: the quaternary ammonium compounds were cleared from the mouth more rapidly than was chlorhexidine.[12] Fridman et al. prepared the cast film composed of ethylcellulose and CPC. The films exhibited sustained inhibition of *Streptococcus mutans* growth *in vitro*. The results of the clinical study proved that a single application of cetylpyridinium films decreased plaque accumulation for a period of 3 days. No changes in the total salivary flora were observed during the study.[13]

The aim of this study is to develop a sustained- release tablet for local application of CPC. This delivery system would supply the drug at an effective level for a long period of time, and thereby overcome the problem of the short retention time of CPC and could be used for buccal delivery as a topical anti-infective agent.

Materials and Methods

Materials

Cetyl pyridinium Chloride, magnesium stearate, potassium hydrogen phosphate and lactose were purchased from Merck Co. (Germany). Carbopol 934P and polycarbophill from BF Goodrich Co. (USA), and HPMC K100M were prepared from Colorcon Co. (UK). All chemicals and solvents were of analytical grade. Freshly double distilled water was used in the experiments.

Preparation of bioadhesive tablets

Six formulations (F1-F6) were directly prepared using 7 mm flat-faced punches on a hydraulic press. The materials for each tablet (Table 1) were weighed, mixed and introduced into the die and compacted at constant compression pressure using 1% (w/w) magnesium stearate.

Table 1. Formulation composition of cetylpyridinium chloride mucoadhesive tablets

Formulation code	Formulation Composition (mg)					
	Drug	Carbopol 974P	Poly carbophill	HPMC K100M	Lactose	Mg stearate
F1	30	30	-	-	-	0.6
F2	30	15	-	-	15	0.6
F3	30	-	30	-	-	0.6
F4	30	-	15	-	15	0.6
F5	30	-	-	30	-	0.6
F6	30	-	-	15	15	0.6

In vitro dissolution

The dissolution tests were performed to the rotation paddle method (USP pharmacopoeia 24). A dissolution apparatus (Caleva 8ST, Germany) was employed with a stirring rate of 100 rpm. The dissolution medium was 900 ml phosphate buffer (pH: 6.8). Samples of the solution were withdrawn at definite time intervals. The dissolution media was then replaced by fresh dissolution fluid to maintain a constant volume. The solution was passed through a filter and then the concentration of CPC in solution was measured with an ultraviolet spectrophotometer (Varian, Australia) at a wavelength of 258 nm after suitable dilution with the dissolution medium when necessary. The experiment was carried out in triplicate.[14]

Kinetic analysis

In order to describe the kinetics of drug release from mucoadhesive tablets, various mathematical equation models (zero-order, first-order, Higuchi) were tested

$Q_t = k_0 t$

$\ln Q_t = \ln Q_0 - k_1 t$

$Q_t = k_H t^{1/2}$

Where Q_t is the amount of drug released in time t, Q_0 is the initial amount of drug in the tablet and k_0, k_1 and k_H are the respective release rate constants for zero-order, first-order and Higuchi models. In order to define a model, that will represent a better fit for the formulations, dissolution data can be further analyzed by the Ritger and peppas and Korsmeyer equation

$M_t/M_\infty = k_p t^n$

Where M_t corresponds to the amount of drug released in time t, M_∞ is the total amount of drug that must be released at infinite time, k_p is a constant and 'n' is the release exponent indicating the type of drug release mechanism.[15]

Determination of bioadhesive strength

To evaluate the bioadhesion strength, a tensile tester apparatus was designed similar to a tensile tester apparatus (Instron model 4301) and the bioadhesive strength of the tablets was measured according to previously published method by a tensile tester apparatus. After isolation of hairless abdominal skin of the rat, the dorsal section of abdominal skin of rat (mucosa part) was fixed on the head of diffusion cell and filled with phosphate buffer with pH 6.8. The same conditions were exactly used according to previously published method.[16]

Statistical analysis

Statistical analysis was carried out by using the analysis of variance (ANOVA) with computer software SPSS 10. Tukey-Kramers multiple comparison tests were used to compare the group data.

Results and Discussion

Bioadhesive preparations are preferred for treatment of diseases of oral cavity because they can adhere to the mucosa, protect the diseased part, and retain the drug for the desired period. Examples of oral cavity diseases for which buccal dosage forms have been designed include: aphthous stomatitis, oral candidiasis, and periodontal disease. In the buccal region, a tablet may be adhered either to the buccal tissue (cheek) or the gingival. For local drug delivery, the highly keratinized epidermis of the gingival will present a barrier to systemic absorption. The buccal tablet must be sufficiently thin (1-2 mm) and of small diameter (6-8 mm), so as to be comfortable and not obtrusive when placed into the oral cavity. Bioadhesion is the phenomenon between two materials, which are held together for extended periods of time by interfacial forces. It is generally referred as bioadhesion when interaction occurs between polymer and epithelial surface, mucoadhesion when occurs with the mucus layer covering a tissue.

The adhesion force of mucoadhesive tablets are shown in Figure 1. The bioadhesion strength of mucoadhesive tablets were evaluated by method that described by Akbari et al. The results of this study clearly demonstrate that the changing the type of polymer can also change the bioadhesive strength of tablets. Maximum bioadhesive strength was seen with F3 (HPMC K100M). Also the results showed that the bioadhesion strength decreased with incorporation of lactose in formulations.

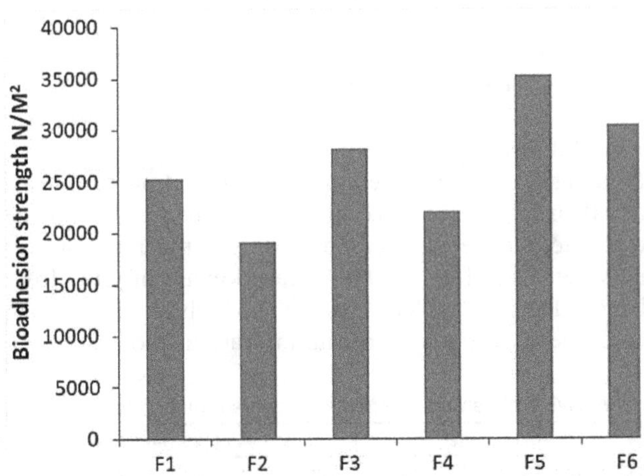

Figure 1. Comparison of the mucoadhesive force of investigated cetylpyridinium buccal tablets containing carbopol 974P, polycarbophyl, and HPMC K100M (n=3).

Bioadhesive force means the force with which tablets bind to buccal mucous membranes. The bioadhesive forces of the tablet are affected by the shape of the tablet, the swelling degree of the tablet and the nature of the tablet components.[17]

Various classes of polymers have been investigated in order to meet the requirements for a mucoadhesive polymer, such as proper hydrogen-bonding functional groups, suitable wetting properties, swelling/water load properties, and sufficient flexibility for entanglement with the tissue mucus network. The mucosal surface is covered with a mucus layer, in which mucins are the major component. Mucins are highly glucosylated glycoproteins with a large peptide backbone and oligosaccharides as side chains. As a result, mucins are negatively charged at physiological pH. Mechanisms of polymer attachment to mucosal surfaces are not yet fully understood. However, certain theories of bioadhesion have suggested that it might occur via physical entanglement (diffusion theory) and/or chemical interactions, such as electrostatic, hydrophobic, hydrogen bonding, and Van der waals interactions (adsorption and electronic theories).[18]

Formulation F2 was having lowest bioadhesive force because the carbopol 974P has a lower viscosity than the other two polymers. While formulation F5 containing HPMC K100M shows higher bioadhesion force due to higher viscosity. HPMC is a long chained, nonionic polymer and so its mucoadhesion is attributable to the formation of physical bonds or hydrogen bonding with the mucus components. HPMC possesses a large number of hydroxyl groups that are responsible for adhesion. Formation of hydrogen bonds between the hydrophilic functional groups of the mucoadhesive polymers and the mucus layer or the mucosal surface is a prerequisite for extensive and longer mucoadhesion. The increased sites for bond formation can explain the increase in bioadhesion with an increase in concentration. The higher mucoadhesive potential observed with formulations containing only HPMC is probably due to the controlled rate of hydration of HPMC as a nonionic polymer. This could in turn prevent the tablet from quick over hydration and formation of slippery and weak mucilage, which could be easily removed from the mucosal surface.[19]

From the above results it was found that polymers having high molecular weight and high viscosity exhibited higher adhesion. Chandira et al. prepared the mucoadhesive tablets of Clarithromycin by using the Carbopol 974P, HPMC K15M and HPMC K4M. They found that polymers having high molecular weight and high viscosity exhibited higher adhesion. HPMC K15M and Carbopol 974P were found to be having good mucoadhesive strength. HPMC and carbopol possesses hydroxy and carboxy groups respectively required for bioadhesion.[20] Akbari et al evaluated the effect of fillers on the bucoadhesive propranolol hydrochloride tablets. The results that they obtained showed bioadhesion force increased with increasing the concentration of polycarbophil. It is clear that the formation of very thin and strong gel layer at the boundary might be necessary for adhesion. The viscosity of this layer is increased by adding polycarbophil and therefore the bioadhesion strength increases.[21]

Also Maniyar et al. stated that the strength of mucoadhesion can be influence by polymer concentration. Physical state of the delivery system defines the polymer concentration, with observational differences between semisolid and solid state platforms. In semisolid state, an optimum concentration exists for each polymer beyond which reduced adhesion occurs because a lower number of polymer chains are available for interpenetration with mucus. On other hand, solid dosage forms such as buccal tablets exhibit increased adhesive strength as the mucoadhesive polymer concentration increases.[22]

In vitro dissolution studies

The effect of polymer type and addition of lactose on release rate are shown in Figure 2. The initial percentage drug release after 2 hour for F1, F2, F3, F4, F5 and F6 were 14.20, 48.48, 14.63, 48.02, 16.12 and 25.52 respectively. The percentage drug release after 8 hour for F1, F2, F3, F4, F5 and F6 were 39.91, 70.66, 35.63, 67.41, 26.87 and 50.59 respectively. The lowest release rate was observed with formulation F5 containing HPMC K100M and the highest release rate was observed with formulation F2 containing Carbopol and Lactose ($P<0.01$). The significant difference was not observed between F1-F3 and F2-F4 but there were the significant differences between the release rate of formulations F1 - F3 with F5 ($p<0.01$) and F2-F4 with F6 ($p<0.001$).

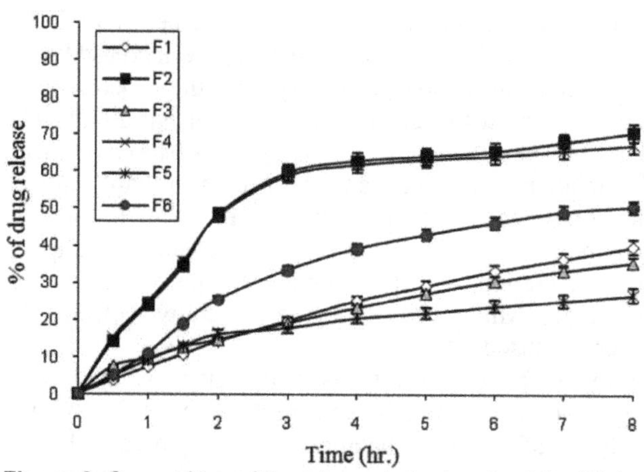

Figure 2. Comparison of the release behavior of cetylpyridinium chloride from buccoadhesive tablets containing carbopol 974P, polycarbophyl, and HPMC K100M (n=3).

It was observed that the type of polymer influences the drug release pattern. Amount of polymer affects the drug release. Drug release from HPMC K100M was lesser owing to its high viscosity and also due to less permeability of water to HPMC K100M. As expected, the drug release rate was dependent on the viscosity grade and the concentration of the polymer used.

Figure 2 shows the effect of replacement of HPMC, Polycarbophil and Carbopol 974P by lactose on the release profile of drug. The figure shows that replacement of polymer by lactose increases the release rate of drug from buccoadhesive tablets. Changing the polymer /filler ratio increases the release rate by altering the diffusivity of drug in gel layer. Water diffusivity depends only on the total concentration of viscosity inducing agents in the system irrespective of their nature or polymerization degree. Replacement of polymer by lactose decreases the concentration of polymer in gel layer and therefore diffusion of water into the tablet is facilitated. Lactose also decreases the tourtosity of the path of diffusion. The results confirmed the finding of Lapidus and Lordi that replacement polymer by either a soluble or an insoluble diluents increased dissolution rate.[21] Also Diasa et al. formulated the mucoadhesive Acyclovir tablet with using the HPMC K100M. Their results showed high HPMC K100M content results in a greater amount of gel being formed. This gel layer increases the diffusion path length of the drug, hence controlling drug release via diffusion through the gel and erosion of the gel barrier. Its viscous nature also affects the diffusion coefficient of the drug. As a result, drug release was found to be decreased as the amount of HPMC K100M was increased.[23]

Kinetic evaluation

Dissolution rate data were analyzed based on Eqs. (1-4) and their results are listed in Table 2. The results showed that altering the type of polymer and the ratio of two polymer, had effect on the release kinetic of CPC from buccoadhesive tablets and the highest correlation coefficient were achieved with the various models.

Table 2. The kinetics of Cetylpyridinium Chloride release from mucoadhesive tablets with different kind and amount of polymer

Formulation code	Zero-order model			First-order model			Higuchi model			Peppas model			
	K_0 (%.min)	r^2	*ss*	K_1 (min^{-1})	r^2	*ss*	K_H ($\%.min^{-1/2}$)	r^2	*ss*	K_p ($\%.min^{-n}$)	*n*	r^2	*ss*
F1	0.0009	0.948	25711	-0.0013	0.978	13961	0.0249	0. 994	1786	0.0155	0. 574	0.991	212
F2	0.0011	0.779	33779	-0.023	0.860	13780	0.033	0. 888	2680	0.0109	0.764	0.960	404
F3	0.0006	0.988	19014	-0.0008	0.995	12146	0.018	0.993	7312	0.0090	0.595	0.992	209
F4	0.0010	0.756	36943	-0.002	0.827	17468	0.0315	0.873	2777	0.0175	0.657	0.967	763
F5	0.0004	0.905	29330	-0.0005	0.926	23470	0.0126	0.972	2326	0.0085	0.554	0.971	1310
F6	0.0010	0.905	15027	-0.0015	0.946	5414	0.0287	0.974	30616	0.0090	0.595	0.951	2718

k_0: zero order release rate constant, k_1: first order release rate constant, k_H: Higuchi model release rate constant, k_p: Peppas model release rate constant, *n*: release exponent in Peppas model, r^2: definition coefficient, *ss*: sum of squares of errors

There are the following possible mechanisms by which drug release from a polymeric matrix may occur: (a) the first and the most often encountered mechanism is drug diffusion through the outside layers of the matrix, also known as ''Fickian'' release or ''Case I'' mechanism (b) non-Fickian or anomalous (c) ''zero-order'' release or ''Case II'' mechanism Another mechanism of release involves devices made from water-soluble or swellable polymers, where matrix swelling and drug diffusion occur concurrently. This mechanism has been described as non-Fickian or anomalous transport and the release is controlled by swelling and diffusion. However, in practice, polymeric matrices release the drug via a combination of mechanisms. The exponent, n, depends on the polymer swelling characteristics and the relaxation rate at the swelling front.[24]

The CPC release from matrix tablets containing different types of polymers showed a good fit into the Peppas equation, indicating combined effect of diffusion and erosion mechanisms for drug release. As shown in Table 2, release data fit well with this model as a correlation coefficient (r^2) greater than 0.951 was obtained in all cases.

According to the criteria for release kinetics from swellable systems, a value of release exponent, $n = 0.45$, $0.45 < n < 0.89$, and $0.89 < n < 1.0$ indicates Fickian (Case I) diffusion, non-Fickian (anomalous) diffusion and zero-order (Case II) transport, respectively.[25]

The value of diffusional coefficient, n, for mucoadhesive matrices was 0.574-0.764 which indicates non-Fickian (anomalous) behaviour and that the drug partially diffuses through the swollen polymer matrix and also partly through the gradually expanding hydrated matrix with increasing diffusional path length.

Conclusion

In this study, the effect of type and amount of polymer on the bioadhesive strength and release rate of Cetylpyridinium Chloride were evaluated. Different mucoadhesive tablets were formulated to adhere to the buccal mucosa for a local CPC release. The dissolution rate, release kinetic and bioadhesion force of tablets were evaluated. The results showed that as the concentration of polymer increased, the release rate decreased. The lowest release rate observed with HPMC K100M. The bioadhesion strength of mucoadhesive tablets were evaluated by method that described by Akbari et al. the results showed that the highest bioadhesion force also was observed with HPMC K100M.

Conflict of Interest

The authors declare that they have no conflict of interest.

References

1. Ahn JS, Choi HK, Chun MK, Ryu JM, Jung JH, Kim YU, et al. Release of triamcinolone acetonide from mucoadhesive polymer composed of chitosan and poly (acrylic acid) *in vitro*. *Biomaterials* 2002;23(6):1411-6.
2. Bernkop-Schnürch A. Mucoadhesive systems in oral drug delivery. *Drug Discov Today Technol* 2005;2(1):83-7.
3. Rathbone MJ, Drummond BK, Tucker IG. The oral cavity as a site for systemic drug delivery. *Adv Drug Del Rev* 1994;13(1-2):1-22.
4. Ameye D, Mus D, Foreman P, Remon JP. Spray-dried Amioca® starch/Carbopol® 974P mixtures as buccal bioadhesive carriers. *Int J Pharm* 2005;301(1–2):170-80.
5. Chun MK, Cho CS, Choi HK. Mucoadhesive drug carrier based on interpolymer complex of poly (vinyl pyrrolidone) and poly (acrylic acid) prepared by template polymerization. *J Control Release* 2002;81(3):327-34.
6. Ameye D, Voorspoels J, Foreman P, Tsai J, Richardson P, Geresh S, et al. *Ex vivo* bioadhesion and in vivo testosterone bioavailability study of different bioadhesive formulations based on starch-g-poly(acrylic acid) copolymers and starch/poly(acrylic acid) mixtures. *J Control Release* 2002;79(1-3):173-82.
7. Kast CE, Bernkop-Schnürch A. Polymer–cysteamine conjugates: new mucoadhesive excipients for drug delivery? *Int J Pharm* 2002;234(1-2):91-9.
8. Wu CD, Savitt ED. Evaluation of the safety and efficacy of over-the-counter oral hygiene products for the reduction and control of plaque and gingivitis. *Periodontol 2000* 2002;28(1):91-105.
9. Pitten FA, Kramer A. Efficacy of cetylpyridinium chloride used as oropharyngeal antiseptic. *Arzneimittelforschung* 2001;51(7):588-95.
10. Quisno R, Foter MJ. Cetyl pyridinium chloride: I. Germicidal properties. *J Bacteriol* 1946;52(1):111.
11. Bereswill S, Vey T, Kist M. Susceptibility in vitro of Helicobacter pylori to cetylpyridinium chloride. *FEMS Immunol Med Microbiol* 1999;24(2):189-92.
12. Bonesvoll P, Gjermo P. A comparison between chlorhexidine and some quaternary ammonium compounds with regard to retention, salivary concentration and plaque-inhibiting effect in the human mouth after mouth rinses. *Arch Oral Biol* 1978;23(4):289-94.
13. Friedman M, Harrari D, Rimer A, Stabholz A. Inhibition of plaque formation by a sustained release delivery system for cetylpyridinium chloride. *Int J Pharm* 1988;44(1-3):243-7.
14. Nafee NA, Boraie MA, Ismail FA, Mortada LM. Design and characterization of mucoadhesive buccal patches containing cetylpyridinium chloride. *Acta pharm* 2003;53(3):199-212.
15. Saeedi M, Morteza-Semnani K, Ansoroudi F, Fallah S, Amin G. Evaluation of binding properties of Plantago psyllium seed mucilage. *Acta Pharm* 2010;60(3):339-48.
16. Akbari J, Saeedi M, Enayatifard R, Sagheb-Doost M. Development and evaluation of mucoadhesive chlorhexidine tablet formulations. *Trop J Pharm Res* 2010;9(4):321-7.
17. Choi HG, Kim CK. Development of omeprazole buccal adhesive tablets with stability enhancement in human saliva. *J Control Release* 2000;68(3):397-404.
18. Salamat-Miller N, Chittchang M, Johnston TP. The use of mucoadhesive polymers in buccal drug delivery. *Adv Drug Deliv Rev* 2005;57(11):1666-91.
19. Majithiya RJ, Raval AJ, Umrethia ML, Ghosh PK, Murthy RSR. Enhancement of Mucoadhesion by Blending Anionic, Cationic and Nonionic Polymers. *Drug Deliv Tech* 2008;8:40-5.
20. Chandira RM, Palanisamy P, Jayakar B, Chatakonda R. Design and Development of Controlled Release

Mucoadhesive Oral tablet of Clarithromycin. *Int J Pharma Recent Res* 2009;1(1):59-66.
21. Akbari J, Nokhodchi A, Farid D, Adrangui M, Siahi-Shadbad MR, Saeedi M. Development and evaluation of buccoadhesive propranolol hydrochloride tablet formulations: effect of fillers. *Farmaco* 2004;59(2):155-61.
22. Maniyar AH, Patil RM, Kale MT, Jain DK, Baviskar DT. Mucoadhesion: A new polymeric controlled drug delivery. *Int J Pharm Sci Rev Res* 2011;8(1):54-60.
23. Jacky Dias R, Shamling Sakhare S, Krishnat Mali K. Design and development of mucoadhesive acyclovir tablet. *Iran J Pharm Res* 2010;8(2):231-9.
24. Sinha Roy D, Rohera BD. Comparative evaluation of rate of hydration and matrix erosion of HEC and HPC and study of drug release from their matrices. *Eur J Pharm Sci* 2002;16(3):193-9.
25. Ritger PL, Peppas NA. A simple equation for description of solute release I. Fickian and non-fickian release from non-swellable devices in the form of slabs, spheres, cylinders or discs. *J Control Release* 1987;5(1):23-36.

12

Nanomedicine in Central Nervous System (CNS) Disorders: A Present and Future Prospective

Shringika Soni, Rakesh Kumar Ruhela, Bikash Medhi*

Department of Pharmacology, Postgraduate Institute of Medical Education & Research, Chandigarh, 160012, India.

Article info

Keywords:
· Blood brain barrier
· CNS therapeutics
· Drug delivery
· Nanotechnology
· Nanomedicine
· Nanocarrier

Abstract

Purpose: For the past few decades central nervous system disorders were considered as a major strike on human health and social system of developing countries. The natural therapeutic methods for CNS disorders limited for many patients. Moreover, nanotechnology-based drug delivery to the brain may an exciting and promising platform to overcome the problem of BBB crossing. In this review, first we focused on the role of the blood-brain barrier in drug delivery; and second, we summarized synthesis methods of nanomedicine and their role in different CNS disorder.

Method: We reviewed the PubMed databases and extracted several kinds of literature on neuro nanomedicines using keywords, CNS disorders, nanomedicine, and nanotechnology. The inclusion criteria included chemical and green synthesis methods for synthesis of nanoparticles encapsulated drugs and, their *in-vivo* and *in-vitro* studies. We excluded nanomedicine gene therapy and nanomaterial in brain imaging.

Results: In this review, we tried to identify a highly efficient method for nanomedicine synthesis and their efficacy in neuronal disorders. SLN and PNP encapsulated drugs reported highly efficient by easily crossing BBB. Although, these neuro-nanomedicine play significant role in therapeutics but some metallic nanoparticles reported the adverse effect on developing the brain.

Conclusion: Although impressive advancement has made via innovative potential drug development, but their efficacy is still moderate due to limited brain permeability. To overcome this constraint,powerful tool in CNS therapeutic intervention provided by nanotechnology-based drug delivery methods. Due to its small and biofunctionalization characteristics, nanomedicine can easily penetrate and facilitate the drug through the barrier. But still, understanding of their toxicity level, optimization and standardization are a long way to go.

Introduction

At present, the large spectrum of brain disorders classified as deficits in bot neurological and psychiatric chapters with short and long-term disabilities.[1] These deficits are the results of intrinsic brain dysfunction or environmental interaction with brain.[2] CNS disorders affect 1.5 million people worldwide and responsible for 1% deaths.[3] Out of any other disease, 11% brain disorder burden is reported[3] which might be increased to 14.7% by 2020.[4]

A variety of potential drugs has discovered to treat several neuronal disorders.[5-8] But, the therapeutic success of these pharmaceuticals is still limited due to the presence of (i) Blood-brain barrier (BBB), and (ii) Blood-cerebrospinal fluid barrier (BCSFB). It acts as anatomical and biochemical dynamic barriers in the brain.[9-11] BBB has made up by specific vascular endothelial cells that tightly bound with neurons, pericytes, and astrocytes.[12-14] Less than 1% of the traditional drug can cross this barrier,[15] therefore, BBB protects the brain from systematic circulatory molecules as well as externally injected molecules and poses a key challenge for drug delivery.[9,16] Although, there are several endogenous transporters are present in the nervous system, BBB makes treatment ineffective by interacting with enzymes and restricts the entry of neuropharmaceutical agents.[17] Hence, large dose of the drug requires to treat CNS disorders and neurotoxic effects observed in the form of physical or mental deformations.[11]

Several researchers are working on a multidisciplinary approach to nanotechnology to overcome these major obstacles in CNS therapeutics. Nanoparticles and combination with therapeutic agents may consider as an effective tool in brain drug targeting for safer therapies in future.[9,18]

In first decades PNPs, SLNS, liposomes, and micelles have used as nanocarriers in the medical field. But, now this nanotechnology approach has shifted towards newer and more advance nano-system e.g. dendrimers, nanoemulsions, nano gels and nanosuspensions.[10]

***Corresponding author:** Bikash Medhi, Email: drbikash11@rediffmail.com, drbikashmedhi@gmail.com

Traditional therapies have very little capacity to penetrate the BBB as well as null capacity for neuronal repair and neuronal regeneration.[19] Hence, functionalized nanomaterial may serve as a potential drug delivery vehicle. It can use as both *in-vivo* and *in-vitro* viz, polysorbate coated poly (butyl cyanoacrylate) (PBCA) nanomaterial interact with endothelial cells of cerebral vessels and stimulate drug delivery via endocytosis.[20] Nanotechnology combined with stem cell therapy is being increasingly used to rebuild the neural circuit and to induce specific cellular response.[18,20-22]
Recently, biofunctionalized carbon nanotubes (CNTs) have become a promising tool due to its cell-penetrating ability, surface chemistry diversity, structural, and mechanical properties.[23] In contrast, instead of having larger structure than CNT, functionalized fullerenes have identified as more efficient in CNS drug delivery[24,25] due to its higher permeability and less excitotoxity.[26]

Normal drug delivery to CNS and their challenges

For effective traditional therapy, the drug should lipid soluble with small molecular weight (400-600 Dalton's).[27] This transport can perform by invasive, non-invasive and miscellaneous techniques,[3,28] but, BBB allows restricted entry of potential drugs.[9,15,16,29] Major reasons for therapeutic failures in the brain are slow drug action, association or conversion of the drug into non-transporting legends and less neuronal absorption.[13] Some catalytic mechanisms in the nervous system also degrade the drug which performs a non-specific action or stay in inactive form in the brain.[29]

Strategies of drug delivery in brain

BBB acts as a capillary endothelial interface, that facilitates transport of essential chemical and ion to the brain.[30] Crossing BBB is always a key obstacle for drug delivery system. Hydrophilic molecules reported transferring via specific carrier-mediated endocytosis, transporter, and paracellular pathway. Lipophilic molecules have transported by diffusion and P-glycoprotein.[31] Routes of drug delivery include:

Invasive approach

This physically breached technique penetrates BBB and directly injects the drug into the brain. It requires craniotomy for intracerebroventricular (ICV) infusion and intracerebral drug administration.[31,32] BBB disruption for drug delivery performs via breaking down the tight junction of endothelial cells.[31,33] This can administer through osmotic disruption[30,34,35] or disruptive plasma solutes.[36,37] ICV drug delivery considered as a very poor approach, because the drug transported in the peripheral blood stream, less to the targeted tissues.[38] Instead of having the advancement of high molecular drug transport, ICV also restricted to limited drug distribution and loss of desired CNS action due to high intracranial pressure during direct drug administration.[39]

Pharmacological approach

This observational approach based on the free passive movement of drugs through BBB.[31,32] These molecules can cross BBB unassisted due to their small molecular size, low hydrogen bonding capacity and lipophilicity.[40] This approach also consists chemical change, e.g. reduction in number of polar groups, which increases drug transfer across the BBB.[41] But, the modified molecule may act as P-glycoprotein efflux pump, if lipophilicity increases by many folds.[31]

Physiological approach

Receptor-mediated and carrier-mediated drug delivery to the brain considered as a most advanced technique in pharmacology.[30,31] Transferrin and insulin receptors are commonly found on the BBB.32 Hence, the drug adjoins with the ligand of these receptors might transport drugs to the targeted brain area. In the case of transporter mediated delivery, the drug needs to mimic to the endogenous carrier substrate.[42] But kinetics and binding capacity of transporter molecule limit the CNS drug delivery through physiological approach.

Nano-formulated drug delivery in CNS

Conventional drug delivery strategies are unable to restore cytoarchitecture and connection pattern in CNS disorders.[43] Nanotechnologies overcome these problems due to its nanoscale quantum effect, small and high surface area to volume ratio.[44,45] Basically, nanotechnology is a convergence of science and engineering, which needs one-dimensional designing and characterization at the nanometric scale.[21] Nanoparticles used in CNS drug delivery should have following promising features:

i. They should biodegradable, non-toxic and biocompatible.[46,47]
ii. Their physical properties should easily manipulate according to mode of delivery.[48]
iii. Different nanoparticles with modified chemical properties should achieve organ- or cell- specific drug delivery.[49]
iv. The formulation should cost-effective.

In summary, all these beneficial considerations enhance CNS drug delivery.

Nano-formulation strategies

For an affecting drug delivery system in CNS treatment, nanoparticle alters the pharmacokinetics of drug48 and enhances drug loading capacity.[50] Drugs need to chemically modify and transported to the brain via loading with different nanomaterial-based vehicles.[45] It also received in the brain via transcytosis through the BBB.[31] Nanobiotechnology has made a revolutionary progress in drug delivery system. We have mentioned the properties, nanotechnology-based drug delivery, and drug release mechanism with few example of patent nanomedicine in Table 1.[51]

Table 1. Properties of different nanocarriers, drug delivery and drug release mechanism with example of patents (partially adapted from reference 51).

Type	Size (nm)	Synthesis technique	Mode of administration	Mechanism for delivery	Drug release mechanism	Example		
						Drug	disease	Patent
PNP	10-1000	• Solvent evaporation • Nanoprecipitation • Dialysis • Supercritical fluid technology • Emulsification/solvent diffusion	Subcutaneous, intravenous and oral	• Receptor-mediated endocytosis • Transcytosis	• Swelling of PNPs via diffusion • Degradation of polymer through enzymatic reaction	Chitosan-coated erythropoietin (HMG-Co-A reductase inhibitors)	Brain targeting	US20070237827
						PLGA encapsulated NMDA-NR1 vaccine	Alzheimer's disease	US20100173004
SLN	50-1000	• High-pressure homogenization • Ultrasonication • Microemulsification • Supercritical fluid technique • Spray drying technique	Nasal, oral, parenteral, rectal and respiratory	• Absorption	• High-pressure homogenization causes dispersed molecular drug in solid solution • Supersaturation of SLN-drug conjugates at high cooling	LDL-cholesterol conjugates	AD, PD, and cancer	US7682627
						LDL nanoparticles	Epilepsy, stroke, Trauma and AD	US20060222716
Micelles	80-100	• Self-assembly • Ring-opening polymerization	Pulmonary delivery	Receptor-mediated transport, absorption, and endocytosis	Bursting, diffusion, and cleavage	doxorubicin, vincristine sulphate loaded poly (L-histidine)-poly(ethylene glycol) block copolymer and PLEG poly micelles	Cancer	US7659314
						Paclitaxel-loaded copolymer micelle	Lung cancer	NCT01023347
Nanoliposomes	Less than 100	• High-pressure homogenization	Pulmonary delivery, intravenous,	Adsorption, fusion and diffusion/ endocytosis	Endocytosis and Adsorption to cell surface Bursting due to environmental stimuli	Glutathione encapsulated liposomes	Myoclonus	US20100166846
						Tempamine loaded liposome	Multiple sclerosis and PD	US20110027351
CNTs	Diameter of 3.5-70nm	• Arc discharge method • Chemical vapors deposition • Laser ablation method • Flame synthesis method	mainly intraperitoneal and intravenous	Endocytosis, diffusion, penetration	Electrically or chemical controlled	Streptavidin-HRP (Horseradish peroxidase) bounded SWCNT-annexin conjugates	Breast cancer	US201001846691 A1
						Stem cell loaded CNT	AD, PD, and ischemia	US20090148417A1
Dendrimers	Diameter range 1.5-13.5	• Divergent method-Micheal reaction • Convergent method • Click chemistry-Diels_alder reactions, azide-alkyne reaction, and thiol-yne reactions • Hypercore & branched monomers	Oral, transdermal, topical, IV	Transcytosis and endocytosis	Degradation and environmental stimuli	Anxiolytic and antipsychotic agents	Psychotic disorder	US20100160299

Nanotechnology-based drug delivery vehicles

The nanotechnology-based drug administration has shown significant advantages over traditional drug delivery. The different nanoformulation carrier has used for targeted drug delivery, some of them are Nanoparticles (NP), lipid-based vehicle, carbon nanostructure-based vehicle and polymer based vehicle; as shown in Figure 1. We are discussing important nano drug carrier in the following section.

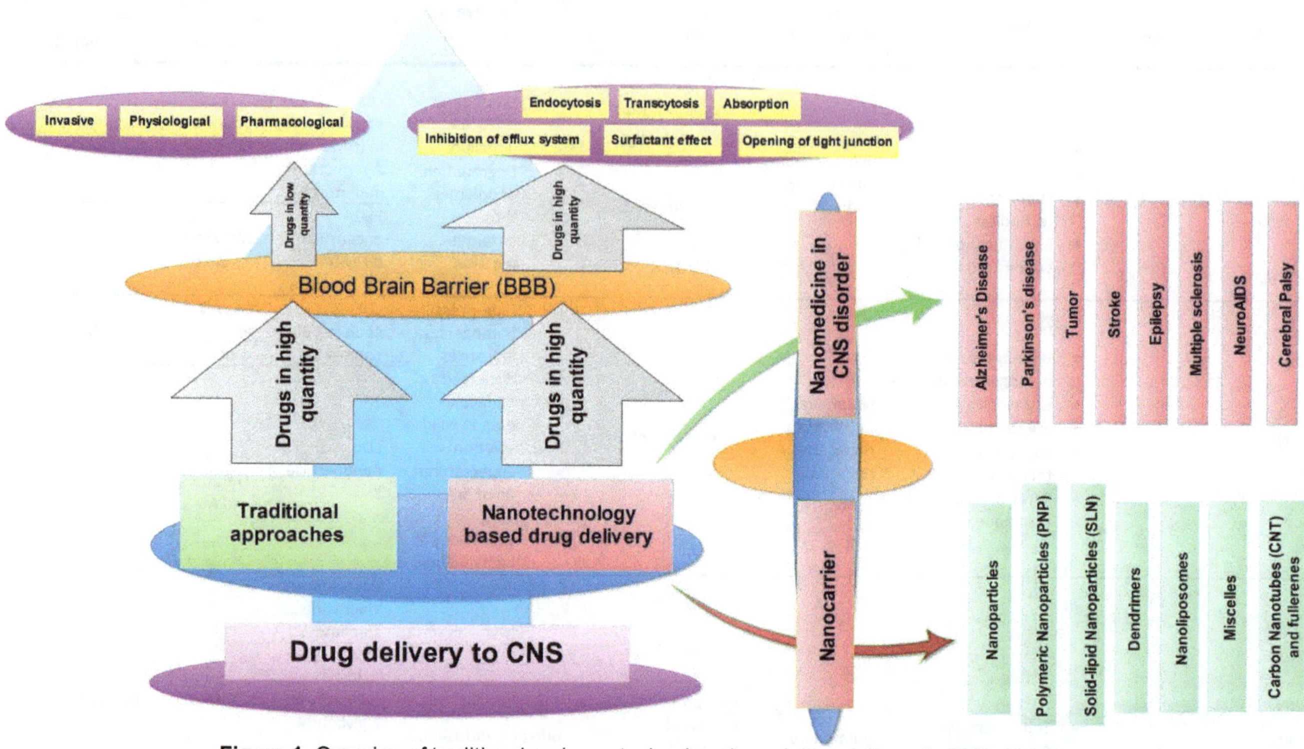

Figure 1. Overview of traditional and nanotechnology based drug delivery in CNS disorders

Nanoparticle

The inorganic nanoparticle of size 10-1000nm recently elicited much interest due to their chemical and biological properties. Several features of nanoparticles show significant advantages to overcome problems associated with traditional drug delivery, which includes: high drug carrying capacity, high stability, controlled release, high specificity and hydrophilic and hydrophobic molecules transportability.[52] Drug-loaded nanoparticles release to target site via diffusion, degradation, erosion or due to external energy input.[53] Protein and ceramic NP are most commonly used in targeted drug delivery.[54]

Easy functionalization property and good biocompatibility of modified molecule are the key requirements to select an effective route for prepare different sized NP.[55] Drug delivery through gold nanoparticles (AuNP) gives a versatile platform for effective drug delivery. Doxorubicin coated AuNP have reported making enhanced drug accumulation by overcoming multidrug resistance (MDR) in cancer treatment.[56] Similarly, curcumin conjugated AuNP also shows haemocompatibility, resulting in antitumor activity in leukemia.[57] Recent research on imatinib mesylate (IM) encapsulated, layer by layer coated functionalized AuNP, demonstrated rapid delivery into murine melanoma cells in mice.[58] This topical application for iontophoretic IM delivery shows effective cancer treatment. Chitosan derived mitochondrial targeted multifunctional NP (MNPs) performs lysosomal escape, multistage pH response, and mitochondrial and hepatocyte targeting for safe and targeted anticancer drug delivery.[59]

Polymeric nanoparticles (PNPs)

Polymeric nanoparticles are a particulate dispersion of biodegradable and biocompatible polymers with size 10-1000nm. The core-shell structure of PNP varies with hydrophilic and hydrophobic blocks present in the polymer chain.[60] The core of these PNP made up of a dense polymer matrix to encapsulate the hydrophobic drug and hydrophilic polymers in corona to serve steric stability and stealth properties to NP.[61] Drug delivery through PNP were also performed via drug encapsulation, absorption or chemically linked to surface.[62]

Availability of polymer choice and drug release from nanoparticle makes them unique candidates for drug delivery. Biologically inert polymers PEG (Polyethylene glycol), PLGA (poly-L- glutamic acid),[43] poly(alkyl cyanoacrylate), and poly(butyl) cyanoacrylate are most common used formulated nanopolymers. Level of drug release is not only controlled by molecular weight & polymer composition, drug-to-polymer ratio also affects as well.[63]

The role of PNP's in drug delivery can also consider non-replaceable. Doxorubicin loaded nanoparticles used to treat glioblastoma[64] and quinoline derivatives loaded polymeric nanoparticles used in Alzheimer's disease (AD).[65] Similarly, nano gels, a crosslinked polymer[66] and nanosuspensions, mixture of crystalline drug and nonionic surfactants[67] provide excellent pharmacokinetics control in CNS disorders.[68]

Solid-lipid nanoparticles (SLN)

SLN is surfactant stabilized lipid oily droplet, which is generally solid at room temperature.[54] It considered as a colloidal nano drug carrier that synthesized by homogenization of melted lipid at high pressure while dispersing in water at 70 ^{0}C with a nanometric range of 50-1000nm.[69,70] It also exhibits physical stability and easy manufacturing; hence it replaces liposomal technology in drug delivery.[71] SLN particles conjugate with lipid emulsions that can stabilize by high-level surfactant inclusions and protect from degradation.[72] The active part or drug to transported is administrated via loading or coating with nanoparticles.[73]

Recently, self-amplifying RNA in SLN nanoparticles has demonstrated the importance of lipid nanoparticle in nucleic acid vaccine development.[74] The effect of different SLN conjugated drug is widely investigated in CNS treatment. Quercetin loaded SLN shows the antioxidant property to treat AD[75] and diminazene aceturate loaded SLN particles used to treat human African trypanosomiasis (HAT).[76] Similarly, 3',5'-dioctanoyl-5-fluoro-2'-deoxyuridine (DO-FUdR) incorporated SLN used to treat neurological disorders.[77] (3H)-atazanavir loaded SLN also crossed the BBB in HIV-encephalitis treatment.[78]

Dendrimers

Highly branched dendrimers made up of a focal core, building blocks with repetitive units in interior layers and peripheral functional units.[79] Other than synthesis routes, the functionality, and efficacy of dendrimers depend on upon the used monomer and targeted polymer structure.[80] Low dispersity and high functionality of these dendrimers offer themselves as a useful therapeutic tool in biomedical and pharmaceutical science.[81] High penetration ability, high density, and peripheral functional group reactivity also considered as featured advantages as a drug vehicle.[82] The terminal surface group, biocompatibility, and multivalency of three-dimensional dendrimers have displayed their importance in emerging with Nanomedicine.[83] Polyamidoamine (PAMAM), polypropylene imine (PPI), and polylysine dendrimers are the most commonly used dendrimeric drug carrier for both hydrophobic and hydrophilic drug molecule.[84] Drug either physically entraps with dendrimer, or covalently bound with peripheral functionalized molecules of dendrimer to form dendrimer-drug conjugates.[79] The complexities of their bounding keep the chemical integrity and pharmaceutical properties of the drug.

In further research, cholesterol loaded poly (amidoamine) dendrimers reported neuroinflammation treatment.[85] Similarly, multi-functionalized CMCht/PAMAM dendrimer nanoparticles incorporation with antibody also played an important role in specific CNS targeting.[86] Different dendrimers such as PAMAM, polyester-copolyester (PEPE) and PPI, shows anticancer and anti-inflammatory properties to treat several neurological disorders.[87]

Nanoliposome

These lipid nanoparticles are the most studied bilayer vehicle, developed in drug delivery in the 70's.[88] Less than 100nm sized nanoliposomes may consider as an advanced form of SLN that includes nanostructured lipid carrier (NLC), nanoemulsions and lipid nanocapsules (LNC).[54] The distorted structure of NLC provides enough space to accommodate active drug molecule which can develop by mixing lipid droplet into solid media at very high temperature.[54] Combination of liposomes and nanoemulsion particle gives rise to LNCs (less than 100nm) with thicker outer wall that allows more functionalization and controlled targeted drug delivery.[89]

The lipid, oily core of LNCs surrounded by lipophilic and hydrophobic surfactant that improves therapeutic drug delivery.[42] Liposomal technique emerged with pegylation for targeted brain drug delivery[41] which optimized the plasma pharmacokinetics. Neurotrophic agents loaded liposomes used in brain disorders.[90] Pegylated liposomes loaded with doxorubicin and (3H)-Prednisolone treats brain tumors[91] and autoimmune encephalitis[92] respectively. OX26 monoclonal antibody-mediated antineoplastic agent, (3H) daunomycin, conjugate with a liposome and exhibit brain drug delivery.[93] Similarly, heat shock protein (HSP) encapsulated liposomes also used in the stroke treatment.[94]

Micelles

Micelles are monolayered spherical lipid nanostructures with inwards facing hydrophobic ends and outwards facing hydrophilic ends with a range of 80-100nm.[95] Due to its small, the micelles shows short circulation time in body compares to liposomes that make them easily transportable elements.[54] Polymeric micelles considered as more stable with longevity and good biodistribution compare to traditional micelles.[96] These modified micelles show improved target penetration due to their nanoscale size, easy transportation to target location, and low critical association concentration (CMC).[97] Physically entrapped and covalently bonded micelles drug conjugate play an important role in controlled drug release system.[98] Drug loading to micelles generally depends on upon the physiochemical property of drug, the chemical composition of core forming polymers, and physical state of micelles core.[99] The release is generally affected by temperature, pH, and environment.[100]

Carbon Nanotubes and fullerenes

CNT exhibits advanced physical, mechanical property, and high aspect ratio at the nanometer scale of less than 100nm.[101] Functionalized CNT shows high solubility and high biocompatibility which generally depends on upon surface property, size and shape of modified molecules.[102] These parameters greatly influence the internalization of therapeutic molecules inside the cell. CNT functionalization strategies include the addition of an organic group at sidewall/tip of CNTs and carboxyl group coupling after oxidation process.[103] Polymers and dendrimer conjugated CNTs also reduces aggregation, increases their solubility and biocompatibility.[104] Very few studies of the CNT in CNS treatment have been reported, yet acetylcholine loaded SWCNT (Single wall carbon nanotube) studied in the AD treatment[105] and CNT with stem cell therapy used in stroke treatment.[106] Amphotericin B loaded CNT showed lower aggregation, high solubility with reduced toxicity, and anti-fungal activity compares to administration of amphotericin B alone.[107]

Carbon nano horns and nanodiamonds modified the form of CNT which reported enhancing the nanotechnology application in biosciences and pharmaceutical industry.[54] Diamond nanoparticles also used as an important therapeutic tool in tumor patches and wound healing.[108] Fullerene has uniquely identified a class of carbon allotropes which described as 60 linked carbon with 60 vertices and 32 faces.[109] The extensive research on nanosized C60 have identified its use in drug delivery.[110] Their antioxidant and radical oxygen quenching character made them more promising than any other nanomaterial.[111] Hydrated C60 fullerene prevents astrocytes and glial fibrillary acidic proteins (GFAP) damage which caused by oxidative stress and improves cognitive function.[112]

Nanoparticle-mediated drug transport mechanism

For effective drug treatment, nanomedicine needs to cross the BBB without losing its properties. There are several possibilities for this translocation: Absorption, opening of tight junctions, endocytosis, transcytosis, surfactant effect, and inhibition of efflux system.[113]

i. Polysorbate coated dalargin nanoparticle reported to induce an antinociceptive effect (surfactant effect) and created high concentration gradient which helps to transport nanomedicine.[47]

ii. Polysorbate-80 coated nanoparticle also unfolded the tight junction and increases inulin space without disrupting BBB.[114]

iii. At present, endocytosis is considered as the most likely mechanism of nanomedicine transport. Polysorbate-80 coated PBCA nanoparticle endocytotic transport studied by laser confocal microscopy and significant and rapid uptake of coated nanoparticles were observed, rather than uncoated nanoparticle.[115]

iv. Dipalmitoyl phosphatidyl choline cholesterol-coated malto-dextrin nanoparticle transcytosis through BBB and upregulated the LDL receptor expression in a cholesterol-depleted model system.[116]

CNS disorder and nanomedicine

Recent trends of nano-therapeutics advance over traditional drug therapy in CNS disorders via its proper property to cross the BBB.[19,117] Nanotechnology used in for both diagnoses (imaging) and treatment, here we will discuss *in-vivo* drug delivery system in CNS disorders.

Alzheimer's disease

Alzheimer's disease (AD) recognized as a progressive neurodegenerative disorder, which characterized by memory loss and dementia.[118] Pieces of evidence support inclined graph of AD patients with prevalence rate 0.62% and 1.07% in people with age +55 and +65 years respectively. Estimated data are much scaring as 24.3 million people globally affected by dementia and each year 4.6 million cases reported.[119,120] Amyloid-β aggregation considered as hallmarks of AD.[121] Other than this, wide spectrum of AD pathology covers genetic change of EpoE protein, mitochondrial abnormalities, oxidative stress, and dysfunction of D-serine.[122-124]

Insufficient use of oral administrated drugs for AD, such as tacrine, memantine, rivastigmine etc, pulls the door open for nanomedicine in neurodegenerative disorders.[125,126] Cerium oxide nanoparticles,[127] SLN of ferulic acid,[128] tempol loaded PLGA nanoparticles,[129] and epigallocatechin-3-gallate (EGCG) phenol coated nanolipids[130] reported to show antioxidant property and degrade amyloid-β.[131] Thioflavin-T (ThT), charged and fluorescent biomarker, detect Aβ in senile plaques. Therefore, ThT encapsulated polymerized but cyanoacrylate NP injected directly into intrahippocampal space, and light microscopy and TEM analysis confirmed Aβ in AD brain.[132] Cu (I) chelator and MBP-PE induced D- penicillamine nanoparticles were also used tauopathies detection in AD brain.[133] Nanofabricated quinoline derivative, clioquinol (5-chloro-7-iodo-8-hydroxyquinoline,CQ), was reported to inhibit Aβ when it was functionalized with n-butyl cyanoacrylate and PBCA nanoparticle.[65] Imbalance in Ach of the cholinergic nervous system also reported in AD and free Ach could not inject into the brain directly, because it is easier to decompose in the blood and high polarities.[134] Curcumin nanoparticles have been also identified as important finding in AD treatment.[135]

Parkinson Disease

Increasing lifespan and demographic changes in population demonstrates increased prevalence of Parkinson disease (PD).[136] 50+ people in world's most 10 populous countries have around 4.6 million PD patients, which might be 9.3 million by 2030 with a rate of 1 per 100.[137,138] A hallmark of PD is gliosis and degeneration of dopaminergic neurons in the substantia nigra are not the only features of PD. It also involves selective denervation,[139] dysfunctions in the mitochondrial and ubiquitin-proteosome system, and oxidative and nitrosative stress.[140] Available drugs for PD neither surpass nor reverse disease progression[141] and BBB causes additional challenge in drug delivery.[142]

Nanotechnologies control and manipulate the drug delivery in PD to overcome these problems. Recent research has demonstrated that nerve growth factor (NGF) bound poly butyl cyanoacrylate nanoparticles[143] and L-Dopa encapsulated nanoparticles[48] crosses BBB and reduces basic symptoms of PD. Physically modified saline RNS60 with charged-stabilized nanobubbles, suppresses the proinflammatory molecules in MPTP-induced animal model of PD.[144] Similarly, coumarin-6 loaded lactoferrin conjugated PEG-PLGA nanoparticle show important role in neuroprotection in Parkinson disease.[145]

Tumor

Upward trends of brain tumor show increased incident rate with 6/100,000 for malignant brain tumors in the adult.[146] Male shows higher susceptibility than female with increasing age at a rate of 8.5 v/s 7.9 per 100,000 that have increased 5-6 folds by now.[147,148] Drug therapy is less effective in brain tumor because of less infiltration of tumor cells from normal cells[149] and less microvascular permeability of BBB.[150]

To overcome these problems, nanoformulation drug therapy is widely used an alternative approach. Gold porphyrin or camptothecin encapsulated lipid nanoparticles enhanced drug delivery to tumor tissue with a low side effect to the liver.[151] Nanotechnology-based drug delivery used in cancer treatment with a combination of gene and radiotherapy.[152] Nanotechnology in chemotherapy enhances efficacy to treat glioblastoma. DOX-loaded nanodiamond exhibit excellent cell biocompatibility and increase apoptosis of glioma cell lines.[153] MWCNTs (Multiwall carbon nanotube) showed a high level of internalization of macromolecules in microglial cells and their molecular modulation helped in immunotherapy of cancer.[154] Folic acid (as targeting agent) and methotrexate conjugated PAMAM dendritic polymers bind to tumor cell which overexpressed for folate receptor in cancer treatment.[155] Boron-enriched nanocomposites of copolymerized acetal-poly(ethylene glycol)-*block*-poly(lactide)-methacrylate with 4-vinylbenzyl substituted *closo*-carborane demonstrated high incorporation and hemocompatibility.[156]

NeuroAIDS

NeuroAIDS drags both infectious and neurological pathophysiologic pathways under one umbrella, in which HIV1 (Human Immunodeficiency Virus 1) enters in the CNS in the early stage of infection.[157] Approximately 15-30% of AIDS patients experiences several neurological and neurocognitive complications in which 7.3-11.3% and 30-60% experienced dementia and encephalopathy respectively.[158,159] BBB disruption is not the only mechanism in neuroAIDS, activated endothelial cells with decreased permeability of the barrier[160] and CD 163, Glut5 & ISG15 genes[161] are also shown deleterious effect. Currently, there are no effective vaccines or specific drug therapy for NeuroAIDS,[162] therefore, multidisciplinary approach to nanotechnology shed light on potential therapeutic approaches in HIV infection.

Nanoformulated antiretroviral therapy (ART) reported increasing blood-brain penetration in neuroAIDS treatment. Indinavir (IDV) NP loaded murine bone marrow macrophages (BMM) cause reduced HIV-1 replication in HIVE (HIV-1 encephalitis) region of the brain.[163] Their research also demonstrated the role of NP loaded BMM in studying targeted migration and antiretroviral responses. Nanotechnology-based, highly active antiretroviral therapy (HAART) also played a significant role in neurosis treatment.[164] Several antiretroviral drugs, zidovudine, delavirdine, saquinavir, and lamivudine, were nanoformulation with PBCA, MMSPM (methylmethacrylate–sulfopropyl methacrylate), polylactide (PLA) and PLGA that increases BBP 10-20 folds.[165] Liposome loaded AZT-myristate and zalcitabine were also reported with improved efficacy and longer half-life compare to traditional ARV drug treatment.[166] SLN loaded ARV drugs recently come into a highlight. Large surface area and high efficacy of SLN coated delavirdine and saquinavir ARV drug replaced MMSPM coated ARV drug treatment in neuroAIDS.[162]

Stroke

With second place, stroke is affecting mortality rates of 6,000,000 deaths annually with estimated susceptibility of 8-10% of lifetime.[167] 1.2% deaths in India reported due to this in which 87% caused by ischemia and the remaining is due to hemorrhage.[168] Glutamate excitotoxity, oxidative stress, lipid peroxidation, BBB dysfunction, leukocyte infiltration and brain injuries play an important role in the pathophysiology of stroke.[169,170] BBB and blood-cerebrospinal-fluid barrier (BCSFB) are the main issues in stroke drug delivery,[171] so optimization and efficiency of drug carriers are needed to improve.

The new, unusual perspective of nanotechnologies in stroke therapy is *'jeevandayani'* (life protecting).[37] One researcher used engineering triiodothyronine (T3) nanoparticle coated with PLGA-PEG and enhanced neuroprotection observed compared to glutathione alone.[172] Cerium oxide nanoparticles also showed neuroprotective naturally in the rodent stroke model. Cerium oxide nanoparticle reduces the 3-nitrotyrosine level, which was generally induced by peroxynitrite radical during the stroke.[173] Similarly, platinum nanoparticles showed their antioxidant property which reported lowering cerebral cortex volume and improved motor function in stroke animal model.[174] Irreversible caspase-3 inhibitor loaded transferrin targeted nanospheres provide a reduction in infarct volume in ischemic brain.[175] SiRNA loaded carbon nanotube also documented as potential therapeutics in stroke treatment.[37] Transferrin-coupled liposomes promote vascular regeneration and neuroprotection via delivering vascular endothelial growth factor (VEGF) in stroke treatment.[176] The stroke damage can also recover by progenitor stem cell differentiation when it impregnated with CNT.[106]

Cerebral palsy

Cerebral palsy (CP) is one of the major neurodevelopmental disorders in children that considered as chronic & non-progressive in nature.[177] It causes motor dysfunction, serve paralysis[178] and musculoskeletal problems in 2-3 per 1000 children[179] with a male/female ratio of 1.4:1.[180] Unfortunately, there is no effective cure available for CP due to unknown molecular and biochemical mechanisms involvement.[181] But researchers show the wide interest to use Nanoscience used drug delivery in CP.

PAMAM dendrimers and dendrimer-based N-acetyl-L-cysteine administration suppress neuroinflammation & motor dysfunction in CP patients.[182] Stem cell therapy with nanomedicine has also come in the limelight recently to cure CP via promoting repair and regeneration of injured neurons.[183]

Epilepsy

Epilepsy is leading in all CNS disorders with a rate of 57 per 1000 people[184] which might increase as in 5.5 million patients by the year 2001 in India.[185] Abnormal neuronal discharges considered linking with oxygen deprivation, trauma, tumors and infections that cause neuronal excitability[186] and neuroinflammatory cytokine dysfunction in epilepsy.[187] The adverse effect of anti-epileptic drugs,[188] promotes the use of nanoparticle-loaded drugs with the ability to cross the BBB and direct drug delivery.[189] Carbamazepine loaded solid lipid nanoparticles of chitosan reported to be more effective than nano emulged loaded carbamazepine.[190] Similarly, poly (d,l-lactide-co-glycolide) nanoparticle loaded β-carotene anticonvulsant considered more effective when it coated with polysorbate-80.[191]

Multiple sclerosis

Multiple sclerosis (MS) considered as an autoimmune neurodegenerative disease with chronic inflammatory processes.[192] Modification of myelin basic protein (MBP) and glial fibrillary acidic protein (GFAP) triggers lesions in white matter[192] that causes MS. Advanced stage of MS causes demyelination and tissue damage due to oxidative stress are found higher in the patients.[193] Ultra sized cerium oxide nanoparticles declines oxidative stress and alleviates motor deficits in MS brain.[194]

Challenges

Emerging nanotechnology with neurosciences is like a game of risk and gain. Currently, Nanomedicine considered as a successful tool in drug delivery via crossing the BBB.[195,196] These nano drugs are in the process of clinical trials, but their proper transport and safety concerns are yet to be determined.[1,45] The composition and properties of nanoparticles may lead to oxidative stress, amino acid disturbance and BBB disruption,[196,197] that causes neurotoxicity in the brain. Although functionalized nanoparticles pose successful drug targeting, but their nano-size structure and the large surface area may result in particle aggregation and limited drug loading.[65,198] State of aggregation and mechanical properties affects nanoparticles toxicity which basically depends on preparation and purification methods. Hence, one should select a proper method to reduce toxicity.

Toxicity concerns of nanomedicine delivery based on their mode of drug administration and a measure of the drug; which causes neuroinflammation, excitotoxicity, DNA damage and allergic responses.[199] Therefore, biocompatibility and biodegradability of nano drug are also needed to understand.

As Nanomedicine need to interact with neurons at a systemic level to show their effect. But, multidimensional cellular interaction at neuronal level and restricted anatomical access increase the challenges in nano-drug delivery system.[21] The primary function of CNS needed to preserve before drug administration which also a big challenge itself.[200]

Conclusion

CNS disorders are a most serious problem in this industrialized world. Nanotechnology has proven very advanced and promising science which provides easily targeted drug delivery to the brain. But, we still need to gain more knowledge about their properties and features to evaluate their dynamic behavior in biomedical science.[201] At present, we don't have any multidimensional drug for different CNS disorders that may result of several individual biochemical pathways.[21] Nanodrugs may lead to solving this problem.

Sometimes, few diseases viz, diabetes, trauma or some of the psychotic diseases, also associated with the neurological disorder. Hence, nanomedicine requires achieving termination of these entire co-morbidity factors with fewer side effects. Other than this, Genetic manipulation in the neuronal cell is also considered as a difficult target, so nanotechnology-based drug delivery should potentially efficacious approach in CNS treatment.

Polymer-based gold nanoparticles and CNT nano drugs have very few clinical trials, but due to their noble physical and mechanical strength, they may useful to carry the drug whose transport is still unidentified.

Although, the nanoparticle-based drug has several advantages, but many aspects are still matters of concern. So far there is no specific method to identify the toxicity level and targeted drug release in the CNS. Hence, the current nanotechnology application needs to improve further, so that it can be safe and target oriented.[68]

In recent years, some nanomedicine registered for patents in complex CNS treatment, which are following: Gold nanoparticle (US2011262546, US2011111040), lipid nanoparticle (WO2008024753, WO2008018932), chitosan nanoparticle (US2010260686) and SLN (US2011208161).[1]

Increasing population and increasing brain disorders are calling for the urgent need of new promising therapies. Involvements of nanotechnology in neurosciences will unmet medical need and give a hope to patients. The new generation nanomedicine might control prolonged and targeted drug delivery in a specific manner. Instead of reduced side effect and increased viability of nano drug, we still need to improve nanotechnological methods in pharmaceuticals for better comprehension and improved life quality. It can not be denied the potential benefit of nanomedicines, but their opportunity and risk formula also point towards hazardous effects. Due to the high ongoing emergence of nanotechnology in today's research, one just cannot throw it away due to its negative points only. Specific guidelines should follow to avoid the most harmful effect of nanotechnology. It can also predict that nanotechnology-based drug delivery can revolutionize the era of traditional drugs delivery and that modified drug will be incredibly efficient from the current standard.

Conflict of Interest

The authors report no conflicts of interest in this work.

References

1. Spuch C, Saida O, Navarro C. Advances in the Treatment of Neurodegenerative Disorders Employing Nanoparticles. *Recent Pat Drug Deliv Formul* 2012;6(1):2-18.
2. Hyman S, Chisholm D, Kessler R, Petal V, Whiteford H. Mental Disorders. In: Jamsion DT, Breman JG, Measham AR, Alleyne G, Claeson M, Evans DB, et al, editors. Disease control priorities in developing countries. New York: Oxford University Press; 2006. P. 605-25.
3. Domínguez A, Álvarez A, Hilario E, Suarez-Merino B, Goñi-de-Cerio F. Central nervous system diseases and the role of the blood-brain barrier in their treatment. *Neurosci Discov* 2013;1(3):1-11. doi: 10.7243/2052-6946-1-3
4. Menken M, Munsat TL, Toole JF. The global burden of disease study: implications for neurology. *Arch Neurol* 2000;57(3):418-20. doi: 10.1001/archneur.57.3.418
5. Whiting PJ. GABA-A receptor subtypes in the brain: A paradigm for CNS drug discovery? *Drug Discov Today* 2003;8(10):445-50. doi: 10.1016/S1359-6446(03)02703-X
6. Alguacil LF, Perez-Garcia C. Histamine H3 receptor: a potential drug target for the treatment of central nervous system disorders. *Curr Drug Targets CNS Neurol Disord* 2003;2(5):303-13. doi: 10.2174/1568007033482760
7. Langmead CJ, Watson J, Reavill C. Muscarinic acetylcholine receptors as CNS drug targets. *Pharmacol Ther* 2008;117(2):232-43. doi: 10.1016/j.pharmthera.2007.09.009
8. Sproule BA, Naranjo CA, Brenmer KE, Hassan PC. Selective serotonin reuptake inhibitors and CNS drug interactions. A critical review of the evidence. *Clin Pharmacokinet* 1997;33(6):454-71. doi: 10.2165/00003088-199733060-00004
9. Jain KK. Nanobiotechnology-based drug delivery to the central nervous system. *Neurodegener Dis* 2007;4(4):287-91. doi: 10.1159/000101884
10. Wong HL, Wu XY, Bendayan R. Nanotechnological advances for the delivery of CNS therapeutics. *Adv Drug Deliv Rev* 2012;64(7):686-700. doi: 10.1016/j.addr.2011.10.007
11. Domínguez A, Álvarez A, Suárez-Merino B, Goñi-de-Cerio F. Neurological disorders and the blood-brain barrier. Strategies and limitations for drug delivery to the brain. *Rev Neurol* 2014;58(5):213-24.
12. Pardridge WM. Strategies for Drug Delivery through the Blood-Brain Barrier. In: Borchardt RT, Repta AJ, Stella VJ, editors. Directed Drug Delivery: A Multidisciplinary Approach. Clifton, NJ: Humana Press; 1985. P. 83-96.
13. Tamai I, Tsuji A. Drug delivery through the blood-brain barrier. *Adv Drug Deliv Rev* 1996;19(3):401-24. doi: 10.1016/0169-409X(96)00011-7
14. Tajes M, Ramos-Fernández E, Weng-Jiang X, Bosch-Morató M, Guivernau B, Eraso-Pichot A, et al. The blood-brain barrier: Structure, function and therapeutic approaches to cross it. *Mol Membr Biol* 2014;31(5):152-67. doi: 10.3109/09687688.2014.937468
15. Stockwell J, Abdi N, Lu X, Maheshwari O, Taghibiglou C. Novel central nervous system drug delivery systems. *Chem Biol Drug Des* 2014;83(5):507-20. doi: 10.1111/cbdd.12268
16. Yi X, Manickam DS, Brynskikh A, Kabanov AV. Agile delivery of protein therapeutics to CNS. *J Control Release* 2014;190:637-63. doi: 10.1016/j.jconrel.2014.06.017
17. Alam MI, Beg S, Samad A, Baboota S, Kohli K, Ali J, et al. Strategy for effective brain drug delivery. *Eur J Pharm Sci* 2010;40(5):385-403. doi: 10.1016/j.ejps.2010.05.003
18. Halberstadt C, Emerich DF, Gonsalves K. Combining cell therapy and nanotechnology. *Expert Opin Biol Ther* 2006;6(10):971-81. doi: 10.1517/14712598.6.10.971
19. Emerich DF, Orive G, Borlongan C. Tales of biomaterials, molecules, and cells for repairing and treating brain dysfunction. *Curr Stem Cell Res Ther* 2011;6(3):171-89. doi: 10.2174/157488811796575350
20. Aliautdin RN, Kreuter J, Kharkevich DA. Drug delivery to the brain with nanoparticles. *Eksp Klin Farmakol* 2003;66(2):65-8.
21. Silva GA. Nanotechnology approaches for the regeneration and neuroprotection of the central

nervous system. *Surg Neurol* 2005;63(4):301-6. doi: 10.1016/j.surneu.2004.06.008
22. Orive G, Anitua E, Pedraz JL, Emerich DF. Biomaterials for promoting brain protection, repair and regeneration. *Nat Rev Neurosci* 2009;10(9):682-92. doi: 10.1038/nrn2685
23. Hwang JY, Shin US, Jang WC, Hyun JK, Wall IB, Kim HW. Biofunctionalized carbon nanotubes in neural regeneration: a mini-review. *Nanoscale* 2013;5(2):487-97. doi: 10.1039/c2nr31581e
24. Matsumura Y, Maeda H. A new concept for macromolecular therapeutics in cancer chemotherapy: mechanism of tumoritropic accumulation of proteins and the antitumor agent smancs. *Cancer Res* 1986;46(12 Pt 1):6387-92.
25. Segal E, Satchi-Fainaro R. Design and development of polymer conjugates as anti-angiogenic agents. *Adv Drug Deliv Rev* 2009;61(13):1159-76. doi: 10.1016/j.addr.2009.06.005
26. Chen YW, Hwang KC, Yen CC, Lai YL. Fullerene derivatives protect against oxidative stress in RAW 264.7 cells and ischemia-reperfused lungs. *Am J Physiol Regul Integr Comp Physiol* 2004;287(1):R21-6. doi: 10.1152/ajpregu.00310.2003
27. Pardridge WM. Drug delivery to the brain. *J Cereb Blood Flow Metab* 1997;17(7):713-31. doi: 10.1097/00004647-199707000-00001
28. Pathan SA, Iqbal Z, Zaidi SM, Talegaonkar S, Vohra D, Jain GK, et al. CNS drug delivery systems: novel approaches. *Recent Pat Drug Deliv Formul* 2009;3(1):71-89. doi: 10.2174/187221109787158355
29. Crone C. The blood-brain barrier: a modified tight epithelium. In: Suckling AJ, Rumsby MG, Bradbury MWB, editors. The blood-brain barrier in health and disease. Chichester: Ellis Horwood Ltd; 1986. P. 17-40.
30. Upadhyay RK. Drug Delivery Systems, CNS Protection, and the Blood Brain Barrier. *Biomed Res Int* 2014;2014:869269. doi: 10.1155/2014/869269
31. Stenehjem DD, Hartz AM, Bauer B, Anderson GW. Novel and emerging strategies in drug delivery for overcoming the blood-brain barrier. *Future Med Chem* 2009;1(9):1623-41. doi: 10.4155/fmc.09.137
32. Gabathuler R. Approaches to transport therapeutic drugs across the blood-brain barrier to treat brain diseases. *Neurobiol Dis* 2010;37(1):48-57. doi: 10.1016/j.nbd.2009.07.028
33. Inamura T, Black KL. Bradykinin selectively opens blood-tumor barrier in experimental brain tumors. *J Cereb Blood Flow Metab* 1994;14(5):862-70. doi: 10.1038/jcbfm.1994.108
34. Neuwelt EA, Goldman DL, Dahlborg SA, Crossen J, Ramsey F, Roman-Goldstein S, et al. Primary CNS lymphoma treated with osmotic blood-brain barrier disruption: prolonged survival and preservation of cognitive function. *J Clin Onc*ol 1991;9(9):1580-90.
35. Rapoport SI. Osmotic opening of the blood-brain barrier: Principles, mechanism, and therapeutic applications. *Cell Mol Neurobiol* 2000;20(2):217-30
36. Erdlenbruch B, Schinkhof C, Kugler W, Heinemann DE, Herms J, Eibl H, et al. Intracarotid administration of short-chain alkylglycerols for increased delivery of methotrexate to the rat brain. *Br J Pharmacol* 2003;139(4):685-94. doi: 10.1038/sj.bjp.0705302
37. Lee HJ, Park J, Yoon OJ, Kim HW, Lee DY, Kim do H, et al. Amine-modified single-walled carbon nanotubes protect neurons from injury in a rat stroke model. *Nat Nanotechnol* 2011;6(2):121-5. doi: 10.1038/nnano.2010.281
38. Aird RB. A study of intrathecal, cerebrospinal fluid-to-brain exchange. *Exp Neurol* 1984;86(2):342-58. doi: 10.1016/0014-4886(84)90192-4
39. Zhang Y, Miller DW. Pathways for drug delivery to the Central nervous system. In: Wang B, Siahaan TJ, Soltero R, editors. Drug delivery: Principles and applications. New Jersey: John Wiley and Sons; 2005. P. 29-56.
40. Lipinski CA, Lombardo F, Dominy BW, Feeney PJ. Experimental and computational approaches to estimate solubility and permeability in drug discovery and development settings. *Adv Drug Deliv Rev* 2001;46(1-3):3-26. doi: 10.1016/S0169-409X(00)00129-0
41. Pardridge WM. CNS drug design based on principles of blood-brain barrier transport. *J Neurochem* 1998;70(5):1781-92. doi: 10.1046/j.1471-4159.1998.70051781.x
42. Allen TM, Cullis PR. Liposomal drug delivery systems: From concept to clinical applications. *Adv Drug Deliv Rev* 2013;65(1):36-48. doi: 10.1016/j.addr.2012.09.037
43. Modi G, Pillay V, Choonara YE, Ndesendo VM, du Toit LC, Naidoo D. Nanotechnological applications for the treatment of neurodegenerative disorders. *Prog Neurobiol* 2009;88(4):272-85. doi: 10.1016/j.pneurobio.2009.05.002
44. Ochekpe NA, Olorunfemi PO, Ngwuluka NC. Nanotechnology and drug delivery part 1: Background and applications. *Trop J Pharm Res* 2009;8(3):265-74. doi: 10.4314/tjpr.v8i3.44546
45. Dinda SC, Pattnaik G. Nanobiotechnology-based drug delivery in brain targeting. *Curr Pharm Biotechnol* 2013;14(15):1264-74. doi: 10.2174/1389201015666140608143719
46. Desai MP, Labhasetwar V, Walter E, Levy RJ, Amidon GL. The mechanism of uptake of biodegradable microparticles in Caco-2 cells is size dependent. *Pharm Res* 1997;14(11):1568-73. doi: 10.1023/A:1012126301290
47. Kreuter J. Influence of the surface properties on nanoparticle-mediated transport of drugs to the brain. *J Nanosci Nanotechnol* 2004;4(5):484-8. doi: 10.1166/jnn.2003.077

48. Mohanraj K, Sethuraman S, Krishnan UM. Development of poly(butylene succinate) microspheres for delivery of levodopa in the treatment of parkinson's disease. *J Biomed Mater Res B Appl Biomater* 2013;101(5):840-7. doi: 10.1002/jbm.b.32888
49. Miller G. Drug targeting. Breaking down barriers. *Science* 2002;297(5584):1116-8. doi: 10.1126/science.297.5584.1116
50. Khanbabaie R, Jahanshahi M. Revolutionary impact of nanodrug delivery on neuroscience. *Curr Neuropharmacol* 2012;10(4):370-92. doi: 10.2174/157015912804143513
51. Haque S, Md S, Intekhab Alam M, Kaur Sahni J, Ali J, Baboota S. Nanomedicines for brain targeting: A patent review. *Recent Pat Nanomed* 2011;1(2):149-61. doi: 10.2174/1877912311101020149
52. Prabha S, Zhou WZ, Panyam J, Labhasetwar V. Size-dependency of nanoparticle-mediated gene transfection: Studies with fractionated nanoparticles. *Int J Pharm* 2002;244(1-2):105-15.
53. Caldorera-Moore M, Peppas NA. Micro- and nanotechnologies for intelligent and responsive biomaterial-based medical systems. *Adv Drug Deliv Rev* 2009;61(15):1391-401. doi: 10.1016/j.addr.2009.09.002
54. Jain N, Jain R, Thakur N, Gupta BP, Jain DK, Banveer J, et al. Nanotechnology: A safe and effective drug delivery system. *Asian J Pharm Clin Res* 2010;3(3):159-65.
55. Liu Q, Cao X, Wang T, Wang C, Zhang Q, Ma L. Synthesis of shape-controllable cobalt nanoparticles and their shape-dependent performance in glycerol hydrogenolysis. *RSC Adv* 2015;5(7):4861-71. doi: 10.1039/c4ra13395a
56. Wang F, Wang YC, Dou S, Xiong MH, Sun TM, Wang J. Doxorubicin-tethered responsive gold nanoparticles facilitate intracellular drug delivery for overcoming multidrug resistance in cancer cells. *ACS Nano* 2011;5(5):3679-92. doi: 10.1021/nn200007z
57. Manju S, Sreenivasan K. Gold nanoparticles generated and stabilized by water soluble curcumin-polymer conjugate: Blood compatibility evaluation and targeted drug delivery onto cancer cells. *J Colloid Interface Sci* 2012;368(1):144-51. doi: 10.1016/j.jcis.2011.11.024
58. Labala S, Mandapalli PK, Kurumaddali A, Venuganti VV. Layer-by-Layer Polymer Coated Gold Nanoparticles for Topical Delivery of Imatinib Mesylate To Treat Melanoma. *Mol Pharm* 2015;12(3):878-88. doi: 10.1021/mp5007163
59. Chen Z, Zhang L, Song Y, He J, Wu L, Zhao C, et al. Hierarchical targeted hepatocyte mitochondrial multifunctional chitosan nanoparticles for anticancer drug delivery. *Biomaterials* 2015;52:240-50. doi: 10.1016/j.biomaterials.2015.02.001
60. Discher DE, Eisenberg A. Polymer vesicles. *Science* 2002;297(5583):967-73. doi: 10.1126/science.1074972
61. Costantino L, Boraschi D. Is there a clinical future for polymeric nanoparticles as brain-targeting drug delivery agents? *Drug Discov Today* 2012;17(7-8):367-78. doi: 10.1016/j.drudis.2011.10.028
62. Parveen S, Misra R, Sahoo SK. Nanoparticles: a boon to drug delivery, therapeutics, diagnostics and imaging. *Nanomedicine* 2012;8(2):147-66. doi: 10.1016/j.nano.2011.05.016
63. Faraji AH, Wipf P. Nanoparticles in cellular drug delivery. *Bioorg Med Chem* 2009;17(8):2950-62. doi: 10.1016/j.bmc.2009.02.043
64. Banks WA, Kastin AJ, Barrera CM. Delivering peptides to the central nervous system: dilemmas and strategies. *Pharm Res* 1991;8(11):1345-50. doi: 10.1023/A:1015884603456
65. Roney C, Kulkarni P, Arora V, Antich P, Bonte F, Wu A, et al. Targeted nanoparticles for drug delivery through the blood-brain barrier for Alzheimer's disease. *J Control Release* 2005;108(2-3):193-214. doi: 10.1016/j.jconrel.2005.07.024
66. Bronich TK, Bontha S, Shlyakhtenko LS, Bromberg L, Hatton TA, Kabanov AV. Template-assisted synthesis of nanogels from Pluronic-modified poly(acrylic acid). *J Drug Target* 2006;14(6):357-66. doi: 10.1080/10611860600833781
67. Friedrich I, Reichl S, Muller-Goymann CC. Drug release and permeation studies of nanosuspensions based on solidified reverse micellar solutions (SRMS). *Int J Pharm* 2005;305(1-2):167-75. doi: 10.1016/j.ijpharm.2005.09.007
68. Dikpati A, Madgulkar AR, Kshirsagar SJ, Bhalekar MR, Singh Chahal A. Targeted Drug Delivery to CNS using Nanoparticles. *J Adv Pharm Sci* 2012;2(1):179-91.
69. Hou D, Xie C, Huang K, Zhu C. The production and characteristics of solid lipid nanoparticles (SLNs). *Biomaterials* 2003;24(10):1781-5. doi: 10.1016/S0142-9612(02)00578-1
70. Saupe A, Rades T. Solid Lipid Nanoparticles. In: Mozafari MR, editor. Solid Lipid Nanoparticles. Frontiers of Nanotherapy. Dordrecht, Netherlands: Springer; 2006. P. 41-50.
71. Onoue S, Yamada S, Chan HK. Nanodrugs: Pharmacokinetics and safety. *Int J Nanomedicine* 2014;9:1025-37. doi: 10.2147/IJN.S38378
72. Esposito E, Fantin M, Marti M, Drechsler M, Paccamiccio L, Mariani P, et al. Solid lipid nanoparticles as delivery systems for bromocriptine. *Pharm Res* 2008;25(7):1521-30. doi: 10.1007/s11095-007-9514-y
73. McClements DJ, Decker EA, Weiss J. Emulsion-based delivery systems for lipophilic bioactive components. *J Food Sci* 2007;72(8):R109-24. doi: 10.1111/j.1750-3841.2007.00507.x
74. Rodríguez-Gascón A, del Pozo-Rodríguez A, Solinís MÁ. Development of nucleic acid vaccines: Use of

self-amplifying RNA in lipid nanoparticles. *Int J Nanomedicine* 2014;9:1833-43. doi: 10.2147/IJN.S39810
75. Dhawan S, Kapil R, Singh B. Formulation development and systematic optimization of solid lipid nanoparticles of quercetin for improved brain delivery. *J Pharm Pharmacol* 2011;63(3):342-51. doi: 10.1111/j.2042-7158.2010.01225.x
76. Olbrich C, Gessner A, Kayser O, Müller RH. Lipid-drug-conjugate (LDC) nanoparticles as novel carrier system for the hydrophilic antitrypanosomal drug diminazenediaceturate. *J Drug Target* 2002;10(5):387-96. doi: 10.1080/10611860210000001832
77. Wang JX, Sun X, Zhang ZR. Enhanced brain targeting by synthesis of 3',5'-dioctanoyl-5-fluoro-2'-deoxyuridine and incorporation into solid lipid nanoparticles. *Eur J Pharm Biopharm* 2002;54(3):285-90. doi: 10.1016/S0939-6411(02)00083-8
78. Chattopadhyay N, Zastre J, Wong HL, Wu XY, Bendayan R. Solid lipid nanoparticles enhance the delivery of the HIV protease inhibitor, atazanavir, by a human brain endothelial cell line. *Pharm Res* 2008;25(10):2262-71. doi: 10.1007/s11095-008-9615-2
79. Cheng Y, Wang J, Rao T, He X, Xu T. Pharmaceutical applications of dendrimers: promising nanocarriers for drug delivery. *Front Biosci* 2008;13:1447-71. doi: 10.2741/2774
80. Safari J, Zarnegar Z. Advanced drug delivery systems: Nanotechnology of health design A review. *J Saudi Chem Soc* 2014;18(2):85-99. doi: 10.1016/j.jscs.2012.12.009
81. Bhadra D, Bhadra S, Jain S, Jain NK. A PEGylated dendritic nanoparticulate carrier of fluorouracil. *Int J Pharm* 2003;257(1-2):111-24. doi: 10.1016/S0378-5173(03)00132-7
82. Martinho N, Florindo H, Silva L, Brocchini S, Zloh M, Barata T. Molecular modeling to study dendrimers for biomedical applications. *Molecules* 2014;19(12):20424-67. doi: 10.3390/molecules191220424
83. Duncan R, Izzo L. Dendrimer biocompatibility and toxicity. *Adv Drug Deliv Rev* 2005;57(15):2215-37. doi: 10.1016/j.addr.2005.09.019
84. Pan S, Wang C, Zeng X, Wen Y, Wu H, Feng M. Short multi-armed polylysine-graft-polyamidoamine copolymer as efficient gene vectors. *Int J Pharm* 2011;420(2):206-15. doi: 10.1016/j.ijpharm.2011.08.036
85. Boridy S, Soliman GM, Maysinger D. Modulation of inflammatory signaling and cytokine release from microglia by celastrol incorporated into dendrimer nanocarriers. *Nanomedicine (Lond)* 2012;7(8):1149-65. doi: 10.2217/nnm.12.16
86. Cerqueira SR, Silva BL, Oliveira JM, Mano JF, Sousa N, Salgado AJ, et al. Multifunctionalized CMCht/PAMAM dendrimer nanoparticles modulate the cellular uptake by astrocytes and oligodendrocytes in primary cultures of glial cells. *Macromol Biosci* 2012;12(5):591-7. doi: 10.1002/mabi.201100294
87. Beg S, Samad A, Alam MI, Nazish I. Dendrimers as novel systems for delivery of neuropharmaceuticals to the brain. *CNS Neurol Disord Drug Targets* 2011;10(5):576-88. doi: 10.2174/187152711796235023
88. Bilia AR, Guccione C, Isacchi B, Righeschi C, Firenzuoli F, Bergonzi MC. Essential oils loaded in nanosystems: A developing strategy for a successful therapeutic approach. *Evid Based Complement Alternat Med* 2014;2014:651593. doi: 10.1155/2014/651593
89. Zucker D, Andriyanov AV, Steiner A, Raviv U, Barenholz Y. Characterization of PEGylated nanoliposomes co-remotely loaded with topotecan and vincristine: Relating structure and pharmacokinetics to therapeutic efficacy. *J Control Release* 2012;160(2):281-9. doi: 10.1016/j.jconrel.2011.10.003
90. Bawa R. Nanoparticle-based therapeutics in humans: A survey. *Nanotechnol Law Bus* 2008;5(2):135-55.
91. Koukourakis MI, Koukouraki S, Giatromanolaki A, Kakolyris S, Georgoulias V, Velidaki A, et al. High intratumoral accumulation of stealth liposomal doxorubicin in sarcomas--rationale for combination with radiotherapy. *Acta Oncol* 2000;39(2):207-11. doi: 10.1080/028418600430789
92. Schmidt J, Metselaar JM, Gold R. Intravenous liposomal prednisolone downregulates in situ TNF-alpha production by T-cells in experimental autoimmune encephalomyelitis. *J Histochem Cytochem* 2003;51(9):1241-4. doi: 10.1177/002215540305100915
93. Huwyler J, Wu D, Pardridge WM. Brain drug delivery of small molecules using immunoliposomes. *Proc Natl Acad Sci U S A* 1996;93(24):14164-9. doi: 10.1073/pnas.93.24.14164
94. Ramos-Cabrer P, Campos F, Sobrino T, Castillo J. Targeting the ischemic penumbra. *Stroke* 2011;42(1 Suppl):S7-11. doi: 10.1161/STROKEAHA.110.596684
95. Ahn J, Miura Y, Yamada N, Chida T, Liu X, Kim A, et al. Antibody fragment-conjugated polymeric micelles incorporating platinum drugs for targeted therapy of pancreatic cancer. *Biomaterials* 2015;39:23-30. doi: 10.1016/j.biomaterials.2014.10.069
96. Mohamed S, Parayath NN, Taurin S, Greish K. Polymeric nano-micelles: versatile platform for targeted delivery in cancer. *Ther Deliv* 2014;5(10):1101-21. doi: 10.4155/tde.14.69
97. Butun S, Ince FG, Erdugan H, Sahiner N. One-step fabrication of biocompatible carboxymethyl cellulose polymeric particles for drug delivery

systems. *Carbohydr Polym* 2011;86(2):636-43. doi: 10.1016/j.carbpol.2011.05.001

98. Akimoto J, Nakayama M, Okano T. Temperature-responsive polymeric micelles for optimizing drug targeting to solid tumors. *J Control Release* 2014;193:2-8. doi: 10.1016/j.jconrel.2014.06.062
99. Zhao BX, Zhao Y, Huang Y, Luo LM, Song P, Wang X, et al. The efficiency of tumor-specific pH-responsive peptide-modified polymeric micelles containing paclitaxel. *Biomaterials* 2012;33(8):2508-20. doi: 10.1016/j.biomaterials.2011.11.078
100. Vigderman L, Zubarev ER. Therapeutic platforms based on gold nanoparticles and their covalent conjugates with drug molecules. *Adv Drug Deliv Rev* 2013;65(5):663-76. doi: 10.1016/j.addr.2012.05.004
101. Sahoo NG, Rana S, Cho JW, Li L, Chan SH. Polymer nanocomposites based on functionalized carbon nanotubes. *Prog Polym Sci* 2010:35(7):837-67. doi: 10.1016/j.progpolymsci.2010.03.002
102. Tran PA, Zhang L, Webster TJ. Carbon nanofibers and carbon nanotubes in regenerative medicine. *Adv Drug Deliv Rev* 2009;61(12):1097-114. doi: 10.1016/j.addr.2009.07.010
103. Dyke CA, Tour JM. Overcoming the insolubility of carbon nanotubes through high degrees of sidewall functionalization. *Chemistry* 2004;10(4):812-7. doi: 10.1002/chem.200305534
104. Zeineldin R, Al-Haik M, Hudson LG. Role of polyethylene glycol integrity in specific receptor targeting of carbon nanotubes to cancer cells. *Nano Lett* 2009;9(2):751-7. doi: 10.1021/nl8033174
105. Yang Z, Zhang Y, Yang Y, Sun L, Han D, Li H, et al. Pharmacological and toxicological target organelles and safe use of single-walled carbon nanotubes as drug carriers in treating alzheimer disease. *Nanomedicine* 2010;6(3):427-41. doi: 10.1016/j.nano.2009.11.007
106. Moon SU, Kim J, Bokara KK, Kim JY, Khang D, Webster TJ, et al. Carbon nanotubes impregnated with subventricular zone neural progenitor cells promotes recovery from stroke. *Int J Nanomedicine* 2012;7:2751-65. doi: 10.2147/IJN.S30273
107. Wu W, Wieckowski S, Pastorin G, Benincasa M, Klumpp C, Briand JP, et al. Targeted delivery of amphotericin b to cells by using functionalized carbon nanotubes. *Angew Chem Int Ed Engl* 2005;44(39):6358-62. doi: 10.1002/anie.200501613
108. Passeri D, Rinaldi F, Ingallina C, Carafa M, Rossi M, Terranova ML, et al. Biomedical applications of nanodiamonds: An overview. *J Nanosci Nanotechnol* 2015;15(2):972-88.
109. Nielsen GD, Roursgaard M, Jensen KA, Poulsen SS, Larsen ST. In vivo biology and toxicology of fullerenes and their derivatives. *Basic Clin Pharmacol Toxicol* 2008;103(3):197-208. doi: 10.1111/j.1742-7843.2008.00266.x
110. Anilkumar P, Lu F, Cao L, Luo PG, Liu JH, Sahu S, et al. Fullerenes for applications in biology and medicine. *Curr Med Chem* 2011;18(14):2045-59.
111. Johnston HJ, Hutchison GR, Christensen FM, Aschberger K, Stone V. The biological mechanisms and physicochemical characteristics responsible for driving fullerene toxicity. *Toxicol Sci* 2010;114(2):162-82. doi: 10.1093/toxsci/kfp265
112. Tykhomyrov AA, Nedzvetsky VS, Klochkov VK, Andrievsky GV. Nanostructures of hydrated c60 fullerene (c60hyfn) protect rat brain against alcohol impact and attenuate behavioral impairments of alcoholized animals. *Toxicology* 2008;246(2-3):158-65. doi: 10.1016/j.tox.2008.01.005
113. Kreuter J. Nanoparticulate systems for brain delivery of drugs. *Adv Drug Deliv Rev* 2001;47(1):65-81.
114. Alyaudtin RN, Reichel A, Lobenberg R, Ramge P, Kreuter J, Begley DJ. Interaction of poly(butylcyanoacrylate) nanoparticles with the blood-brain barrier in vivo and in vitro. *J Drug Target* 2001;9(3):209-21.
115. Ramge P, Unger RE, Oltrogge JB, Zenker D, Begley D, Kreuter J, et al. Polysorbate-80 coating enhances uptake of polybutylcyanoacrylate (PBCA)-nanoparticles by human and bovine primary brain capillary endothelial cells. *Eur J Neurosci* 2000;12(6):1931-40.
116. Fenart L, Casanova A, Dehouck B, Duhem C, Slupek S, Cecchelli R, et al. Evaluation of effect of charge and lipid coating on ability of 60-nm nanoparticles to cross an in vitro model of the blood-brain barrier. *J Pharmacol Exp Ther* 1999;291(3):1017-22.
117. Hwang SR, Kim K. Nano-enabled delivery systems across the blood-brain barrier. *Arch Pharm Res* 2014;37(1):24-30. doi: 10.1007/s12272-013-0272-6
118. Mucke L. Neuroscience: Alzheimer's disease. *Nature* 2009;461(7266):895-7. doi: 10.1038/461895a
119. Sloane PD, Zimmerman S, Suchindran C, Reed P, Wang L, Boustani M, et al. The public health impact of alzheimer's disease, 2000-2050: Potential implication of treatment advances. *Annu Rev Public Health* 2002;23:213-31. doi: 10.1146/annurev.publhealth.23.100901.140525
120. Ferri CP, Prince M, Brayne C, Brodaty H, Fratiglioni L, Ganguli M, et al. Global prevalence of dementia: A delphi consensus study. *Lancet* 2005;366(9503):2112-7. doi: 10.1016/S0140-6736(05)67889-0
121. Drolle E, Hane F, Lee B, Leonenko Z. Atomic force microscopy to study molecular mechanisms of amyloid fibril formation and toxicity in alzheimer's disease. *Drug Metab Rev* 2014;46(2):207-23. doi: 10.3109/03602532.2014.882354
122. Munoz DG, Feldman H. Causes of alzheimer's disease. *CMAJ* 2000;162(1):65-72.

123. Hirai K, Aliev G, Nunomura A, Fujioka H, Russell RL, Atwood CS, et al. Mitochondrial abnormalities in alzheimer's disease. *J Neurosci* 2001;21(9):3017-23.
124. Hashimoto K, Fukushima T, Shimizu E, Okada S, Komatsu N, Okamura N, et al. Possible role of d-serine in the pathophysiology of alzheimer's disease. *Prog Neuropsychopharmacol Biol Psychiatry* 2004;28(2):385-8.
125. Fazil M, Shadab, Baboota S, Sahni JK, Ali J. Nanotherapeutics for alzheimer's disease (ad): Past, present and future. *J Drug Target* 2012;20(2):97-113. doi: 10.3109/1061186X.2011.607499
126. Goldsmith M, Abramovitz L, Peer D. Precision nanomedicine in neurodegenerative diseases. *ACS Nano* 2014;8(3):1958-65. doi: 10.1021/nn501292z
127. D'Angelo B, Santucci S, Benedetti E, Di Loreto S, Phani RA, Falone S, et al. Cerium Oxide nanoparticles trigger neuronal survival in a human Alzheimer disease model by modulating BDNF pathway. *Curr Nanosci* 2009;5(2):167-76. doi: 10.2174/157341309788185523
128. Picone P, Bondi ML, Montana G, Bruno A, Pitarresi G, Giammona G, et al. Ferulic acid inhibits oxidative stress and cell death induced by Ab oligomers: Improved delivery by solid lipid nanoparticles. *Free Radic Res* 2009;43(11):1133-45.
129. Carroll RT, Bhatia D, Geldenhuys W, Bhatia R, Miladore N, Bishayee A, et al. Brain-targeted delivery of tempol-loaded nanoparticles for neurological disorders. *J Drug Target* 2010;18(9):665-74. doi: 10.3109/10611861003639796
130. Smith A, Giunta B, Bickford PC, Fountain M, Tan J, Shytle RD. Nanolipidic particles improve the bioavailability and alpha-secretase inducing ability of epigallocatechin-3-gallate (egcg) for the treatment of alzheimer's disease. *Int J Pharm* 2010;389(1-2):207-12. doi: 10.1016/j.ijpharm.2010.01.012
131. Giordano C, Albani D, Gloria A, Tunesi M, Rodilossi S, Russo T, et al. Nanocomposites for neurodegenerative diseases: Hydrogel-nanoparticle combinations for a challenging drug delivery. *Int J Artif Organs* 2011;34(12):1115-27. doi: 10.5301/IJAO.2011.8915
132. Hartig W, Paulke BR, Varga C, Seeger J, Harkany T, Kacza J. Electron microscopic analysis of nanoparticles delivering thioflavin-t after intrahippocampal injection in mouse: Implications for targeting beta-amyloid in alzheimer's disease. *Neurosci Lett* 2003;338(2):174-6.
133. Cui D, Gao H. Advance and prospect of bionanomaterials. *Biotechnol Prog* 2003;19(3):683-92. doi: 10.1021/bp025791i
134. Herholz K. Acetylcholine esterase activity in mild cognitive impairment and alzheimer's disease. *Eur J Nucl Med Mol Imaging* 2008;35 Suppl 1:S25-9. doi: 10.1007/s00259-007-0699-4
135. Cheng KK, Yeung CF, Ho SW, Chow SF, Chow AH, Baum L. Highly stabilized curcumin nanoparticles tested in an in vitro blood-brain barrier model and in alzheimer's disease Tg2576 mice. *AAPS J* 2013;15(2):324-36. doi: 10.1208/s12248-012-9444-4
136. Fernandes C, Soni U, Patravale V. Nano-interventions for neurodegenerative disorders. *Pharmacol Res* 2010;62(2):166-78. doi: 10.1016/j.phrs.2010.02.004
137. Dorsey ER, Constantinescu R, Thompson JP, Biglan KM, Holloway RG, Kieburtz K, et al. Projected number of people with parkinson disease in the most populous nations, 2005 through 2030. *Neurology* 2007;68(5):384-6. doi: 10.1212/01.wnl.0000247740.47667.03
138. Singh N, Pillay V, Choonara YE. Advances in the treatment of parkinson's disease. *Prog Neurobiol* 2007;81(1):29-44. doi: 10.1016/j.pneurobio.2006.11.009
139. Moore RY. Organization of midbrain dopamine systems and the pathophysiology of parkinson's disease. *Parkinsonism Relat Disord* 2003;9 Suppl 2:S65-71.
140. Moore DJ, West AB, Dawson VL, Dawson TM. Molecular pathophysiology of parkinson's disease. *Annu Rev Neurosci* 2005;28:57-87. doi: 10.1146/annurev.neuro.28.061604.135718
141. Lewitt PA. Levodopa for the treatment of parkinson's disease. *N Engl J Med* 2008;359(23):2468-76. doi: 10.1056/NEJMct0800326
142. Pardridge WM. Blood-brain barrier delivery. *Drug Discov Today* 2007;12(1-2):54-61. doi: 10.1016/j.drudis.2006.10.013
143. Kurakhmaeva KB, Djindjikhashvili IA, Petrov VE, Balabanyan VU, Voronina TA, Trofimov SS, et al. Brain targeting of nerve growth factor using poly(butyl cyanoacrylate) nanoparticles. *J Drug Target* 2009;17(8):564-74. doi: 10.1080/10611860903112842
144. Khasnavis S, Ghosh A, Roy A, Pahan K. Castration induces parkinson disease pathologies in young male mice via inducible nitric-oxide synthase. *J Biol Chem* 2013;288(29):20843-55. doi: 10.1074/jbc.M112.443556
145. Hu K, Shi Y, Jiang W, Han J, Huang S, Jiang X. Lactoferrin conjugated peg-plga nanoparticles for brain delivery: Preparation, characterization and efficacy in parkinson's disease. *Int J Pharm* 2011;415(1-2):273-83. doi: 10.1016/j.ijpharm.2011.05.062
146. Ricard D, Idbaih A, Ducray F, Lahutte M, Hoang-Xuan K, Delattre JY. Primary brain tumours in adults. *Lancet* 2012;379(9830):1984-96. doi: 10.1016/S0140-6736(11)61346-9
147. Walker AE, Robins M, Weinfeld FD. Epidemiology of brain tumors: The national survey of intracranial neoplasms. *Neurology* 1985;35(2):219-26.

148. Wrensch M, Minn Y, Chew T, Bondy M, Berger MS. Epidemiology of primary brain tumors: Current concepts and review of the literature. *Neuro Oncol* 2002;4(4):278-99.
149. Bidros DS, Vogelbaum MA. Novel drug delivery strategies in neuro-oncology. *Neurotherapeutics* 2009;6(3):539-46. doi: 10.1016/j.nurt.2009.04.004
150. Zhan C, Lu W. The blood-brain/tumor barriers: Challenges and chances for malignant gliomas targeted drug delivery. *Curr Pharm Biotechnol* 2012;13(12):2380-7.
151. Lee P, Zhang R, Li V, Liu X, Sun RW, Che CM, et al. Enhancement of anticancer efficacy using modified lipophilic nanoparticle drug encapsulation. *Int J Nanomedicine* 2012;7:731-7. doi: 10.2147/IJN.S28783
152. Jain KK. Nanotechnology-based drug delivery for cancer. *Technol Cancer Res Treat* 2005;4(4):407-16. doi: 10.1177/153303460500400408
153. Xi G, Robinson E, Mania-Farnell B, Vanin EF, Shim KW, Takao T, et al. Convection-enhanced delivery of nanodiamond drug delivery platforms for intracranial tumor treatment. *Nanomedicine* 2014;10(2):381-91. doi: 10.1016/j.nano.2013.07.013
154. Kateb B, Van Handel M, Zhang L, Bronikowski MJ, Manohara H, Badie B. Internalization of mwcnts by microglia: Possible application in immunotherapy of brain tumors. *NeuroImage* 2007;37 Suppl 1:S9-17. doi: 10.1016/j.neuroimage.2007.03.078
155. Kukowska-Latallo JF, Candido KA, Cao Z, Nigavekar SS, Majoros IJ, Thomas TP, et al. Nanoparticle targeting of anticancer drug improves therapeutic response in animal model of human epithelial cancer. *Cancer Res* 2005;65(12):5317-24. doi: 10.1158/0008-5472.CAN-04-392
156. Yinghuai Z, Hosmane NS. Applications and perspectives of boron-enriched nanocomposites in cancer therapy. *Future Med Chem* 2013;5(6):705-14. doi: 10.4155/fmc.13.47
157. Shapshak P, Chiappelli F, Commins D, Singer E, Levine AJ, Somboonwit C, et al. Molecular epigenetics, chromatin, and NeuroAIDS/HIV: translational implications. *Bioinformation* 2008;3(1):53-7. doi: 10.6026/97320630003053
158. Mintz M. Clinical comparison of adult and pediatric NeuroAIDS. *Adv Neuroimmunol* 1994;4(3):207-21. doi: 10.1016/S0960-5428(06)80259-7
159. Bloom FE, Rausch DM. HIV in the brain: pathology and neurobehavioral consequences. *J Neurovirol* 1997;3(2):102-9. doi: 10.3109/13550289709015800
160. Banks WA, Ercal N, Price TO. The blood-brain barrier in neuroAIDS. *Curr HIV Res* 2006;4(3):259-66. doi: 10.2174/157016206777709447
161. Roberts ES, Zandonatti MA, Watry DD, Madden LJ, Henriksen SJ, Taffe MA, et al. Induction of pathogenic sets of genes in macrophages and neurons in NeuroAIDS. *Am J Pathol* 2003;162(6):2041-57. doi: 10.1016/S0002-9440(10)64336-2
162. Doualla-Bell F, Turner D, Loemba H, Petrella M, Brenner B, Wainberg MA. HIV drug resistance and optimization of antiviral treatment in resource-poor countries. *Med Sci (Paris)* 2004;20(10):882-6. doi: 10.1051/medsci/200420100882
163. Dou H, Destache CJ, Morehead JR, Mosley RL, Boska MD, Kingsley J, et al. Development of a macrophage-based nanoparticle platform for antiretroviral drug delivery. *Blood* 2006;108(8):2827-35. doi: 10.1182/blood-2006-03-012534
164. Sagar V, Pilakka-Kanthikeel S, Pottathil R, Saxena SK, Nair M. Towards nanomedicines for neuroAIDS. *Rev Med Virol* 2014;24(2):103-24. doi: 10.1002/rmv.1778
165. Omar RF, Dusserre N, Desormeaux A, Poulin L, Tremblay M, Beauchamp D, et al. Liposomal encapsulation of foscarnet protects against hypocalcemia induced by free foscarnet. *Antimicrob Agents Chemother* 1995;39(9):1973-8. doi: 10.1128/AAC.39.9.1973
166. Kuo YC, Su FL. Transport of stavudine, delavirdine, and saquinavir across the blood-brain barrier by polybutylcyanoacrylate, methylmethacrylate-sulfopropylmethacrylate, and solid lipid nanoparticles. *Int J Pharm* 2007;340(1-2):143-52. doi: 10.1016/j.ijpharm.2007.03.012
167. Seshadri S, Beiser A, Kelly-Hayes M, Kase CS, Au R, Kannel WB, et al. The lifetime risk of stroke: estimates from the Framingham Study. *Stroke* 2006;37(2):345-50. doi: 10.1161/01.STR.0000199613.38911.b2
168. Shcharbina N, Shcharbin D, Bryszewska M. Nanomaterials in stroke treatment: perspectives. *Stroke* 2013;44(8):2351-5. doi: 10.1161/STROKEAHA.113.001298
169. Allen CL, Bayraktutan U. Oxidative stress and its role in the pathogenesis of ischaemic stroke. *Int J Stroke* 2009;4(6):461-70. doi: 10.1111/j.1747-4949.2009.00387.x
170. Martin HG, Wang YT. Blocking the Deadly Effects of the NMDA Receptor in Stroke. *Cell* 2010;140(2):174-6. doi: 10.1016/j.cell.2010.01.014
171. Weiss N, Miller F, Cazaubon S, Couraud PO. Blood-brain barrier part III: therapeutic approaches to cross the blood-brain barrier and target the brain. *Rev Neurol (Paris)* 2010;166(3):284-8. doi: 10.1016/j.neurol.2009.06.005
172. Mdzinarishvili A, Sutariya V, Talasila PK, Geldenhuys WJ, Sadana P. Engineering triiodothyronine (T3) nanoparticle for use in ischemic brain stroke. *Drug Deliv Transl Res* 2013;3(4):309-17. doi: 10.1007/s13346-012-0117-8
173. Estevez AY, Pritchard S, Harper K, Aston JW, Lynch A, Lucky JJ, et al. Neuroprotective mechanisms of cerium oxide nanoparticles in a mouse hippocampal brain slice model of ischemia. *Free Radic Biol Med* 2011;51(6):1155-63. doi: 10.1016/j.freeradbiomed.2011.06.006

174. Takamiya M, Miyamoto Y, Yamashita T, Deguchi K, Ohta Y, Abe K. Strong neuroprotection with a novel platinum nanoparticle against ischemic stroke- and tissue plasminogen activator-related brain damages in mice. *Neuroscience* 2012;221:47-55. doi: 10.1016/j.neuroscience.2012.06.060
175. Karatas H, Aktas Y, Gursoy-Ozdemir Y, Bodur E, Yemisci M, Caban S, et al. A nanomedicine transports a peptide caspase-3 inhibitor across the blood-brain barrier and provides neuroprotection. *J Neurosci* 2009;29(44):13761-9. doi: 10.1523/JNEUROSCI.4246-09.2009
176. Zhao H, Bao XJ, Wang RZ, Li GL, Gao J, Ma SH, et al. Postacute ischemia vascular endothelial growth factor transfer by transferrin-targeted liposomes attenuates ischemic brain injury after experimental stroke in rats. *Hum Gene Ther* 2011;22(2):207-15. doi: 10.1089/hum.2010.111
177. Beckung E, Hagberg G. Neuroimpairments, activity limitations, and participation restrictions in children with cerebral palsy. *Dev Med Child Neurol* 2002;44(5):309-16. doi: 10.1111/j.1469-8749.2002.tb00816.x
178. Li MH, Choi SK, Thomas TP, Desai A, Lee KH, Kotlyar A, et al. Dendrimer-based multivalent methotrexates as dual acting nanoconjugates for cancer cell targeting. *Eur J Med Chem* 2012;47(1):560-72. doi: 10.1016/j.ejmech.2011.11.027
179. Odding E, Roebroeck ME, Stam HJ. The epidemiology of cerebral palsy: incidence, impairments and risk factors. *Disabil Rehabil* 2006;28(4):183-91. doi: 10.1080/09638280500158422
180. Arneson CL, Durkin MS, Benedict RE, Kirby RS, Yeargin-Allsopp M, Van Naarden Braun K, et al. Prevalence of cerebral palsy: Autism and Developmental Disabilities Monitoring Network, three sites, United States, 2004. *Disabil Health J* 2009;2(1):45-8. doi: 10.1016/j.dhjo.2008.08.001
181. Robinson KG, Mendonca JL, Militar JL, Theroux MC, Dabney KW, Shah SA, et al. Disruption of basal lamina components in neuromotor synapses of children with spastic quadriplegic cerebral palsy. *PLoS One* 2013;8(8):e70288. doi: 10.1371/journal.pone.0070288
182. Kannan S, Dai H, Navath RS, Balakrishnan B, Jyoti A, Janisse J, et al. Dendrimer-based postnatal therapy for neuroinflammation and cerebral palsy in a rabbit model. *Sci Transl Med* 2012;4(130):130ra46. doi: 10.1126/scitranslmed.3003162
183. Huang DM, Chung TH, Hung Y, Lu F, Wu SH, Mou CY, et al. Internalization of mesoporous silica nanoparticles induces transient but not sufficient osteogenic signals in human mesenchymal stem cells. *Toxicol Appl Pharmacol* 2008;231(2):208-15. doi: 10.1016/j.taap.2008.04.009
184. Senanayake N, Roman GC. Epidemiology of epilepsy in developing countries. *Bull World Health Organ* 1993;71(2):247-58.
185. Sridharan R, Murthy BN. Prevalence and pattern of epilepsy in India. *Epilepsia* 1999;40(5):631-6. doi: 10.1111/j.1528-1157.1999.tb05566.x
186. Berg AT, Berkovic SF, Brodie MJ, Buchhalter J, Cross JH, Van Emde Boas W, et al. Revised terminology and concepts for organization of seizures and epilepsies: Report of the ILAE Commission on Classification and Terminology, 2005-2009. *Epilepsia* 2010;51(4):676-85. doi: 10.1111/j.1528-1167.2010.02522.x
187. Vezzani A, Balosso S, Ravizza T. The role of cytokines in the pathophysiology of epilepsy. *Brain Behav Immun* 2008;22(6):797-803. doi: 10.1016/j.bbi.2008.03.009
188. Lee HS, Wang SY, Salter DM, Wang CC, Chen SJ, Fan HC. The impact of the use of antiepileptic drugs on the growth of children. *BMC Pediatr* 2013;13:211. doi: 10.1186/1471-2431-13-211
189. Eskandari S, Varshosaz J, Minaiyan M, Tabbakhian M. Brain delivery of valproic acid via intranasal administration of nanostructured lipid carriers: in vivo pharmacodynamic studies using rat electroshock model. *Int J Nanomedicine* 2011;6:363-71. doi: 10.2147/IJN.S15881
190. Samia O, Hanan R, Kamal el T. Carbamazepine mucoadhesive nanoemulgel (MNEG) as brain targeting delivery system via the olfactory mucosa. *Drug Deliv* 2012;19(1):58-67. doi: 10.3109/10717544.2011.644349
191. Yusuf M, Khan RA, Khan M, Ahmed B. Plausible antioxidant biomechanics and anticonvulsant pharmacological activity of brain-targeted β-carotene nanoparticles. *Int J Nanomedicine* 2012;7:4311-21. doi: 10.2147/IJN.S34588
192. Bradford CM, Ramos I, Cross AK, Haddock G, McQuaid S, Nicholas AP, et al. Localisation of citrullinated proteins in normal appearing white matter and lesions in the central nervous system in multiple sclerosis. *J Neuroimmunol* 2014;273(1-2):85-95. doi: 10.1016/j.jneuroim.2014.05.007
193. Gironi M, Borgiani B, Mariani E, Cursano C, Mendozzi L, Cavarretta R, et al. Oxidative stress is differentially present in multiple sclerosis courses, early evident, and unrelated to treatment. *J Immunol Res* 2014;2014:961863. doi: 10.1155/2014/961863
194. Heckman KL, Decoteau W, Estevez A, Reed KJ, Costanzo W, Sanford D, et al. Custom cerium oxide nanoparticles protect against a free radical mediated autoimmune degenerative disease in the brain. *ACS Nano* 2013;7(12):10582-96. doi: 10.1021/nn403743b
195. Menon PK, Muresanu DF, Sharma A, Mössler H, Sharma HS. Cerebrolysin, a Mixture of Neurotrophic Factors Induces Marked Neuroprotection in Spinal Cord Injury Following Intoxication of Engineered Nanoparticles from

Metals. *CNS Neurol Disord Drug Targets* 2012;11(1):40-9. doi: 10.2174/187152712799960781

196. Sharma HS, Sharma A. Nanoparticles aggravate heat stress induced cognitive deficits, blood-brain barrier disruption, edema formation and brain pathology. *Prog Brain Res* 2007;162:245-73. doi: 10.1016/S0079-6123(06)62013-X

197. Sharma HS, Ali SF, Tian ZR, Hussain SM, Schlager JJ, Sjöquist PO, et al. Chronic treatment with nanoparticles exacerbate hyperthermia induced blood-brain barrier breakdown, cognitive dysfunction and brain pathology in the rat. Neuroprotective effects of nanowired-antioxidant compound H-290/51. *J Nanosci Nanotechnol* 2009;9(8):5073-90. doi: 10.1166/jnn.2009.gr10

198. Kaur IP, Bhandari R, Bhandari S, Kakkar V. Potential of solid lipid nanoparticles in brain targeting. *J Control Release* 2008;127(2):97-109. doi: 10.1016/j.jconrel.2007.12.018

199. Vega-Villa KR, Takemoto JK, Yáñez JA, Remsberg CM, Forrest ML, Davies NM. Clinical toxicities of nanocarrier systems. *Adv Drug Deliv Rev* 2008;60(8):929-38. doi: 10.1016/j.addr.2007.11.007

200. Krol S. Challenges in drug delivery to the brain: Nature is against us. *J Control Release* 2012;164(2):145-55. doi: 10.1016/j.jconrel.2012.04.044

201. Gloria A, De Santis R, Ambrosio L, Causa F, Tanner KE. A multi-component fiber-reinforced PHEMA-based hydrogel/HAPEX^{TM} device for customized intervertebral disc prosthesis. *J Biomater Appl* 2011;25(8):795-810. doi: 10.1177/0885328209360933

Experimental Design to Predict Process Variables in the Microcrystals of Celecoxib for Dissolution Rate Enhancement Using Response Surface Methodology

Mitra Jelvehgari[1,2], Hadi Valizadeh[1,2]*, Seyed Hassan Montazam[3], Sanam Abbaszadeh[4,5]

[1] *Drug Applied Research Center, Tabriz University of Medical Sciences, Tabriz, Iran.*
[2] *Faculty of Pharmacy, Tabriz University of Medical Sciences, Tabriz, Iran.*
[3] *Islamic Azad University of Bonab Unit, Bonab, Iran.*
[4] *Biotechnology Research Center, Tabriz University of Medical Sciences, Tabriz, Iran.*
[5] *Student Research Committee, Tabriz University of Medical Sciences, Tabriz, Iran.*

Article info

Keywords:
- Celecoxib
- Brij 35
- Microcrystal
- Dissolution
- Release

Abstract

Purpose: The purpose of the present investigation was to increase the solubility and dissolution rate of celecoxib (CLX) by preparing microcrystals of drug by solvent change precipitation.

Methods: This procedure was optimized in order to obtain stable and homogeneous particles with a small particle size, high yield and fast dissolution rate. CLX agglomerates were prepared with brij35 (stabilizer agent) using acetone as solvent, water as non-solvent, respectively. The agglomerates were characterized by DSC, XRD, FTIR studies. A full-factorial design was employed to study the effect of independent variables, the amounts of stirring rate (X1), volume of organic solvent (X2), volume of aqueous solvent (X3), time of stirring (X4), concentration of Brij (X5), concentration of Tween 80 (X6), concentration of HPMC (X7) on dependent variables, particle size (PS), drug content (DC), drug released after 15 min (Q15), crystal yield (CY), Gibbs free energy change (ΔG°tr), antalpy change (ΔH) and saturated solubility (Ss).

Results: The DSC and FTIR results indicated the absence of any interactions between drug and stabilizers. These studies showed a decrease in crystalinity in agglomerates. The crystals exhibited significantly improved micromeritic properties compared to pure drug. The drug content and crystal yield were in the range of 32.84-48.22% and 64.55-83.33% with all formulations, respectively. The solubility and drug release rates increased with an increase in concentration of stabilizer.

Conclusion: The results show that microcrystals of the drug in stabilizer considerably enhanced the dissolution rate.

Introduction

Micronization is the common method to increase specific surface area. Various types of mechanical mills are used to reduce the large crystals into smaller. Micronization means transfer of the coarse drug powder to an ultrafine powder with a mean particle size being typically in the range of 2-5 µm, size distributions normally ranges from approximately 0.1 to 25 µm. It is basically applied to class II drugs of the BCS classification system, i.e. drugs having a good permeability but a low bioavailability due to their poor solubility and low dissolution velocity. But, very recently micronization doesn't lead to a very effective increment in the bioavailability.[1]

The bioavailability intrinsically related to drug particle size. By reducing particle size, increased surface area improves the dissolution properties. In this method, typically, low excipient to drug ratios is required. Formulations are generally well tolerated provided that strong surfactants are not required for stabilization. Generally, crystal forms are chemically and physically more stable than amorphous particles.

There are certain disadvantages for the micronization caused by mills. Few of them include extreme inefficiency in reducing size disruption in crystal lattice which may lead thermodynamic imbalance and thus recrystalize when it absorbs atmospheric moisture.[2] Microcrystals can be produced using milling by high pressure homogenizer. The drug crystals with a starting size as small as possible are suspended in an aqueous stabilized surfactant solution.[3,4]

Response surface methodology is a useful tool in the development and optimization of controlled release microcrystals.[5] Different steps involved in response surface methodology include experimental design, regression analysis, constraint optimization and validation. Response surface methodology (RSM) is widely practiced approach in the development and optimization of drug

***Corresponding author:** Hadi Valizadeh, Email: valizadeh@tbzmed.ac.ir

delivery devices. Based on the principle of design of experiments (DoEs), the methodology encompasses the use of various types of experimental designs, generation of polymonal equations, and mapping of the response over the experimental domain to determine the optimum formulation(s).[5] The technique requires minimum experimentation and time, thus proving to be far more effective and cost-effective than the conventional methods of formulating dosage forms.

Celecoxib (CLX), a non-steroidal anti-inflammatory drug (NSAID), is the first selective cyclooxygenase-2 inhibitor used in the treatment of osteoarthritis and rheumatoid arthritis in adult patients.[6] CLX exhibits poor flow and compression characteristics and is hence a suitable candidate for *in situ* micronization process to improve the flow properties and compressibility. Also, CLX shows incomplete and poor oral bioavailability due to low aqueous solubility.[7] Hence, the improvement of aqueous solubility in such a case is a valuable goal to improve therapeutic efficacy.[8]

CLX is a highly permeable drug that can be absorbed throughout the GI tract and that dissolution may be a rate-limiting factor for absorption from solid dosage forms. Although these changes would likely result in delayed drug absorption due to delayed gastric emptying, the longer gastric residence time would allow more time for dispersion and dissolution of a poorly soluble, lipophilic drug such as CLX thereby increasing the extent of absorption.

In the present investigation, the effect of factors (RPM, volume of solvent of CLX, volume of non-solvent of CLX, time and rate of stirring, type and concentration stabilizer) that can influence the drug dissolution rate, particle size, crystal yield, and dissolution efficiency of microcrystals CLX was investigated.

Materials and Methods

CLX was obtained from Jaber Ebne Hyane Pharmaceutical Company, Iran, Hydrxypropylmethyl Cellulose (HPMC) low viscosity (Merck, Darmstadt, Germany), Brij 35, Tween 80 and acetone, sodium lauryl sulfate (SLS) (Merck, Darmstadt, Germany) were used.

Micronization

Preparation of microcrystals

In preliminary studies, three different stabilizing agents (HPMC and Brij 35, Tween 80 and HPMC) with different concentrations of CLX (0.5–1g) and stabilizers (0.05–0.1%) were studied by a full factorial design to give the most stable microcrystals with the least particle size.[9,10] Details of the preparation methods of microcrystals are reported previously.[9] Briefly, in solvent-change method, 0.75 g of CLX was dissolved in 15 ml of acetone. One hundred milliliters of water (as the non-solvent of CLX) containing 0.1% of Brij35 (as stabilizer) was poured rapidly into the drug solution under stirring at 26,000 rpm by an ultra-homogenizer (Heidolph Silent Crusher M, Germany) at ice bath temperature. A micron-sized dispersion was formed spontaneously. The mixture was allowed to be mixed for further 15 min, and then aqueous suspension was freeze dried (Christ ALPHA-4, Germany).[9]

Micromeritic Properties

The microcrystals size analysis was performed by laser light scattering particle size analyzer (SALD-2101, Shimadzu, Japan). Samples were suspended in distilled water contained in a 1 cm cuvette and stirred continuously during the particle size analysis. The particle size distribution of the microspheres for all formulations was determined and the results were the mean of three determinations.

Solubility study

The solubility of CLX in various organic solvents was measured by adding excess amount of drug to 10 ml of solvents. The resulting drug suspension was agitated for 24 h at 37°C in glass vials sealed with Teflon-lined closure. These samples were centrifuged and filtered (0.45 μ nylon filter millipore). An aliquot of the filtrate was weighted and diluted appropriately for UV spectrophotometer (Shimatzu-160, Japan) measurement. The Gibbs-free energy of change (ΔG°tr°) of microcrystal occurred during formation of microcrystals from un-treated CLX powder was calculated using equation 1.

$$\Delta G^{\circ}_{tr} = -2.303RT\log\frac{S_0}{S_s} \qquad (1)$$

Where S_0/Ss, is the ratio of the molar solubility of CLX microcrystals in distilled water to that of the untreated CLX powder. R is gas constant (8.31 J $k^{-1}mol^{-1}$) and T is temperature (310.15°K).

Determination of crystal yield

The crystal yield of the microcrystals was determined by calculating accurately the initial weight of the raw materials and the final weight of the polymeric particles obtained. All the experiments were performed in triplicate (Table 1).

Table 1. Effect of drug concentration on the drug content, production yield and particle size and flowability characteristics of CLX microcrystal formulations

Formulation code	Production Yield (%)	Drug Content (%)	Mean particle Size (μm)	Bulk Density (g/cm³± SD)	Tapped Density (g/cm³± SD)	Carr's index (%±SD)	Hausner ratio(±SD)	Angle of repose (°θ ±SD)
F_1	73.33±7.3	2.84±46.10	7.11±0.55	0.069±0.00	0.100 ±0.00	35.00±0.02	11.54 ± 0.0	29.68±0.71
F_2	76.55±5.2	46.55±1.89	7.31±0.52	0.080±0.00	0.099 ±0.00	19.19 ± 0.01	1.14 ± 0.01	30.54 ±0.84
F_3	74.71±6.2	48.22±5.01	7.73±0.56	0.055±0.01	0.070 ±0.01	21.43 ± 0.01	1.27 ± 0.00	30.40 ±0.89

X-ray powder diffractometry (X-RPD)
X-ray diffraction analysis was performed with an apparatus (Siemens D5000, Munich, Germany), using nickel-filtered CuKα radiation (a voltage of 40 KV and a current of 20 mA). The scanning rate was 2° /min over a range of 20-70° and with an interval of 0.02°. Each measurement was repeated three times.

Fourier transforms infrared spectroscopy (FT-IR)
A computerized FT-IR (Bomem, Quebec, Canada) was used to obtain the spectra of various CLX samples. The microcrystal sample (about 10 mg) in potassium bromide discs (0.5% w/w) was placed on the plate of the machine and the handle was placed on the powder sample to generate enough pressure for compression. The spectrum for each sample showed the wavelength of absorbed light, which is a characteristic of the chemical bonds in the sample. The scanning range was 400-4000 cm^{-1} and the resolution was 1 cm^{-1}.

Differential scanning calorimetry (DSC)
A differential scanning calorimeter (DSC 60, Shimadzu, Japan) was used to monitor the thermal events during heating. The DSC was calibrated by the melting point of aluminium oxide (2072°C) standard. Samples weighing 5 mg were placed in open aluminium pans and heated from 30 to 300° C at a rate of 10°C per min. Nitrogen gas was purged at a flux rate of 10 ml/min. The onsets of the melting points and enthalpies of fusion were calculated.

Flow property study
The bulk density and tapped bulk densities were determined by using density apparatus (the apparatus was locally assembled). The Carr's index (%) and the Hausner's ratio were calculated by using CLX. The angle of repose of untreated CLX powder and the microcrystals were assessed by fixed funnel method (Table 1).

In vitro release studies
The *in vitro* release studies of drug-loaded microcrystals were carried out at 37°C in 500 mL of distilled water contain 1%, *m*/*V* sodium lauryl sulfate (SLS). Each batch of microcrystals containing 100 mg of drug was individually added to 500 mL of dissolution medium in flask. The dissolution media was stirred at 75 rpm according to USP basket method. Three mL of samples were withdrawn at regular time intervals and the same volume of fresh medium was replaced. After suitable dilution, the drug content of each sample was estimated by using a UV spectrophotometer analysis at 277.6 nm, respectively. Each experiment was repeated three times. In order to have a better comparison between different formulations dissolution efficiency (DE), $t_{50}\%$ (dissolution time for 50% fraction of drug); and difference factor, f_1 (used to compare multipoint dissolution profiles) were calculated and the results are listed in Table 2. DE is defined as the area under the dissolution curve up to a certain time, *t*, expressed as a percentage of the area of the rectangle arising from 100% dissolution in the same time. The areas under the curve (AUC) were calculated for each dissolution profile by the trapezoidal rule. DE can be calculated by the following:

$$\text{DE} = \int y \frac{dt}{100t}$$

Where *y* is the drug percent dissolved at time *t*. All dissolution efficiencies were obtained with *t* equal to 1440min.The *in vitro* release profiles of different micrystals formulations were compared with physical mixture formulation using difference factor (f_1), as defined by:[11]

$$f_1 = \frac{\{[\Sigma_t = 1^n |R_t - T_t|]}{[\Sigma_t = 1^n\, R_t]\}} \times 100$$

Where *n* is the number of time points at which % dissolved was determined, R_t is the % dissolved of one formulation at a given time point and T_t is the % dissolved of the formulation to be compared at the same time point. The difference factor fits the result between 0 and 15 when the test and reference profiles are identical, and approaches above 15 as the dissimilarity increases.

Table 2. Comparison of various release characteristics of CLX from different microcrystal formulations, untreated CLX powder and commercial® capsules

Formulations	Rel_{15}[a](%±SD)	Rel_{30}[b](%±SD)	Rel_{60}[c](%±SD)	DE[d]	$t_{50\%}$[e](min)	f_1[f]
F_1	1.39 ± 35.65	0.48±39.65	59.29±0.79	40.10	19.42	15>
F_2	38.26±1.15	1.15± 45.78	61.99±0.48	44.84	16.60	15>
F_3	0.77±54.21	0.58±61.46	72.68±3.64	56.30	13.53	15>
Cap celecoxib®	6.62±0.67	21.54±1.13	43.01±0.53	22.36	28.81	15>
Untreated celecoxib	1.84±0.34	4.47±0.88	14.62±1.37	5.94	35.61	0

[a] Rel_{15} = amount of drug release after 15 min; [b] Rel_{30} = amount of drug release after 30 min; [c] Rel_{60} = amount of drug release after 60 min ;[d]DE = dissolution efficiency; [e]t 50% = dissolution time for 50% fractions; [f] f_1 = Differential factor ($0<f_1<15$).

Optimization of the CLX microcrystals
The experimental design was a modified Box-Behnken design for seven variables. This design was suitable for exploring quadratic response surfaces and constructing second-order polynomial models. Response surface methodology (RSM) is a very useful statistical technique for optimization of CLX formulations. In this design 7 factors were evaluated, each at 3 levels, and

experimental trials were performed at all 17 possible combinations. The rate of stirring (X_1), volume of organic solvent (X_2), dispersing medium (volume of aqueous solvent) (X_3), time of stirring (X4), concentration of stabilizer (brij) (X_5), concentration of stabilizer (Tween 80) (X_6) and concentration of e stabilizer (HPMC) (X_7) were selected as independent variables. The particle size (PS, Y_1), drug content (DC, Y_2), amount of drug release after 15 minute (Q_{15}, Y_3), crystal yield (CY, Y4), Gibbs free energy change (ΔG°, Y_5), enthalpy change (ΔH, y_6) and saturated solubility (Ss, Y_7) were dependent variables (Table 3).

Table 3. Effect of agitation speed, volume of solvent, volume of non-solvent, time and rate of stirring, type and concentration stabilizer on particle size (PS), drug content (DC), amount of drug release after 15 minute (Q_{15}), crystal yield (CY), Gibbs free energy change ($\Delta G°_{tr}$), enthalpy Change (ΔH) and saturated solubility (Ss) of CLX microcrystals

Formulation code	Variable levels in coded form							PS(μm)	DC(%)	Q_{15}(%)	CY(%)	ΔG_{tr} ($Jmol^{-1}$)	ΔH (J/g)	S_s (mg/ml)
	X1	X2	X3	X4	X5	X6	X7							
F_2	26000	15	100	10	0.1	0	0	7.31	46.55	38.26	66.55	-2933.12	-54.52	1.56
F_{2-1}	26000	10	100	10	0.1	0	0	7.33	25.99	30.06	57.65	-2492.96	-41.71	1.29
F_{2-2}	26000	20	100	10	0.1	0	0	10.31	43.70	4.27	82.35	-2911.55	-86.57	1.55
F_{2-3}	26000	15	50	10	0.1	0	0	8.15	13.18	0.60	61.18	-2191.53	-82.72	1.17
F_{2-4}	26000	15	150	10	0.1	0	0	8.34	26.70	8.39	72.94	-2521.94	-29.15	1.33
F_{2-5}	26000	15	100	10	0.05	0	0	7.9	29.76	1.78	51.25	-2463.13	-60.84	1.3
F_{2-6}	26000	15	100	10	0.15	0	0	5.75	42.92	38.26	80	-2916.54	-48.60	1.54
F_{2-7}	26000	15	100	5	0.1	0	0	8.88	26.23	1.55	61.25	-2672.51	0.716	1.41
F_{2-8}	26000	15	100	15	0.1	0	0	13.82	28.62	36.69	66.25	-2866.16	-10.73	1.52
F_{2-9}	20000	15	100	10	0.1	0	0	4.99	26.49	27.37	57.65	-2789.75	-18.52	1.47
F_{2-10}	14000	15	100	10	0.1	0	0	4.30	19.21	4.43	60	-2032.49	-3.87	1.10
F_{2-11}	26000	15	100	10	0	0.05	0	7.53	17.45	6.06	90.59	-2382.57	-80.98	1.26
F_{2-12}	26000	15	100	10	0	0.1	0	7.84	27.33	1.6	67.78	-2443.22	-19.18	1.29
F_{2-13}	26000	15	100	10	0	0.15	0	4.27	18.58	7.3	73.75	-2341.32	-11.25	1.24
F_{2-14}	26000	15	100	10	0	0	0.05	6.89	22.22	2.18	60	-2101.86	-52.63	1.13
F_{2-15}	26000	15	100	10	0	0	0.1	5.08	15.43	19.88	45.56	-2101.85	-45.11	1.13
F_{2-16}	26000	15	100	10	0	0	0.15	7.26	28.08	1.11	98.75	-2008.95	-67.09	1.09
F_{2-17}	26000	15	100	10	0	0	0	9.31	8.03	0.29	76	-512.60	-1.58	0.61

Formulations contained 750 mg CLX and 100 mg Brij 35. 100 ml water, 15 ml acetone, †X_1 is RPM and; X_2 is volume of organic solvent; X_3 is volume of non-solvent; X_4 is time of stirring; X5, X6 and X7 is concentration of stabilizing agents as Brij 35, HPMC and Tween 80. PS particle size; DC drug content; $Q_{15\%}$ indicates drug release after 15 min; CY indicates crystal yield; ΔG° indicates Gibbs free energy change; ΔH indicates enthalpy change; Ss indicates saturated solubility.
X_1 = RPM, X_2 = volume of organic solvent, X_3 = dispersing medium (volume of aqueous solvent), X4 = time of stirring
X5 = concentration of stabilizer (brij), X6= concentration of stabilizer (Tween 80), X7= concentration of e stabilizer (HPMC), PS= particle size, DC = drug content, Q_{15}= amount of drug release after 15 minute, CY= Crystal yield, $\Delta G°_{tr}$ = Gibbs free energy change, ΔH = enthalpy change, Ss = saturated solubility

Various batches of the selected formulation (F_2) were made, but the stirring rate was the only parameter that was varied between 14000, 20000 and 26000 rpm. Concentration of stabilizers (as brij, HPMC and Tween 80) was shifted between 0.05, 0.075, 0.1 g. Also, while keeping the other parameter constant, time of homogenizer stirring was changed (5, 10 and 15 min). Volume of organic solvent and dispersing medium was changed 5-15 ml and 50-150ml, respectively. After drying, the weighed batch of microcrystals was subjected to particle size, drug content, amount of drug release after 15 minute, crystal yield, Gibbs free energy change, enthalpy change and saturated solubility experiments. The influence of process variables on microcrystals formation, micromeritics and drug release characteristics was investigated.

Regression analysis

The targeted response parameters were statistically analyzed by applying one-way ANOVA at 0.05 levels. Individual response parameters were evaluated using the *F*-test and quadratic models of the form given below were generated for each response parameter using the multiple linear regression analysis.[12]

Results

CLX microcrystals were prepared by solvent change method using Brij 35 as a hydrophilic stabilizing agent. Solvent ratio (acetone/water) 1:6.7 and 0.1% Brij 35 were optimum parameters for microcrystallization of CLX. Drug was dissolved in organic solvent and then non-solvent was poured rapidly into the drug solution under stirring by an ultrahomogenizer. Microcrystals produced using Brij 35 showed narrow particle size distribution and change in the crystal habit. Higher crystal yield 76.55% was obtained in case of CLX microcrystals prepared using 0.1% Brij 35 (F_1 formulation with 1g CLX) (Table 1).

Measurement of powder flow

According of Table 1, angle of repose for microcrystals was between 29.68° to 30.54°, thus indicating poor flow property for microcrystals. The findings were supported by Carr's (compressibility) index, which was > 20 indicating poor flow characterizes (F_1, F_2 and F_3) (Table 1).

The physical state of the CLX in the Brij 35was studied by classical techniques such as DSC,

XRPD and FTIR. DSC analyses were carried out for CLX, Brij 35, microcrystals (F_1, F_2 and F_3) and physical mixtures (Figure 1). Any abrupt or drastic change in the thermal behavior of rather the drug or polymer may indicate a possible drug-polymer interaction (9). CLX and Brij 35 exhibited crystalline state (Figure 1). In the thermogram of the microcrystals containing Brij 35, endothermic peaks at 155.80°C (F_1), 158.01°C (F_2) and 158.41°C (F_3) corresponds to the melting point of CLX.

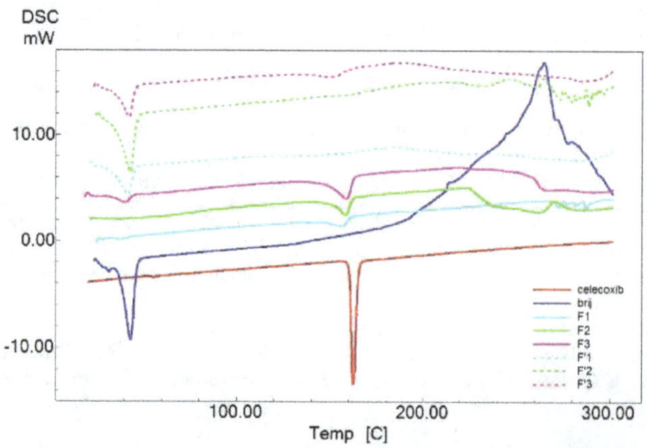

Figure 1. DSC thermogram of CLX powder; Brij35; microcrystals of F_1 , F_2, F_3 and physical mixtures of F'_1, F'_2 and F'_3, respectively.

The X-ray diffraction patterns of pure CLX and Brij 35 showed that the pure drug is crystalline in nature nearly 16 to 20 at 2θ scale (Figure 2). XRPD is a powerful tool to identify any changes in crystallinity of the drug. When the microcrystals were prepared with different drug/stabilizer agent ratios (F_1, F_2 and F_3) it is clear that the samples with lower drug concentration showed similar peaks as the physical mixture.

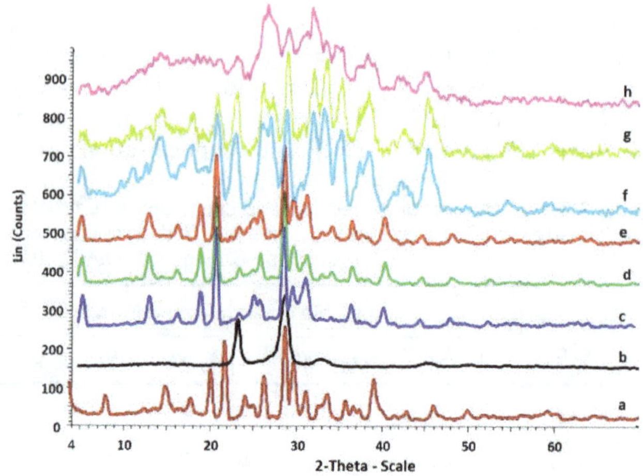

Figure 2. Thermogram of CLX powder (a); brij35 (b); microcrystals of F_1 (c) , F_2 (d), F_3 (e) and physical mixtures of F'_1 (f), F'_2 (g) and F'_3 (h), respectively.

In order to investigate any changes in molecular levels of CLX during the micronization process, FT-IR spectrum was obtained for all formulations and their spectra are shown in Figure 3. FTIR spectra are assigned as follows: (1) CLX: first type amine at 341.51 cm^{-1}, S=O stretching asymmetric band at 1164.58 cm^{-1} and S=O stretching symmetric band 1347.75 cm^{-1}; CF3 band at 1229.99, 1274.96 cm^{-1}, (2) microcrystals F_1, F_2 and F_3: first type amine at 3343.3 cm^{-1}, S=O stretching asymmetric band at 1133.4 cm^{-1} and S=O stretching symmetric band 1345.76 cm^{-1}; CF3 band at 1257.2, 1202.8 cm^{-1} ,respectively (Figure 3). After CLX was micronized and covered with brij, the characteristic peaks for CLX showed by the smaller intensity peaks than pure drug and stabilizer agent. On the other hand, the S=O stretching bands of CLX in microcrystal systems were merged, thus leading to a peak shifting from 1164.58 cm^{-1} to 1133.4 cm^{-1}.

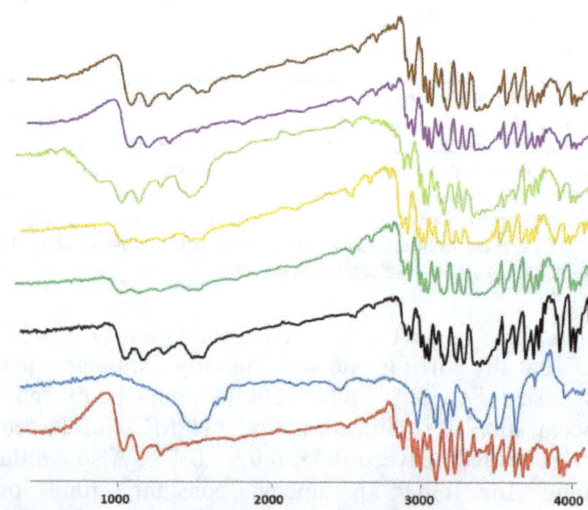

Figure 3. FTIR thermogram of CLX powder (a); brij35 (b); microcrystals of F_1 (c) , F_2 (d), F_3 (e) and physical mixtures of F'_1 (f), F'_2 (g) and F'_3 (h), respectively.

The micronized CLX formulations showed a dramatic enhancement in dissolution rate than CLX powder untreated as illustrated in Figure 4. DE of the studied microcrystals in comparison with the pure CLX powder and commercial capsule CLX was presented in Table 2. Results suggested that dissolution profile of microcrystals was significantly differ (p<0.05) from untreated CLX powder. CLX crystals prepared without stabilizing agent did not show significant improvement in drug release when compared with pure CLX drug powder (Figure 4).

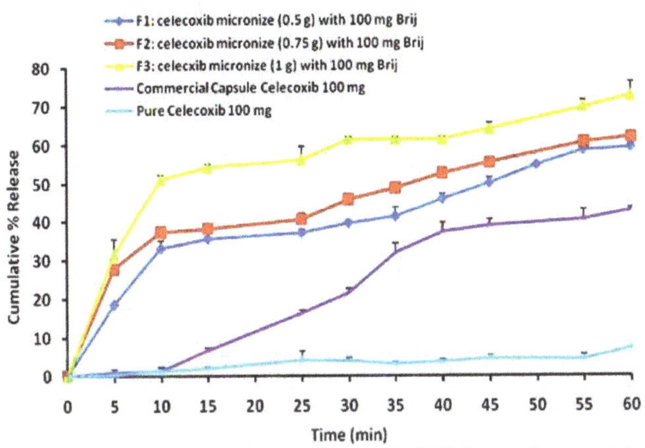

Figure 4. Cumulative percent release of CLX from microcrystals, untreated CLX powder and commercial capsule.

Higher drug release (38.26% for F_2 formulation) after 15 min obtained in case of 0.1% Brij 35 as compared to CLX microcrystals prepared using other concentration of Brij 35 (0.05 and 0.075g). Results of drug release was observed highly significant difference for CLX microcrystals prepared using 0.1 g of Brij 35 with different amounts of drug as compared to untreated CLX powder and commercial capsule CLX (100 mg) (p<0.05).

According of Table 2 and 3, CLX microcrystals prepared using 0.1% Brij 35 as stabilizing agent showed small particle size (7.31 μm), higher crystal yield (66.55%), high water solubility (1.56 mg/ml), great reduction in Gibb's free energy (-2933.12 $Jmol^{-1}$), and higher dissolution efficiency (44.84%) as compared to other CLX microcrystals. Therefore, 0.1% concentration was optimum concentration of Brij 35 for microcrystallization of CLX.

The tendency of the solid phase to exhibit solubility is best described by the Gibbs free energy change ($\Delta G^{\circ}tr$). Negative Gibbs free energy values indicate favorable conditions. The $\Delta G^{\circ}tr$ values were all negative at various concentrations, thus indicating that CLX microcrystals had higher aqueous solubility. These values decreased with increasing concentration of Brij 35 up to 0.1 g, thereby demonstrating that drug solubility increased as the concentration of Brij 35 increased up to 0.1 g.

F_1, F_2 and F_3 microcrystals showed higher dissolution efficiency i.e. rapidly dissolution in comparison to respective CLX powder (untreated) and commercial capsule of CLX (p< 0.05), (Table 2). According of Table 2 the lowest DE was observed for F_1 (40.10%) and dissolution efficiency of CLX powder (untreated was 5.94% (p< 0.05). The value of $t_{50\%}$ varied between 13.53 (F_3 formulation) to 19.42 min (F_1 formulation). The results of difference factor (f_1) showed that the release profile of microcrystals formulations is different from that of CLX powder (untreated) and commercial capsule of CLX (Table 2).

The independent variables and their levels were selected based on the preliminary trials undertaken. The PS, DC, Q_{15}, CY, ΔG°, ΔH and Ss for the formulations (F_1 to F_{17}) showed a wide variation. The data clearly indicated that the PS, DC, CY, ΔG° and Ss values are strongly dependent on the selected independent variables. The fitted equations (full and reduced) relating the responses PS, DC, Q_{15}, CY, ΔG°, ΔH, Ss and %F to the transformed factors are shown in Table 3. The polynomial equations can be used to draw conclusions after considering the magnitude of coefficient and the mathematical sign it carries (i.e., positive or negative). Table 4 & 5 shows the results of the analysis of variance (ANOVA), which was performed to identify insignificant factors. The high values of correlation coefficient for PS, DC, CY, ΔG° and Ss indicate a good fit i.e., good agreement between the dependent and independent variables. The equations may be used to obtain estimates of the response as a small error of variance was noticed in the replicates. The significance test regression coefficient was performed by applying the student F test.

The results of statistical analysis are shown in Table 4. The coefficients b_1, b_2, and b_{11} were found to be significant at $p < 0.05$; hence they were retained in the reduced model.

The reduced model was tested in portions to determine whether the coefficients b_{12} and b_{22} contribute significant information for the prediction of PS, DC, CY, ΔG° and Ss or not. The results for testing the model in portions are. The results of multiple linear regression analysis (response surface regression) reveal that, on increasing the amount of rate of stirring, volume of organic phase, volume of aqueous phase, volume of aqueous phase, time of stirring, type of stabilizer agent (Brij 35, Tween 80 and HPMC) decreased PS is observed; the coefficients b_1 to b_7 are negative sign. The results of statistical analysis are shown in Table 4. The reduced model was tested in portions to determine whether the coefficients b_{11}, b_{12}, and b_{22} contribute significant information for the prediction of %F or not. The results for testing the model in portions are depicted in Table 4. Hence, conclusions can be drawn considering the magnitude of the coefficient and the mathematical sign (positive or negative) it carries. According to Figure 5, particle size is dependent on major independent factors such as RPM, volume of aqueous solvent and i.e.

Table 4. Model equations obtained from response surface regression analysis

Term	Equation of regression coefficients
PS versus X1, X2, X3, X4, X5, X6, X7	PS = 38.26 - 5.36X1 -1.81X2 – 0.09X3 – 2.93X4 – 17.86X5 – 4.96X6 – 76.78X7 + 0.07X2X2 + 0.00047X3X3 + 0.17X4X4 – 26.53X5X5 – 168.53X6X6 + 421.25X7X7
DC versus X1, X2, X3, X4, X5, X6, X7	DC = 47.98 + 12.42X1 + 8.85X2 + 6.76X3 + 1.19X4 + 17.72X5 + 5.65X6 + 8.83X7 + 5.14X1X1 – 9.21X2X2 – 24.12X3X3 – 16.63X4X4 – 13.64X5X5 – 9.49X6X6 – 1.90X7X7
Q_{15} versus X1, X2, X3, X4, X5, X6, X7	Q_{15}= 45.93 + 12.19X1 – 12.89X2 + 3.89X3 + 17.57X4 + 23.37X5 + 5.32X6 + 4.14X7 – 10.74X1X1 – 11.64X2X2 – 24.31X3X3 – 9.69X4X4 – 2.61X5X5 – 2.61X5X5 – 3.58X6X6 – 13.01X7X7
PY versus X1, X2, X3, X4, X5, X6, X7	PY = 16.24 – 5.83X1 + 12.35X2 + 5.88X3 + 2.5X4 – 1.71X5 – 6.10X6 + 6.39X7 – 3.48X1X1 + 21.67X2X2 + 18.73X3X3 + 15.42X4X4 + 36.24X5X5 – 2.76X6X6 + 41.01X7X7
$\Delta G°_{tr}$ versus X1, X2, X3, X4, X5, X6, X7	ΔG_{tr} = -1749.97 – 528.36X1 – 209.29X2 – 165.20X3 – 96.82X4 – 1173.25X5 – 868.46X6 + 1196X7 + 228.90X1X1 + 386.95X2X2 + 732.47X3X3 + 319.87X4X4 + 1154.72X6X6 – 1600.75X7X7
ΔH versus X1, X2, X3, X4, X5, X6, X7	ΔH = -87.18 – 29.28X1 – 22.43X2 + 26.78X3 – 5.73X4 – 14.25X5 + 7.81X6 – 22.92X7 – 14.63X1X1 – 1.70X2X2 + 6.49X3X3 + 57.42X4X4 + 29.22X5X5 + 45.50X6X6 + 9.56X7X7
Ss versus X1, X2, X3, X4, X5, X6, X7	Ss = 2.51 + 0.23X1 + 0.13X2 + .08X3 + 0.55X4 + 0.43X5 + 0.27X6 + 0.20X7 – 0.13X1X1 – 0.15X2X2 – 0.32X3X3 – 0.11X4X4 – 0.37X5X5 – 0.37X6X6 -0.29X7X7

Table 5. Results obtained from the model evaluation

Response/coefficients	DF	SS	MS	F(cal)	R2	p	MPE(%)
PS	14	88.21	6.30	7.27	97.14	0.05	6.29
DC	14	1719.48	122.82	3.13	93.59	0.18	7.48
Q_{15}	14	3246.33	231.881	1.54	87.75	0.40	32.02
PY	14	3173.80	226.70	1.61	88.23	0.38	8.46
$\Delta G°_{tr}$	14	55168743	3440625	22.33	99.05	0.013	8.64
ΔH	14	12099	864.24	1.10	83.75	0.53	28.11
Ss	14	0.88	0.063	7.46	97.21	0.05	5.12

Discussion

According to Noyes–Whitney equation, the dissolution rat is proportional to the surface area exposed to the dissolution medium.[13] In addition to the general solubility enhancement techniques described above; drug particle size reduction has often been used, in regards to the Noyes–Whitney and Ostwald–Freundlich equations, to enhance dissolution of poorly water-soluble compounds.[14]

Disruptions in the crystal lattice can cause physical or chemical instability. Micronized powders with a higher energetic surface show poor flow property and broad size distribution.[15]

The Hausner ratio is correlated to the flowability of a powder or microcrystals. A Hausner ratio greater than 1.25 is considered to be an indication of poor flowability for microcrystals.

XRD, DSC and FTIR studies

The FTIR, DSC, and XRD results showed no chemical interaction between the drug and the stabilizer, and crystalline habit modification has occurred in the microcrystals without any polymorphic changes.

The XRD revealed that crystallinity was reduced significantly in microcrystals. Negative Gibb's free energy change represented higher aqueous solubility of microcrystals. The enhanced dissolution rates attributed to the reduction of the particle size, change in crystal habit, formation of hydrophilic surface and the increased wettability due to adsorption of stabilizer agent and reduction in crystallinity of CLX during microcrystallization.

In vitro studies

Dissolution enhancement effect of CLX microcrystals explained by the reduction in the particle size and as a consequence the increment in the surface area, which is additionally hydrophilized by the adsorbed hydrophilic stabilizing agent. Moreover, the natural crystalline growth creates particles with no electrostatic charge and with better wettability properties.[16]

The *in vitro* release profiles of CLX from microcrystals (Table 2) exhibited initial burst effect, which may be due to the presence of some drug particles on the surface of the microcrystals. In most cases, a biphasic dissolution profile was observed: the initial rapid drug leakage generally ended very early and for the remaining time, nearly linear behavior was observed. The first portion of the dissolution curves is due to CLX dissolution, which starts immediately after the beginning of the test for the portion of drug on the surface of microcrystals. After such a phase, two phenomena can combine in enhancing in the diffusion of the remaining dispersed drug into the bulk phase as well as the formation of pores within the matrix due to the initial drug dissolution; particle wetting and swelling which enhances the permeability of the microcrystals to the drug (Table 2). Drug release rates were decreased with increasing amounts of drug in the formulation (Table 2). Higher level of CLX corresponding to higher level of the Brij 35 in the formulation resulted in an increase in the drug release rate (F_3). As more drugs are released from the microcrystals, more channels are probably produced, contributing to faster drug release rates. CLX microcrystals of each formulation displayed an immediate and important initial drug release in the first 30 min (22-40%), followed by an 84-87% during 60 min (Table 2).

During the crystal precipitation, surface energy of the system increases. Here, stabilizer agent (Brij 35) adsorbed onto the newly created surface of the precipitated drug in order to lower the interfacial tension. Thereby, the surface energy and consequently the enthalpy of the system are lowered. The formed small particles, which normally would aggregate in order to lower the surface energy, are stabilized sterically against crystal growth by an adsorbed layer of Brij 35. Micron sized particle formed and simultaneously stabilized in the formed dispersion by stabilizer agent.

CLX microcrystals were prepared by solvent change method using Brij 35 as a hydrophilic stabilizing agent. Solvent ratio (acetone/water) 0.1% Brij 35, 15 ml acetone, 100 ml water and 26000 RPM were optimum parameters for microcrystallization of CLX. Microcrystals produced using Brij 35 showed narrow particle size distribution and change in the crystal habit to small crystal type. A volume-based size distribution of drug, stabilizer agent, and drug loaded microcrystals indicated a log–probability distribution.

The results show that linear and interaction components in the proposed model are significant (R^2= 97.14). The optimum condition for CLX microcrystals preparation was 1:7.5 (w/w) drug to stabilizer agent ratio, 0.1 g amount of stabilizer agent, 15 ml (volume of organic phase), 100 ml (volume of aqueous phase), 5 min (time of stirring) and 26000 RPM. RPM, volume of organic phase and aqueous phase and stabilizer agent concentrations were the most effective factors on the particles size, drug content, crystal yield, free energy Gibbs change and solubility (MPE<10%) (Table 5). The results obtained from the predicted model were used to create a contour plot for particle size with rate of stirring and volume of aqueous solvent (Figure 5).

An increase in the rate of stirring, volume of organic phase, volume of dispersing medium, time of stirring and concentration of stabilizer agents leads to a decrease in particle size because the coefficient b_2 bears a negative sign (r^2=97.14, p=0.05 and MPE=6.24%).

An increase in the rate of stirring, volume of organic phase, volume of dispersing medium, time of stirring and concentration of stabilizer agents leads to an increase in drug content because the coefficient b_2 bears a positive sign (r^2=93.95, p=0.18 and MPE=7.48%).

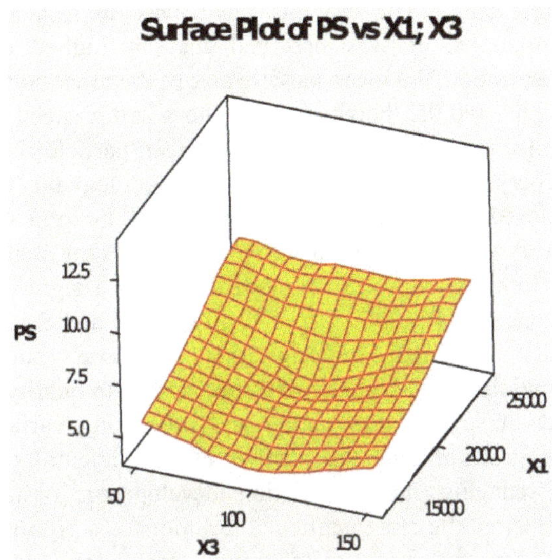

Figure 5. Response surface plot showing the effect of formulation variables (X1=RPM and X3=volume of aqueous phase) on particle size.

An increase in the rate of stirring, volume of dispersing medium, time of stirring and concentration of stabilizer agents (except volume of organic phase) leads to an increase in drug content because the coefficient b_2 bears a positive sign (r^2=87.75, p=0.4 and MPE=32.02%).

An increase in the volume of organic phase, volume of dispersing medium, time of stirring and concentration of stabilizer agent as HPMC (except rate of stirring, concentration of stabilizer agents as Brij 35 and Tween 80) leads to an increase in drug content because the coefficient b_2 bears a positive sign (r^2=88.23, p=0.38 and MPE=8.46%).

An increase in the rate of stirring, volume of organic phase, volume of dispersing medium, time of stirring and concentration of stabilizer agent as Brij 35 and Tween80 (except concentration of stabilizer agents as HPMC) leads to a decrease in drug content because the coefficient b_2 bears a positive sign (r^2=99.05, p=0.013 and MPE=8.64%).

An increase in the rate of stirring, volume of organic phase, volume of dispersing medium, time of stirring and concentration of stabilizer agent as brij35 and HPMC (except concentration of stabilizer agents as Tween80) leads to a decrease in drug content because the coefficient b_2 bears a positive sign (r^2=83.75, p=0.53 and MPE=28.11%).

An increase in the rate of stirring, volume of organic phase, volume of dispersing medium, time of stirring and concentration of stabilizer agents leads to an increase in drug content because the coefficient b_2 bears a positive sign (r^2=97.21, p=0.05 and MPE=5.12%) (Table 5).

Conclusion

CLX microcrystals were prepared using solvent change method (*insitu* micronization). Stirring speed, time of stirring, volume of solvent, volume of non-solvent and stabilizer agent influenced the characteristics of the microcrystals. The crystal Yield was high for all formulations. It was observed that at higher drug concentration, the mean particle size of the microcrystals is high (p>0.05) but increasing the stirring speed and stabilizer agent resulted in smaller mean particle size of microcrystals. A response surface methodology has been employed to produce CLX microcrystals for oral drug delivery with stabilizer agent by change solvent method. The formulation variables studied exerted a significant influence on PS, DC, Q_{15}, CY, $\Delta G°_{tr}$, ΔH and Ss. The results obtained indicate that response surface methodology can be employed successfully to qualify the effect of several formulation and processing variables thereby minimizing the number of experimental trials and reducing the formulation development cost. In conclusion, the aforementioned technique is a promising tool for effective microcrystal formation during pharmaceutical development in order to increase dissolution rate of poorly water soluble active ingredient.

Conflict of Interest

The authors report no conflicts of interest.

References

1. Rawat N, Senthil M, Mahadevan N. Solubility: Particle size reduction is a promising approach to improve the bioavailability of lipophillic drugs. *Int J Recent Adv Pharm Res* 2011;1(1):8-18.
2. Feeley JC, York P, Sumby BS, Dicks H. Determination of surface properties and flow characteristics of salbutamol sulphate, before and after micronisation. *Int J pharm* 1998;172(1):89-96. doi: 10.1016/s0378-5173(98)00179-3
3. Jacobs C, Kayser O, Möller RH. Nanosuspensions as a new approach for the formulation for the poorly soluble drug tarazepide. *Int J pharm* 2000;196(2):161-4. doi: 10.1016/s0378-5173(99)00412-3
4. Rasenack N, Hartenhauer H, Muller BW. Microcrystals for dissolution rate enhancement of poorly water-soluble drugs. *Int J Pharm* 2003;254(2):137-45. doi: 10.1016/s0378-5173(03)00005-x
5. Hans ML, Lowman AM. Biodegradable nanoparticles for drug delivery and targeting. *Curr Opin Solid St M* 2002;6(4):319-27. doi: 10.1016/s1359-0286(02)00117-1
6. Reynolds JEF, Parfitt K, Parsons A, Sweetman SC. Martindale. The Extra Pharma-copoeia 31 ed. London: Pharmaceutical Society; 1996.
7. Gupta VR, Mutalik S, Patel MM, Jani GK. Spherical crystals of celecoxib to improve solubility, dissolution rate and micromeritic properties. *Acta Pharm* 2007;57(2):173-84. doi: 10.2478/v10007-007-0014-8
8. Nagarsenker MS, Joshi MS. Celecoxib-cyclodextrin systems: characterization and evaluation of in vitro and in vivo advantage. *Drug Dev Ind Pharm* 2005;31(2):169-78. doi: 10.1081/DDC-200047795
9. Talari R, Varshosaz J, Mostafavi SA, Nokhodchi A. Gliclazide microcrystals prepared by two methods of in situ micronization: pharmacokinetic studies in diabetic and normal rats. *AAPS PharmSciTech* 2010;11(2):786-92. doi: 10.1208/s12249-010-9441-9
10. Talari R, Varshosaz J, Mostafavi SA, Nokhodchi A. Dissolution enhancement of gliclazide using pH change approach in presence of twelve stabilizers with various physico-chemical properties. *J Pharm Pharm Sci* 2009;12(3):250-65.
11. Azeredo HMC. Encapsulation: application technologia de alimentos. *Aliment Nutr Araraquara* 2005;16(1):89-97.
12. Narendra C, Srinath MS, Prakash Rao B. Development of three layered buccal compact containing metoprolol tartrate by statistical optimization technique. *Int J Pharm* 2005;304(1-2):102-14. doi: 10.1016/j.ijpharm.2005.07.021
13. Mansouri M, Pouretedal HR, Vosoughi V. Preparation and Characterization of Ibuprofen Nanoparticles by using Solvent/Antisolvent Precipitation. *Open Conf Proc J* 2011;2(1):88-94. doi: 10.2174/2210289201102010088
14. Mosharraf M, Nyström C. The effect of particle size and shape on the surface specific dissolution rate of microsized practically insoluble drugs. *Int J pharm* 1995;122(1):35-47. doi: 10.1016/0378-5173(95)00033-f
15. Möller RH, Peters K. Nanosuspensions for the formulation of poorly soluble drugs: I. Preparation by a size-reduction technique. *Int J Pharm* 1998;160(2):229-37. doi: 10.1016/s0378-5173(97)00311-6
16. Cunha-Filho MSS, Martínez-Pacheco R, Landin M. Dissolution rate enhancement of the novel antitumoral β-lapachone by solvent change precipitation of microparticles. *Eur J Pharm Biopharm* 2008;69(3):871-7. doi: 10.1016/j.ejpb.2008.02.014

Development of Floating-Mucoadhesive Microsphere for Site Specific Release of Metronidazole

Md. Lutful Amin*, Tajnin Ahmed, Md. Abdul Mannan

Department of Pharmacy, Stamford University Bangladesh.

Article info

Keywords:
- Alginate
- Guar gum
- Floating microsphere
- Metronidazole
- Mucoadhesive microsphere
- Eudragit

Abstract

Purpose: The purpose of this study was to develop and evaluate metronidazole loaded floating-mucoadhesive microsphere for sustained drug release at the gastric mucosa.

Methods: Alginate gastroretentive microspheres containing metronidazole were prepared by ionic gelation method using sodium bicarbonate as gas forming agent, guar gum as mucoadhesive polymer, and Eudragit L100 as drug release modifier. Carbopol was used for increasing the bead strength. The microspheres were characterized by scanning electron microscopy and evaluated by means of drug entrapment efficiency, *in vitro* buoyancy, and swelling studies. *In vitro* mucoadhesion and drug release studies were carried out in order to evaluate site specific sustained drug release.

Results: All formulations showed 100% buoyancy *in vitro* for a prolonged period of time. Amount of guar gum influenced the properties of different formulations. The formulation containing drug and guar gum at a ratio of 1:0.5 showed the best results with 76.3% drug entrapment efficiency, 61.21% mucoadhesion, and sustained drug release. Carbopol was found to increase surface smoothness of the microspheres.

Conclusion: Metronidazole mucoadhesive-floating microspheres can be effectively used for sustained drug release to the gastric mucosa in treatment of upper GIT infection.

Introduction

Metronidazole is a nitroimidazole antimicrobial which is effective against a variety of anaerobic bacteria.[1,2] It is actively used as an adjunct in the treatment of *H.pylori* infection, responsible for developing gastric ulcers.[3] Treatment of upper gastro-intestinal tract (GIT) infection is challenging due to the location of the infection site in stomach mucus lining.[4] Treatment of local gastric infection with conventional formulations becomes ineffective due to their short gastric residence time and non-targeted drug release. Gastric emptying, which is highly variable, transfer the conventional formulation quickly to the intestine without significant release of drug to the mucous site. Thus frequent dosing is required.[5,6]

Gastroretentive drug delivery systems favor prolonged drug release in the stomach.[7] Unlike traditional controlled release formulations, they bypass the gastric emptying process which interferes with drug delivery to the upper GIT.[8] Gastroretentive drug delivery systems have been developed employing floating technique. Asnaashari et al. developed HPMC based metronidazole floating tablet and showed gastric buoyancy for a prolonged period.[9] In general, these floating dosage forms release drugs at multidirections and cannot selectively release drugs on the mucosal surface. Consequently, small amount of drug reaches the target site from multidirectional drug release. Release of drug to the specific site is important for effective treatment.[10] It is particularly necessary for eradicating the local infection at the mucous layer where drugs from conventional formulations may not reach.[11] Previous studies mainly focused on developing floating formulations. However, site specific metronidazole delivery system was not explored. Mucoadhesive drug delivery systems have recently been explored for sustained release at the mucosa and increasing bioavailability of drugs.[12] Indeed, drug delivery systems with floating and mucoadhesive properties may ideally maximize drug release to the specific site, adhering to the mucous layer, in treatment of upper GIT infection.

This study was aimed to develop metronidazole loaded floating-mucoadhesive microsphere for drug release at the mucous layer of upper GIT. Metronidazole microsphere was developed by ionic gelation method using sodium alginate and calcium chloride. Sodium bicarbonate was used to incorporate floating property in the microsphere. Eudragit L100, which dissolves at a pH greater than 6, was used for sustained drug release. Guar gum, a natural viscous polymer having adhesive property, was used for mucoadhesion. Additionally, guar gum was reported to be useful as a gastroprotective agent against peptic ulcer. It reduces gastric acid, and promotes ulcer healing.[13] Besides, alginate has *in situ* gel forming ability, and good mucoadhesive property.[14] Mucoadhesive property of guar gum and sodium alginate was compared.

***Corresponding author:** Md. Lutful Amin, Email: lutful_amin@yahoo.com

Materials and Methods

Materials

Eudragit L100 and Carbopol 940 were purchased from Evonik Industries and Lubrizol Corporation, respectively. Metronidazole was provided as a gift sample from Beximco Pharmaceuticals Ltd. Sodium alginate and guar gum were supplied by Sigma-Aldrich. Sodium bicarbonate and calcium chloride (crosslinking agent) were obtained from Merck KGaA, Germany, and Wilfrid Smith Ltd., UK, respectively. Deionized water was locally produced in the laboratory, and used for all the experiments. All chemicals used were of analytical grade.

Methods

Preparation of microsphere

Metronidazole floating-mucoadhesive microspheres were prepared by ionic gelation method[15] varying the ratio of guar gum and Eudragit (Table 1). Sodium alginate was dissolved in deionized (DI) water (3% w/v). Carbopol (0.06:1 with alginate) was dissolved separately in DI water, and Euragit L100 was mixed in the thick Carbopol solution. In case of formulations containing guar gum, guar gum was added to the Eudragit-Carbopol mixture. Metronidazole (0.6:1 with alginate) was added in the Carbopol-Eudragit matrix and stirred vigorously. Then the gas forming agent sodium bicarbonate (0.2:1 with alginate) was mixed. The prepared slurry was added to sodium alginate solution and mixed continuously. Crosslinking solution was prepared by dissolving calcium chloride in DI water (5% w/v) containing 10% v/v glacial acetic acid. Then the mixture, free from air bubbles, was added drop-wise to the crosslinking solution through a syringe containing 26G needle. The immediately formed beads were collected by filtration and air dried for 8-10 hours. Spherical dried microspheres were stored in air tight vials for further evaluation. All experiments were performed in triplicate, and the data are shown as mean±standard deviations.

Table 1. Polymer ratio (with alginate), particle size, DEE, and swelling index of the developed microspheres.

Formulations	Eudragit L100	Guar gum	Avg. Size of Microsphere (µm)	DEE (%)	Swelling Index
M1	0.15	-	725.34± 17.4	39.67±3.21	0.53±0.01
M2	0.3	-	739.91± 23.3	46.75±4.19	1.20±0.02
M3	0.15	0.15	847.44± 29.7	65.12±3.87	2.18±0.03
M4	0.15	0.3	901.70± 13.3	76.30±2.56	2.59±0.01

Morphology and size

The morphology of the microspheres was studied by electron scanning microscopy (SEM). Microspheres from each formulation were sputter coated with gold under the vacuum. The images were taken at an acceleration voltage (20 kV) by a scanning electron microscope (JEOL JSM – 6490 LA, Japan). Shape and surface texture of the microspheres were analyzed.

Standard sieving method was used to determine the particle size of the microspheres.[16] Microspheres from each formulation were spread on the upper sieve of an automatic sieve shaker (AS 200, Germany) and sieved. The amount passed and retained on each sieve was weighed and the average particle size was calculated using the following equation;

$$\text{Mean particle size} = \frac{\Sigma\ (\text{mean particle size of the fraction} \times \text{weight fraction})}{\Sigma\ (weigt\ fraction)}$$

Drug entrapment efficiency (DEE)

Microspheres, containing 50 mg of metronidazole, were crushed and immersed into 100mL of simulated gastric fluid (SGF) (0.1N HCl; pH 1.2, without pepsin). The suspension was kept oscillating overnight and filtered through a 0.22 mm filter. The drug concentration was determined by a UV spectrophotometer (Hatch 4000) at the wavelength of 278 nm. DEE was calculated according to the following equation:

$$\text{DEE\%} = \frac{\text{Actual drug content}}{\text{Theoretical amount of drug}} \times 100$$

In vitro buoyancy

In vitro floating properties of the metronidazole loaded microspheres were evaluated in a USP dissolution apparatus II (paddle type).[7] 50 individual microspheres from each formulation were immersed into the vessel filled with 500 mL of SGF. The paddles were rotated at 50 RPM and the temperature was maintained at 37±0.5°C. The number of floating microspheres was counted at hourly intervals up to 8 hours. *In vitro* buoyancy was expressed as a percentage and was calculated from the following equation:

$$\text{F (\%)} = \frac{\text{Number of floating beads}}{\text{Total number of beads immersed}} \times 100$$

Swelling measurement

Swelling study was conducted using the dissolution test apparatus II. Accurately weighed amount of beads were placed in the vessels containing SGF and allowed to swell. Rotation speed was set at 50 rpm. The microspheres were withdrawn at predetermined time intervals and blotted with filter paper to remove excess amount of water. The changes in weight were measured at different time intervals until maximum weight was gained. The swelling index was then calculated using the following equation:
Swelling index (S):

$$S = \frac{W_m - W_t}{W_t}$$

Where, W_t denotes the initial weight of the microspheres, and W_m denotes the weight at equilibrium.

In vitro mucoadhesion study

Mucoadhesion property was evaluated using rat stomach mucosa.[17] The tissue specimen was collected and cut into required size (2cm × 1cm). Microspheres from each formulation were spread onto the rinsed stomach mucosa and kept inside a humidity chamber at 80% relative humidity and 25°C for 20 minutes. Then those were rinsed with SGF placing at an angle of 45°. The number of microspheres adhering to the tissue was calculated and mucoadhession was expressed as the percentage.

In vitro drug release study

Drug release from the floating microspheres was investigated using the USP dissolution apparatus I (basket type). SGF (0.1M HCl; pH 1.2) was used as the dissolution medium and 500mL of it was poured into each dissolution vessel. Microspheres, equivalent to 50 mg of metronidazole, were placed inside the baskets and they were rotated at a speed of 50 rpm, maintained at a temperature of 37±0.5°C. An aliquot of 5mL was withdrawn at hourly intervals up to 8 hours and the volume was replaced with 5mL of fresh medium. The aliquots were diluted and the concentration of metronidazole was determined spectrophotometrically at 278 nm.

Results and Discussion

Metronidazole microsphere, with floating and mucoadhesive properties, was successfully developed by ionic gelation method. The underlying mechanism involves crosslinking of the carboxylate groups of the alginate molecules by divalent calcium ions.[18] Sodium bicarbonate was used as the gas forming substance to incorporate floating property, which reacted with glacial acetic acid and formed CO_2 [equation 1]. Four different formulations (M1-M4) were developed varying the ratio of Eudragit L100 and guar gum, keeping the amount of alginate, metronidazole, Carbopol, and sodium bicarbonate constant. The amount of sodium bicarbonate was determined by formulating microspheres with lower amounts. The specified amount was found to be optimal for developing floating microsphere.

Equation 1:

$$NaHCO_3 + CH_3COOH = CH_3COONa + CO_2 + H_2O \text{ ------------- } (1)$$

Production of carbon dioxide by sodium bicarbonate usually impedes the crosslinking of the alginate molecules. As Carbopol is viscous and possesses free carboxylate groups,[19] it was used for additional crosslinking by calcium ions to increase bead strength and surface smoothness.

All microspheres were discrete and acceptably spherical. The formulations M1 and M2 were relatively smoother than the microspheres containing guar gum (M3 and M4). Figure 1 shows the shape and surface topography of the microspheres. The SEM images showed that the surface of M2 was smoother than that of M4 (Figure 1). Presence of guar gum on the surface of the microspheres might cause a slightly rough surface as guar gum can interfere with the crosslinking process of alginate by calcium ions.

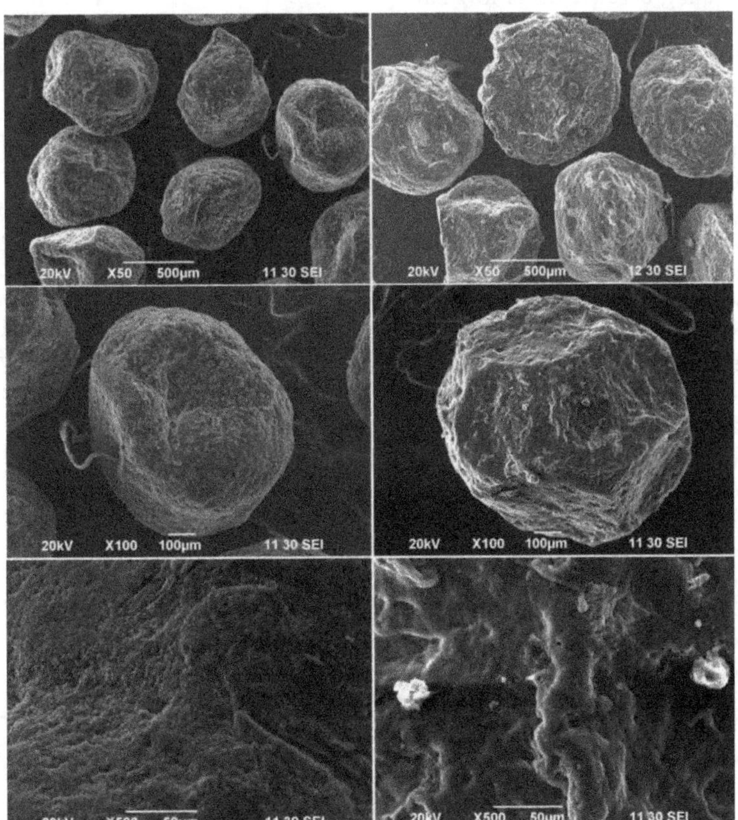

Figure 1. Shape and surface texture of the prepared microspheres: left: formulation M2, right: formulation M4.

Table 1 summarizes the formulation variables, size, swelling index, and DEE of the formulations. The sizes of formulation M1 and M2 were smaller than that of M3 and M4. Addition of guar gum increased the viscosity of the slurry resulting in an increase in droplet volume which caused larger particle size. Thus, the size of the microspheres also increased with increasing polymer ratio. Swelling study was performed in order to evaluate solvent uptake by different formulations. It can also be correlated with drug diffusion. Result showed that swelling ability of M3 and M4 was higher than that of other formulations (Table 1). Greater hydrophilicity and high water retaining capacity of guar gum facilitated increased swelling. Moreover, surface guar gum provided rapid hydration. In contrast, swelling of M1 and M2 was low due to lower hydration rate and lack of polymer solubility.

The DEE was affected by both polymer ratio and the type of polymer. Formulations M3 and M4 possessed higher DEE (65.12% and 76.3%, respectively) than that of formulations M1 and M2. Addition of guar gum increased viscosity and prevented diffusion of drug to the crosslinking solution more than Carbopol alone during carbon dioxide formation by sodium bicarbonate. The entrapment efficiency of M1 and M2 was low due to the diffusion of drug into the crosslinking solution as a result of CO_2 production. DEE increased with increasing polymer ratio due to increase of viscosity. *In vitro* floating test revealed that all the formulations had excellent floating ability. 100% floating was observed for all the batches (M1-M4) after 8 hours of study. Eudragit might have aided for prolonged floating because of its low bulk density as previously reported.[20]

Figure 2 illustrates the *in vitro* mucoadhesion properties of different formulations. The formulations were compared with the control spheres (prepared with alginate, Eudragit (0.3), and sodium bicarbonate). The formulations M3 and M4 showed higher mucoadhesion than that of formulations M1 and M2. M4 demonstrated the highest mucoadhesion ability (61.21%) among all formulations. According to the mechanism of mucoadhesion, wetting and swelling of the polymer is the initial step employing intimate contact with the mucosa which results in interpenetration and entanglement between the polymer and the mucin chains, promoting hydrogen bond formation.[21] Rapid hydration of guar gum present on the microsphere surface facilitated expansion of polymer chain and formation of hydrogen bond with the mucous layer. Linear relationship was observed between swelling index and mucoadhesion. In contrast, lack of surface hydration resulted in reduced solvent transfer which might cause low mucoadhesion of formulations M1 and M2. Hence, alginate alone could not sufficiently provide mucoadhesion. Combination of alginate and guar gum can work well to form adhesion bond with the gastric mucosa. This result showed that the developed formulation can provide drug release at the gastric mucosa having both floating and mucoadhesive properties. Previously reported studies focused on floating formulation of metronidazole. However, for treating local infection at the gastric mucosa, site specific drug release would be more beneficial. Moreover, Formulations with only floating property provides multidirectional drug release. Combination of floating and mucoadhesive properties maximizes drug release at the mucus membrane.

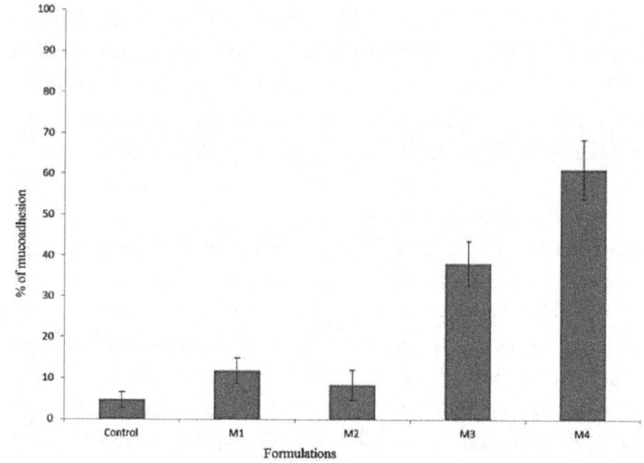

Figure 2. *In vitro* mucoadhesion property of different formulations. Control: alginate microsphere with Eudragit and sodium bicarbonate only.

Drug release was affected by polymer solubility and surface hydration of the microspheres. Figure 3 shows the drug release profile of different formulations. The release of metronidazole from the formulations M1 and M2 was very low (~ 31% and 29% release, respectively after 8 h). Acid insoluble property of Eudragit L100 and lack of hydration resulted in poor solvent transfer and very slow drug release. A large quantity of drugs might be embedded in Eudragit and could not diffuse out of the microspheres, leading to the low cumulative release of the drug. However, formulations M3 and M4 provided steady and sustained drug release (~ 62% and 73%, respectively, after 8 h). Hydration and swelling of guar gum attributed to the steady drug release. Guar gum is thixotropic in nature which can facilitate solvent transfer into the microspheres. A little faster release in the first hour was possibly associated with the amount of drug present on the particle surface. Mechanism of drug release was determined by fitting the dissolution data in different kinetic models. It revealed that the release of drug followed Higuchi's model where non-Fickian diffusion was the primary mechanism.

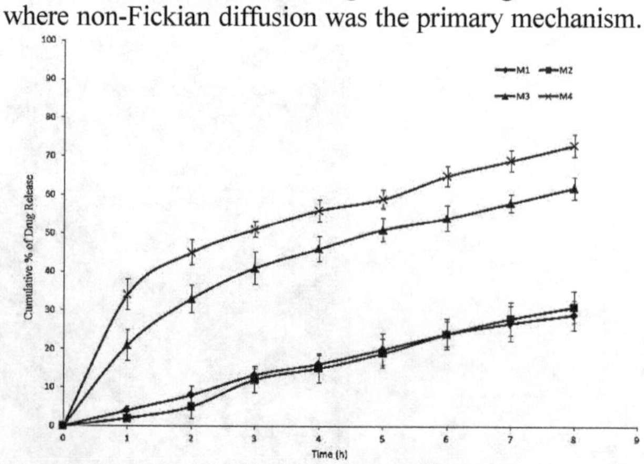

Figure 3. Drug release profile of the metronidazole loaded floating microspheres in SGF.

Among all the formulations, M4 showed the best results in terms of floating, DEE, mucoadhesion, and drug release. The effect of guar gum was prominent in the formulation. The results substantiate the primary hypothesis for providing specific drug release to the gastric mucosa with prolonged floating and good mucoadhesive property.

Conclusion

In this study, metronidazole loaded floating-mucoadhesive microsphere was developed for drug delivery to the mucous layer in upper GIT. Microspheres were successfully developed with the combination of natural and synthetic polymers. Guar gum was found to be important for DEE, mucoadhesion, and drug release of the microspheres. Formulation M4 showed the best results which contained maximum amount of guar gum among all other formulations. It provided longer floating, good mucoadhesion, and steady drug release implying its potential for the treatment of upper GIT infections.

Acknowledgments

The authors are thankful to the Department of Pharmacy, Stamford University Bangladesh for providing materials and support.

Conflict of Interest

Authors declare no conflict of interest in this study.

References

1. Cohen-Wolkowiez M, Sampson M, Bloom BT, Arrieta A, Wynn JL, Martz K, et al. Determining population and developmental pharmacokinetics of metronidazole using plasma and dried blood spot samples from premature infants. *Pediatr Infect Dis J* 2013;32(9):956-61. doi: 10.1097/INF.0b013e3182947cf8
2. de CBC, Berto LA, Venancio PC, Cogo K, Franz-Montan M, Motta RH, et al. Concentrations of metronidazole in human plasma and saliva after tablet or gel administration. *J Pharm Pharmacol* 2014;66(1):40-7. doi: 10.1111/jphp.12161
3. Kusters JG, van Vliet AH, Kuipers EJ. Pathogenesis of helicobacter pylori infection. *Clin Microbiol Rev* 2006;19(3):449-90. doi: 10.1128/CMR.00054-05
4. Romano M, Cuomo A. Eradication of helicobacter pylori: A clinical update. *MedGenMed* 2004;6(1):19.
5. Sahasathian T, Praphairaksit N, Muangsin N. Mucoadhesive and floating chitosan-coated alginate beads for the controlled gastric release of amoxicillin. *Arch Pharm Res* 2010;33(6):889-99. doi: 10.1007/s12272-010-0612-8
6. Chun MK, Sah H, Choi HK. Preparation of mucoadhesive microspheres containing antimicrobial agents for eradication of h. Pylori. *Int J Pharm* 2005;297(1-2):172-9. doi: 10.1016/j.ijpharm.2005.03.011
7. Ishak RA, Awad GA, Mortada ND, Nour SA. Preparation, in vitro and in vivo evaluation of stomach-specific metronidazole-loaded alginate beads as local anti-helicobacter pylori therapy. *J Control Release* 2007;119(2):207-14. doi: 10.1016/j.jconrel.2007.02.012
8. Chen YC, Ho HO, Liu DZ, Siow WS, Sheu MT. Swelling/floating capability and drug release characterizations of gastroretentive drug delivery system based on a combination of hydroxyethyl cellulose and sodium carboxymethyl cellulose. *PLoS One* 2015;10(1):e0116914. doi: 10.1371/journal.pone.0116914
9. Asnaashari S, Khoei NS, Zarrintan MH, Adibkia K, Javadzadeh Y. Preparation and evaluation of novel metronidazole sustained release and floating matrix tablets. *Pharm Dev Technol* 2011;16(4):400-7. doi: 10.3109/10837451003774393
10. Bakowsky H, Richter T, Kneuer C, Hoekstra D, Rothe U, Bendas G, et al. Adhesion characteristics and stability assessment of lectin-modified liposomes for site-specific drug delivery. *Biochim Biophys Acta* 2008;1778(1):242-9. doi: 10.1016/j.bbamem.2007.09.033
11. Bytzer P, O'Morain C. Treatment of helicobacter pylori. *Helicobacter* 2005;10 Suppl 1:40-6. doi: 10.1111/j.1523-5378.2005.00333.x
12. Shaikh R, Raj Singh TR, Garland MJ, Woolfson AD, Donnelly RF. Mucoadhesive drug delivery systems. *J Pharm Bioallied Sci* 2011;3(1):89-100. doi: 10.4103/0975-7406.76478
13. Borrelli F, Izzo AA. The plant kingdom as a source of anti-ulcer remedies. *Phytother Res* 2000;14(8):581-91.
14. Kesavan K, Nath G, Pandit JK. Sodium alginate based mucoadhesive system for gatifloxacin and its in vitro antibacterial activity. *Sci Pharm* 2010;78(4):941-57. doi: 10.3797/scipharm.1004-24
15. Choi BY, Park HJ, Hwang SJ, Park JB. Preparation of alginate beads for floating drug delivery system: Effects of co(2) gas-forming agents. *Int J Pharm* 2002;239(1-2):81-91.
16. Mateovic-Rojnik T, Frlan R, Bogataj M, Bukovec P, Mrhar A. Effect of preparation temperature in solvent evaporation process on eudragit rs microsphere properties. *Chem Pharm Bull (Tokyo)* 2005;53(1):143-6.
17. Rajinikanth PS, Karunagaran LN, Balasubramaniam J, Mishra B. Formulation and evaluation of clarithromycin microspheres for eradication of helicobacter pylori. *Chem Pharm Bull (Tokyo)* 2008;56(12):1658-64.
18. Amin ML, Jesmeen T, Sutradhar KB, Mannan MA. Development and in vitro evaluation of diclofenac sodium loaded mucoadhesive microsphere with natural gum for sustained delivery. *Curr Drug Deliv* 2013;10(6):765-70.

19. Neutralizing Carbopol® and Pemulen™ Polymers in Aqueous and Hydroalcoholic Systems. Lubrizol. Technical Data Sheet. https://www.lubrizol.com/Home-Care/Documents/Technical-Data-Sheets/TDS-237-Neutralizing-Carbopol-Pemulen-in-Aqueous-Hydroalcoholic-Systems--HC.pdf. 2015
20. El-Kamel AH, Sokar MS, Al Gamal SS, Naggar VF. Preparation and evaluation of ketoprofen floating oral delivery system. *Int J Pharm* 2001;220(1-2):13-21.
21. Serra L, Domenech J, Peppas NA. Engineering design and molecular dynamics of mucoadhesive drug delivery systems as targeting agents. *Eur J Pharm Biopharm* 2009;71(3):519-28. doi: 10.1016/j.ejpb.2008.09.022

15

pH-Triggered Magnetic-Chitosan Nanogels (MCNs) For Doxorubicin Delivery: Physically vs. Chemically Cross Linking Approach

Somayeh Sadighian[1], Hassan Hosseini-Monfared[1]*, Kobra Rostamizadeh[2,3], Mehrdad Hamidi[2,4]

[1] *Faculty of Science, Department of Chemistry, University of Zanjan, Zanjan, Iran.*
[2] *Zanjan Pharmaceutical Nanotechnology Research Center, Zanjan University of Medical Sciences, Zanjan, Iran.*
[3] *Department of Medicinal Chemistry, School of Pharmacy, Zanjan University of Medical Sciences, Zanjan, Iran.*
[4] *Department of Pharmaceutics, School of Pharmacy, Zanjan University of Medical Sciences, Zanjan, Iran.*

Article info

Keywords:
- Magnetite
- Chitosan
- Doxorubicin
- Nanocomposites

Abstract

Purpose: This paper evaluates the impact of cross linking strategy on the characteristics of magnetic chitosan nanogels (MCNs) as targeted drug delivery system for doxorubicin.
Methods: Sodium tripolyphosphate (TPP) and glutaraldehyde were used as physical (electrostatic) and chemical (covalent binding) cross-linker agents, respectively. MCNs were characterized by means of X-ray diffraction (XRD), Scanning electron microscopy (SEM), fourier transform infrared (FT-IR) spectroscopy and vibrating sample magnetometer (VSM). Scanning electron microscopy (SEM) indicated the formation of spherical nanostructures with the final average particle size of around 35-40 nm.
Results: The finding proved the superparamagnetic properties of the MCNs with relatively high-magnetization values which indicate that the MCNs were enough sensitive to external magnetic fields as a magnetic drug carrier. To understand the differences between the drug delivery properties of chemically and physically cross linked MCNs, the drug release studies were also conducted. Altogether, the results of this study clearly indicate that, however, both MCNs exhibited sustained drug release behaviour, the chemically cross linked MCNs provided enhanced controlled drug release characteristics in comparison to physically cross linked MCNs. Besides, according to the drug release behaviour of MCNs in buffer solutions in two different medium with the pH values of 5.3 and 7.4, it was clear that both nanoparticles exhibited pH sensitivity where the extent of drug release in the acidic media was significantly higher than neutral media.
Conclusion: It can be concluded that chemically cross linked MCNs may serve as an ideal carrier for stimuli-triggered and controlled anticancer drug delivery.

Introduction

Polymeric nanocomposites consisting of inorganic nanoparticles and organic polymers as a new class of materials have attracted wide attention in different fields. They offer unique features with the combination of both inorganic nanoparticles and organic polymers characteristics, which are not available in each individual constituent.[1] The nanocomposites provide significant improvements in several properties, such as optical, mechanical, and magnetic properties.[2] Magnetic nanoparticles (MNPs) are a rapidly evolving materials contributing to their multifunctional properties including small size, superparamagnetism and low toxicity.[3] Particularly in the pharmaceutical field, they have now attracted a lot of interests owing to their intrinsic magnetic properties for guided delivery of drugs.[4] In order to improve MNPs characteristics for drug delivery propose such as colloidal stability and prolong circulation kinetics, it is demonstrated that their coatings with hydrophilic polymers, namely chitosan, could be considered as an adequate strategy. Chitosan, a naturally-derived co-polymer of N-acetyglucosamine and d -glucosamine, has been extensively studied as a biodegradable and biocompatible polymer in drug delivery systems, gene therapy, and membranes for ultrafiltration.[5,6] It seems that chitosan-encapsulated Fe_3O_4 nanoparticles would most likely improve magnetite nanoparticles characteristics in terms of biodegradability and long circulation time. Moreover, the amino groups on the chitosan structure can also be used for further functionalization with specific components, such as targeting agents, various drugs, or other functional groups for the purpose of achieving carriers with advanced characteristics. We reported on our recent study the synthesis and in vitro characterization of a dual targeted drug delivery system using a core–shell magnetite nanoparticulate system conjugated with doxorubicin. In order to enhance the biocompatibility of carrier and minimize unwanted side effects of doxorubicin and Fe_3O_4 nanoparticles, conjugated magnetite core–shell nanoparticles were encapsulated within chitosan.[7]
Doxorubicin and its bioactive derivatives are among the

***Corresponding author:** Hassan Hosseini-Monfared, Email: monfared@znu.ac.ir most widely used anticancer drugs in chemotherapy treatment,[8] however, it suffers from disadvantageous side effects. Drug targeting, therefore, shows an interesting motivation to prevent side effects and enhance cytotoxicity of doxorubicin. The majority of attempts to associate doxorubicin to nanoparticulate carriers have used anionic or neutral polymers. For instance, Janes et al.[9] synthesized chitosan/ TPP nanoparticles to encapsulate doxorubicin as an efficient drug carrier with possibility of targeting to specific site, reduced side effects and controlled drug release.

Following our previous results, in this contribution we aimed to investigate the impact of crosslinking strategy on the chitosan modified magnetic nanoparticles characteristics for the purpose of designing novel drug carrier with improved properties in terms of targeting to specific site, reduced side effects and controlled drug release. To achieve the goal, chitosan modified magnetic nanoparticles were prepared by two different cross linking methods; (1) physically by ionotropic gelation method using tripolyphosphate (TPP) and (2) chemically via glutaraldehyde.[10]

Materials and Methods

Materials

Ferric chloride hexahydrate ($FeCl_3 \cdot 6H_2O$), ferrous chloride tetrahydrate ($FeCl_2 \cdot 4H_2O$), sodium tripolyphosphate (TPP), glutaraldehyde and glacial acetic acid were from Merck and purchased locally. Chitosan of molecular weight in the range of $10^5 - 3\times10^5$ g/mol and degree of deacetylation ≥75% was obtained from Sigma. Doxorubicin hydrochloride was purchased from Celonlabs (Andhra Pradesh, India).

Preparation of TPP cross linked magnetic chitosan nanogels (TPP/MCNs)

TPP cross linked magnetic chitosan nanogels (TPP/MCNs) were prepared by the co-precipitating method. Briefly, ferric chloride hexahydrate (2 mmol) and ferrous sulfate heptahydrate (1 mmol) were dissolved in 50 ml of acetic acid buffer solution of chitosan (chitosan solution was prepared by dissolving 0.5 g chitosan powder in acetate buffer (100 mL, pH=4.8) at room temperature). Next, 3 mL of NH_4OH solution (25%) was added to the solution under vigorous stirring at 80 °C. The synthesis process was followed by the addition of 12.5 ml of 1 mg/ml TPP solution as cross-linker. Then, the black product was separated by an external magnet and washed three times with distilled water to remove the excess ammonia and finally the product were dried in vacuum conditions at 60 °C for 12 h.

Preparation of glutaraldehyde cross linked magnetic chitosan nanogels (GA/MCNs)

Glutaraldehyde cross-linked magnetic chitosan nanogels (GA/MCNs) were prepared as follows: Typically, ferric chloride hexahydrate (2 mmol) and ferrous sulfate heptahydrate (1 mmol) were dissolved in 50 ml of acetic acid buffer solution of chitosan (1 w/v%) and followed by the addition of 0.5 ml glutaraldehyde solution (25%) under vigorous stirring to obtain a homogeneous solution. Then, the solution was held until the chitosan hydrogel was formed completely due to the cross-linking effect of glutaraldehyde. The product was separated by an external magnet and washed several times with distilled water and lastly dried at 60 °C for 12 h.

Drug loading and release study

The drug loading was accomplished by dissolving 5 mg of doxorubicin in 25mL of deionized water containing 8 mg/mL of nanogels, and stirring for 24 h under dark condition at room temperature. Next, the drug loaded suspended nanoparticles were separated from the dispersion by centrifugation at 12000 rpm and then washed twice with deionized water to remove any loosely adsorbed drug on the surface of nanoparticles. Afterwards, the doxorubicin entrapped MCNs were dried in vacuumed oven at 30 °C for 12 h. To determine the extent of unloaded drug (free doxorubicin), the centrifuged solution was collected and analyzed for drug content by UV–Vis spectrophotometry at wavelength of 480 nm. The Entrapment efficiency was calculated from the following expression:

$$Entrapment\ efficiency(\%)=\frac{total\ amount\ of\ drug - free\ amount\ of\ drug}{total\ amount\ of\ drug}\times 100$$

The drug release behavior of MCNs was studied in physiological pH of 7.4. Typically, 2.0 mg of MCNs were placed into a dialysis bag (cut off 12 kDa) and introduced to 15 mL of phosphate buffered saline (PBS) with desired pH under stirring (100 rpm) at 37 °C. At predetermined time intervals, in order to determine the extent of released drug, and thereby time dependent drug release profile, 1.0 mL of solution was taken out and replaced with 1.0 mL of fresh buffer solution maintained at 37 °C and assayed by UV–Vis spectroscopy at wavelength of 480 nm. To evaluate the pH dependency of drug release from MCNs, the release study was also conducted in acidic media with pH value of 5.3.

Characterization techniques

FT-IR spectra of nanoparticles were taken with a Matson FT–IR spectrophotomer in the range of 400–4000 cm^{-1} as KBr disks at room temperature. The XRD patterns of nanoparticles were recorded on an x-ray diffractometer (Bruker D8 Advence). The samples were irradiated with monochromatized Cu Kα radiation (0.154060 nm). The voltage and current used were 40 kV and 30 mA, respectively. Vibrating sample magnetometer (VSM, Meghnatis Daghigh Kavir Co, Iran) was used to characterize the magnetic properties of MCNs. The hysteresis of the magnetization was obtained by changing H between +8500 Oe and −8500 Oe. The zeta potential and particle size distribution of the prepared nanoparticles were determined by photon correlation spectroscopy (PCS) using a Nano/zetasizer (Malvern Instruments, Nano ZS, Worcestershire, UK) working on the dynamic light scattering (DLS) platform. Scanning electron microscopy (SEM), Hitachi f 4160 was used to examine the morphology and size distribution of the carriers.

Results and Discussion

FT-IR analysis

The chemical structure and functional groups of TPP/MCNs and GA/MCNs were investigated by FT-IR (Figure 1). As it can be seen, the appearance of characteristic peak of Fe–O stretching band at 577 cm^{-1} could evidence formation of magnetite nanopartcles. In chitosan, the broad band at 3430 cm^{-1} corresponds to the stretching vibration of –NH and –OH groups and the bands at 2920 cm^{-1} and 1600 cm^{-1} represent the presence of sreching and bending vibration of –CH and $–CH_2$ groups, respectively. The bands at 1026 and 1061 cm^{-1} (Figure 1a) were attributed to the ν(C-O) of chitosan and ν(P=O) of TPP/MCNs, respectively. In Figure 1c and d, the peak at 880 cm^{-1} can be clearly attributed to the presence of $=C–O–CH_3$ in the doxorubicin structure, which is indicative of the successful drug entrapment by the nanocarriers.

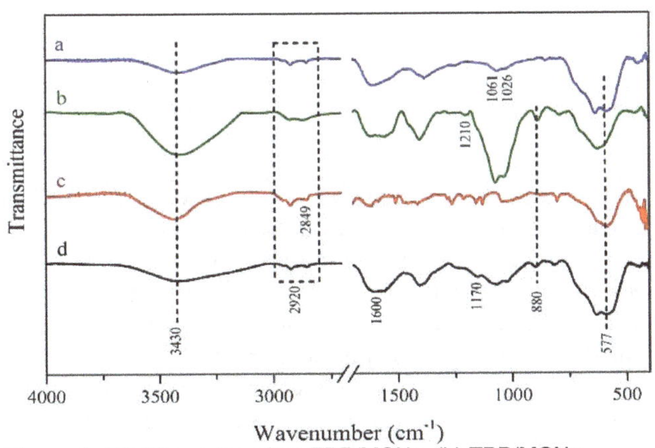

Figure 1. FT–IR spectra of (a) TPP/MCNs, (b) TPP/MCNs -doxorubicin, (c) GA/MCNs, (d) GA/MCNs -doxorubicin nanocomposites

Size and zeta potential measurements

The size of all nanoparticles was analyzed by DLS technique (Table 1). Particle size distribution curves exhibited only one peak with a relatively low polydispersity index. As it is clear, there was no significant difference between the particle size of TPP/MCNs and GA/MCNs. From the results, it can be concluded that type of crosslinking method has no influence on particle size of nanogels. The measurement of zeta potential provides valuable insight into the stability of colloidal aqueous dispersions. Usually, particle aggregation is less likely to occur for charged particles with optimum zeta potential because of electrostatic repulsions. The zeta potential and standard deviation values of nanogels are shown in Table 1. From the data presented in Table 1, higher negative charge of TPP/MCNs compared to the GA/MCNs can be related to the presence of TPP with negative charge in the nanogels structure.

Table 1. Average particle diameter, polydispersity index, and the surface zeta potential of chitosan nanogels, magnetite nanoparticles, and magnetic composites

Composite	Z-Average (nm)	PDI[a]	Zeta potential (mV)
Fe_3O_4 nanoparticles	186.0 ± 2.4	0.100	-31.00
TPP/MCNs	68.7 ± 4.6	0.466	-15.20
GA/MCNs	65.5 ± 2.3	0.250	-7.35

[a]Polydispersity index

Figure 2 shows the typical SEM images and corresponding histograms for TPP/MCNs and GA/MCNs. The histograms shows the average size of nanogels were about 40 and 35 nm for TPP/MCNs and GA/MCNs, respectively. Difference between the results of particle size of nanogels Size of particles from DLS technique was slightly larger than the ones from SEM technique which can be arise from measurement condition. Indeed, DLS analysis measures hydrodynamic diameter, while SEM results corresponds to the particle size in dry condition.

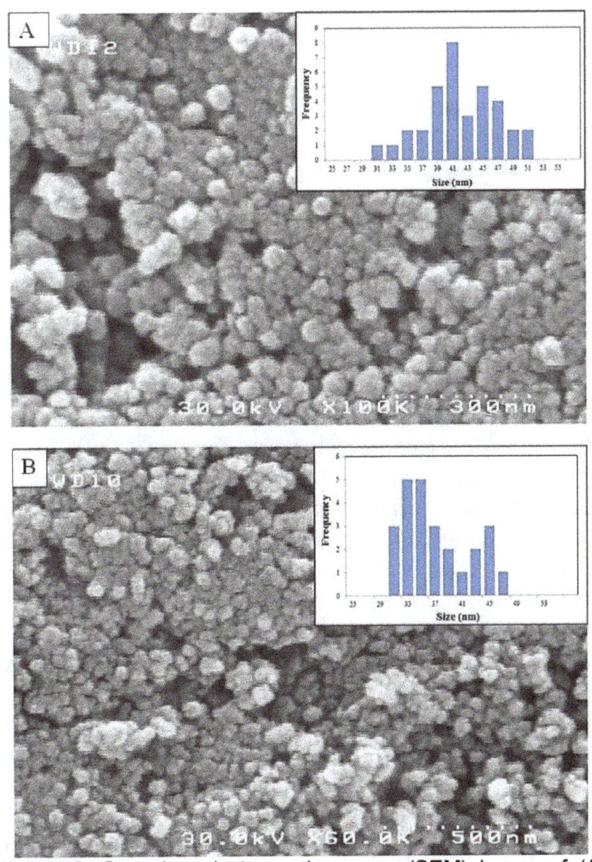

Figure 2. Scanning electron microscopy (SEM) image of (A) TPP/MCNs and (B) GA/MCNs

Magnetic properties of MCNs

High saturation magnetization is required so as to maximize the ability to target the particles using an external magnetic field. A representative hysteresis curve of the TPP/MCNs and GA/MCNs were studied by vibrating sample magnetometer as illustrated in Figure 3 by plotting of magnetization versus applied magnetic field (M–H loop) at 300 K. The saturation magnetization were 47.62 emu/g and 30.28 emu/g for TPP/MCNs and GA/MCNs, respectively. Giving consideration to the magnetization curve, it is clear that they exhibited neither remanence nor coercivity indicating that both MCNs show superparamagnetism. It was not surprising in the light of the size of nanoparticles, since it has been demonstrated that particles at a size in nanometer scale exhibit superparamagnetism.[11] The saturation magnetization of TPP/MCNs was slightly lesser than that of GA/MCNs probably due to their size.[12] Generally, it can be concluded that both nanoparticles have adequate superparamagnetic properties and could respond well to magnetic fields without any permanent magnetization as a magnetic drug carrier for targeted delivery.

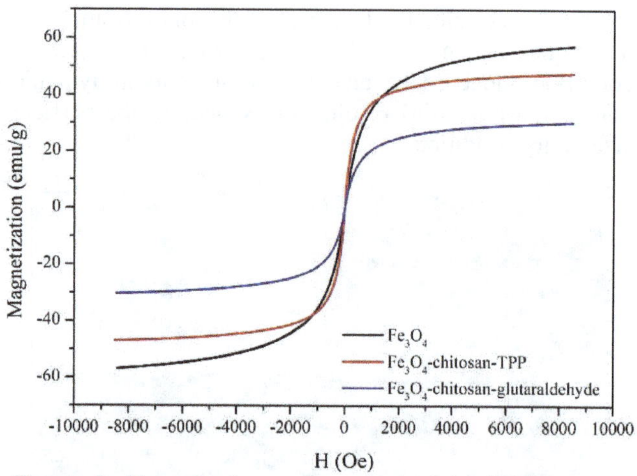

Figure 3. Magnetization curves obtained by VSM at room temperature

Figure 4 shows X-ray diffraction (XRD) patterns of TPP/MCNs and GA/MCNs nanogels. A series of characteristic peaks which correspond to (220), (311), (400), (422), (511) and (440) Bragg reflections of magnetite nanoparticles were observed for nanogels. The low intensity and broaden peaks indicates the presence of chitosan on the surface of Fe_3O_4 nanoparticles.

Drug loading and "In vitro" drug release studies

The results revealed that the drug loading for TPP/MCNs and GA/MCNs nanogels were 71% and 58%, respectively. Low drug loading for GA/MCNs can be related to the reaction of amino functional group of chitosan with carbonyl group of glutaraldehyde which consequently limits their possible interaction with carbonyl group of doxorubicin. Figure 5 illustrates the drug release response of the MCNs in PBS with two different pH values of 5.3 and 7.4 at the physiological temperature of 37 °C. Clearly, the drug release profiles of doxorubicin from both MCNs were approximately steady-linear throughout the time evaluated. Surprisingly in spite of common physically drug loading carrier in which generally there are a high extent of burst drug release, the results demonstrated that both variants showed a considerable sustained drug release behavior with no significant initial burst release in all media. Such behavior can be explained in view of various effective parameters on drug release behavior. Indeed, it is believed that the rate of drug release from the nanogels is theoretically affected by many factors such as rate of polymer degradation, diffusion of the drug through the nanogels particles, and extent of swelling of nanogels in aqueous media. As a results, sustained drug release profile of both MCNs can be presumably originate from high cross linking efficiency of nanogels which in turn restricts corresponding swelling ratio.

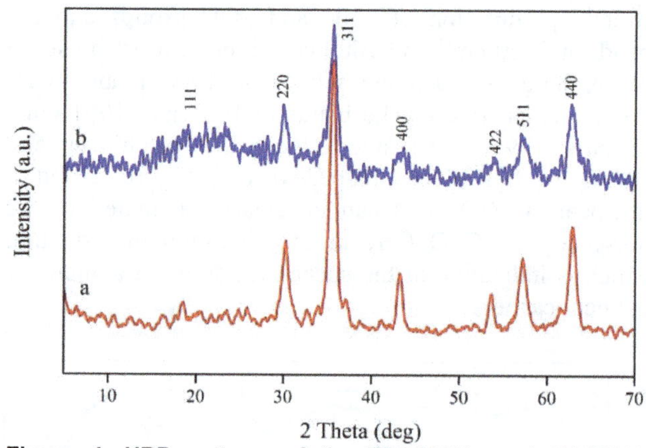

Figure 4. XRD patterns of the TPP/MCNs and GA/MCNs nanogels

From Figure 5, it is obvious that in case of TPP/MCNs about 34.5% of payload drug was released over 72 h, while for GA/MCNs it was close to 26% during the same period of time (pH=7.4). A possible explanation for this behavior could be the high stability of chemical cross linking compared to the physical cross linking. In fact, as the cross linking degrades the structure might become loose which, in turn, lead to high rate of drug release.

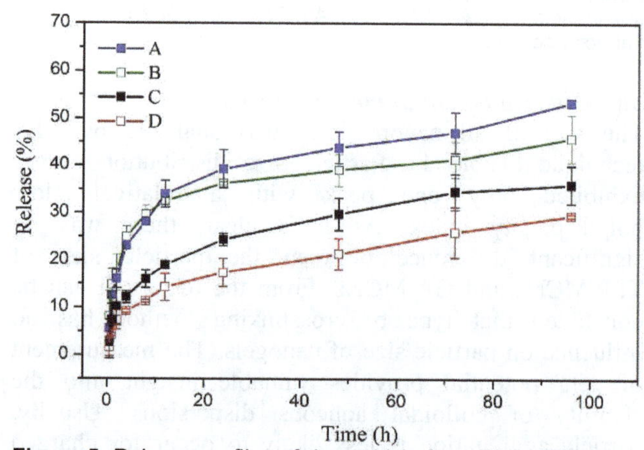

Figure 5. Release profiles of doxorubicin from TPP/MCNs (A in pH=5.3, C in pH=7.4) and GA/MCNs (B in pH=5.3, D in pH=7.4). Each data point represents the mean ±S.D. (n=3).

Additionally, another important and surprising feature of both carriers was pH dependency of drug release where it was high rate of drug release in acidic media (pH, 5.3) compared to the neutral pH (7.4). We believe that there are presumably two impetuses behind such observation. First, formation of pH sensitive imine bonds between amine functional group of chitosan and carbonyl group of doxorubicin in the course of drug loading. This hypothesis is supported by the appearance of imine characteristic peaks at 880 cm-1 in the FT-IR spectrum both MCNs (Figure 1). Secondly, acidic medium may enhance the swelling properties of chitosan and increasing the size of pores, and consequently increase the extent of drug diffusion from chitosan. There were similar reports in the literature to support this explanation.[13]

Drug release kinetic

To understand the factors that control the drug release from MCNs-doxorubicin nanogels, the release data were fitted with mathematical model. Drug release kinetics analyzed by fitting the cumulative release data to an exponential equation using the equation proposed by Korsmeyer-Peppas.

$$M_t/M_\infty = kt^n$$

Where M_t/M_∞ is a fraction of drug release at time t, n is the release exponent and k is the release rate constant. To find out the mechanism of drug release, first 60% drug release data were fitted in Korsmeyer-Peppas model. From TPP/MCNs and GA/MCNs (R^2=0.9473 and R^2=0.9694), respectively. A scattering plot of Ln-Ln fit is shown in Figure 6 for our experimental data. Using the least squares procedure, the values of n for TPP/MCNs and GA/MCNs were estimated to be 0.30 and 0.23 which indicate that for both nanogels the majority of drug release study (about 60%), the release mechanism is mainly dominated by the diffusion control mechanism.

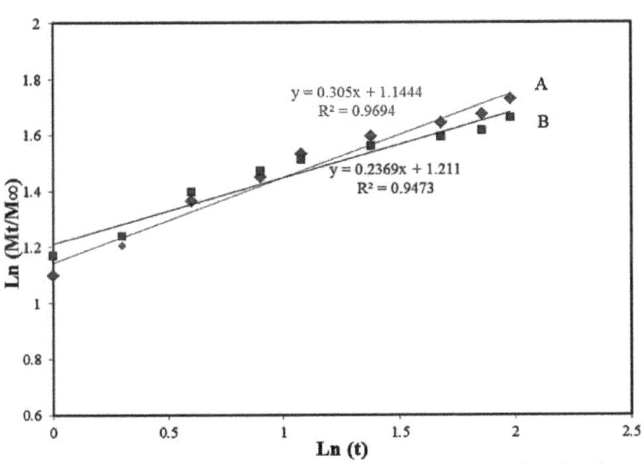

Figure 6. The data scattering plot showing the Ln-Ln fit of our experimental data according to the Korsmeyer and Peppas model (A=. TPP/MCNs-Doxorubicin, B= GA/MCNs-Doxorubicin)

Conclusion

In the present contribution, a novel pH sensitive magnetic chitosan nanogels (MCNs) composed were prepared using two different crosslinkers, i.e. tripolyphosphate (for physical crosslinking) (TPP/MCNs) and glutraldehyde (for chemical crosslinking, GA/MCNs). The FT-IR confirmed the successful synthesis of both MCNs. Scanning electron microscopy (SEM) and particle size analysis (DLS) confirmed the formation of spherical nanoparticles with the final average particle size about 35-40 nm (SEM). The VSM analysis showed saturation magnetization values of 47.62 and 30.28 emu/g for TPP/MCNs and GA/MCNs, respectively. Both MCNs possessed outstanding Entrapment efficiency for doxorubicin (76.6, 65.0%, for TPP/MCNs and GA/MCNs, respectively). The finding revealed that both MCNs provide a sustained release pattern. It was found that the maximum drug release attainable for TPP/MCNs was higher than the one for GA/MCNs, probably due to the high stability of chemically cross linking compared to the physically cross linking method. The release study of doxorubicin also revealed that the extent of drug release at pH=5.3 was promisingly more than drug release at pH=7.4 for both MCNs. Generally, it can be concluded that type of drug cross linking provide an opportunity to tune drug release pattern of MCNs according to the specific drug delivery purpose.

Acknowledgments

We are most grateful for the continuing financial support of this research project by University of Zanjan and Zanjan University of Medical Sciences.

Conflict of Interest

The authors report no conflicts of interest.

References

1. Lassalle V, Zysler R, Ferreira M. Novel and facile synthesis of magnetic composites by a modified co-precipitation method. *Mater Chem Phys* 2011;130(1-2):624-34.
2. Kango S, Kalia S, Celli A, Njuguna J, Habibi Y, Kumar R. Surface modification of inorganic nanoparticles for development of organic–inorganic nanocomposites—A review. *Prog Polym Sci* 2013;38(8):1232-61.
3. Ko JA, Park HJ, Hwang SJ, Park JB, Lee JS. Preparation and characterization of chitosan microparticles intended for controlled drug delivery. *Int J Pharm* 2002;249(1-2):165-74.
4. Sahu SK, Maiti S, Pramanik A, Ghosh SK, Pramanik P. Controlling the thickness of polymeric shell on magnetic nanoparticles loaded with doxorubicin for targeted delivery and MRI contrast agent. *Carbohydr Polym* 2012;87(4):2593-604.
5. Chen R, Chen Q, Huo D, Ding Y, Hu Y, Jiang X. In situ formation of chitosan-gold hybrid hydrogel and

its application for drug delivery. *Colloids Surf B Biointerfaces* 2012;97:132-7.
6. Liu YL, Hsu CY, Su YH, Lai JY. Chitosan-silica complex membranes from sulfonic acid functionalized silica nanoparticles for pervaporation dehydration of ethanol-water solutions. *Biomacromolecules* 2005;6(1):368-73.
7. Sadighian S, Rostamizadeh K, Hosseini-Monfared H, Hamidi M. Doxorubicin-conjugated core-shell magnetite nanoparticles as dual-targeting carriers for anticancer drug delivery. *Colloids Surf B Biointerfaces* 2014;117:406-13.
8. Azevedo J, Sizilio R, Brito M, Costa AM, Serafini M, Araújo AA, et al. Physical and chemical characterization insulin-loaded chitosan-TPP nanoparticles. *J Therm Anal Calorim* 2011;106(3):685-9.
9. Janes KA, Fresneau MP, Marazuela A, Fabra A, Alonso MJ. Chitosan nanoparticles as delivery systems for doxorubicin. *J Control Release* 2001;73(2-3):255-67.
10. Morales MA, de Souza Rodrigues EC, de Amorim AS, Soares JM, Galembeck F. Size selected synthesis of magnetite nanoparticles in chitosan matrix. *Appl Surf Sci* 2013;275:71-4.
11. Sun S, Zeng H. Size-controlled synthesis of magnetite nanoparticles. *J Am Chem Soc* 2002;124(28):8204-5.
12. Ahmadi R, Hosseini HRM. An investigation on the optimum conditions of synthesizing a magnetite based ferrofluid as MRI contrast agent using Taguchi method. *Mater Sci-Poland* 2013;31(2):253-8.
13. Lin CL, Chiu WY, Lee CF. Thermal/pH-sensitive core-shell copolymer latex and its potential for targeting drug carrier application. *Polymer* 2005;46(23):10092-101.

Comparison of Different Nanosuspensions as Potential Ophthalmic Delivery Systems for Ketotifen Fumarate

Saieede Soltani[1,2], Parvin Zakeri-Milani[3,4], Mohammad Barzegar-Jalali[4], Mitra Jelvehgari[1,4]*

[1] Drug Applied Research Center, Tabriz University of Medical Sciences, Tabriz, Iran.
[2] Student Research Committee, Tabriz University of Medical Sciences, Tabriz, Iran.
[3] Liver and Gastrointestinal Diseases Research Center, Tabriz University of Medical Sciences, Tabriz, Iran.
[4] Department of Pharmaceutics, Faculty of Pharmacy, Tabriz University of Medical Sciences, Tabriz, Iran.

Article info

Keywords:
- Ketotifen fumarate
- Nanosuspension
- Transcorneal
- Permeability

Abstract

Purpose: The objective of this study was to develop, characterize, and comparatively investigate the ketotifen fumarate (KF) nanosuspensions (NS_S) to enhance the permeability of KF.

Methods: In the present work, the NS_P and NS_E were prepared by double-emulsion solvent evaporation/nanoprecipitation methods with poly (D,Llactide-co-glycolide) and Eudragit RL100 polymers, respectively. The loading efficiency, particle size, and polydispersity index of prepared different NSs were evaluated with scanning electron microscopy (SEM), X-ray diffraction, differential scanning calorimetry (DSC), Fourier transform infrared spectroscopy (FTIR), and in vitro release and transcorneal permeation . NSs were also compared on the basis of particle size and polydispersity index.

Results: Particle size, polydispersity index, and loading efficiency of NS_{P1} and NS_{E3} showed the best value (158 nm, 117 nm, 0.21, 0.43 and 43%, 95.23%, respectively). SEM showed spherical globules and DSC results showed the reduction in crystallinity. The NS_{E3} formulations demonstrated significantly ($p<0.05$) higher drug release rates than the NS_{P1} due to increases in the surface area. Comparative studies showed that NS_E release and permeability are higher than NS_P.

Conclusion: It is concluded that both NS_P and NS_E provide a useful dosage form for the ocular drug delivery which can enhance the permeability of KF.

Introduction

Eye is the most exclusive organ of the body and a wide range of drug delivery systems are employed to deliver the drug into the eye. Presently, conventional eye drops encompass more than 90% of the marketed ophthalmic formulations. However, after using an eye drop, normally up to 5% of the instilled drug passes the cornea and reaches the intraocular tissues. This happens because of quick and vast precorneal drop loss afforded by blinking and high tear fluid output. To this end, controlled drug delivery to the eye has been suggested as one of the remarkable fields of pharmaceutical research. The major problems associated with conventional systems consist of low drug contact time and poor ocular bioavailability as a result of drainage of drug solution, tear turnover and dilution or lacrimation. Moreover, the anatomical barriers and physiological conditions of the eye are also considerable criteria which dominate designing of drug delivery systems. Numerous novel ocular drug delivery systems such as nanoparticles (NPs), nanoemulsions (NEs), nanosuspensions (NSs) have been developed to achieve higher bioavailability, controlled ocular delivery, patient compliance, and less side effects.[1,2]

NSs and polymeric NPs are more valuable approaches over the current methods in delivering the highly hydrophilic or highly lipophilic molecules across the ocular mucosa. For instance, nanocrystal drug suspensions (NS) entitle an increased dissolution velocity along with saturation solubility of poorly water soluble drugs which is accompanied by an increase in ocular bioavailability.[3]

As a colloidal dispersion of nanosized particles, NSs are stabilized by other excipients like surfactants (as polyvinyl alcohol), viscosity enhancers, or charge modifiers.[4] NSs can also be described as a biphasic system consisting poorly water soluble drug particles dispersed in an aqueous media in which the diameter of the dispersed particles is below 1μm. Size reduction of drug particles conducts to increasing the dissolution rate (enhanced surface area and saturation solubility). The increment in the saturation solubility rate of nanoparticles is related to increase of vapour pressure of the particles.[5] A nanosuspension formulation like this can be prepared by pearl milling, high-pressure homogenization, and precipitation techniques.[6,7]

The precipitation method is the most currently used technique in which the drug is solved in an organic solvent

***Corresponding author:** Mitra Jelvehgari, Email: jelvehgri@tbzmed.ac.ir

and this solution is admixed with a miscible anti-solvent. In this method, mixing leads to precipitation of drug in the solution, and producing a very fine amorphous or crystalline drug. Precipitation has also been accompanied with the high shear proceeding.[5,8] Several NS formulations have been developed and successfully used for topical ocular drug delivery.[9,10]

Kassem *et al.* formulated NSs for prednisolone, hydrocortisone, and dexamethasone for topical ocular delivery and evaluated them.[11] Studies on the *in vivo* tissue distribution of the glucocorticoid NSs certified remarkably higher levels in anterior chamber tissues in comparison with solution and microcrystalline suspension of similar compounds.[12]

Aksungur *et al.* demonstrated NPs of cyclosporine (CsA) loaded PLGA and /or Eudragit RL-100 and PLGA coated with Carbopol for intensive dry eye syndrome therapy. The ultrafine NPs were supplied with Eudragit RL polymer. It was obtained that the NPs size reduction with Eudragit RL concentration increasing resulted from physicochemical characteristics of the polymer.[13] Mandal *et al.* showed that cloricromene loaded Eudragit RL100 polymeric NPs enhance the ocular bioavailability. They suggested cloricromene-loaded NPs system for clinical trial.[14]

Gupta *et al.* supplied PLGA nanoparticles containing sparfloxacin for ophthalmic delivery using nanoprecipitation technique and showed modified precorneal residence time and ocular penetration for NPs. The improved lyophilized NPs were stable for longer period of time than traditional commercial formulation.[15]

The use of ketotifen fumarate (KF) for the treatment of allergic conjunctivitis behaves as a histamine H1-receptor antagonist, mast cell stabilizer, and eosinophil inhibitor in that it decreases the chemotaxis and activation of eosinophils. Eudragit RL 100 polymers are referred to as ammonium methacrylate copolymers, which are synthesized from acrylic acid and methacrylic acid esters with 10% of functional quaternary ammonium groups.[16] Biodegradable poly (DL-lactic-co-glycolic acid) (PLGA) copolymers have been broadly used as carriers of bioactive molecules.[17] The biocompatibility and biodegradability of PLGA have been proved, and also approved by the FDA for specific human clinical applications.[18] Polymeric carrier systems using Eudragit and PLGA have been investigated for the ophthalmic release of gentamicin,[19] cloricromene,[20] acetazolamide[21] and non-steroidal anti-inflammatory drugs such as ibuprofen.[22] These carrier systems showed good stabilizing properties and narrow size distribution.

NSs of KF may overcome the problems observed in conventional drops. These nanocarriers may prolong the corneal contact time (higher bioavailability), controlled ocular delivery, rapid penetration of active ingredients, patient compliance, and ocular effect of KF.

The preparation of KF-loaded NS systems and evaluating the effect of polymer type and composition of formulations on the nanocarriers formation have targeted in this study. The feasibility of using the KF-loaded nanoparticulate system as an ocular formulation was demonstrated through extensive characterization of the size, charge, loading efficiency, drug release, and transcorneal permeability.

Materials and Methods

Materials

For this study, the KF was supplied by Behansar Co. (Iran). Eudragit RL 100 was kindly a gift from Akbarie Co. (from RÖhm Pharma GMBh, Weiterstadt, Germany). PLGA polymer Resomer® 502 H (MW 7000-17000) was purchased from Sigma-Aldrich (Sigma-Aldrich Co. US). Polyvinyl alcohol (MW 72000), D-mannitol, dichloromethane (DCM), ethanol, sodium chloride, calcium chloride, and potassium chloride were obtained from Merck (Germany). All solvents and reagents were of analytical grade. Commercial eye drop (Zaditen®, 0.025%) was purchased from Thea pharma (France).

Methods

Preparation of KF-NS_P and KF-NS_E

Two nanocarriers, NS_P (Nanosuspension of PLGA polymer) and NS_E (Nanosuspension of Eudragit RL100 polymer) were produced using PLGA and Eudragit RL 100, described polymers.[23] Briefly, NS_E and NS_P were prepared by nanoprecipitation method and double emulsion solvent evaporation technique ($W_1/O/W_2$) at different drug to polymer ratios, respectively (Table 1).

Table 1. Selected preparation parameters and their investigated range

Preparation parameter	Selected formulation		Investigation range	
	NS_{P1}	NS_{E3}	NS_P	NS_E
Polymer type	PLGA	Eudragit RL100	PLGA	Eudragit RL100
Drug to polymer ratio	1:5	1:15	1:5 - 1:10	1:7.5 - 1:15
Amount of drug (mg)	10	10	10	10
Concentration of polymer (mg/ml)	5	12.5	5-10	6.25-12.5
PVA (1%w/v)/ NaCl (0.8 %w/v) (ml)	25	-	25	-
PVA (1%w/v) (ml)	-	25	-	25
Theoretical drug content (%)	16.67	6.25	9.10-16.67	6.25-11.76
Mean drug entrapped (%±SD)	10.58±0.85	9.52±6.35	4.07-10.58	9.39-9.52
Drug loading efficiency (%±SD)	43.00±8.00	95.23±8.45	43-55	93.95-95.23
Mean particle size (nm)	158±2.24	117±16.00	158-754.6	117-182
Zeta Potential (mV±SD)	-3.30±3.21	+13.40±0.28	-3.30 - -2.99	+6.58-13.40
Polydispersity Index (±SD)	0.21±0.29	0.43±0.18	0.21-0.83	0.34-0.73

Formulation of KF-NS_P: An aqueous 0.5 % w/v KF solution was added to 10 ml PLGA in organic solvent (dichloromethane) by using an ultrasound probe (Hielscher, UP200H, amplitude 80%) in an ice bath for 3 min. This solution was added drop by drop using syringe needle to 25 ml aqueous phase of PVA (1%w/v), NaCl (0.8% w/v) and sonicated for 3 min. Then this emulsion was diluted in 50 ml distilled water. The organic solvent was allowed to evaporate at room temperature under magnetic stirring and NS_P were collected by centrifugation (Eppendorf, Centrifuge 5810 R, Germany) at 12000 rpm, 4°C for 60 min and washed and freeze-dried .

Formulation of KF-NS_E: KF and Edragit RL 100 were dissolved in 12 ml ethanol. The solution was mixed with 25 ml of 1% w/v PVA aqueous solution using ultrasound probe (Hielscher, UP200H) for 3 min. Then the mixture of drug and polymer was diluted in 50 ml distilled water. Finally, the resulted nanosuspension was stirred at room temperature to extract the organic solvent. NS_E was separated under the same conditions of NS_P. Prepared NPs were mixed with 10ml 5%w/v mannitol solution as a cryoprotectant and then lyophilized.

Characterization of NS_P and NS_E

Particle size and zeta potential

Particle size and zeta potential of freshly prepared NS_P and NS_E were determined by Dynamic Light Scattering (Malvern, UK) using a Zetasizer. The zeta potential is used to measure the electric charge at the surface of the particles, showing the physical stability of colloidal systems. For this study, the formulated NS_P and NS_E were diluted with distilled water. Visual observations were made immediately after dilution for evaluation of NS_P and NS_E efficiency, appearance (transparency), phase separation, and precipitation of drug. The polydispersity index of the resulting NS_P and NS_E were determined by dynamic light scattering with Zeta sizer.

Morphology

The outer macroscopic structure of NS_P and NS_E were investigated by scanning electron microscopy (SEM). SEM (MIRA3 TESCAN, Czech Republic) was used to examine the surface morphology of Eudragit and PLGA nanoparticles. The samples were stationed on a metal stub with a double adhesive tape and coated with the platinum/palladium alloy under the vacuum.

Drug loading and production yield of NS_P and NS_E

To determine the amount of drug loaded in prepared nanocarriers, NS_P and NS_E, the supernatant was UV analyzed for the unloaded drug at wavelength 298 nm. Calibration curve was performed by means of KF in 1% PVA aqueous solution. The drug loading efficiency was determined using the following equations:[24]

$$\text{Drug loading efficiency} = \frac{\text{Total amount of drug} - \text{unincorporated drug amount}}{\text{Total amount of drug}} \times 100$$

Evaluation of physical state and polymer-drug interaction of NS_P and NS_E

Physical state and polymer-drug interaction of NS_P and NS_E were examined by XRD, DSC and FTIR analyses.

X-ray diffraction (XRD): XRD analysis was performed using Bruker Axs, D8 Advance diffractometer with nickel-filtered CuKα radiation (operating at 40KV, 20mA). The scanning rate was 4 °C/min over a 2θ range of 10°-90°.

Differential scanning calorimetry: Differential scanning calorimetry (DSC) (Shimadzu, Japan) measurements were carried out on drug, polymers and different formulations. The weighed samples were put in aluminum pans and scanned for 30°C-300°C with heating rate of 10°C/min.

Fourier transform infrared spectroscopy: The Fourier transform infrared spectroscopy (FT-IR) spectra for KF loaded nanocarriers, blank NPs, polymer and drug were obtained by a computerized FT-IR (Bruker, Tensor 27, and USA) operating in the scanning wavenumber range of 400-4000 cm^{-1} at 1 cm^{-1} resolution.

***In vitro* release study**

In vitro release

In vitro release experiments were performed on the NS_P and NS_E using dialysis bag diffusion method.[20] Fifty milligrams of particles were suspended in 4 ml SLF (simulated lacrimal fluid) buffer (pH 6.8) in the dialysis bag (cutoff 12,000 Da), which was immersed in 300 ml of the same buffer as dissolution medium. The medium was preheated to 32±1°C and stirred at 100 rpm. At preset intervals, 3.5 ml of medium were withdrawn and replaced with 3.5 ml of fresh SLF to keep the sink condition. The amount of KF in the samples was determined by UV spectrophotometer (Shimadzu, Japan) analysis at wavelength 298 nm. The experiments were repeated for each formulation in triplicate.

Ex-vivo transcorneal permeation studies

The *in vitro* permeation study of the KF-loaded NS_P and NS_E through the bovine cornea was performed using Franz diffusion cell at 32 °C. Freshly obtained scleral layer was mounted between the donor and the recipient compartments. The nanocarriers suspended in 5 ml distilled water were placed on the epithelial faced surface and the compartments were clamped together. The NS_P and NS_E was stationed on the cornea, and the opening of the donor compartment was sealed with a glass coverslip and soaked with simulated lacrimal fluid (SLF, composition: 8.3 g of NaCl, 0.084g of $CaCl2{\cdot}2H\ 2O$, 1.4g of KCl, and distilled deionized water to 1000 mL). The recipient compartment was filled with 22-25 ml SLF at pH 6.8 and stirred with a magnetic bead at 200 rpm.[25] Three milliliters of the sample were withdrawn at predetermined time intervals and analyzed for drugs at 298 nm.

Permeability coefficient was calculated using the following equation:

$$Kp = \frac{Jss}{C_0}$$

Where Jss is the steady state flux per unit area, Kp is the permeability coefficient for a given solute in a given vehicle (cm h^{-1}), and C_0 is the concentration of the solute in the donor compartment.

Statistical analysis

Where appropriate, all results were evaluated using a one-way ANOVA or t-test at the 0.05 level of error.

Results & Discussion

The composition of NS_P and NS_E formulations are listed in Table1, where the amount of the different compounds is expressed as % (w/w). As shown in the table, NS_P was prepared by using PLGA and DCM as the organic phase, PVA as stabilizer and sodium chloride as osmosis pressure agent.[26] NS_E was produced by using Eudragit RL100 and ethanol as organic phase and PVA as emulsifier. Both formulations, NS_P and NS_E, were loaded with the same amount of KF (10 mg) and stabilized with the same surfactant in the same concentration (1% w/v).

In the NS, water was used as an anti-solvent whereas polyvinyl alcohol was used as the surfactant. Nanoprecipitation occurs at the interface of the organic phase (ethanol) and anti-solvent phase (water) due to diffusion of the solvent by forming local disturbances followed by precipitation of nanoparticles which were governed by surfactant system.

Under the sonication, the mixture of ethanolic was injected into the aqueous phase so the nanosuspension (polymeric solutes become aggregated to produce nanosized particles) was formed by precipitation with diluted organic solution in the aqueous phase leading to the production of nanoparticles. The sonication was operated for several minutes to let the system reach equilibrium. The solvent displacement method for fabrication of NS was adopted from the nanoprecipitation method applied for polymeric nanoparticles. The organic phase (O) was poured into an aqueous phase (W) containing a surfactant to yield nanosuspension.[4]

The highest loading efficiency for NS_P and NS_E formulations were 43% and 95.23%, respectively. The results showed that the drug was uniformly distributed throughout the NS_E formulations (Table 2).

Table 2. Comparison of various release characteristics, flux and permeability coefficient of KF from different NPs formulations and commercial® drop

Formulation code	$^a Rel_{0.25}$ (%)	$^b Rel_8$ (%)	^{c}DE	$^d T_{50\%}$ (min)	$^e f_1$	^{f}Flux (mg/cm^2.min)*10^{-3}	^{g}Kp (cm/min) *10^{-4}
NS_{P1}	15.81±3.04	82.57±4.87	74.49	248.84	44.68	0.2	5.82
NS_{P2}	12.30±0.52	65.15±7.75	62.72	352.61	54.72	0.06	3.44
NS_{P3}	10.67±0.26	58.77±8.53	54.04	383.74	63.38	0.06	4
NS_{E1}	30.67±1.54	65.51±4.10	61.28	93	49.24	0.6	10.7
NS_{E2}	55.74±5.28	80.31±3.48	77.77	45.64	28.19	0.6	16.78
NS_{E3}	65.14±1.44	88.82±3.33	85.88	46.61	20.22	0.5	17.30
KF drop®	97.77±0.00	101.62±1.81	101.03	8.31	0	0.1	28.99

^{a} $Rel_{0.25}$ = amount of drug release after 0.25 h; ^{b} Rel_8 = amount of drug release after 8 h; ^{c}DE = dissolution efficiency; ^{d}t 50% = dissolution time for 50% fractions; ^{e} f_1 = Differential factor ($0<f_1<15$), ^{f}flux and ^{g}permeability coefficient.

Particle size diameter (Z-Ave), polydispersity index (PI), and zeta potential of NS_P and NS_E were determined just after preparation (reported in Table 1). Freshly prepared NS_{P1} showed a Z-Ave of 158 nm (0.21 PI) and a zeta potential of −3.30 mV while freshly prepared NS_{E3} presented a Z-Ave of 117 nm (0.43 PI) and a zeta potential of +13.40 mV. As can be observed, NS_P and NS_E, showed negative and positive zeta potential values, respectively. The positive zeta potential of NS_E may a longer residence time of NPs on the corneal surface. As shown in Table 2, freshly prepared NS_{P1} was well homogeneously dispersed with reduced particle size and PI, compared to the NP_{E3} that was briefly homogeneously dispersed. However, Table 2 clearly shows that NS_E was less stable than the NS_P. The low stability of this formulation (NS_E) was also confirmed by the increasing of polydispersity index value from 0.34 to 0.73. On the basis of PDI, we found that KF-loaded NS_P was better than KF-loaded NS_E. A higher value of polydispersity index indicates a broad particle size distribution.[27] NS_P and NS_E data were confirmed by SEM images (Figure 1).

SEM is used to assess the microscopic surface morphology of the formulations. Prepared formulations were present in the form of a rough surface which might have led to the enhanced dissolution rate.[27] Moreover, the particle showed a satisfactory regular spherical shape in the case of NS_P, which is probably the reason for its best results even in the dissolution.

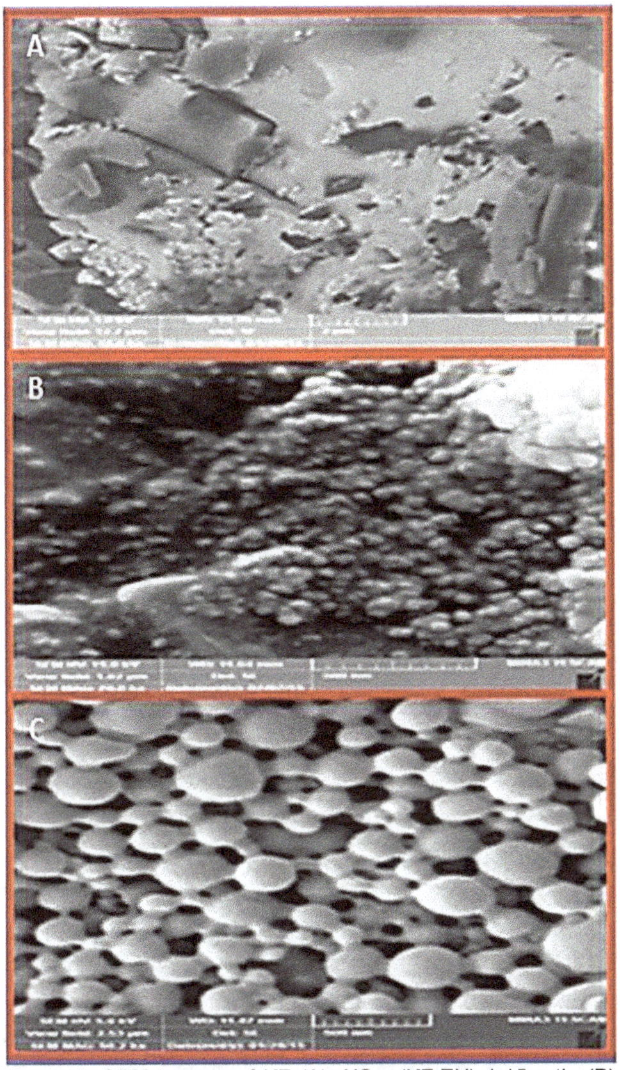

Figure 1. SEM images of KF (A); NS_{E3} (KF:EU) 1:15 ratio (B); NS_{P1} (KF:PLGA) 1:5 ratio (C) at 1000× magnification.

The influence of preparation method on the KF degree of crystallinity and melting point was evaluated by DSC characterization of NS_P and NS_E. The freeze dried drug loaded NS_E exhibited a sharp melting endotherm at an onset temperature of 197.69 °C, a peak temperature of 201.09 °C, and a heat of fusion of 176.14 J/g (Figure 2). The freeze dried drug loaded NS_E showed a broad endothermic transition at an onset of 216.68 °C, a peak at an onset of 197.93°C, and a peak at 213.96°C (from F_1 to F_3). Eudragit RL 100 and PLGA polymers are found as an utterly amorphous form with a glass transition temperature (Tg) of about 60°C.[28] No fusion peak or phase transition was observed in the amorphous polymer, apart from a broad signal around 55–60°C owing to a partial loss of residual humidity.[29] The thermal behavior of the freeze dried NPs proposed that the polymer prevented the melting of drug crystals. The ionic interaction may have occurred in the NPs as observed for the KF and Eudragit RL 100 system.[30] However, the NPs of KF shows drug melting peak. The thermal profile comparison between NS_P and NS_E KF confirmed that the solid state transition that occurred during NS preparation did not influence the drug behavior.

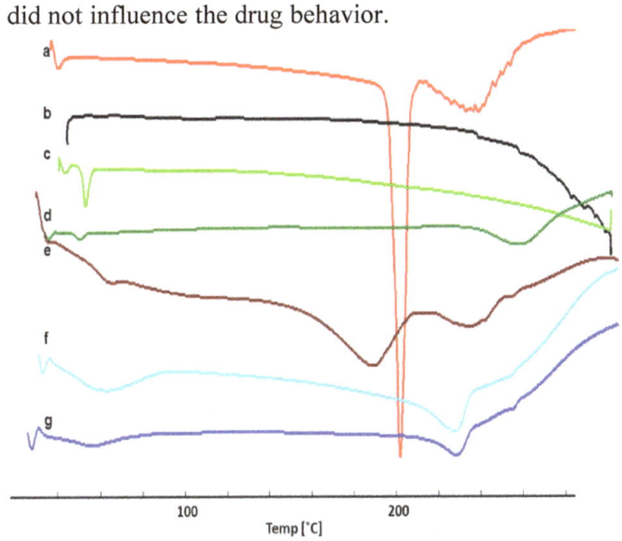

Figure 2. DSC thermogram of KF (a); PLGA (b); NS_{P1} (KF:PLGA) 1:5 ratio (c); blank NS_{P1} (d); Eudragit RL100 (e); NS_{E3} (KF:EU) 1:15 ratio (f); blank NS_{E3} (g), respectively.

In the XRD, spectra are obvious and the NS_P with lower polymer concentration would show similar peaks as the blank NS_P. For NS_P, some of the identifying peaks for KF are detectable at a high concentration of polymer; though these peaks hold very low intensity due to the presence of lower concentration of drug in the sample compared to pure KF sample (Figure 3). Eudragit RL polymer is completely amorphous in nature, and entrapment of crystalline KF (sharp intense peaks as seen in Figure 3) into the polymeric NS_E reduced its crystallinity to a greater extent. This is evident from the disappearance of most peaks in the NS_E compared to the drug. There may also be the possibility of overlapping of drug peaks by the background diffraction pattern of the amorphous structure.

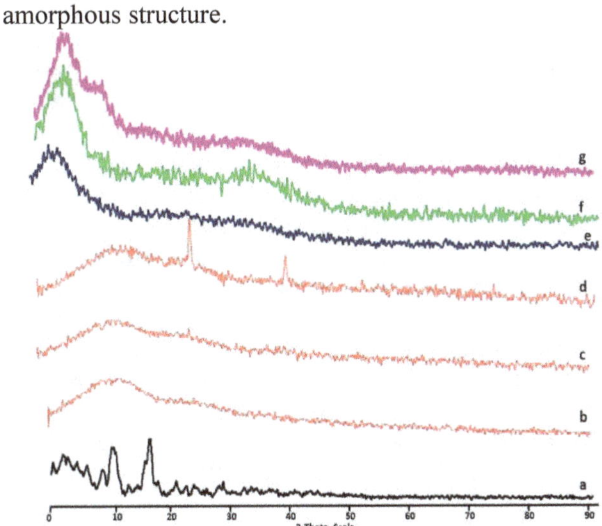

Figure 3. XRD thermogram of KF (a); PLGA (b); NS_{P1} (KF:PLGA) 1:5 ratio (c); blank NS_{P1} (d); Eudragit RL100 (e); NS_{E3} (KF:EU) 1:15 ratio (f); blank NS_{E3} (g), respectively.

The FT-IR spectrum of KF alone showed that the principal peaks were observed at wave numbers stretching vibration N-H at 3424.64 cm−[1], aromatic stretching vibration C=C at 1649.70 cm−[1], bending vibration CH3 at 1476.99 cm-[1], bending vibration phenolic OH at 1397.14, and CH out of plane bending vibrations in substituted ethylenic system (-C=CH- (cis) at 754.15 cm^{-1} (Figure 4). The spectra obtained by FT-IR for the PLGA are presented in Figure 4. The strong bands in the region between 1760 and 1750 cm^{-1} could be observed, in the spectra, due to the stretch of the carbonyl groups within the PLGA. Moreover, stretching bands are observed because of asymmetric and symmetric C-C(=O)-O vibrations between 1300 and 1150 cm^{-1}. The presence of bands in these regions is of benefit in the characterization of esters. The 3525 and 3459 cm^{-1} bands in the FT-IR spectra for lactide and glycolide are ascribed to moisture in the sample (OH group). The absorption bands between 3600 and 3400 cm^{-1} in the spectra presented in Figure 4, showing the hydroxyl group, indicate that the PLGA copolymers are hydrous. FT-IR studies showed characteristic peaks of KF, confirming the purity of the drug. For NS_P, stretching vibration N-H is seen at 3400-3423, a stretch of the carbonyl groups at 1760, asymmetric and symmetric C-C(=O)-O vibrations at 1390 and bending vibrations in substituted ethylenic system (-C=CH- (cis) at 725-752 cm^{-1}.

For Eudragit RL 100, in the spectra, the strong bands are observed in the region between 1150-1190 cm^{-1} and 1240-1270 cm^{-1}, due to the stretch of carbonyl (ester) groups present in the Eudragit (Figure 4). There are also stretching bands in view of the C (=O) ester vibration at 1734.01 cm^{-1}. The 1388.22, 1449.97, 2953, and 2992.11 cm^{-1} bands in the FT-IR spectra can be discerned to CHx vibration. IR absorption frequency at 3437.91cm-1 (OH stretch) presented in Figure 3 and showing the hydroxyl group, indicates that the Eudragit RL100 is hydrous.[29,31]

FT-IR spectral studies showed that there was an interaction between KF and polymers used. For NS_E, stretching strong band C-H (alkyne group) are seen at 3293.88-3298cm^{-1}, stretch band strong C-H (alkane group) at 2936.61, 2937.50 and 2939.24 cm^{-1}, N-H stretch band of the amine group at 3000 cm^{-1}, stretch band of carbonyl group at 1728.54, 1728.79, and 1729.01 cm^{-1}, bending vibrations in -C-H at 1436.12, 1436.62, and 1438.91 cm^{-1}, stretch band of ester group C-O at 1089.41, 1089.61, and 1090.74 cm^{-1}, and stretch band in -C-Cl at 844.76, 845.12, and 845.57 cm^{-1} (Figure 4). The available differences in the positions of the absorption bands of KF were seen in spectra of the prepared formulations, proving the presence of chemical interactions in the solid state between the drug and the polymers (PLGA and Eudragit RL100).

In vitro dissolution studies

In vitro dissolution data of all best formulations (NS_P and NS_E) were compared together. The NS_P formulation showed that 82.57% of drug was released in 480 min (NS_{P1}). NaCl increased the solubility of drug by entrapping the KF in the network interstitial spaces of NaCl molecule and also reducing the particle size. In NSs, increasing the osmotic pressure of W_2 (external phase of second emulsion) directs water migration from W_1 to W_2 as well as a rapid shrinkage of the droplets. This phenomenon results in smaller nanoparticles and increases drug release.

In the NS_E formulation 88.82% drug was released in 480 min (NS_{E3}). Increasing the dissolution kinetics of KF from NS_E may be due to the conversion of the drug from crystalline to amorphous state. Also presence of surfactant (PVA) and co-surfactant (ethanol) in NS_E reduces the interfacial tension and helps to solubilize the drug in the formulation of NS_E. According to the literature, the drug release amount and behavior as well as the drug absorption are influenced by the particle size. The particle size of NS_{E3} (117 nm) and NS_{P1} (158 nm) are the smallest which may be the reason for their highest releases (Figure 5).

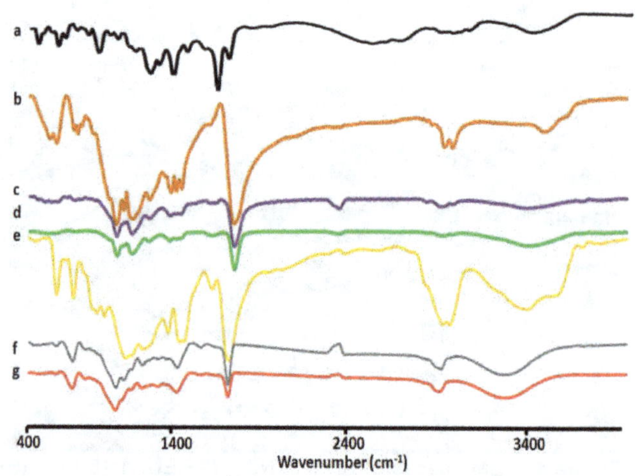

Figure 4. FT-IR thermogram of KF (a); PLGA (b); NS_{P1} (KF:PLGA) 1:5 ratio (c); blank NS_{P1} (d); Eudragit RL100 (e); NS_{E3} (KF:EU) 1:15 ratio (f); blank NS_{E3} (g), respectively.

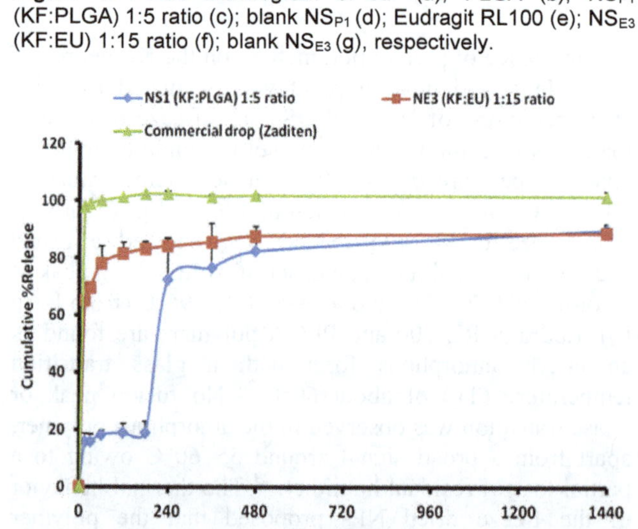

Figure 5. Cumulative percent release of KF from naoparticles with different polymer ratios and KF commercial drop.

KF delivery into and through the bovine cornea was evaluated in *ex vivo* conditions, by the use of Franz vertical diffusion cells. During this study, transcorneal delivery of prepared KF nanosuspensions was compared with commercial (Zaditen®) eye drop as control. Comparison of data obtained from NS_P and NS_E (Table 2) highlights a different KF delivery into and through the bovine cornea. As expected, the NS_E showed a higher drug permeation and transcorneal delivery than the NS_P. However, differences of drug permeability in two types of formulations (as NS_P and NS_E) were statistically significant ($p < 0.05$). Comparison of data obtained from NS_P and NS_E underlines the influence of different formulations on the *ex vivo* drug availability; NS_E is useful for improving the transcorneal delivery. NS_E is able to favor KF permeation into the eye and at the same time to prolong the contact time with the cornea and increase the efficacy of drug delivery.

In NSs, solid drug is dissolved in the vehicle (lacrimal fluid) and diffuses through the vehicle to the cornea. On the other side, when a nanocarrier is applied onto the eye, two consecutive physical events may limit corneal absorption, namely, the drug release (from nanocarrier) into lacrimal fluid and its penetration through the corneal barrier. These two processes are intimately intertwined, and both are due to the physicochemical properties of drug (type of nanocarrier) and barrier.

The degree of partitioning of the drug into the cornea relies on the relative affinity for the vehicle and for the intercellular environment. In the present investigation, the higher drug permeability may be due to the polymer type (Table 2), surfactant, and the method of preparation, which taken together act as penetration enhancers.[32,33] In addition, as shown for NS_E, the small particle size of the NS_E (in comparison with NS_p) makes it an excellent carrier for promoting *ex vivo* corneal KF permeation. Overall results show that NS_E is suitable nanoparticles for corneal delivery of KF. NSs are almost exclusively formed from drug nanoparticles with small amounts of biocompatible and safe surfactants, such as PVA used in this work. This leads to a highly fast dissolution process that favors drug penetration into the cornea. Moreover, compared to other colloidal carriers, NSs show extra advantages such as simplicity, biodegradability of polymer (PLGA), and scalable preparation methods.[34,35]

Conclusion

On the whole, this work showed the high potential of NS_P and NS_E in ocular drug delivery of KF. Indeed, NS_s has been established to be able to localize the drug into the cornea *ex vivo*. Besides, the NS_P was shown to give comparable ocular KF delivery as the NS_E, which strongly enhanced *in vitro* ocular drug delivery. Furthermore, the application of NS_E in ocular KF delivery showed the advantage of increasing permeability and retention time of the drug in comparison with the NS_P. To conclude, results of this work evinces that NS_E formulation approach could be a potentially valuable tool of use in the design of new KF nanomedicines for the treatment of eye diseases.

Acknowledgments

The authors report that they have no conflicts of interests. The financial support from the Drug Applied Research Center of Tabriz University of Medical Sciences under the grant No. 42 is greatly acknowledged. Mitra Jelvehgari received the research grant from Drug Applied Research Center, Tabriz University of Medical Sciences, Tabriz, Iran.

Conflict of Interest

The authors declare that there is no conflict of interests regarding the publication of this article.

References

1. Sahoo SK, Dilnawaz F, Krishnakumar S. Nanotechnology in ocular drug delivery. *Drug Discov Today* 2008;13(3-4):144-51. doi: 10.1016/j.drudis.2007.10.021
2. Patel A, Cholkar K, Agrahari V, Mitra AK. Ocular drug delivery systems: An overview. *World J Pharmacol* 2013;2(2):47-64. doi: 10.5497/wjp.v2.i2.47
3. Ganta S, Paxton JW, Baguley BC, Garg S. Formulation and pharmacokinetic evaluation of an asulacrine nanocrystalline suspension for intravenous delivery. *Int J Pharm* 2009;367(1-2):179-86. doi: 10.1016/j.ijpharm.2008.09.022
4. Adamczak M. Surfactants, polyelectrolytes and nanoparticles as building blocks for nanocarriers. Poland : AGH University of Science and Technology in Krakow; 2013.
5. Jay KT. Nanosuspensions: Types of nanosuspension methods and various applications. Available from: http://www.biotecharticles.com/Nanotech/2011/May/Nanotechnology-Article/Nanosuspensions-Types-of-Nanosuspension-Methods-and-Various-Applications-893.htmlArticle. 2011.
6. Kumari A, Yadav SK, Yadav SC. Biodegradable polymeric nanoparticles based drug delivery systems. *Colloids Surf B Biointerfaces* 2010;75(1):1-18. doi: 10.1016/j.colsurfb.2009.09.001
7. Nagarwal RC, Kant S, Singh PN, Maiti P, Pandit JK. Polymeric nanoparticulate system: A potential approach for ocular drug delivery. *J Control Release* 2009;136(1):2-13. doi: 10.1016/j.jconrel.2008.12.018
8. Patel VR, Agrawal YK. Nanosuspension: An approach to enhance solubility of drugs. *J Adv Pharm Technol Res* 2011;2(2):81-7. doi: 10.4103/2231-4040.82950
9. Mudgil M, Gupta N, Nagpal M, Pawar P. Nanotechnology: a new approach for ocular drug delivery system. *Int J Pharm Pharm Sci* 2012;4(2):105-12.
10. Bangia JK, Om H. Nanoemulsions: a versatile drug delivery tool. *Int J Pharm Sci Res* 2015;6(4):1363-72 doi: 10.13040/IJPSR.0975-8232.6(4).1363-72
11. Mygind T, Stiehler M, Baatrup A, Li H, Zou X, Flyvbjerg A, et al. Mesenchymal stem cell ingrowth

and differentiation on coralline hydroxyapatite scaffolds. *Biomaterials* 2007;28(6):1036-47. doi: 10.1016/j.biomaterials.2006.10.003

12. James D. Pipkin, Rupert O. Zimmerer, John M. Siebert, inventors; Cydex Pharmaceuticals, Inc., assignee. Nasal and ophthalmic delivery of aqueous corticosteroid solutions. United States patent US20090312724 A1.2009
13. Aksungur P, Demirbilek M, Denkbas EB, Vandervoort J, Ludwig A, Unlu N. Development and characterization of cyclosporine a loaded nanoparticles for ocular drug delivery: Cellular toxicity, uptake, and kinetic studies. *J Control Release* 2011;151(3):286-94. doi: 10.1016/j.jconrel.2011.01.010
14. Mandal B, Alexander KS, Riga AT. Sulfacetamide loaded eudragit(r) rl100 nanosuspension with potential for ocular delivery. *J Pharm Pharm Sci* 2010;13(4):510-23.
15. Gupta H, Aqil M, Khar RK, Ali A, Bhatnagar A, Mittal G. Sparfloxacin-loaded plga nanoparticles for sustained ocular drug delivery. *Nanomedicine* 2010;6(2):324-33. doi: 10.1016/j.nano.2009.10.004
16. Oshlack B, Pedi Jr F, Chasin M., Inventors; Euro-Celtique SA, assignee. Controlled release formulations coated with aqueous dispersions of acrylic polymers. United States patent US5580578 A. 1996
17. Mundargi RC, Babu VR, Rangaswamy V, Patel P, Aminabhavi TM. Nano/micro technologies for delivering macromolecular therapeutics using poly(d,l-lactide-co-glycolide) and its derivatives. *J Control Release* 2008;125(3):193-209. doi: 10.1016/j.jconrel.2007.09.013
18. Danhier F, Ansorena E, Silva JM, Coco R, Le Breton A, Preat V. Plga-based nanoparticles: An overview of biomedical applications. *J Control Release* 2012;161(2):505-22. doi: 10.1016/j.jconrel.2012.01.043
19. Al-Kassas R. Design and in vitro evaluation of gentamicin-eudragit microspheres intended for intra-ocular administration. *J Microencapsul* 2004;21(1):71-81. doi: 10.1080/02652040310001619992
20. Pignatello JJ, Oliveros E, MacKay A. Advanced oxidation processes for organic contaminant destruction based on the Fenton reaction and related chemistry. *Crit Rev Environ Sci Tech* 2006;36(1):1-84. doi:10.1080/10643380500326564
21. Haznedar S, Dortunc B. Preparation and in vitro evaluation of eudragit microspheres containing acetazolamide. *Int J Pharm* 2004;269(1):131-40.
22. Pignatello R, Bucolo C, Ferrara P, et al. Eudragit RS100® nanosuspensions for the ophthalmic controlled delivery of ibuprofen. *Eur J Pharm Sci* 2002;16(1):53-61. doi:10.1016/S0928-0987(02)00057-X
23. Dillen K, Vandervoort J, Van den Mooter G, Ludwig A. Evaluation of ciprofloxacin-loaded eudragit rs100 or rl100/plga nanoparticles. *Int J Pharm* 2006;314(1):72-82. doi: 10.1016/j.ijpharm.2006.01.041
24. Muthu MS, Rawat MK, Mishra A, Singh S. Plga nanoparticle formulations of risperidone: Preparation and neuropharmacological evaluation. *Nanomedicine* 2009;5(3):323-33. doi: 10.1016/j.nano.2008.12.003
25. Jantarat C. Application of Molecularly Imprinted Polymer for Drug Delivery and Membrane Separation of Chiral Drugs (PhD thesis). Southern Thailand: Prince of Songkla University; 2009.
26. Meinel L, Illi OE, Zapf J, Malfanti M, Peter Merkle H, Gander B. Stabilizing insulin-like growth factor-i in poly(d,l-lactide-co-glycolide) microspheres. *J Control Release* 2001;70(1-2):193-202.
27. Hu J, Johnston KP, Williams RO, 3rd. Spray freezing into liquid (sfl) particle engineering technology to enhance dissolution of poorly water soluble drugs: Organic solvent versus organic/aqueous co-solvent systems. *Eur J Pharm Sci* 2003;20(3):295-303.
28. Ignatious F, Sun L, inventors; Ignatious F, Sun L, assignee. Electrospun amorphous pharmaceutical compositions. United States patent US 20060013869A1. 2006.
29. Mandal B. Preparation and physicochemical characterization of Eudragit® RL100 Nanosuspension with potential for Ocular Delivery of Sulfacetamide (PhD thesis). Ohio: The University of Toledo Digital Respository; 2010.
30. Swarnakar NK, Jain AK, Singh RP, Godugu C, Das M, Jain S. Oral bioavailability, therapeutic efficacy and reactive oxygen species scavenging properties of coenzyme q10-loaded polymeric nanoparticles. *Biomaterials* 2011;32(28):6860-74. doi: 10.1016/j.biomaterials.2011.05.079
31. Basu SK, Adhiyaman R. Preparation and characterization of nitrendipine-loaded Eudragit RL 100 microspheres prepared by an emulsion-solvent evaporation method. *Trop J Pharm Res* 2008;7(3):1033-41.
32. Kaur IP, Kanwar M. Ocular preparations: The formulation approach. *Drug Dev Ind Pharm* 2002;28(5):473-93. doi: 10.1081/DDC-120003445
33. Ye T, Yuan K, Zhang W, Song S, Chen F, Yang X, et al. Prodrugs incorporated into nanotechnology-based drug delivery systems for possible improvement in bioavailability of ocular drugs delivery. *Asian J Pharm Sci* 2013;8(4):207-17. doi:10.1016/j.ajps.2013.09.002
34. Champion JA, Katare YK, Mitragotri S. Particle shape: a new design parameter for micro-and nanoscale drug delivery carriers. *J Control Rel* 2007;121(1):3-9. doi:10.1016/j.jconrel.2007.03.022
35. Reis CP, Neufeld RJ, Ribeiro AJ, et al. Nanoencapsulation I. Methods for preparation of drug-loaded polymeric nanoparticles. *Nanomed: Nanotech, Bio Med* 2006;2(1):8-21. doi:10.1016/j.nano.2005.12.003

Synthesis of *Bis*(Isoxazol-4-Ylmethylsulfanyl)Alkanes and Some Metal Complexes as a Hepatoprotective Agents

Vnira Rakhimovna Akhmetova[1*], Rozalia Akramovna Galimova[2], Nail Salavatovich Akhmadiev[1], Albina Midkhatovna Galimova[2], Ravil Akhmetzyanovich Khisamutdinov[3], Galiya Maratovna Nurtdinova[1], Eduard Feliksovich Agletdinov[2], Valery Alekseevich Kataev[2]

[1] *Institute of Petrochemistry and Catalysis, Russian Academy of Sciences, 141 Prospekt Oktyabrya, 450075 Ufa, Russia.*
[2] *Bashkir State Medical University, 3 Lenin Str., 450008 Ufa, Russia.*
[3] *Ufa Institute of Chemistry, Russian Academy of Sciences, 71 Prospekt Oktyabrya, 450054 Ufa, Russia.*

Article info

Keywords:
· Metal-organic frameworks
· Isoxazoles
· Hepatoprotector
· *In vivo*
· Liver
· Hepatitis

Abstract
Purpose: This research is devoted to designing the synthesis of sulfanyl-substituted 3,5-dimethylisoxazoles, which contain structural analogues of the SAM drug in the molecule. SAM (S-adenosyl-L-methionine), formed in the biosynthetic process, is used as an effective hepatoprotective drug. Complexation and hepatoprotective properties of the combinatorial series of bis(isoxazolylsulfanyl)ethane have been studied.
Methods: Bis(isoxazol-4-ylmethylsulfanyl)alkanes were synthesized using the *one-pot* method. The structures of compounds were established by one-dimensional (^{1}H,^{13}C) and two-dimensional (COSY, HCQS, HMBC) NMR spectroscopy, mass-spectrometry and X-ray diffraction. The biological activity of the combinatorial series of sulfanyl derivatives of diketones, azoles and their metal complexes has been studied by *in vivo* method. Simulation of the animal associated processes was carried out in accordance with the principles of bioethics. Screening studies of hepatoprotective activity were carried out in a model of acute CCl_4 intoxication after a single injection intraperitoneally as a 50% solution in olive oil. The pharmacologically known hepatoprotective drug SAM served as a control.
Results: Two-step synthesis of novel α,ω-*bis*(isoxazol-4-ylmethylsulfanyl)alkanes was carried out via the multicomponent reaction between 2,4-pentandione, CH_2O and α,ω-dithiols, then the resulting α,ω-*bis*(1,3-diketone-2-ylmethylsulfanyl)alkanes were transformed by hydroxyl amine to obtain *bis*-isoxasole derivatives. Promising precursor 1,2-*bis*(isoxazol-4-ylmethylsulfanyl)ethane was converted to metal complexes by interaction with $PdCl_2$ or CuCl. The obtained compounds were found to be practically non-toxic compounds (1001 – 3000 mg/kg) according to the classification of K.K. Sidorov, but copper complex refers to low-toxic compounds substances (165 mg/kg). Compounds of sulfanyl ethane series demonstrate hepatoprotective activity.
Conclusion: Palladium(II) complex being almost non-toxic possesses hepatoprotective activity comparable to the drug like SAM.

Introduction

Currently the use of organometallic complexes in medicine is considered as an innovative approach, due to their unusual activity in biological systems.[1-3] From the standpoint of metal-ligand homeostasis, organic complexes with essential metals forming part of the active site of many enzymes,[4-7] are very promising for the treatment of pathological states.[8] Recently[9] it has been found that baicolin-copper complex is effective hepatoprotective agent unlike baicalin itself.

Breakthrough event was the discovery in the late 20th-century therapeutic properties of cisplatin,[10] and other platinum complexes against cancer,[11,12] which, unfortunately, have significant toxic side effects.[13,14] Later it was shown that the less toxic palladium(II) complexes were also effective for the treatment of cancer. Nowadays there is the interest of researchers to look for low-toxic organometallic complexes with an effective anti-tumor[15-18] or hepatoprotective activity.[19]

We have previously reported the one-pot effective synthesis of α,ω-*bis*(1,3-diketone-2-ylmethylsulfanyl)alkanes,[20] which are promising precursors for methylsulfanyl substituted α,ω-*bis*-pyrazoles with pronounced inhibitory effects on alpha-amylase activity.[21-23]

Taking into account, that isoxazoles exhibit pharmacological properties,[24-27] and sulfanyl substituted isoxazoles are polydentate ligands,[28,29] our aim was to carry out the synthesis of novel complexes of Pd(II) and Cu(I) with 1,2-*bis*[(3,5-dimethylisoxazol-4-yl)methylsulfanyl] ligands and examine the toxicological and hepatoprotective properties of metallo-complexes and precursors thereof.

Materials and Methods

General procedures and materials

The reaction products were characterized by ^1H and ^{13}C NMR spectra that were recorded on spectrometers Bruker Avance 400 NMR (400.13 MHz and 100.62 MHz) and Bruker Ascend III HD 500 (500.17 MHz and 125.78 MHz), internal standard TMS, solvent DMSO-d_6. The homo- and heteronuclear 2D experiments were performed by the standard pulse sequences of Bruker. IR spectra were recorded on a Bruker Vertex-70V FTIR and Specord M80 spectrometers. Electrospray ionization (ESI) mass spectra were obtained on a HPLC massspectrometer LCMS-2010EV (Shimadzu) in positive and negative ions mode at the corona discharge needle ionizing electrode and ionizing capillary potential of – 3.5 kV. Sample solution (direct syringe sample inlet) under ESI conditions was in methanol (acetonitrile), mobile phase was acetonitrile/water, 95/5. Mass-spectra was recorded on a device MALDI TOF Autoflex III firm Bruker (compounds **2a-e**) with sinapinic acid as a matrix (see *Supplementary data*). Elemental analysis was performed on a Carlo Erba 1106 elemental analyzer. Melting points were determined on a Kofler hot-stage microscope and utilized uncorrected. Individuality and purity of synthesized compounds were controlled by means of TLC on Silufol UV-254 plates; I_2 was used as developer.

*General procedure of thiomethylation of 2,4-pentanedione with formaldehyde and a,ω-dithiols. 1,2-Bis[(pentane-2,4-dione-3-yl)methylsulfanyl]alkanes (**1a-e**)*

In Schlenk vessel using a magnetic stir bar was added with formaldehyde (37% aqueous solution, 20 mmol, 1.47 mL) and α,ω-dithiol (10 mmol) stirred for 30 min in argon atmosphere. Then 2,4-pentanedione (20 mmol) and the promoter BuONa (10 mmol) in 5 mL $CHCl_3$-C_2H_5OH (1:1) were added. The mixture was stirred for 1 h at r.t. The precipitate was filtered, washed with alcohol to give the target product **1a**: (81%, 2.58 g) as a white crystals, mp 139–141°C (data lit. 138–140°C). The spectra of other sulfanyl derivatives of bis-diketones are similar to those previously obtained.[21]

*Synthesis of 1,2-bis[(3,5-dimethylisoxazol-4-yl)methylsulfanyl]alkanes (**2a-e**) (General method)*

Sulfanyl-substituted bis-diketones (10 mmol), 15 mL of ethanol were charged into the glass vessel, was added with small portions of hydroxylamine (25 mmol, 1.74 g). The reaction mixture was heated up to 60 °C and stirred for 2 h. Then formed precipitate was filtered, washed with water (2 × 15 mL), and dried in open air.

1,2-Bis[(3,5-dimethylisoxazol-4-yl)methylsulfanyl]ethane (**2a**) Yield: 97%; white crystals, mp: 155–156°C (data lit. 154-156°C[21]).

1,3-Bis[(3,5-dimethylisoxazol-4-yl)methylsulfanyl]propane (**2b**) white solide (56%): R_f=0.59 (1:2:10 cyclohexane/CH_2Cl_2/EtOAc); mp 84–86 °C; IR (thin film) ν_{max} 1632, 1190, 1034, 886, 738 cm^{-1}; ^1H NMR (DMSO-d_6, 500 MHz) δ=3.53 (4H, s, CH_2); 2.48 (4H, t, ^3J = 7.2 Hz, H-9, -11); 2.33 (6H, s, CH_3); 2.20 (6H, s, CH_3); 1.77 (2H, p, ^3J = 7.2 Hz, CH_2); ^{13}C NMR (DMSO-d_6, 125 MHz,) δ=166.1 (C, C-3, -15), 159.6 (C, C-5, -18), 111.3 (C, C-4, -14), 30.2 (CH_2, C-9, -11), 28.9 (CH_2, C-10), 22.8 (CH_2, C-7, -13), 10.9 (CH_3, C-21, -19), 10.1 (CH_3, C-6, -20); MALDI TOF *m/z* 327.327 $C_{15}H_{23}N_2O_2S_2$ (calcd. 327.485); 349.267 $C_{15}H_{22}N_2O_2S_2Na$ (calcd. 349.467); Anal. Calcd. for $C_{15}H_{22}N_2O_2S_2$: C, 55.18; H, 6.79; N, 8.58; S, 19.64. Found: C, 55.34; H, 6.85; N, 8.42; S, 19.71.

1,4-Bis[(3,5-dimethylisoxazol-4-yl)methylsulfanyl]butane (**2c**): white solide (94%): R_f=0.61 (1:2:10 cyclohexane/CH_2Cl_2/EtOAc); mp 68–70 °C; IR (thin film) ν_{max} 1637, 1192, 1032, 893, 719 cm^{-1}; ^1H NMR (DMSO-d_6, 500 MHz) δ=3.45 (4H, s, CH_2); 2.40 (4H, m, CH_2); 2.32 (6H, s, CH_3); 2.19 (6H, s, CH_3); 1.57 (4H, m, CH_2); ^{13}C NMR (DMSO-d_6, 125 MHz) δ=166.0 (C, C-3, -15), 159.7 (C, C-5, -19), 111.4 (C, C-4, -15), 30.7 (CH_2, C-9, -12), 28.4 (CH_2, C-10, -11), 22.7 (CH_2, C-7, -14), 10.9 (CH_3, C-20, -22), 10.1 (CH_3, C-6, -21); MALDI TOF *m/z* 363.341 $C_{16}H_{24}N_2O_2S_2Na$ (calcd. 363.494); Anal. Calcd. for $C_{16}H_{24}N_2O_2S_2$: C, 56.44; H, 7.10; N, 8.23; S, 18.83. Found: C, 56.49; H, 7.21; N, 8.19; S, 18.97.

1,5-Bis[(3,5-dimethylisoxazol-4-yl)methylsulfanyl]-3-thiapentane (**2d**): white solide (74%): R_f= 0.66 (1:2:10 cyclohexane/CH_2Cl_2/EtOAc); mp 71–73 °C; IR (thin film) ν_{max} 3421 (N–H), 1633 (C=N), 1192 (C–N), 726 (C–S) cm^{-1}; ^1H NMR (DMSO-d_6, 500 MHz) δ=3.61 (4H, s, CH_2); 2.74 – 2.61 (8H, m, $SC_2H_4SC_2H_4S$) 2.34 (6H, s, CH_3); 2.20 (6H, s, CH_3); ^{13}C NMR (DMSO-d_6, 125 MHz) δ=166.2 (C, C-3, -17), 159.7 (C, C-5, -20), 111.3 (C, C-4, -16), 31.6 (CH_2, C-10, -12), 31.5 (CH_2, C-9, -13), 22.7 (CH_2, C-7, -15), 10.9 (CH_3, C-21, -23), 10.1 (CH_3, C-6, -22); MALDI TOF *m/z* 395.041 $C_{16}H_{24}N_2O_2S_3Na$ (calcd. 395.558); 411.004 $C_{16}H_{24}N_2O_2S_3K$ (calcd. 411.667); Anal. Calcd. for $C_{16}H_{24}N_2O_2S_3$: C, 51.58; H, 6.49; N, 7.52 S, 25.82. Found: C, 51.67; H, 6.53; N, 7.64; S, 26.13.

1,6-Bis[(3,5-dimethylisoxazol-4-yl)methylsulfanyl]hexane (**2e**): white solide (69%): R_f= 0.59 (1:2:10 cyclohexanes/CH_2Cl_2/EtOAc); mp 76–78 °C; IR (thin film) ν_{max} 3436, 1634, 1196, 1038, 721 cm^{-1}; ^1H NMR (DMSO-d_6, 500 MHz) δ=3.52 (4H, s, CH_2); 2.39 (4H, t, ^3J = 7.2 Hz, CH_2S); 2.33 (6H, s, CH_3); 2.20 (6H, s, CH_3); 1.49 (4H, m, CH_2); 1.30 (4H, m, CH_2); ^{13}C NMR (DMSO-d_6, 125 MHz) δ=165.9 (C, C-3, -18), 159.6 (C, C-5, -21), 111.4 (C, C-4, -17), 31.1 (CH_2, C-9, -14), 29.2 (CH_2, C-10, -13), 28.3 (CH_2, C-11, -12), 22.8 (CH_2, C-7, -16), 10.9 (CH_3, C-22, -24); 10.1 (CH_3, C-6, 23); MALDI TOF *m/z* calculated for 369.316 $C_{18}H_{29}N_2O_2S_2$ (calcd. 369.565); $C_{18}H_{28}N_2S_2Na$ 391.267 (calcd. 391.547); 407.222 $C_{18}H_{28}N_2S_2K$ (calcd. 407.655);

Anal. Calcd. for $C_{18}H_{28}N_2S_2$: C, 58.66; H, 7.66; N, 7.60; S, 17.40. Found: C, 58.87; H, 7.81; N, 7.54; S, 17.62.

*Cis-S,S-dichloride-1,6-(3,5-dimethylisoxazol-4-yl)-2,5-dithiahexane palladium(II) complex (**3**)*

In the glass vessel (1.405 mmol, 0.25 g) palladium(II) chloride was dissolved in 15 mL of acetonitrile by stirring at 60 °C. After cooling up to r.t. 1,2-*bis*[(3,5-dimethylisoxazol-4-yl)methylsulfanil]ethane (1.405 mmol, 0.44 g) was added and reaction mixture was stirred for 3 h. The resulting bright yellow precipitate was filtered through filter paper (blue ribbon) and washed by acetonitrile, water and dried in open air with formation yellow powder **3** (54%); mp > 250°C (dec.); IR (thin film) ν_{max} 1635 (br), 1274, 1250, 1193, 883, 829, 715, 661, 334, 307 cm^{-1}; ^1H NMR (DMSO-d_6, 500 MHz) of diastereomeric mixture (AB system): δ=4.63 ($2H_a$, dd, ^2J 14.4, Hz, $C\underline{H_2}$), 4.33 ($2H_a$, dd, ^2J 14.4 Hz, $IzC\underline{H_2}S$), 4.47 ($2H_b$, dd, ^2J 14.0 Hz, $C\underline{H_2}$), 4.18 ($2H_b$, dd, ^2J 14.0 Hz, $C\underline{H_2}$), 3.51 ($2H_a$, dd, ^2J = 9.2 Hz, SCH_2CH_2S), 3.15 and 3.09 ($2H_b$, br s, SCH_2CH_2S), 2.93 ($2H_a$, dd, ^2J = 9.2 Hz, SCH_2CH_2S), 2.43 (6H, s, CH_3), 2.26 (6H, s, CH_3); ^{13}C NMR (DMSO-d_6, 125 MHz) δ=168.9 (C, C-3, -16), 159.6 (C, C-5, -19), 107.8 (C-4, -15), 37.5 and 37.3 (CH_2, C-9, -10), 30.4 and 29.7 (CH_2, C-7, -14), 11.5 (CH_3, C-13,23), 10.3 (CH_3, C-6,22); ESI *m/z* 527 $[M+Cl]^-$ (100); Anal. Calcd. for $C_{14}H_{20}Cl_2N_2O_2PdS_2$: C, 34.33; H, 4.12; Cl, 14.48; N, 5.72; Pd, 21.73, S, 13.09. Found: C, 34.07; H, 3.84; Cl, 14.74; N, 5.82; Pd, 22.12, S, 13.10.

*Cis-S,S-dichloride-1,6-(3,5-dimethylisoxazol-4-yl)-2,5-dithiahexane copper(I) complex (**4**)*

In a three-necked flask equipped with thermometer, refluxer and argon was charged with 1,2-bis[(3,5-dimethylisoxazol-4-yl)methylsulfanyl]ethane in 4 mL CH3CN 0.28 g (2.81 mmol) and copper(I) chloride was added (1.405 mmol, 0.44 g). Than reaction mixture was stirred for 3 h at 60 °C. The resulting white precipitate was filtered through filter paper (blue ribbon) and washed with acetonitrile. The complex **4** was received as white powder (0.43 g, 60%); mp 221–223 °C; IR (thin film): ν 1629, 1196, 884, 724, 480, 398, 320. ^1H NMR (DMSO-d_6, 500 MHz) δ=3.53 (4H, s, CH_2), 2.57 (4H, m, $SC_2\underline{H_4}S$), 2.24 (6H, s, CH_3), 2.10 (6H, s, CH_3); ^{13}C NMR (DMSO-d_6, 125 MHz) δ=166.0 (C, C-3, -19), 160.1 (C, C-5, -22), 111.5 (C, C-4, -18), 31.2 (CH_2, C-9, -10), 22.8 (CH_2, C-7, -17), 11.0 (CH_3, C-16, -24), 10.2 (CH_3, C-6, -23). Anal. Calcd. for $C_{14}H_{20}N_2O_2S_2Cu_2Cl_2$: C, 32.94; H, 3.95; Cl, 13.89; Cu, 24.90; N, 5.49; S, 12.56. Found, %: C, 32.58; H, 3.82; Cl, 13.51; Cu, 24.78; N, 5.43; S, 12.87.

Crystal Structure Determination and Refinement

The X-ray diffraction experiments of **2c** and **2d** single-crystals were carried out by a Bruker SMART 1000 CCD area detector using graphite monochromated MoeKa radiation at 100 K. All calculations were performed on an IBM PC/AT using the SHELXTL software Atomic coordinates, bond lengths, bond angles, and thermal parameters have been deposited at the Cambridge Crystallographic Data Centre (CCDC). X-ray diffraction data of **2c** and **2d** single-crystal was collected on a XCalibur Eos diffractometer with graphite monochromated Mo-Kα radiation (λ=0.71073 Å). Collection and processing of data performed with using the program CrysAlis^{Pro} Oxford Diffraction Ltd., Version 1.171.36.20. The structure was solved by direct methods as implemented in the program SHELXS-97.[30,31] The refinement was carried out using SHELXL-97. The structure was refined by a fullmatrix least-square technique using anisotropic thermal parameters for non-hydrogen atoms and a riding model for hydrogen atoms.

Crystallographic data for the structure of **2c** have been deposited in the Cambridge Crystallographic Data Centre as a CIF deposition with file number CCDC 1545010. Copies of these data can be obtained free of change on application to CCDC, 12, Union Road, Cambridge, CB2 1EZ, UK (fax: 44 1223 336033, e-mail: deposit@ccdc.cam.ac.uk) or from http://www.ccdc.cam.ac.uk/data_request/cif.

Crystallographic data for the structure of **2d** have been deposited in the Cambridge Crystallographic Data Centre as a CIF deposition with file number CCDC 1545008. Copies of these data can be obtained free of change on application to CCDC, 12, Union Road, Cambridge, CB2 1EZ, UK (fax: 44 1223 336033, e-mail: deposit@ccdc.cam.ac.uk) or from http://www.ccdc.cam.ac.uk/data_request/cif.

Biological assay

Simulation of animal-related processes was carried out in accordance with rules of laboratory practice (GLP) and the ethical norms of the Geneva Convention (1971). Conditions of experiment and keeping animals were carried out according to modern requirements.[32] The tissue was fixed in a 10% solution of neutral formalin for light-optical examination of the liver. For further histological treatment it was used samples of 5-7 mm thickness which were cut from a large proportion of the liver by cross-sectional dissection and subjected to standard treatment on the histological complex MICROM (Carl Zeiss, Germany). Samples were dehydrated in alcohols with increasing concentration, followed by pouring into paraffin blocks.

The studies were carried out on mice with a line BALB/CJ weighing 20 – 23 g (mice are provided by the Bashkir State Medical University Vivarium, Ufa, Russia). The animals were kept in 10 cells in a cage in standard vivarium conditions at an air temperature of 18 – 22 °C and a relative humidity of 50 to 65%. During the process there were free access to water and feed (~ 5 g/day).

Results and Discussion

Chemistry

The key substrates for the three step synthesis of target metallo-complexes of Pd(II) and Cu(I) was α,ω-

bis[(pentane-2,4-dione-3-yl)methylsulfanyl]alkanes **1a-e** produced by a *n*-BuONa *mediated* multicomponent reaction (MCR) between 2,4-pentanedion, CH_2O and α,ω-dithiols.[20] The yield of products **1a-e** was decreased with increasing the aliphatic chain of α,ω-dithiols from 97 to 54%. Substrates **1a-e** was successfully converted into α,ω-*bis*[sulfanylmethyl(3,5-methylisoxazol-4-yl)]alkanes **2a-e** with high yields through the interaction between **1a-e** and hydroxylamine hydrochloride in refluxing ethanol during 2 h (Figure 1).

It should be noted, that in the indicated above two-step sequence, the total yield of **2a** is higher than in the case of *one-pot* four-component reaction between 2,4-pentandione, CH_2O, 1,2-ethanedithiol and $NH_2OH \cdot HCl$.[21]

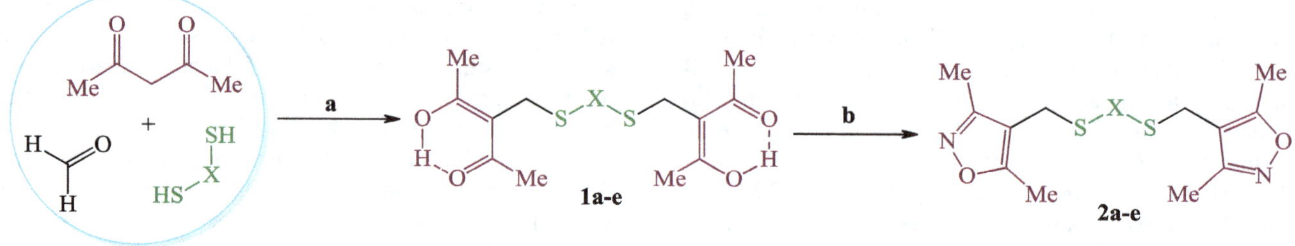

1a, 2a: X = C_2H_4 **1d, 2d**: X = $C_2H_4SC_2H_4$
1b, 2b: X = C_3H_6 **1e, 2e**: X = C_6H_{12}
1c, 2c: X = C_4H_8

Figure 1. Reagents and conditions: a) BuONa, RT, 1.5 h, C_2H_5OH:$CHCl_3$ (1:1); b) NH_2-OH · HCl, 70 °C, C_2H_5OH

According to X-ray data (Figure 2), compound **2c** is crystallized in the monoclinic and **2d** - in orthorhombic crystalline system. It was found that *bis*(3,5-dimethylizoxazol) rings are in the *cis*-conformation with respect to S-$(C)_n$-S fragment for compound **2c** and *trans*-configuration for compound **2d**. The crystallographic data for compounds **2c** and **2d** are collected in Table 1.

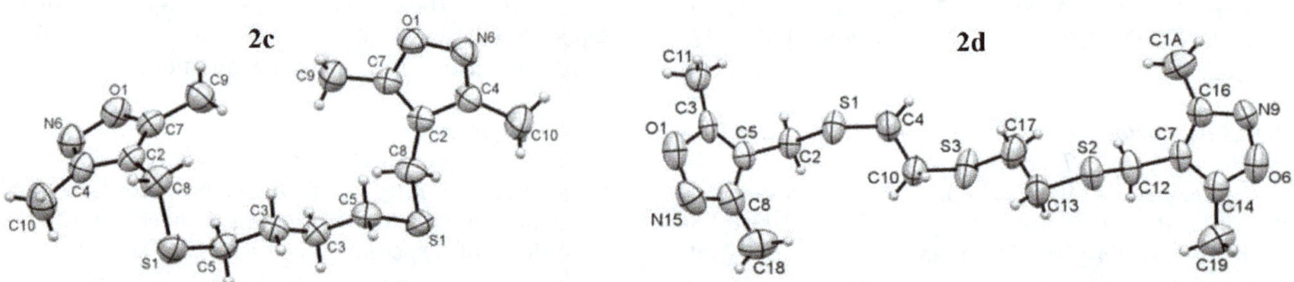

Figure 2. The geometry of molecules of compounds **2c** and **2f** in a crystal. Atoms are represented by thermal ellipsoids (p = 50%).

Among the synthesized 1,2-*bis*[sulfanylmethyl(3,5-dimethylisoxazol-4-yl)]alkanes **2a-e, 2a** is the most promising for practical application taking into account the production efficiency and availability of the starting reagents.

So that, 1,2-*bis*[sulfanylmethyl(3,5-dimethylisoxazol-4-yl)]ethane **2a** was then transformed to Pd(II) complex **3** by reaction with $PdCl_2$ in CH_3CN. According NMR analysis, Pd(II) complex **3** in solution is the mixture of diastereomers (see *Supplementary data*). Using CuCl under the same reaction conditions Cu(I) complex **4** was also produced in 97% yield (Figure 3). According elemental analysis for complex **3** the ligand-metal ratio was 1:1 and for 4 as 1:2. In IR spectra of complexes **3** and **4** there are signals of M-S: bonds is Pd-S in region 334 cm^{-1} and Cu-S in region 320 cm^{-1}

Biology

Combinatorial series of compounds **1a**, **2a**, **3**, and **4** having the same alkylsulfanyl chain and different cyclic fragments of substitutes were assessed as hepatoprotective agents. They were used as solutions in TWIN oil.

As known, the SAM drug (S-adenosyl-L-methionine **5**, Figure 4) being produced via biosynthetic process is used for treatment of large group of diseases associated with the hepatotoxic action of the chemicals or the alcohol causing morphological changes in liver tissue, metabolism disorder or the toxic liver damages[33-35] SAM drug is considered as non-toxic sulfanyl-containing hepatoprotectors.[36] It provides a stability of hepatocytes.[37] Moreover, the transsulfuration (synthesis and turnover of glutathione and taurine, as well as conjugation and detoxication of bile acids and other xenobiotics), aminoproliliration and transmethylation processes are activated.

Obviously SAM is a powerful antioxidant due to its sulfur atoms and heterocyclic fragments in the structure.[38,39] As seen, compounds **2a-e, 3, 4** also contain these units.

Thus, we have used SAM as the object of comparison to study toxicity and hepatoprotective activity of the compounds **1a**, **2a**, **3** and **4**.

Table 1. Crystallographic and structure refinement data for **2c** and **2d**

Compounds	2c	2d
Empirical formula	$C_{16}H_{24}N_2O_2S_2$	$C_{16}H_{24}N_2O_2S_3$
Formula weight	340.49	372.55
T/K	298	298
Crystal system	orthorhombic	monoclinic
Space group	Pbcn	$P2_1/c$
a/Å	17.514(2)	5.0140(7)
b/Å	7.8852(9)	11.6177(7)
c/Å	13.027(2)	33.308(9)
α/°	90	90
β/°	90	93.45(2)
γ/°	90	90
V/Å^3	1799.1(4)	1936.7(6)
Z	4	4
ρ_{calc}mg/cm^3	1.257	1.278
μ/mm^{-1}	0.304	0.392
F(000)	728.0	792.0
Crystal size/mm^3	0.54 × 0.26 × 0.22	0.71 × 0.30 × 0.28
2Θ range for data collection	4.66 to 62.82°	6.03 to 62.04°
Index ranges	$-25 \le h \le 22$, $-11 \le k \le 10$, $-18 \le l \le 17$	$-7 \le h \le 3$, $-16 \le k \le 15$, $-36 \le l \le 29$
Reflections collected	9025	4900
Independent reflections	2712[R_{int} = 0.0737, R_{sigma} = 0.0479]	3079[R_{int} = 0.0198, R_{sigma} = 0.0331]
Data/restraints/parameters	2712/0/126	3079/0/212
Goodness-of-fit on F^2	1.057	1.050
Final R indexes [I>=2σ (I)]	R_1 = 0.0570, wR_2 = 0.1524	R_1 = 0.0744, wR_2 = 0.1750
Final R indexes [all data]	R_1 = 0.0898, wR_2 = 0.1934	R_1 = 0.1034, wR_2 = 0.1943
Largest diff. peak/hole / e Å^{-3}	0.32/-0.29	0.40/-0.22

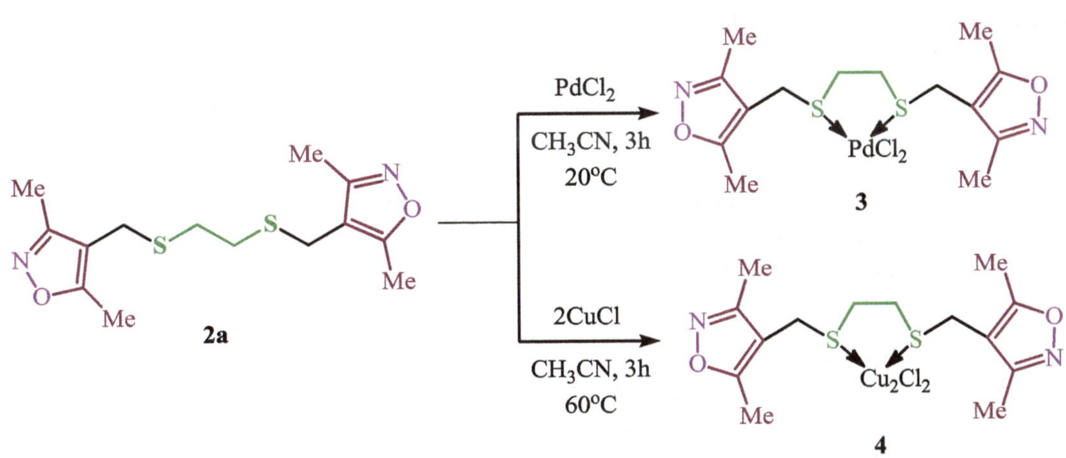

Figure 3. Reagents and conditions: a) $PdCl_2$, CH_3CN, 20 °C, 3h; b) CuCl, CH_3CN, 60 °C, 3h.

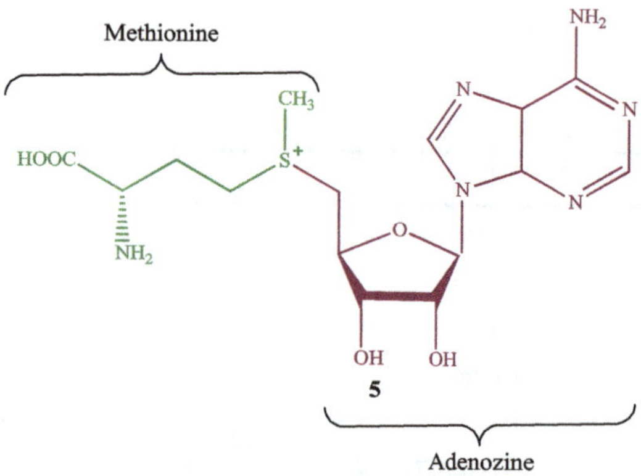

Figure 4. Structure of S-adenosyl-L-methionine **5**

Parameters of acute toxicity

To get reliable results acute toxicity was determined with Litchfield and Wilcoxon method modified by Prozorovskiy.[40] As a result of determining the comparative evaluation of acute toxicity in albino mice after intraperitoneal injection and oral administration, it was established that compounds **1a**, **2a** and **3** are assigned to the group of virtually non-toxic compounds (1001 – 3000 mg/kg) according to the Sidorov classification (Table 2).[40] After oral administration, LD_{50} value does not differ essentially from those of intraperitoneal administration.

Thus, structure-activity relationship shows that sulphanyl *bis*-diketone **1a** is less toxical compound (Sidorov classification, non-toxic group). It is not trivial fact that Pd(II) *cis*-chelate S,S-complex **3** also refers to group being not toxic. As seen from the Table 1, Cu(I) *cis*-chelate S,S-complex **4** is more toxical compound (Sidorov classification, low-toxic group). For this reason, compound **4** is not promising to treat liver diseases.

The model of acute hepatitis

Screening studies of compounds **1a** and **3** were carried out on a model of acute toxicity *in vivo*. Simulation of animal-related processes was carried out with the principles of bioethics. The animals received single dose of CCl_4 0.2 mL/kg intraperitoneally as a 50 percent solution of olive oil. The compound was administered intraperitoneally in a dose of 25 mg/kg 1 hour before the injection of CCl_4. As control was used SAM **5** (ademetionine), a pharmacologically known hepatoprotective drug in a dose of 25 mg/kg. The control group received 0.2 mL of saline solution (Table 3).

Thus, compound **3** in dose of 25 mg/kg has a strong antitoxic effect on the model of acute intoxication of CCl_4. In other words the compound 3 in the dose of 25 mg/kg causes significant lowering of lethality from 50 percent to 0 percent, compared with untreated animals in control group.

Biochemical analysis of blood were taken on the 10-th day of observation of acute hepatitis, caused with CCl_4, to control the development of cytolytic syndrome and evaluate degree of liver injury.

The complex **3** at dose 25 mg/kg resulted in a significant lowering ($p<0.05$) alanine aminotransferase by 70% comparing with untreated group of animals. At the same time the reference preparation ademetionine at the same dose resulted a significant lowering only by 53% ($p<0.05$) (Table 4).

Compounds **1a** and **2a** are less active according to this indicator. A significant lowering of aspartate aminotransferase between control and experimental groups was not recorded. By the 10 day of observation in all groups with an acute hepatitis the level of conjugated bilirubin raised. Compared to the intact group of animals figures receiving compound **3** – by 20.2%, **2a** – at 55.9%, **1a** – 58.8%, SAM – 25.9% in the group with the drug **3** - less often.

Table 2. Acute toxicity study of derivatives of 1,2-*bis*[(pentane-2,4-dione-3-yl)methylsulfanyl]}ethane

Entry	Test compound LD_{50}, mg/kg	LD_{50}, mg/kg
1	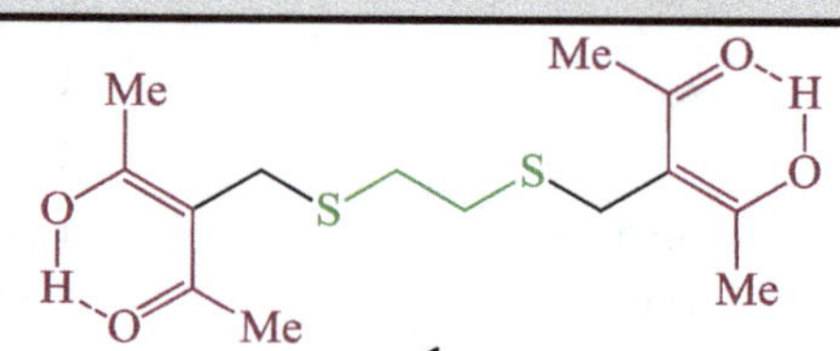 **1a**	1580.0
2	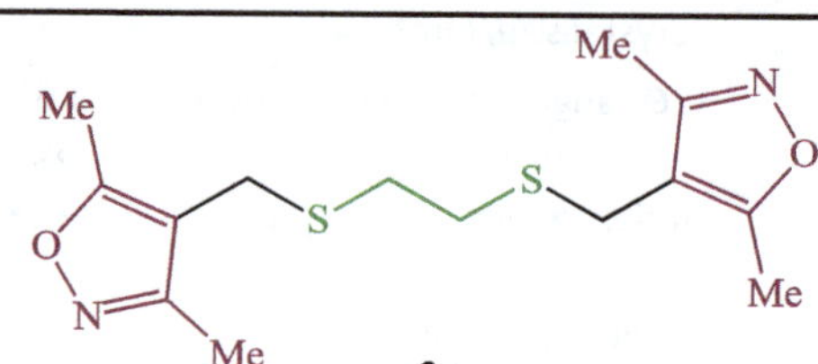 **2a**	1050.0
3	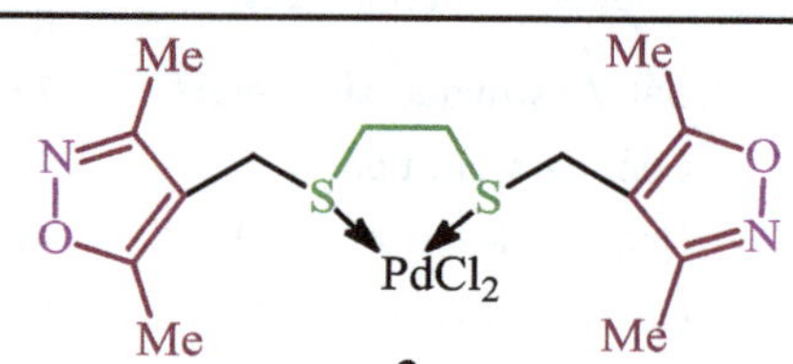 **3**	1240.0
4	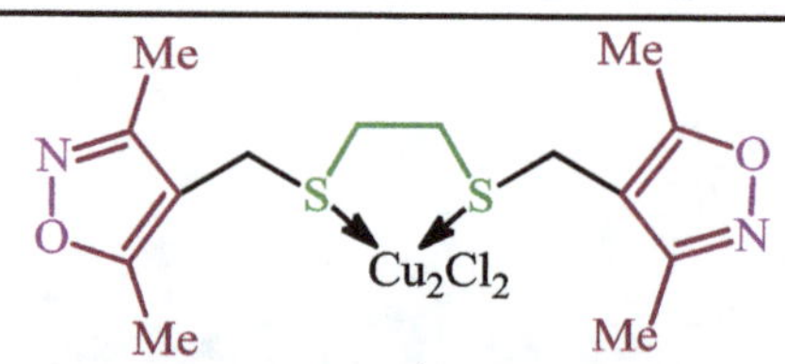 **4**	74.5
5	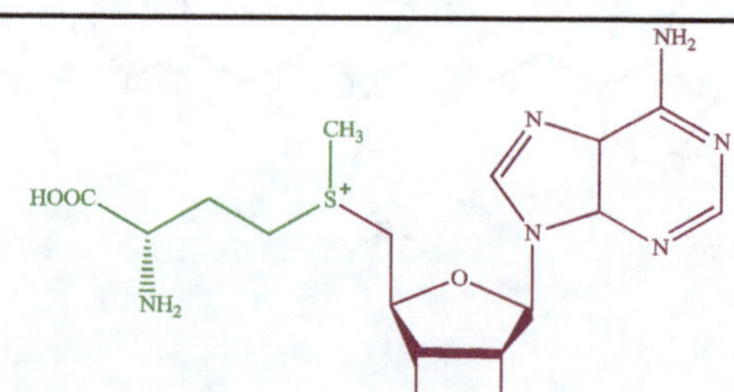 **5**	4650.0[41]

Table 3. Effects of compounds **1a, 2a, 3** and SAM **5** survival of white mice with acute toxic hepatitis

Administering compounds	Number of animals in groups	Surviaval rate on the 10 day of observation, %
Saline solution 0.2 mL/kg (intact group)	10	100
CCl_4 0.2 mL/kg (control group)	10	50
SAM 25 mg/kg + CCl_4 0.2 mg/kg	10	80
1a 25 mg/kg + CCl_4 0.2 mg/kg	10	70
2a 25 mg/kg + CCl_4 0.2 mg/kg	10	60
3 25 mg/kg + CCl_4 0.2 mg/kg	10	100

Table 4. Effects of compounds **1a, 2a, 3** and SAM on indicators AST, ALT, and direct bilirubin serum white mice with acute toxic hepatitis

Groups of animals	ALT, mcmol/mL/h	AST, mcmol/mL/h	Bilirubin direct serum, mcmol/L
Control intact	1.49 ± 0.22	1.09 ± 0.07	8.3 ± 2.2
Control (CCl_4)	4.72 ± 0.57*	1.71 ± 0.14*	19.5 ± 5.1*
SAM+ CCl_4	2.21 ± 0.21	0.92 ± 0.06	11.2 ± 3.2
3+ CCl_4	1.51 ± 0.31**	0.98 ± 0.02**	10.4 ± 2.6**
2a+ CCl_4	2.32 ± 0.48**	0.94 ± 0.06**	20.1 ± 4.5
1a+ CCl_4	2.68 ± 0.64	0.93 ± 0.07	18.8 ± 5.1

Note: * - significant differences between indicators of intact animals, ** - significant differences from that of group CCl_4

Histological examination

Staining with hematoxylin, eosin, by standard methods on histological complex MICROM. Histological activity index (HAI) was defined. Evaluation System indicators protein dystrophy, inflammatory infiltration, hyaline drop dystrophy - a 4-point scale.

Administering CCl_4 without treatment led to gross structural changes in the form of large-drop dystrophy of hepatocytes, lymphohistiocytic infiltration of the liver structure.

Compounds pretreatment and heptral at dose 25 mg/kg led to less expression of morphological changes of liver structures: reduction of inflammatory infiltration, necrosis of hepatocytes, hepatocyte degeneration reduction degree.

Semi-quantitative method for assessing the degree of activity of pathological processes in the liver showed:

1) Significant reduction in HAI compared with results of control group was observed during therapy with Compound 3 and heptral. Compounds **1a** and **2a** had no significant digits.
2) The degree of fatty liver among white mice, treated with Compound **3** was minimal, hepatocytes with fatty inclusions are located only on the periphery of the hepatic lobule. Other animal groups **1a** and **2a** had moderate degree – 1/3 – 1/4 the length of the hepatic beams, hearths cirrhosis, liver tissue was sealed.

A new sensibly nontoxic (IV class) compound *cis*-S,S-dichloride-1,6-(3,5-dimethylisoxazol-4-yl)-2,5-dithiahexane palladium(II) complex **3** with hepatoprotective activity in laboratory animals (white mice) at a dose of 25 mg/kg intraperitoneally on acute hepatitis model induced by carbon tetrachloride was discovered. Compound **3** exeled the reference preparation ademetionine (SAM) for indications:

a) animal survival (100%, SAM – 80%);

b) biochemical (ALT, AST, bilirubin direct) parameters;

c) histological (liver parenchyma lesions are minimal) parameters.

On the basis of biochemical tests (ALT, AST, bilirubin) and histological compounds displayed hepatoprotective activity which decreased in the number of **3** > **1a** > **2a**.

Conclusion

In summary, we have developed a two step effective synthesis of α,ω-*bis*(3,5-dimethylisoxazol-4-ylmethylsulfanyl)alkanes via the interaction between 2,4-pentandione, CH_2O, α,ω-dithiols and next with hydroxyl amine. It was shown, that new Pd(II) and Cu(I) complexes are efficiently formed when using 1,2-*bis*(isoxazol-4-ylmethylsulfanyl)ethane as ligand. The *in vivo* method has demonstrated, that combinatorial row - 1,2-*bis*[(pentane-2,4-dione-3-yl)methylsulfanyl]ethane **1a**, 1,2-*bis*[sulfanylmethyl(3,5-dimethylisoxazol-4-yl)]ethane **2a** and its complex with $PdCl_2$ dichlorodi(3,5-dimethylisoxazol-4-yl)-1,2-dithiaethane palladium(II)) **3** are virtally non-toxic and exhibit hepatoprotective activity. The leader among them is palladium(II) complex dichlorodi(3,5-dimethylisoxazol-4-yl)-1,2-dithiaethane **3**, whose activity is comparable to SAM.

Acknowledgments

This work was partially financially supported by the Grant of the republic of Bashkortostan young scientists and youth research teams. The reported study was funded by Russian Foundation for Basic Research and Academy of Sciences of the Republic of Bashkortostan according to the research project № 17-43-020292 p_a and project part 4.6007.2017/8.9. Structural studies of the compounds obtained were performed using unique equipment in "Agidel" collective usage centre (state assignment *AAAA-A17-117012610060-7*).

Conflict of Interest

The authors declare that they have no conflict of interest.

References

1. Jaouen G, Salmain M, Vessieres A. Bioorganicmetallics: Biomolecules, labeling, medicine. Weinheim: Willey-VCH Verlag GmbH and KGaA; 2006.
2. Crisponi G, Nurchi VM, Lachowicz JI, Crespo-Alonso M, Zoroddu MA, Peana M. Kill or cure: misuse of chelation therapy for human diseases. *Coord Chem Rev* 2015;284:329-50. doi: 10.1016/j.ccr.2014.04.023
3. Allardyce CS, Dorcier A, Scolaro C, Dyson PJ. Development of organometallic (organo-transition metal) pharmaceuticals. *Appl Organomet Chem* 2005;19(1):1-10. doi: 10.1002/aoc.725
4. Barashkov GK, Zaitseva LI. Use of laws of interelement interactions for understanding of mechanisms of various human diseases. *Biomed Khim* 2008;54(3):266-77.
5. Osredkar J, Sustar N. Copper and zinc, biological role and significance of copper/zinc imbalance. *J Clin Toxicol* 2011;S3(1):1-19. doi: 10.4172/2161-0495.S3-001
6. Krupanidhi S, Sreekumar A, Sanjeevi CB. Copper & biological health. *Indian J Med Res* 2008;128(4):448-61.
7. Blackburn NJ, Yan N, Lutsenko S. Copper in Eukaryotes. In: Maret W, Wedd A, editors. Binding, transport and storage of metal ions in biological cells. Royal Society of Chemistry; 2014. PP. 524-55.
8. Zheng W, Monnot AD. Regulation of brain iron and copper homeostasis by brain barrier systems: Implication in neurodegenerative diseases. *Pharmacol Ther* 2012;133(2):177-88. doi: 10.1016/j.pharmthera.2011.10.006
9. Hu M, Li X, Du Q, He X, Zhou K, Li D, et al. Effect of baicalin-copper complex against carbon tetrachloride-induced hepatic injury in mice. *Int J Adv Pharm* 2014;4:187-94.
10. Siddik ZH. Cisplatin: mode of cytotoxic action and molecular basis of resistance. *Oncogene* 2003;22(47):7265-79. doi: 10.1038/sj.onc.1206933
11. Hannon MJ. Metal-based anticancer drugs: From a past anchored in platinum chemistry to a post-genomic future of diverse chemistry and biology. *Pure Appl Chem* 2007;79(12):2243-61.doi: 10.1351/pac200779122243
12. Coluccia M, Natile G. Trans-platinum complexes in cancer therapy. *Anticancer Agents Med Chem* 2007;7(1):111-23. doi: 10.2174/187152007779314080
13. Bano N, Najam R, Qazi F. Adverse cardiac manifestations of cisplatin - A review. *Int J Pharm Sci Rev Res* 2013;18(1):80-5.
14. Yao X, Panichpisal K, Kurtzman N, Nugent K. Cisplatin nephrotoxicity: A review. *Am J Med Sci* 2007;334(2):115-24. doi: 10.1097/MAJ.0b013e31812dfe1e
15. Prudhomme M. Advances in anticancer agents in medicinal chemistry. France: Bentham Science Publishers; 2013.
16. Wang, Guo Z. The role of sulfur in platinum anticancer chemotherapy. *Anticancer Agents Med Chem* 2007;7(1):19-34. doi: 10.2174/187152007779314062
17. Kapdi AR, Fairlamb IJ. Anti-cancer palladium complexes: A focus on PdX_2L_2, palladacycles and related complexes. *Chem Soc Rev* 2014;43(13):4751-77. doi: 10.1039/c4cs00063c
18. Amoke OA. Synthesis, characterization, in-vitro antibacterial and anticancer studies on some metal(II) complexes of (methylsulfanyl)chromenol Schiff base. *Elixir Appl Chem* 2011;39:4827-31.
19. Grigorieva AS, Drogovoz SM, Kirichek LM, Konahovich NF, Kuzmenko II, Mokhort NA, et al. Method of treating liver diseases of various origins. Patent RU 2035906. 1995.
20. Akhmetova VR, Akhmadiev NS, Starikova ZA, Tulyabaev AR, Mescheryakova ES, Ibragimov AG. Catalytic multicomponent thiomethylation of aliphatic 1,3-diketones as efficient one-pot synthesis of novel bis(1,3-diketone-2-ylmethylsulphanyl)alkanes. *Tetrahedron* 2015;71(40):7722-8. doi: 10.1016/j.tet.2015.07.055
21. Akhmetova VR, Akhmadiev NS, Meshcheryakova ES, Khalilov LM, Ibragimov AG. Multicomponent synthesis and biological activity of (sulfanylalkyl)-substituted azaheterocycles. *Chem Heterocycl Compd* 2014;50(5):742-51. doi: 10.1007/s10593-014-1529-9
22. Maksimov V, Zaynullin R, Akhmadiev N, Segura-Ceniceros EP, Martınez Hernandez JL, Bikbulatova E, et al. Inhibitory effect of 4,4′-[ethane-1,2-diylbis(sulfandiylmethanediyl)]bis(3,5-dimethyl-1H-pyrazole) and its derivatives on alpha-amylase activity. *Med Chem Res* 2016;25(7):1384-9. doi: 10.1007/s00044-016-1574-2
23. Akhmetova VR, Akhmadiev NS, Ibragimov AG. Catalytic multimolecular reactions of 1,3-dicarbonyl CH-acids with CH_2O and S- and N-nucleophiles. *Russ Chem Bull* 2016;65(7):1653-66. doi: 10.1007/s11172-017-1495-3
24. Galenko AV, Khlebnikov AF, Novikov MS, Pakalnis VV, Rostovskii NV. Recent advances in isoxazole

chemistry. *Russ Chem Rev* 2015;84(4):335-77. doi: 10.1070/RCR4503

25. Kumar KA, Jayaroopa P. Pyrazoles: synthetic strategies and their pharmaceutical applications-an overview. *Int J Pharm Tech Res* 2013;5(4):1473-86.
26. Pradeepkumar Y, Ruthu M, Madhusudhana chetty C, Prasanthi G, Jaya Sankar Reddy V. Pharmacological activities of isoxazole derivatives. *J Global Trends Pharm Sci* 2011;2(1):55-62.
27. Pinto A, Tamborini L, Cullia G, Conti P, De Micheli C. Inspired by Nature: The 3-Halo-4,5-dihydroisoxazole Moiety as a Novel Molecular Warhead for the Design of Covalent Inhibitors. *ChemMedChem* 2016;11(1):10-4. doi: 10.1002/cmdc.201500496
28. Urdaneta N, Landaeta VR, Rodríguez-Lugo RE, Díaz C, Santiso-Quinones G, Quiroga J, et al. Synthesis and characterization of Cu(I) and Zn(II) complexes with new sulfur-bearing isoxazole- or pyrazole-based ligands. *Inorg Chem Commun* 2015;55:43-7. doi: 10.1016/j.inoche.2015.03.007
29. Munsey MS, Natale NR. The coordination chemistry of isoxazoles. *Coord Chem Rev* 1991;109(2):251-81. doi: 10.1016/0010-8545(91)80019-A
30. Sheldrick GM. A short history of SHELX. *Acta Crystallogr A* 2008;64(Pt 1):112-22. doi: 10.1107/S0108767307043930
31. Dolomanov OV, Bourhis LJ, Gildea RJ, Howard JAK, Puschmann H. OLEX2: a complete structure solution, refinement and analysis program. *J Appl Cryst* 2009;42:339-41. doi: 10.1107/S0021889808042726
32. Mironov AN. A guide to preclinical drug research. Moscow: Grif and K; 2012.
33. Singh A, Bhat TK, Sharma OP. Clinical biochemistry of hepatotoxicity. *J Clin Toxicol* 2011;S4:2-19. doi: 10.4172/2161-0495.S4-001
34. Pandit A, Sachdeva T, Bafna P. Drug-induced hepatotoxicity: a review. *J Appl Pharm Sci* 2012;2(5):233-43.
35. Bigoniya P, Singh CS, Shukla A. A comprehensive review of different liver toxicants used in experimental pharmacology. *Int J Pharm Sci Drug Res* 2009;1(3):124-35.
36. Lu SC. S-Adenosylmethionine. *Int J Biochem Cell Biol* 2000;32(4):391-5. doi: 10.1016/s1357-2725(99)00139-9
37. Anstee QM, Day CP. S-Adenosylmethionine (SAMe) therapy in liver disease: a review of current evidence and clinical utility. *J Hepatol* 2012;57(5):1097-109. doi: 10.1016/j.jhep.2012.04.041
38. Kucheryavy YuA, Morozov SV. Hepatoprotectors: rational aspects of the application. Moscow: Fort Drum(Russia); 2012.
39. Okovity SV, Sukhanov DS, Petrov AYu, Romantsov MG. Hepatotropic medicines: current status. *Ther Arch* 2012;84(2):62-8.
40. Berezovskaya IV. Classification of substances with respect to acute toxicity for parenteral administration. *Pharm Chem J* 2003;37(3):139-41. doi: 10.1023/A:1024586630954
41. Center SA. S-adenosyl-methionine (SAMe) an antioxidant and anti-inflammatory nutraceutical. 18th ed. Seattle, WA: ACVIM; 2000.

18

Pharmaceutical Cocrystals: Regulatory and Strategic Aspects, Design and Development

Dipak Dilip Gadade*, Sanjay Sudhakar Pekamwar

School of Pharmacy, S.R.T.M. University, Vishnupuri, Nanded – 431606, India.

Article info

Keywords:

- Cocrystal
- Crystal engineering
- Solubility
- Drug Stability
- Crystallization polymorphism
- Salt

Abstract

Cocrystal is a concept of the supramolecular chemistry which is gaining the extensive interest of researchers from pharmaceutical and chemical sciences and of drug regulatory agencies. The prominent reason of which is its ability to modify physicochemical properties of active pharmaceutical ingredients. During the development of the pharmaceutical product, formulators have to optimize the physicochemical properties of active pharmaceutical ingredients. Pharmaceutical cocrystals can be employed to improve vital physicochemical characteristics of a drug, including solubility, dissolution, bioavailability and stability of pharmaceutical compounds while maintaining its therapeutic activity. It is advantageous being a green synthesis approach for production of pharmaceutical compounds. The formation polymorphic forms, solvates, hydrates and salts of cocrystals during the synthesis reported in the literature which can be a potential issue in the development of pharmaceutical cocrystals. The approaches like hydrogen bonding rules, solubility parameters, screening through the CSD database or thermodynamic characteristics can be utilized for the rational design of cocrystals and selection of coformers for synthesis multi-component cocrystals. Considering the significance of pharmaceutical cocrystals pharmaceutical regulatory authorities in the United States and Europe issued guidance documents which may be helpful for pharmaceutical product registration in these regions. In this article, we deal with the design, synthesis, strategic aspects and characteristics of cocrystals along perspectives on its regulatory and intellectual property considerations.

Introduction

During the last few years, a plethora of drug products has reached the market. The poorly water-soluble drug candidates are becoming more prevalent in the pharmaceutical industry (Lipinski, 2000).[1] Approximately 40% of the marketed immediate release oral products are categorized as practically insoluble (Takagi2006).[2] It was estimated that 70% and more new chemical entities (NCE) are being identified by combinatorial screening program are poorly water-soluble.[3]

The supramolecular chemistry was defined by Lehn JM, as "chemistry beyond the molecule" is the organization of entities that results from the association of two or more chemical species held together by non-covalent interactions.[4] The selective binding through molecular interactions was depicted by lock and key model of Emil Fischer.[5] The chemical systems under study are classified into two major categories organized self-assembly in the solid state as crystal engineering and molecular recognition in solution which is commonly referred to as supramolecular chemistry.[6]

The concept of crystal engineering in solid state chemistry was introduced by Pepinsky R, in 1955.[7] A work on photochemical reactions was reported by Schmidt (1971), provides learning for crystal engineering.[8] Desiraju G, defined crystal engineering as "the understanding of intermolecular interactions in the context of crystal packing and in the utilization of such understanding in the design of new solids with desired physical and chemical properties".[9] Pioneering work in prediction and interpretations of non-covalent bonding interaction using a Cambridge structural database (CSD) was carried out by Etter and Desiraju.[10,11]

Physicochemical properties of a drug govern solubility and dissolution profile which is indicative of drug bioavailability, which in turn can affect the biological activity of the drug. Solubility, dissolution, stability, micromeritics and mechanical characteristics of an active pharmaceutical ingredient (API) are common barriers in pharmaceutical drug development. The aqueous solubility of an API is a vital physicochemical parameter determining various aspects related to the formulation and delivery of a drug. During discovery and development stages the solubility data is required at various stages. It is used to characterize drug through structure-activity relationship, for assessment of

***Corresponding author:** Dipak D. Gadade, Email: deeps_cpn@yahoo.co.in

absorption, distribution, metabolism and elimination constraints and to develop a formulation for early preclinical and clinical screening.[1] Formulation plays a major role in overcoming problems associated with drug delivery and it determines the biological availability of an API in terms the rate and extent of absorption from the gut.[3]

Physical modification often aims to enlarge the particle surface area, improve solubility and/or wetting of the powder and improving the stability of an API. The poorly water-soluble drugs can be formulated as amorphous forms, crystalline solid formulations, or by lipid formulations to improve their solubility. Crystal engineering through cocrystallization is a promising approach to address problems associated with the drug. Although definitions of cocrystals are available in the literature, it is still a topic of debate.[12,13] Broadly cocrystals can be defined as crystalline materials consist of two or more different components (or commonly called multi-component crystals). For the pharmaceutical cocrystals, one component is an API and other components are called as crystals former or conformers. Cocrystals have gained considerable interest in pharmaceutical research due to its ability to improve physicochemical characteristics of an API. Several papers have been published in the recent past which gives an overview of cocrystals[14-17] and some which show its clinical relevance.[18] Design strategies, synthesis procedures, cocrystal characteristics with an emphasis on its applications, regulatory, strategic and patentability considerations are discussed in this review. The process for cocrystal development is depicted in Figure 1.

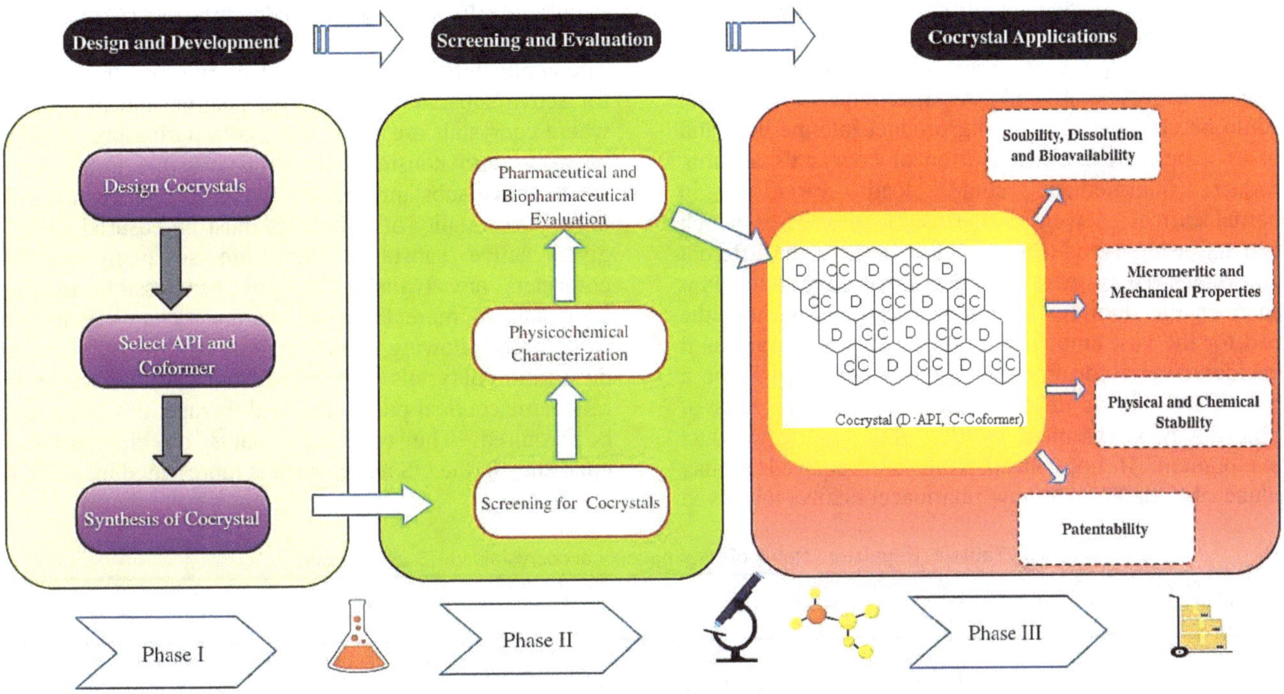

Figure 1. Process for cocrystal development, screening and applications

Regulatory and Strategic Aspects of Cocrystals

The formulation of cocrystals through crystal engineering has emerged as a promising approach in the formulation of poorly water soluble compounds. It has become a topic interest in the pharmaceutical industry, which can be traced from regulatory documents published by United States food and drug administration (USFDA) and European Medicine Agency (EMA).

USFDA defines cocrystals under 'Regulatory Classification of Pharmaceutical Co-Crystals' as, *Crystalline materials composed of two or more molecules within the same crystal lattice'*. The alteration of desired pharmaceutical properties viz. solid state properties, solution behavior, and dissolution, etc. is possible through crystal engineering of the drug with coformers without modifying the chemical structure of drug molecule. According to this guidance an API and excipients which are having Δpka (pKa (base) - pKa (acid)) ≥1 then there will be the formation of salts because there will be complete proton transfer which results in absolute ionization, which is an ionic reaction. If Δpka <1, then there will be negligible proton transfer and cocrystals are formed which is a result of the non-ionic interaction. Any of numerous compounds that result from partial or complete replacement of the acid hydrogen of an acid by a metal or a radical forming metal: an ionic or electrovalent crystalline compound are referred as salt. *Per se* the current regulatory scheme, different salt forms of the same API are considered as dissimilar active ingredients. Polymorphs are different crystalline forms of the same chemical substance. This may include hydration or solvation products (which is also known as pseudo-polymorphs) and amorphous forms. *Per se* the current regulatory scheme, unlike

polymorphic forms of the same compound is considered the same active moiety.[19]
The possible effects of adopting to this definition will be drug products with cocrystals will be considered as drug product intermediates, applications to FDA claiming to contain cocrystals will be required to prove the extent of proton transfer, the cocrystal must be revealed to dissociate in vivo prior it reaches active site (much ambiguous in case of topical formulations), the API cocrystal by definition seems to be physical mixture of API and excipients.[20] In FDA's view the cocrystal considered as a drug product intermediate that is expected to enhance pharmaceutical product performance, such as enhanced solubility and/or dissolution rate. It is less problematic to show dissociation of API and excipient before its pharmacological action. Brittain HG, has suggested that dilutions of cocrystal solutions can demonstrate a dissociation of cocrystal components[15] while recent study reported pH-dependent dissociation of cocrystal.[21] Another aspect that USFDA determines a cocrystal should be considered as a drug product intermediate and not as a new API. Consideration of cocrystals as drug product intermediate could lead variation in pharmaceutical as well as therapeutic properties which need to be analyzed case by case basis with different conformers. This aspect is may of great importance as it can open the door to the use of cocrystals without the need for the vast amount of clinical trials necessary as it considered as it drug product intermediate and not a drug. It may be as an opportunity to use cocrystals of APIs for new chemical entities and generic product development. If no clinical trials are required it may reduce the time taken by pharmaceutically improved cocrystals of the active chemical moiety with GRAS listed coformers to enter into the market, obliviously also cutting expenditure on pharmaceutical development.
Reflection paper released by the European Medicines agency has given subdivision of solid state materials based on the internal structure. It defined cocrystals as, homogeneous (single phase) crystalline structures made up of two or more components in a specific stoichiometric ratio where the arrangement in the crystal lattice is not based on ionic bonds (as with salts).[22] Further, it discussed the regulatory implications of cocrystals understanding and other solid forms of API which may be of great value to the point of view to get a generic drug status for such forms as cocrystals are formed by non-covalent bonding. Cocrystals are not considered as a new drug if the applicant is able to demonstrate its safety and efficacy equivalent to parent API . An applicant can have the opportunity to claim for consideration of cocrystals with same approval or market authorization as given to an API. The applicability of good manufacturing practices (GMP) for active substances or finished pharmaceutical products where cocrystals are produced *in situ* during process shall be taken into consideration. It is possible to present a single active substance master file for cocrystals and API. Safety and quality of coformers must be ensured as for a given active substance there are so many possible coformers are available. It may be possible to form cocrystals of more than one therapeutic moiety in such cases proof showing on the careful rationalization of the dose ratio cocrystals components and its influence on the biopharmaceutical parameters and therapeutics effect shall be required. The regulatory status of Pharmaceutical cocrystals in the US and Europe is represented in Table 1.

Table 1. Regulatory status of Pharmaceutical cocrystals in US and Europe

Cocrystal Parameters	USFDA[19]	EMA[22]
Definition	Solids that are crystalline materials composed of two or more molecules in the same crystal lattice.	Homogenous (single phase) crystalline structures made up of two or more components in a definite stoichiometric ratio where the arrangement in the crystal lattice is not based on ionic bonds (as with salts).
Regulatory status	Drug product intermediate (DPI), not regarded as a new API	New Active Substance status dependent upon demonstration of efficacy and/or safety
Sameness with parent API	Yes	Dependent upon demonstration of efficacy and/or safety
Coformers	Neutral guest compound (excipient)	Non-active components/Regeants (excipient)
Regulatory Consideration	Similar to Polymorph of same API	Similar to salts of same API
Chemical interactions	Nonionic	Nonionic
US-Drug master files (DMF)/EMA-Active substance master file (ASMF)	Not feasible being DPI	Can be filed
Applicable Good manufacturing practice (GMP) regulations/guide	cGMP for drug product	Part II of EU GMP Guide (active substances) and ICH Q7 and in rare cases Part I of EU GMP Guide (finished drug product)

Physical Forms of Solids Associated with Cocrystals

The chemical structure of an API in solution and its ability to interact with its targets determines its intrinsic activity. Depending upon a chemical nature and three-dimensional arrangement of the molecule, a compound can exist in single component systems known as the amorphous state or in several different crystalline states, which are polymorphic forms of the parent chemical moiety. The crystalline, multi-component systems which include a complex with ion or molecules are salts, hydrates, solvates, or cocrystals.[23] The solid forms may exist in multiple crystalline forms as shown in Figure 2 and Figure 3. The identification of particular solid form is important with the view of the formulation of an optimal drug delivery system which will be associated desired biopharmaceutical parameters and it also decides its value as intellectual property.

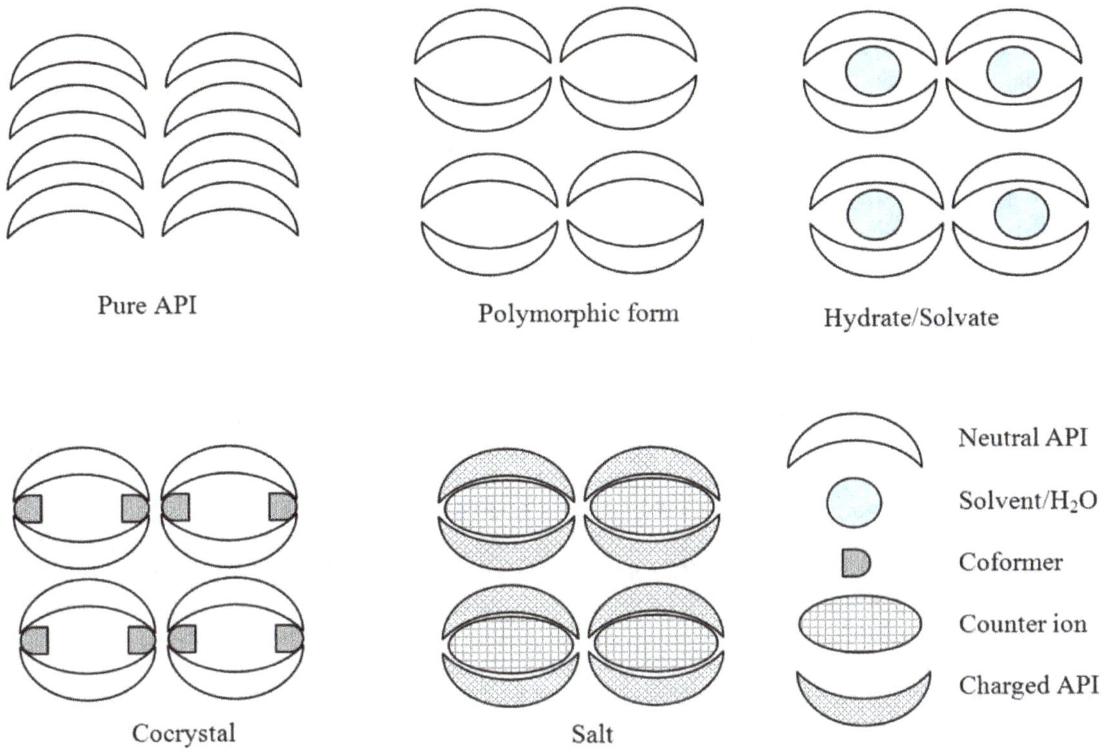

Figure 2. Schematics of salt, cocrystal and polymorphs

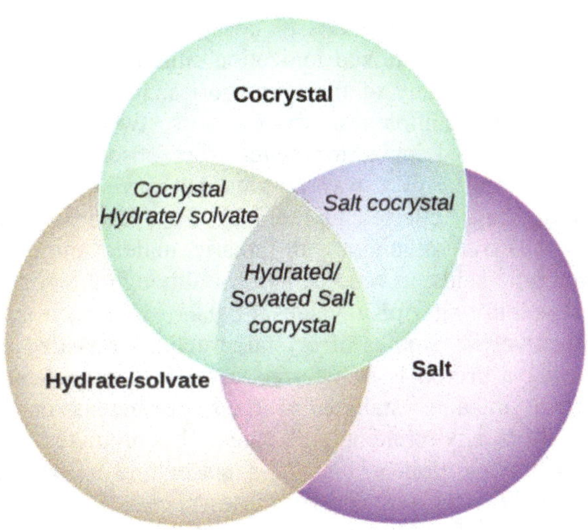

Figure 3. Multiple physical forms of solid with physical state continuum

Polymorphism and Cocrystals

Pharmaceutical polymorphic solids of the same chemical compound having a distinct internal solid-state structure and, have the ability of to crystallize as more than one distinct crystal species. Therefore, polymorphs possess different physical and chemical characteristics, including packing, thermodynamic, melting point, density, hardness, crystal shape, optical and electrical properties, spectroscopic properties, kinetic parameters, interfacial, and mechanical properties.[24,25] Polymorphs offer a unique opportunity to study the structure–property relationships of the same compound formed in different supramolecular environments. Investigating the polymorphic behavior of an API is a critical part of the drug development process.[26] Other crystal variations can be encountered where the crystal structure of the substance is defined by still other unit cells, where these unit cells vary in their elemental composition through the inclusion of one or more molecules of solvent which referred as solvatomorphism.[27] Polymorphism may result in differences in the physicochemical properties of the API and difference in these properties may result in a drug product variable bioequivalence, and hence in a product that is not considered as a therapeutically equivalent to the innovator product. This is because polymorphism can greatly influence pharmaceutical properties, such as solubility, bioavailability, stability, hygroscopicity, etc., and the economic significance of novel polymorphs as intellectual property. Therefore, in the context of the ANDA review, careful attention should be given to the effect that polymorphism may have on a generic drug product equivalent as required by FDA with the innovator brand.[28]

During the search for and prevalence of Polymorphs and Cocrystals, about 90% of the screened compounds found to exist in multiple solid crystalline and noncrystalline forms. There were half of the compounds amongst screened compounds were polymorphic. The percentage of compounds that exist in multiple solid forms was the same for salts and non-salts (91%). Non-salts have been more frequently polymorphic than were salts (55% compared to 39%). Salts were found to exist as hydrates more frequently than did non-salts (48% compared to 30%). The tendency of forming cocrystal was found to be 61%.[29]

Polymorphism in cocrystals is being reported in the literature has significantly increased in the recent past. A detailed review of polymorphic cocrystals has been published by Aitipamula S, et al. which provides a classification of cocrystal polymorphs. Cocrystal polymorphs are classified as Synthon polymorphs, conformational polymorphs, packing polymorphs, tautomeric polymorphs, polymorphic cocrystal hydrates and solvates, ternary cocrystals polymorphs.[30] A summary of representative cocrystals polymorphs reported in the various literature is presented in Table 2. It was demonstrated by Aitipamula S, et al that generation of polymorphic forms of cocrystals is possible by the selection of solvents or mixture of solvents.[36] In an another study reported by same research group metastable polymorphs, EA-GA-II and III eventually convert to stable polymorphic form-I upon solid state grinding which enables the control of polymorphic form. EA-GA and Caffeine-GA cocrystals have relevance to the context of a combination of drugs.[37] The effect of milling experiments was demonstrated by Limwikrant, et al which suggests that polymorphic transformations could occur during processing of raw materials.[33] Stable polymorphic cocrystals of antitubercular drug Isoniazid (INH) tested as per ICH stability guidelines were reported by Swapna B.et al. Interestingly polymorphic cocrystals of INH with fumaric acid and hydroxyl benzoic acid had shown lower solubility and dissolution rate which is in contrast ability of cocrystals to enhance pharmaceutical characteristics of API.[43] Although polymorphic cocrystals of furosemide with nicotinamide and iso-nicotinamide improve solubility of API but their stability is in question as demonstrated through slurry experiment.[46] Interesting chiral and achiral polymorphic cocrystals of tryptamine with hydrocinnamic acid were reported by Koshima, et al.[52] In an attempt to search for stable cocrystals of hydrate-forming compounds, anhydrous caffeine–oxalic acid cocrystals form was reported to be thermodynamically stable in an aqueous environment. It confirmed that hydrate of caffeine can be converted to anhydrous form improving its physical stability.[55] The fact reported that cocrystals could be formed during the phase transition of the low-temperature stable polymorph of furosemide if coformer is available in close contact with the transforming component suggesting increased mass transfer rate can trigger cocrystal formation.[56]

In the summary polymorphic transformation of cocrystals has the ability to alter various pharmaceutical aspects related to an API, including but not limited to solubility, dissolution, bioavailability, and stability. It was also reported in the literature that processing parameters could lead to polymorphic transformations of cocrystals while some metastable polymorphic forms are converted to the stable form after storage. A careful and cautious selection of the specific form of cocrystals of API shall be required to maintain the quality of a pharmaceutical product within specified standards.

Salt-Cocrystal Continuum

A salt contains a single ionic compound, but multiple ions. Formation of salts of organic compounds involves the proton transfer from an acid to a base.[29] If any pair of molecules are ionized, and disordered solid form where the crystallography does not unambiguously locate the protons are called as salt.[57] It is generally accepted that reaction of an acid with a base will be expected to form a salt. Although as discussed above the USFDA guidance defined that API and excipients which are having $\Delta pka \geq 1$ then there will be the formation of salts and if $\Delta pka < 1$, then there will be cocrystals are formed. There are papers reporting the cases that which deviate from this definition in the guidance document.[58-61] At the same time, one shall consider the fact reported by Child SL, et al. that prediction power of cocrystal formation is poor when Δpka is 0 to 3. When the ΔpKa is negative, it correctly predicts the cocrystals formation. In this range, complexes between acids and bases can still form, although they can be salts or cocrystals or can contain shared protons or mixed ionization situation that cannot be assigned to any of these categories. In a study with theophylline complexes, sixteen salts, two cocrystals, and two mixed ionization states were observed, where the transition ΔpKa was ranging between 0 to 2.5.[60] Another case reported in literature for 5-fluorocytosine only salts were obtained with fumaric, maleic, and oxalic carboxylic acids, in water solutions, although the systems were exhibiting ΔpKa values of 0.23, 1.35, and 2.01, respectively.[61] Studies of crystal structures revealed that whether a proton is transferred from one component to another in a crystalline solid is dependent on the crystalline environment and cannot be predicted from ΔpKa values alone. Thus, it is reasonable to consider crystalline salts and cocrystals as species that exist at either end of a continuum of multicomponent crystal structures. At the salt end proton transfer is complete, and at the cocrystal end, proton transfer is absent. When a pair of ionizable components crystallizes, both the ΔpKa value and the crystalline environment, determine the extent of proton transfer and therefore the placement of the structure on the continuum.[27]

Table 2. Pharmaceutical Cocrystals and its Polymorphic forms

Sr. No.	API	Coformer	Polymorphs/hydrate	Stable Polymorph	Melting Point (ºC)	Phase Transition Temp.(ºC)	Ref.
1	Carbamazepine (CBZ)	Nicotinamide (NCT)	CBZ-NCT-I and II,	CBZ-NCT-I	158º	83–90º	Seefeldt, K. et al.[31]
		Nicotinamide	PN-CBZ-NCT and CBZ-NCT I	CBZ-NCT I	--	124-128º	William W. et al.[32]
		Saccharin (SAC)	CBZ-SAC I and II	CBZ-SAC I	173.8º	168º	William W. et al.[32]
		Malonic acid	Form A,B and C	Form A	192º	140-160º	Limwrilant W. et al.[33]
		Isonicotinamide (INA)	CBZ-INA I and II	CBZ-INA I	--	--	Horst J.H.T. et al.[34]
2	5-methoxy sulfadiazine (SMD)	Homosynthon	SMD-I and II	Isomeric forms	---	---	Caira, M. R.[35]
3	Ethenzamide (EA)	Gentisic acid (GNA)	EA-GNA-I,II,III	EA-GNA-I,	100.65º	98.5º	Aitipamula S., et al.[36]
		Ethylmalonic acid (EMA)	EA-EMA I and II	EA-EMA II	85.60º	77º	Aitipamula S., et al.[37]
		Saccharin	EA-SAC I and II	EA-SAC I	122.50º	--	Aitipamula S., et al.[38]
		3,5-Dinitro benzoic acid (DNBA)	EA-DNBA I and II, Solvates	EA-DNBA I	148.73º	--	Aitipamula S., et al.[39]
4	Caffeine	Gallic Acid (GA)	Caffeine–GA form I and II	*	--	--	Trask A.V, et al.[40]
		Trifluoroacetic Acid	Caffeine–TA I and II	Caffeine–TA I	--	--	Trask A.V, et al.[41]
5	Nalidixic acid	Pyrogallol	Hemihydrate	--	--	--	Gangavaram, S. et al.[42]
		Phloroglucinol	Hydrate	--	--	--	
6	Isoniazid (INH)	Vanillic acid (VLA)	INH-VLA 1,2 and 3	INH-VLA2	153.2º	142–144° (Form1)	Swapna, B. et al.[43]
		Ferulic acid (FRA)	INH-FRA 1,2 and 3	INH-FRA1	168.4º	--	
		Caffeic acid (CFA)	INH-CFA 1,2 and 3	INH-CFA2	153.1º	129º (Form-1)	
		Hydroxybenzoic acid (HBA)	INH-HBA I and II	INH-HBA II	123.0º	--	Aitipamula S.[44]
		Fumaric acid (FA)	INH-FA I and II	INH-FA I	169.4º	--	
7	Furosemide (FS)	Nicotinamide	FS-NCT forms I–V and hydrate [45] FS-NIC 1 and 2, [46]	FS-NCT-I > III > II > V > IV	154.9º (FS-NCT-I)	--	Ueto T. et al[45] Goud N.R. et al.[46]
		Isonicotinamide (INIC)	FUROS–INIC I and II	--	--	--	
8	Sulfacetamide (SACT)	Acetamide (ACT)	SACT–ACT I and II	SACT–ACT I	106.5º	79º	Goud N.R. et al.[47]
9	Sulfadimidine (SD)	4-Amino salicylic Acid (ASA)	SD:4-ASA I and II	SD: 4-ASA-I	175º	--	Grossjohan C.et al.[48]
10	Celecoxib	δ-valerolactam	Form –I, II and III	Form –I	106.0º	71.0º (Form-III)	Bolla G. et al.[49]
11	Temozolamide (TMZ)	4,4′-bipyridine-N,N′-dioxide(BPNO)	TMZ-BPNO I, II, and III	TMZ-BPNO I	--	--	Babu N.J. et al.[50]
12	Piroxicam	4-hydroxy benzoic acid	Form 1 and 2	Tautomeric forms	--	--	Childs S.L. et al.[51]
13	Tryptamine	Hydrocinnamic Acid	Chiral and achiral forms	Chiral form	--	--	Koshima H. et al.[52]
14	Chlorzoxazone	2,4-dihydroxybenzoic acid	Form 1 and 2	Form 2	177.4º	--	Child S.L. et al.[53]
15	p-Coumaric Acid	Nicotinamide	Form 1, 2 and 3	Form 1	154.0º	--	Bevill M.J. et al.[54]

*When **caffeine** and **GA** are ground together in the absence of solvent, cocrystal form I predominantly results. Similarly, the addition of four drops from a pipette of a nonpolar solvent, such as n-hexane, cyclohexane, or heptane also produces form I. Conversely, upon addition of four drops of a more polar solvent, including chloroform, dichloromethane, acetonitrile, and water, the grinding experiment results in predominantly form II.

In a study to synthesize the multicomponent solid forms involving pyridine included both salts and cocrystals, while 4-dimethylaminopyridine (DMAP) crystallized exclusively as a salt, in agreement with the differences in the pKa values. During a crystallization of pyridine with carboxylic acids interestingly *cis-trans* isomers, maleic acid and fumaric acid resulted in same cocrystals solid form while DMAP formed a salt with these carboxylic acids. A similar case was demonstrated when terephthalic acid was used as coformer to form a multicomponent crystal with pyridine, resulted in cocrystal formation and with DAMP, a salt was formed.[57] In a study reporting cocrystals of fluoroquinolone salts, ciprofloxacin hydrochloride hydrate (CiHCl·1.34H2O) and 4-hydroxybenzoic acid (4-BHA) cocrystals lead to lower thermodynamic solubility and dissolution rate due to dense crystal packing. (S, S)-moxifloxacin hydrochloride hemihydrate (MoHCl·0.5H2O) formed cocrystals with 4-BHA but interestingly it improved solubility and dissolution as compared to parent salt which was contradictory to the behavior of CiHCl-4BHA cocrystals.[62] Hybrid salt-cocrystals solvate case was disclosed by Jacob A. et al. where the tertiary amine is protonated forming a charge-assisted hydrogen-bond ($N^{+}\cdots OH^{-}$) to the *p*-Coumaric acid (*p*-CA^{-}) anion and the quinoline nitrogen forms a hydrogen-bond (N···OH) to the neutral *p*-Coumaric acid molecule. The methanol molecules occupy voids as the system does not allow for the easy escape of the solvent molecules.[63]

It should be noted that as discussed above different salts of same compound are considered to be chemical moiety other than original compounds in regulatory aspect. It makes necessary to clarify for a multi-component crystal, component is either coformer which lead to cocrystals formation or complementary ion forming a salt. The experimental evidences produced here brings us to conclusion that USFDA's guidance document- 'Regulatory Classification of Pharmaceutical Co-Crystals' is still topic of debate in the field.

Cocrystal Design and Coformer Selection

Hydrogen-Bonding Rules

One can design cocrystals based on empirical understanding hydrogen-bonds patterns can be determined using guidelines provided by Etter M.C[10] and Donohue J.[64] These rules are (a) all acidic hydrogen present in a molecule will be utilized in hydrogen bonding in the crystal structure of that compound, (b) all good acceptors will be used in hydrogen-bonding when there hydrogen-bond donors are available, (c) Preferentially hydrogen bonds are formed between the best hydrogen-bond donor and the best hydrogen-bond acceptor. The important systems which can form hydrogen bonds are N-H...N, N-H...C1, N-H...O, O-H...N, O-H...O, where dash indicates covalent and dots indicates non-covalent contacts with acceptor atom.[62]

Cambridge Structural Database (CSD)

The understanding intermolecular interaction is necessary for syntheses of supramolecular synthons. The study of hydrogen bond patterns in crystalline solids provide information about promising synthons that can be designed.[65] It is possible to determine the frequency of hydrogen-bond motifs and other interactions using CSD. CSD is the repository for small-molecule organic and metal-organic crystal structures developed in 1965 which is continuously updated after extensive validation and verification by experts. CSD provides a way for 'the systematic analysis of large numbers of related structures is a powerful research tool, capable of output results that could not be obtained by any other method'.[66] It is based predominantly on shape and polarity of cocrystal formers.[67] CSD provides the information common functional groups that engage in supramolecular synthon formation.[68] H-bond donor and acceptor counts showed no obvious statistical relationship. A potential drawback of the model is that it was trained on cocrystal observations in the CSD database, ignoring potential failures in realistic cocrystal screenings.[69]

Hansen Solubility Parameter (HSP)

Mohammad MA, et al reported the use of Hansen solubility parameter (HSP) for prediction of cocrystal formation.[70] The concept was originally proposed for predicting polymer solubility in paints by Hansen C.M. The basis of these so-called HSPs is that the total energy of vaporization of a liquid comprising of several individual component forces. These forces arise from (atomic) dispersion forces, (molecular) hydrogen bonding (electron exchange) and (molecular) permanent dipole–permanent dipole forces.[71] The difference in total solubility parameters (Δδt) of the API and conformer is calculated for the purpose of prediction of cocrystal formation. Δδt values less than $7MP^{0.5}$ indicates likely cocrystal may be formed and values greater than 10 $MP^{0.5}$ fewer chances of cocrystal formation. The result reported in the study indicates limited application of this approach in cocrystal prediction as only a few coformer formed cocrystals although $\Delta\delta_t$ was less than $7MP^{0.5}$.[68]

Cocrystal Design Based On Thermodynamic Characteristics

COSMO-RS (Conductor-like Screening Model for Real Solvents) is a universal theory to envisage the thermodynamic equilibrium properties of liquids, which was originally developed by Andreas Klamt.[72,73] The statistical physics of interacting molecular surface segments is the basis for COSMO-RS thermodynamics. The polar and H-bond interaction energies are quantified based on the surface screening charge densities, which result from a quantum chemical continuum solvation calculation. Because of its ability to treat mixtures at variable temperatures and to calculate accurate solvation energies using first principles, it has become very useful in the chemical engineering and in areas of physical and medicinal chemistry. It is possible to compute a virtually supercooled liquid mixture of the cocrystallization components and to compute the excess enthalpy (*H*ex) of stoichiometric *m:n* mixtures created out of the pure components A and B: by using following equation

$$Hex = (HAB - xm\ H pure,\ A - xn\ H pure,\ B) \text{ ------ } Eqn.1$$

*H*pure and *H*AB represent the molar enthalpies in the pure reference state and in the *m*:*n* mixture, with mole fractions $xm = m/(m + n)$ and $xn = n/(m + n)$. *H*ex contains all enthalpy contributions and is not limited to H-bonding interactions, although those may be separated from the overall enthalpy by utilizing COSMO*therm* software.[72] Virtual screening using COSMO-RS approach can be useful for hydrates and for coformer selection.[74,75]

Perlovich G.L. reported methodology for analysis thermodynamic functions for cocrystals formation. Prediction of cocrystal melting points by correlating it with conformer (CF) melting parameter and by using API melting parameters was attempted in the reported study, although good correlations were not obtained between the melting points and the descriptors. Thermodynamic functions of 79 cocrystals have been obtained through SciFinder and analyzed by the diagram method. Gibbs energy of cocrystal formation with the stoichiometric ratio (API)n(CF)m $\Delta G^{298}{}_{f}$(CC), and was calculated by following equations-

$$\Delta G^{298}{}_{sub}(PM) = X_{1}.\,\Delta G^{298}{}_{sub}(API) + X_{2}\,\Delta G^{298}{}_{sub}(CF) \text{----- Eqn.2}$$

where for (API)n(CF)m: X1 = n/(n + m) and X2 = m/(n + m). $\Delta G^{298}{}_{f}$ (PM), $\Delta G^{298}{}_{sub}$(API) and $\Delta G^{298}{}_{sub}$(CF) are the Gibbs energies of sublimation of the physical mixture, API, and CF, respectively.

$$\Delta G^{298}{}_{f}(PM) = \Delta G^{298}{}_{sub}(CC) - \Delta G^{298}{}_{sub}(PM) \text{------- Eqn.3}$$

and enthalpy(API)n(CF)m $\Delta H^{298}{}_{f}$(CC) was calculated by using following equations-

$$\Delta H^{298}{}_{sub}(PM) = X_{1}.\,\Delta H^{298}{}_{sub}(API) + X_{2}\,\Delta H^{298}{}_{sub}(CF) \text{------Eqn.4}$$

$\Delta H^{298}{}_{f}$ (PM), $\Delta H^{298}{}_{sub}$(API) and $\Delta H^{298}{}_{sub}$(CF) are the enthalpies of the physical mixture, API and CF, respectively.

$$\Delta H^{298}{}_{f}(PM) = \Delta H^{298}{}_{sub}(CC) - \Delta H^{298}{}_{sub}(PM) \text{ -------Eqn.5}$$

It was further reported that most of the cocrystals belong to the $\Delta G^{0}{}_{f}$(CC) value interval between 5 and −10 kJ mol^{-1}, i.e. the region of thermodynamically stable cocrystals. This fact signifies that stabilization of the cocrystal crystal lattice compared to that of the physical mixture leads to ordering of molecules (entropy reduction).[76]

Cocrystal Synthesis

Cocrystals can be prepared by solid or liquid based methods. The only summary of cocrystals synthesis methods is presented below; interested readers may see review by Qiao N. et al[17] for details of various methods.

Solid-Based Methods

Solid-based methods include solid state grinding, melt extrusion, and melt crystallization. Solid state grinding or neat grinding is consists of mixing of API with coformers in a specific stoichiometric ratio and grinding them either manually or mechanically.[77] In hot melt extrusion (HME) stoichiometric blends of API and conformers are passed at controlled temperatures with determined residence time. Advantages of these methods are solvent-free process, continuous and scalable green techniques.[78]

Liquid-based methods

Liquid-based methods comprise of liquid assisted grinding (LAG), solvent evaporation, solution crystallization, slurry screening, reaction crystallization, cooling crystallization, spray drying, supercritical fluid assisted crystallization, planetary milling, and ultrasound assisted crystallization.[17]

Solution crystallization offers advantages of particle size and crystal habit control, as well as possible chemical purification and ability to prepare new cocrystal via solution growth.[38] It was demonstrated that use solvent mixtures is advantageous in increasing chances of cocrystal formation and further it also possible to thermodynamically suppress the solvate formation by a competing reaction in solution mediated cocrystallization trials.[79] Friscic T, et al. devised a parameter η, which is the ratio of solvent volume to sample weight. It can be utilized differentiate conditions that distinguish LAG from slurry sonication or slurrying additionally they reported that LAG would require lower amounts of solvent than Sonic Slurry experiments.[80]

Cocrystals Ability to Improve Physicochemical Characteristics of API

Alteration of Thermal Characteristics

The melting point of a substance is a fundamental physicochemical property, which is the temperature at which solid state substance is converted to a liquid state at atmospheric pressure. The melting point can be determined using a capillary method, Kofler bench or differential scanning calorimetry (DSC). DSC data also provide information about enthalpy.

The factors which affect this physical constant are the arrangement of molecules within the crystal lattice, molecular symmetry, intermolecular interactions, conformational degrees of freedom for a molecule, and composition, etc.[81,82] The melting point of cocrystal was either less than or greater than or between the melting points of components of cocrystal. It was demonstrated for carbamazepine cocrystals experimental solubility's shows poor correlation with ideal solubility values derived from enthalpy and melting temperature of crystals.[83] The relation between solubility curves and melting properties has been established by Nordström FL, et al. for predicting melting temperatures from solubility.[84]

Improvement in Micromeritics and Mechanical Properties

The micromeritics and mechanical properties of pharmaceuticals are of utmost importance in the pharmaceutical industry. The understanding of their flow properties is of critical significance in operations such as blending of raw materials, tablet compression, capsule filling, transport, and in scale-up operations. Crystal engineering provides an opportunity for improvement of physical properties especially flow property of pharmaceutical powders.

The etravirine and nicotinamide co-crystal with better flow properties, showing better physical stability, was disclosed by Sansone M, et al.[85] It was demonstrated by Alhalaweh A, et al. that spray drying could produce cocrystal material with smaller surface energies as compared to milled theophylline cocrystal and ability to control particle physicochemical properties.[86] The mechanical properties of paracetamol were improved by cocrystallization with theophylline.[87] The improvement of physicochemical nature of ezetimibe was achieved by its cocrystallization with salicylic acid and benzoic acid.[88] It was demonstrated that Lamivudine: zidovudine cocrystal monohydrate improves flow properties as compared to component mixture.[89]

Enhancement of Solubility, Dissolution, and Bioavailability

The solubility improvement of drugs remains one of the trickiest challenges in formulation and development.[90] The drug dissolution is rate-limiting step in the absorption of a drug from the gastrointestinal tract. The poor aqueous solubility of drug potentially limits bioavailability of drug.[91] The greater understanding of a dissolution and absorption behavior of drugs with low aqueous solubility is necessary to effectively formulate them into bioavailable pharmaceutical drug products.

Several reports have shown that cocrystal is an emerging approach to address low drug solubility poor dissolution and bioavailability. Brittain HG, et al. developed intravenous water soluble cocrystal formulation of aspirin-theanine which has improved stability and bioactivity as compared previously available composition.[92] Buschman HH, et al. had identified drug-drug cocrystals of tramadol and paracetamol which improve pharmacokinetics and pharmacodynamics of components synergistically.[93] Bethune SJ, et al. had reported cocrystals of pterostilbene (neutraceutical antioxidant compound) with caffeine, carbamazepine, glutaric acid and piperazine as coformers showing improved solubility.[94] Zotepine HCl:Benzoic acid cocrystals were reported to amplify aqueous solubility and dissolution rates by several folds compared with a free base.[95] Solubility and bioavailability of quercetin were reported to improve by more than 10 folds by its cocrystallization with caffeine, caffeine: methanol, iso-nicotinamide, and theobromine as coformers.[96] It was demonstrated that solubility of sildenafil, 6-mercaptopurine and clotrimazole can be potentially increased by cocrystals and salt formation with mono and dicarboxylic acids and amides.[97-100] Bioavailability of 6-mercaptopurine was reported to remarkably enhanced by 168.7% as compared to the parent compound.[100] Prolonged mean resident time (MRT) of its parent compound Fluoxetine HCl forms cocrystals with benzoic acid as a co-former having low solubility and dissolution rate while its cocrystals succinic acid was with more solubility and dissolution rate showing contradictory behavior. The former cocrystal of Fluoxetine HCl with benzoic can be potentially used for slow release.[101] Recent studies with various pharmaceutical compounds with diverse chemical and pharmacological nature which includes myricetin (anticancer flavonol), itraconazole (antifungal), adefovir (antiviral), aceclofenac (nonsteroidal anti-inflammatory) and mirtazapine (antidepressant) reemphasize the solubility advantage of cocrystals exhibiting potential to improve bioavailability.[102-106]

Effect of pH and pKa on eutectic point or transition concentrations cocrystal was shown by Bethune SJ, et al.[107] It was demonstrated how cocrystal solubility of nonionizable API can be influenced by pH, pKa, and coformer concentration through mathematical prediction tools. This study was carried out for cocrystals carbamazepine with salicylic acid and p-aminobenzoic acid coformers, which can be exploited to study the behavior of other API's with acidic and basic nature. The unlike crystal forms of an API possess different solubility and permeability behavior which may alter the bioavailability. The correlation of crystal structure of cocrystals with solubility and permeability needs to be addressed with an exploration into aspects of the Biopharmaceutic Drug Classification system (BCS).[108,109] Cocrystals form of an API expected to enhance the solubility of the pharmaceutical compound as demonstrated in various reports cited above. If cocrystals enhance the solubility of pharmaceutical compounds then BCS class II and class IV compounds can be potentially converted to BCS class I and class III. Such studies addressing with the Biopharmaceutical class of cocrystals of pharmaceutical compounds may be helpful practically get bio-waivers from the FDA minimizing need of human involvement.

Impact on Physical Stability

The sorption of moisture can create a hydrated form or new polymorphic forms of drug which may potentially affect the quality of the drug. The hydrolysis of some drugs due to moisture is well documented in literature.[110,111] It can affect adversely on drug release from formulation, shelf life, handling and transportation of formulations.[26,112]

Cocrystals embodiments of tramadol and paracetamol possess the ability to reduce hygroscopicity of each other.[113] Cocrystal of c-glycoside derivative and l-proline were found to be optimally stable at various temperature conditions during ambient and accelerated stability studies with humidity stress.[114] Almarsson O. et al. disclosed that cocrystals prepared by solid and solution based methods either with or without heating have ability to decrease hygroscopicity of the parent compound.[115] The hygroscopic stability *S*-Oxiracetam was improved by cocrystallization with gallic acid. This enhanced stability was assigned to extended hydrogen-bonded network in cocrystal.[116]

The mechanism for moisture generated cocrystals was established by Jayashankar A. et al which can be advantageously utilized formulation development and predict stability conditions. Amount and rate of water uptake by cocrystal components decides the supersaturation which has its effect on the nucleation and growth rate of cocrystal.[117] Although reports for *in situ* formation of cocrystals during pharmaceutical processing, manufacturing and storage are available,[118-120] likelihood of phase separation and polymorphic transformations in cocrystals during storage shall be the challenge to the researchers working in crystal engineering.

Impact on Chemical Stability

Cocrystallization causes a change in the molecular arrangement in crystal lattice which may modify the chemical stability of the compound. The solubility of niclosamide was improved by theophylline cocrystals but at the expense of reduced stability.[121] The reported stability studies of mefloquine hydrochloride shows no significant differences in stability during storage at intermediate ICH stability conditions.[122] It was reported that propiconazole: oxalic acid cocrystal forms stable cocrystal polymorphic forms during stability studies.[123]

A study by Jayasankar A, et al. which revealed reactant solution composition and identification isothermal invariant points (cocrystal pHmax) are crucial for the stability of cocrystals.[124] The effectiveness of a surfactant to stabilize cocrystals is related to the differential solubilization of cocrystal components (Ks) which also applicable to other processes involving differential affinities of components such as complexation, adsorption, etc.[125] It was reported that solution stability of carbamazepine-cinnamic Acid cocrystal depends upon solubility of coformers while further shown that carbamazepine-nicotinamide cocrystal was unstable in water, addition of ethanol could improve stability.[126,127] These understandings can serve as a guide for the selection of coformers and surfactants to control its solubility and transformation during manufacturing, storage, and evaluation.

Cocrystal Patentability and Evergreening Motivation

Evergreening is an aspect of patents that leads to a patent life cycle management of drug or drug product. It can be done in an artful manner by protecting a large number of inventive aspects over basic invention, by avoiding imminent double patent rejection and extending patent term of the same drug product.[128] Innovators can erect 'picket fences' or families of dozens of patents around single drug molecule evergreening innovator domain retaining market monopoly.[129] Cocrystals are gaining interest in pharmaceutical field as it provides an opportunity for new and useful physical property modifications in API, which is demonstrated through recent research literature.[130,131]

As cocrystals are novel crystal form of an API, they possess particular practical regulatory advantages which have the sound scientific base. It provides a lucrative way for patent portfolio management through provisions under Drug Price Competition and Patent Term Restoration Act 1984 and by multiple patent filing.[132] The unique combination of API and a coformer and unique chemical bonding with stoichiometry distinguishing them from the simple physical mixture satisfying novelty requirements for cocrystals.[133] The relative paucity of patents with the keyword search for "pharmaceutically acceptable cocrystal" could suggest that the field is laden with opportunities for novel cocrystal inventions. The challenges in cocrystal prediction suggest obligation of trial and error experimentation rendering them non-obvious from a general patentability perspective.[134] The focus in both European inventive step approach and American obviousness analysis is ultimately the differences in claimed invention and the prior art. Often the prior art has been an API itself or salt or crystalline form of an API. The bonding combination of an API and conformer can provide a platform for the establishment of inventive step or non-obviousness.[133]

Latest Patents issued for cocrystal agomelatine and metaxalone with carboxylic acids shows improved dissolution characteristics and bioavailability of the pure drug.[135] A co-crystalline form of meloxicam with coformers which includes GRAS listed chemicals and others approved API's has shown to improve the bioavailability of pure meloxicam.[136] These patents further underline the impact of cocrystals as intellectual property and can serve as motivation for research on cocrystallization.

The improvements in micromeritics properties, solubility, dissolution rate, bioavailability and stability of API as discussed earlier offer effective pieces of evidence for utility and industrial application of cocrystals.

Conclusion

The importance of crystal engineering through cocrystallization in pharmaceutical field can be understood by looking at regulatory cocrystal considerations and CSD database growth. On the one hand, cocrystals are unexpectedly formed during processing[118-120] while on the other researchers will require the cautious selection of cocrystal design approach as in some cases, cocrystals are not formed as per predictions which indicate challenges in formulating cocrystals.[137] Cocrystal's ability to flourish desired physicochemical and biopharmaceutical properties of API to the optimal extent open a new landscape to Cocrystals of multiple active ingredients can be formulated as fixed dose combinations for better therapeutic applications. It will stimulate investigation of old API's to see new benefits. There is a need to explore into an understanding of cocrystallization mechanism, in vivo behavior of cocrystal for better therapeutics and other unanswered questions like polymorphic transformation. It is an opportunity to capture for patenting new cocrystal forms of API.

Acknowledgments
Authors are thankful to the Secretary, Bhagwan Shikshan Prasarak Mandal, Aurangabad for providing the library facility and remote access services of e-resources of the library.

Conflict of Interest
We declare that there are no potential competing interests related to this manuscript.

References

1. Lipinski CA. Drug-like properties and the causes of poor solubility and poor permeability. *J Pharmacol Toxicol Methods* 2000;44(1):235-49. doi: 10.1016/s1056-8719(00)00107-6
2. Takagi T, Ramachandran C, Bermejo M, Yamashita S, Yu LX, Amidon GL. A provisional biopharmaceutical classification of the top 200 oral drug products in the United States, Great Britain, Spain, and Japan. *Mol Pharm* 2006;3(6):631-43. doi: 10.1021/mp0600182
3. Pouton CW. Formulation of poorly water-soluble drugs for oral administration: physicochemical and physiological issues and the lipid formulation classification system. *Eur J Pharm Sci* 2006;29(3-4):278-87. doi: 10.1016/j.ejps.2006.04.016
4. Lehn JM, Atwood JL. Comprehensive Supramolecular Chemistry. Pergamon: Oxford; 1996.
5. Ball P. The shape of things to come. *Nat* 1994;371(6494):202-3. doi: 10.1038/371202a0
6. Nangia A. Supramolecular chemistry and crystal engineering. *J Chem Sci* 2010;122(3):295-310. doi: 10.1007/s12039-010-0035-6
7. Datta S, Grant DJ. Crystal structures of drugs: advances in determination, prediction and engineering. *Nat Rev Drug Discov* 2004;3(1):42-57. doi: 10.1038/nrd1280
8. Schmidt GM. Photodimerization in the solid state. *Pure Appl Chem* 1971;27(4):647-78. doi: 10.1351/pac197127040647
9. Desiraju GR. Crystal engineering: a holistic view. *Angew Chem Int Ed Engl* 2007;46(44):8342-56. doi: 10.1002/anie.200700534
10. Etter MC. Encoding and decoding hydrogen-bond patterns of organic compounds. *Acc Chem Res* 1990;23(4):120-6. doi: 10.1021/ar00172a005
11. Desiraju GR. Supramolecular synthons in crystal engineering—a new organic synthesis. *Angew Chem Int Ed* 1995;34(21):2311-27. doi: 10.1002/anie.199523111
12. Lara-Ochoa F, Espinosa-Pérez G. Cocrystals definitions. *Supramol Chem* 2007;19(8):553-7. doi: 10.1080/10610270701501652
13. Schultheiss N, Newman A. Pharmaceutical cocrystals and their physicochemical properties. *Cryst Growth Des* 2009;9(6):2950-67. doi: 10.1021/cg900129f
14. Qiao N, Li M, Schlindwein W, Malek N, Davies A, Trappitt G. Pharmaceutical cocrystals: an overview. *Int J Pharm* 2011;419(1-2):1-11. doi: 10.1016/j.ijpharm.2011.07.037
15. Brittain HG. Pharmaceutical cocrystals: The coming wave of new drug substances. *J Pharm Sci* 2013;102(2):311-7. doi: 10.1002/jps.23402
16. Thakuria R, Delori A, Jones W, Lipert MP, Roy L, Rodríguez-Hornedo N. Pharmaceutical cocrystals and poorly soluble drugs. *Int J Pharm* 2013;453(1):101-25. doi: 10.1016/j.ijpharm.2012.10.043
17. Sun CC. Cocrystallization for successful drug delivery. *Expert Opin Drug Deliv* 2013;10(2):201-13. doi: 10.1517/17425247.2013.747508
18. Shan N, Perry ML, Weyna DR, Zaworotko MJ. Impact of pharmaceutical cocrystals: the effects on drug pharmacokinetics. *Expert Opin Drug Metab Toxicol* 2014;10(9):1255-71. doi: 10.1517/17425255.2014.942281
19. US Food and Drug Administration. Guidance for Industry: Regulatory Classification of Pharmaceutical Co-Crystals. US: Center for Drug Evaluation and Research, Silver Spring; 2013.
20. Aitipamula S, Banerjee R, Bansal AK, Biradha K, Cheney ML, Choudhury AR, et al. Polymorphs, salts, and cocrystals: What's in a name? *Cryst Growth Des* 2012;12(5):2147-52. doi: 10.1021/cg3002948
21. Lange L, Lehmkemper K, Sadowski G. Predicting the Aqueous Solubility of Pharmaceutical Cocrystals As a Function of pH and Temperature. *Cryst Growth Des* 2016;16(5):2726-40. doi: 10.1021/acs.cgd.6b00024
22. Reflection paper on the use of cocrystals and other solid state forms of active substances in medicinal products. European Medicines Agency; 2014.
23. Gardner CR, Walsh CT, Almarsson Ö. Drugs as materials: valuing physical form in drug discovery. *Nat Rev Drug Discov* 2004;3(11):926-34. doi: 10.1038/nrd1550
24. Haleblian J, McCrone W. Pharmaceutical applications of polymorphism. *J Pharm Sci* 1969;58(8):911-29. doi: 10.1002/jps.2600580802
25. Grant DJW. Theory and origin of polymorphism. In: Brittain HG, editor. *Polymorphism in Pharmaceutical Solids*. New York: Marcel Dekker;1999. P. 1-34.
26. Bernstein J. Polymorphism in Molecular Crystals. Oxford: Clarendon; 2002.
27. Brittain HG. Polymorphism and Solvatomorphism 2005. *J Pharm Sci* 2007;96(4):705-28. doi: 10.1002/jps.20772
28. Raw AS, Furness MS, Gill DS, Adams RC, Holcombe FO Jr, Yu LX. Regulatory considerations of pharmaceutical solid polymorphism in Abbreviated New Drug Applications (ANDAs). *Adv*

Drug Deliv Rev 2004;56(3):397-414. doi: 10.1016/j.addr.2003.10.011

29. Stahly GP. A survey of cocrystals reported prior to 2000. *Cryst Growth Des* 2009;9(10):4212-29. doi: 10.1021/cg900873t
30. Aitipamula S, Chow PS, Tan RB. Polymorphism in cocrystals: a review and assessment of its significance. *CrystEngComm* 2014;16(17):3451-65. doi: 10.1039/c3ce42008f
31. Seefeldt K, Miller J, Alvarez-Nunez F, Rodriguez-Hornedo N. Crystallization pathways and kinetics of carbamazepine-nicotinamide cocrystals from the amorphous state by in situ thermomicroscopy, spectroscopy, and calorimetry studies. *J Pharm Sci* 2007;96(5):1147-58. doi: 10.1002/jps.20945
32. Porter WW 3rd, Elie SC, Matzger AJ. Polymorphism in carbamazepine cocrystals. *Cryst Growth Des* 2008;8(1):14-6. doi: 10.1021/cg701022e
33. Limwikrant W, Nagai A, Hagiwara Y, Higashi K, Yamamoto K, Moribe K. Formation mechanism of a new carbamazepine/malonic acid cocrystal polymorph. *Int J Pharm* 2012;431(1-2):237-40. doi: 10.1016/j.ijpharm.2012.04.027
34. Horst JH, Cains PW. Co-crystal polymorphs from a solvent-mediated transformation. *Cryst Growth Des* 2008;8(7):2537-42. doi: 10.1021/cg800183v
35. Caira MR, Nassimbeni LR, Van Oudtshoorn B. X-ray structural characterization of anhydrous metronidazole benzoate and metronidazole benzoate monohydrate. *J Pharm Sci* 1993;82(10):1006-9.
36. Aitipamula S, Chow PS, Tan RB. Trimorphs of a pharmaceutical cocrystal involving two active pharmaceutical ingredients: potential relevance to combination drugs. *CrystEngComm* 2009;11(9):1823-7. doi: 10.1039/b904616j
37. Aitipamula S, Chow PS, Tan RB. Conformational and enantiotropic polymorphism of a 1 : 1 cocrystal involving ethenzamide and ethylmalonic acid. *CrystEngComm* 2010;12(11):3691-7. doi: 10.1039/c004491a
38. Aitipamula S, Chow PS, Tan RB. Dimorphs of a 1 : 1 cocrystal of ethenzamide and saccharin: solid-state grinding methods result in metastable polymorph. *CrystEngComm* 2009;11(5):889-95. doi: 10.1039/b821373a
39. Aitipamula S, Chow PS, Tan RB. Polymorphs and solvates of a cocrystal involving an analgesic drug, ethenzamide, and 3,5-dinitrobenzoic acid. *Cryst Growth Des* 2010;10(5):2229-38. doi: 10.1021/cg9015178
40. Trask AV, Motherwell WD, Jones W. Solvent-drop grinding: green polymorph control of cocrystallisation. *Chem Commun (Camb)* 2004(7):890-1. doi: 10.1039/b400978a
41. Trask AV, van de Streek J, Motherwell WD, Jones W. Achieving polymorphic and stoichiometric diversity in cocrystal formation: importance of solid-state grinding, powder X-ray structure determination, and seeding. *Cryst Growth Des* 2005;5(6):2233-41. doi: 10.1021/cg0501682
42. Gangavaram S, Raghavender S, Sanphui P, Pal S, Manjunatha SG, Nambiar S, et al. Polymorphs and cocrystals of nalidixic acid. *Cryst Growth Des* 2012;12(10):4963-71. doi: 10.1021/cg300895c
43. Swapna B, Maddileti D, Nangia A. Cocrystals of the Tuberculosis Drug Isoniazid: Polymorphism, Isostructurality, and Stability. *Cryst Growth Des* 2014;14(11):5991-6005. doi: 10.1021/cg501182t
44. Aitipamula S, Wong AB, Chow PS, Tan RB. Novel solid forms of the anti-tuberculosis drug, Isoniazid: ternary and polymorphic cocrystals. *CrystEngComm* 2013;15(29):5877-87. doi: 10.1039/c3ce40729b
45. Ueto T, Takata N, Muroyama N, Nedu A, Sasaki A, Tanida S, et al. Polymorphs and a hydrate of furosemide–nicotinamide 1:1 cocrystal. *Cryst Growth Des* 2012;12(1):485-94. doi: 10.1021/cg2013232
46. Goud NR, Gangavaram S, Suresh K, Pal S, Manjunatha SG, Nambiar S, et al. Novel furosemide cocrystals and selection of high solubility drug forms. *J Pharm Sci* 2012;101(2):664-80. doi: 10.1002/jps.22805
47. Goud NR, Nangia A. Synthon polymorphs of sulfacetamide–acetamide cocrystal based on N–H··· O [double bond, length as m-dash] S and N–H··· O [double bond, length as m-dash] C hydrogen bonding. *CrystEngComm* 2013;15(37):7456-61. doi: 10.1039/C3CE41179F
48. Grossjohann C, Serrano DR, Paluch KJ, O'Connell P, Vella-Zarb L, Manesiotis P, et al. Polymorphism in Sulfadimidine/4-Aminosalicylic Acid Cocrystals: Solid-State Characterization and Physicochemical Properties. *J Pharm Sci* 2015;104(4):1385-98. doi: 10.1002/jps.24345
49. Bolla G, Mittapalli S, Nangia A. Celecoxib cocrystal polymorphs with cyclic amides: synthons of a sulfonamide drug with carboxamide coformers. *CrystEngComm* 2014;16(1):24-7. doi: 10.1039/C3CE41885E
50. Babu NJ, Sanphui P, Nangia A. Crystal engineering of stable temozolomide cocrystals. *Chem Asian J* 2012;7(10):2274-85. doi: 10.1002/asia.201200205
51. Childs SL, Hardcastle KI. Cocrystals of piroxicam with carboxylic acids. *Cryst Growth Des* 2007;7(7):1291-304. doi: 10.1021/cg060742p
52. Koshima H, Miyauchi M. Polymorphs of a cocrystal with achiral and chiral structures prepared by pseudoseeding: tryptamine/hydrocinnamic acid. *Cryst Growth Des* 2001;1(5):355-7. doi: 10.1021/cg0155189
53. Childs SL, Hardcastle KI. Cocrystals of chlorzoxazone with carboxylic acids. *CrystEngComm* 2007;9(5):364-7. doi: 10.1039/b703292g
54. Bevill MJ, Vlahova PI, Smit JP. Polymorphic cocrystals of nutraceutical compound p-coumaric acid with nicotinamide: Characterization, relative

solid-state stability, and conversion to alternate stoichiometries. *Cryst Growth Des* 2014;14(3):1438-48. doi: 10.1021/cg4019037
55. Eddleston MD, Madusanka N, Jones W. Cocrystal dissociation in the presence of water: A general approach for identifying stable cocrystal forms. *J Pharm Sci* 2014;103(9):2865-70. doi: 10.1002/jps.24003
56. Pal S, Roopa BN, Abu K, Manjunath SG, Nambiar S. Thermal studies of furosemide–caffeine binary system that forms a cocrystal. *J Therm Anal Calorim* 2014;115(3):2261-8. doi: 10.1007/s10973-013-3031-5
57. Mohamed S, Tocher DA, Vickers M, Karamertzanis PG, Price SL. Salt or cocrystal? A new series of crystal structures formed from simple pyridines and carboxylic acids. *Cryst Growth Des* 2009;9(6):2881-9. doi: 10.1021/cg9001994
58. Johnson SL, Rumon KA. Infrared spectra of solid 1:1 pyridine-benzoic acid complexes; the nature of the hydrogen bond as a function of the acid-base levels in the complex1. *J Phys Chem* 1965;69(1):74-86. doi: 10.1021/j100885a013
59. Black SN, Collier EA, Davey RJ, Roberts RJ. Structure, solubility, screening, and synthesis of molecular salts. *J Pharm Sci* 2007;96(5):1053-68. doi: 10.1002/jps.20927
60. Childs SL, Stahly GP, Park A. The salt-cocrystal continuum: the influence of crystal structure on ionization state. *Mol Pharm* 2007;4(3):323-38. doi: 10.1021/mp0601345
61. da Silva CC, de Oliveira R, Tenorio JC, Honorato SB, Ayala AP, Ellena J. The continuum in 5-fluorocytosine. Toward salt formation. *Cryst Growth Des* 2013;13(10):4315-22. doi: 10.1021/cg400662n
62. Martínez-Alejo JM, Domínguez-Chávez JG, Rivera-Islas J, Herrera-Ruiz D, Höpfl H, Morales-Rojas H, et al. A twist in cocrystals of salts: changes in packing and chloride coordination lead to opposite trends in the biopharmaceutical performance of fluoroquinolone hydrochloride cocrystals. *Cryst Growth Des* 2014;14(6):3078-95. doi: 10.1021/cg500345a
63. Jacobs A, Noa FM. Hybrid salt–cocrystal solvate: p-coumaric acid and quinine system. *J Chem Crystallogr* 2014;44(2):57-62. doi: 10.1007/s10870-013-0480-4
64. Donohue J. The hydrogen bond in organic crystals. *J Phys Chem* 1952;56(4):502-10. doi: 10.1021/j150496a023
65. Rodríguez-Hornedo N, Nehm SJ, Jayasankar A. Cocrystals: Design, Properties and Formation Mechanisms. In: Swarbrick J, editor. *Encyclopedia of Pharmaceutical Technology.* 4th ed. New York: Informa Healthcare; 2007. P. 615-35.
66. Allen FH, Kennard O, Taylor R. Systematic analysis of structural data as a research technique in organic chemistry. *Acc Chem Res* 1983;16(5):146-53. doi: 10.1021/ar00089a001
67. Allen FH. The cambridge structural database: A quarter of a million crystal structures and rising. *Acta Crystallogr B* 2002;58(Pt 3 Pt 1):380-8.
68. Haynes DA, Chisholm JA, Jones W, Motherwell WS. Supramolecular synthon competition in organic sulfonates: A CSD survey. *CrystEngComm* 2004;6(95):584-8. doi: 10.1039/b413797c
69. Abramov YA, Loschen C, Klamt A. Rational coformer or solvent selection for pharmaceutical cocrystallization or desolvation. *J Pharm Sci* 2012;101(10):3687-97. doi: 10.1002/jps.23227
70. Mohammad MA, Alhalaweh A, Velaga SP. Hansen solubility parameter as a tool to predict cocrystal formation. *Int J Pharm* 2011;407(1-2):63-71. doi: 10.1016/j.ijpharm.2011.01.030
71. Hansen CM. Hansen solubility parameters: a user's handbook. 2nd Ed. Boca Raton: CRC press; 2007.
72. Klamt A. The COSMO and COSMO-RS solvation models. *WIREs Comput Mol Sci* 2011;1(5):699-709. doi: 10.1002/WCMS.56
73. Klamt A. COSMO-RS: From Quantum Chemistry to Fluid Phase Thermodynamics and Drug Design. 1st Ed. Amsterdam: Elsevier; 2005.
74. Abramov YA. Virtual hydrate screening and coformer selection for improved relative humidity stability. *CrystEngComm* 2015;17(28):5216-24. doi: 10.1039/C4CE02523G
75. Musumeci D, Hunter CA, Prohens R, Scuderi S, McCabe JF. Virtual cocrystal screening. *Chem Sci* 2011;2(5):883-90. doi: 10.1039/c0sc00555j
76. Perlovich GL. Thermodynamic characteristics of cocrystal formation and melting points for rational design of pharmaceutical two-component systems. *CrystEngComm* 2015;17(37):7019-28. doi: 10.1039/C5CE00992H
77. Trask AV, Jones W. Crystal engineering of organic cocrystals by the solid-state grinding approach. *Top Curr Chem* 2005;254:41-70. doi: 10.1007/b100995
78. Dhumal RS, Kelly AL, York P, Coates PD, Paradkar A. Cocrystalization and simultaneous agglomeration using hot melt extrusion. *Pharm Res* 2010;27(12):2725-33. doi: 10.1007/s11095-010-0273-9
79. Rager T, Hilfiker R. Cocrystal formation from solvent mixtures. *Cryst Growth Des* 2010;10(7):3237-41. doi: 10.1021/cg100361y
80. Friščić T, Childs SL, Rizvi SA, Jones W. The role of solvent in mechanochemical and sonochemical cocrystal formation: a solubility-based approach for predicting cocrystallisation outcome. *CrystEngComm* 2009;11(3):418-26. doi: 10.1039/B815174A
81. Pinal R. Effect of molecular symmetry on melting temperature and solubility. *Org Biomol Chem* 2004;2(18):2692-9. doi: 10.1039/B407105K
82. Rao SP, Sunkada S. Making sense of boiling points and melting points. *Resonance* 2007;12(6):43-57. doi: 10.1007/s12045-007-0059-5

83. Good DJ, Rodríguez-Hornedo N. Solubility advantage of pharmaceutical cocrystals. *Cryst Growth Des* 2009;9(5):2252-64. doi: 10.1021/cg801039j
84. Nordstrom FL, Rasmuson AC. Prediction of solubility curves and melting properties of organic and pharmaceutical compounds. *Eur J Pharm Sci* 2009;36(2-3):330-44. doi: 10.1016/j.ejps.2008.10.009
85. Sansone MF, Tawa M, Remenar JF, Baert LE, inventors; Janssen R&D Ireland, assignee. Co-crystal of etravirine and nicotinamide. United States patent US 8,754,093, 2014.
86. Alhalaweh A, Kaialy W, Buckton G, Gill H, Nokhodchi A, Velaga SP. Theophylline cocrystals prepared by spray drying: Physicochemical properties and aerosolization performance. *AAPS PharmSciTech* 2013;14(1):265-76. doi: 10.1208/s12249-012-9883-3
87. Karki S, Friščić T, Fábián L, Laity PR, Day GM, Jones W, et al. Improving Mechanical Properties of Crystalline Solids by Cocrystal Formation: New Compressible Forms of Paracetamol. *Adv Mater* 2009;21(38-39):3905-9. doi: 10.1002/adma.200900533
88. Mulye SP, Jamadar SA, Karekar PS, Pore YV, Dhawale SC. Improvement in physicochemical properties of ezetimibe using a crystal engineering technique. *Powder Technol* 2012; 222:131-8. doi: 10.1016/j.powtec.2012.02.020
89. Roy BN, Singh GP, Srivastava D, Jadhav HS, Desiraju GR, Bhatt PM, inventors; Lupin Ltd, assignee. Lamivudine : zidovudine : water 1 : 1 : 1 cocrystal, PCT/IN2008/000276, 2009.
90. Leuner C, Dressman J. Improving drug solubility for oral delivery using solid dispersions. *Eur J Pharm Biopharm* 2000;50(1):47-60. doi: 10.1016/S0939-6411(00)00076-X
91. Kesisoglou F, Panmai S, Wu Y. Nanosizing--oral formulation development and biopharmaceutical evaluation. *Adv Drug Deliv Rev* 2007;59(7):631-44. doi: 10.1016/j.addr.2007.05.003
92. Brittain HG, Felice PV, inventors; Theaprin Pharmaceuticals Inc., assignee. Intravenous formulation with water-soluble cocrystals of acetylsalicylic acid and theanine. United States patent US 8,173,625, 2012.
93. Buschmann HH, Carandell LS, Buchholz JB, Bertran JC, Salaman CR, Tesson N, inventors; Laboratorios Del Dr. Esteve, SA, assignee. Co-crystals of tramadol and NSAIDS. United States patent application US 14/324,448, 2014.
94. Schultheiss NC, Bethune SJ, inventors; Laurus Labs Private Limited, assignee. Pterostilbene cocrystals. United States patent US 8,318,807, 2012.
95. Kalofonos I, Kalofonos D, Martin-Doyle W, Hanko J, Hagen EJ, inventors; Bionevia Pharmaceuticals, Inc., assignee. Crystalline forms of zotepine hydrochloride. United States patent application US 12/997,499, 2009.
96. Smith AJ, Kavuru P, Wojtas L, Zaworotko MJ, Shytle RD. Cocrystals of quercetin with improved solubility and oral bioavailability. *Mol Pharm* 2011;8(5):1867-76. doi: 10.1021/mp200209j
97. Sanphui P, Tothadi S, Ganguly S, Desiraju GR. Salt and cocrystals of sildenafil with dicarboxylic acids: solubility and pharmacokinetic advantage of the glutarate salt. *Mol Pharm* 2013;10(12):4687-97. doi: 10.1021/mp400516b
98. Xu LL, Chen JM, Yan Y, Lu TB. Improving the solubility of 6-Mercaptopurine via cocrystals and salts. *Cryst Growth Des* 2012;12(12):6004-11. doi: 10.1021/cg3010745
99. Mittapalli S, Mannava MC, Khandavilli UR, Allu S, Nangia A. Soluble salts and cocrystals of clotrimazole. *Cryst Growth Des* 2015;15(5):2493-504. doi: 10.1021/acs.cgd.5b00268
100. Wang JR, Yu X, Zhou C, Lin Y, Chen C, Pan G, et al. Improving the dissolution and bioavailability of 6-mercaptopurine via co-crystallization with isonicotinamide. *Bioorg Med Chem lett* 2015;25(5):1036-9. doi: 10.1016/j.bmcl.2015.01.022
101. Childs SL, inventor; SSCI, Inc., assignee. Cocrystallization. United States patent US 7,452,555, 2008.
102. Hong C, Xie Y, Yao Y, Li G, Yuan X, Shen H. A novel strategy for pharmaceutical cocrystal generation without knowledge of stoichiometric ratio: myricetin cocrystals and a ternary phase diagram. *Pharm Res* 2015;32(1):47-60. doi: 10.1007/s11095-014-1443-y
103. Zhang X, Sun F, Zhang T, Jia J, Su H, Wang C, et al. Three pharmaceuticals cocrystals of adefovir: Syntheses, structures and dissolution study. *J Mol Struct* 2015;1100:395-400. doi: 10.1016/j.molstruc.2015.07.033
104. Shete A, Murthy S, Korpale S, Yadav A, Sajane S, Sakhare S, et al. Cocrystals of itraconazole with amino acids: Screening, synthesis, solid state characterization, in vitro drug release and antifungal activity. *J Drug Deliv Sci Technol* 2015;28:46-55. doi: 10.1016/j.jddst.2015.05.006
105. Ganesh M, Jeon UJ, Ubaidulla U, Hemalatha P, Saravanakumar A, Peng MM, et al. Chitosan cocrystals embedded alginate beads for enhancing the solubility and bioavailability of aceclofenac. *Int J Biol Macromol* 2015;74:310-7. doi: 10.1016/j.ijbiomac.2014.12.038
106. Sarkar A, Rohani S. Molecular salts and co-crystals of mirtazapine with promising physicochemical properties. *J Pharm Biomed Anal* 2015;110:93-9. doi: 10.1016/j.jpba.2015.03.003
107. Bethune SJ, Huang N, Jayasankar A, Rodríguez-Hornedo N. Understanding and predicting the effect of cocrystal components and pH on cocrystal solubility. *Cryst Growth Des* 2009;9(9):3976-88. doi: 10.1021/cg9001187

108. Amidon GL, Lennernäs H, Shah VP, Crison JR. A theoretical basis for a biopharmaceutic drug classification: the correlation of in vitro drug product dissolution and in vivo bioavailability. *Pharm Res* 1995;12(3):413-20.
109. Yu LX, Amidon GL, Polli JE, Zhao H, Mehta MU, Conner DP, et al. Biopharmaceutics classification system: the scientific basis for biowaiver extensions. *Pharm Res* 2002;19(7):921-5.
110. Waterman KC, Adami RC, Alsante KM, Antipas AS, Arenson DR, Carrier R, et al. Hydrolysis in pharmaceutical formulations. *Pharm Dev Technol* 2002;7(2):113-46. doi: 10.1081/PDT-120003494
111. Chen WL, Guo DW, Shen YY, Guo SR, Ruan KP. Effects of highly hygroscopic excipients on the hydrolysis of simvastatin in tablet at high relative humidity. *Indian J Pharm Sci* 2012;74(6):527-34. doi: 10.4103/0250-474X.110587
112. Airaksinen S, Karjalainen M, Kivikero N, Westermarck S, Shevchenko A, Rantanen J, et al. Excipient selection can significantly affect solid-state phase transformation in formulation during wet granulation. *AAPS PharmSciTech* 2005;6(2):E311-22. doi: 10.1208/pt060241
113. Gao D, Czyzewski A, inventors; Czyzewski Ann M., assignee. Acceptably non-hygroscopic formulation intermediate comprising a hygroscopic drug. United States patent application US 10/741,530, 2003.
114. Imamura M, Nakanishi K, Shiraki, R, Onda, K, Sasuga D, Yuda M, inventors; Astellas Pharma Inc. and Kotobuki Pharmaceutical Co. Ltd., assignee. Cocrystal of C-glycoside derivative and L-proline. U.S. Patent 8,097,592, 2012.
115. Almarsson Ö, Hickey MB, Peterson M, Zaworotko M, Moulton B, Rodriguez-Hornedo N, inventors; Almarsson Oern, Zaworotko Michael J, assignee. Pharmaceutical co-crystal compositions of drugs such as carbamazepine, celecoxib, olanzapine, itraconazole, topiramate, modafinil, 5-fluorouracil, hydrochlorothiazide, acetaminophen, aspirin, flurbiprofen, phenytoin and ibuprofen. United States patent application US 10/546,963, 2004.
116. Wang ZZ, Chen JM, Lu TB. Enhancing the hygroscopic stability of S-oxiracetam via pharmaceutical cocrystals. *Cryst Growth Des* 2012;12(9):4562-6. doi: 10.1021/cg300757k
117. Jayasankar A, Good DJ, Rodríguez-Hornedo N. Mechanisms by which moisture generates cocrystals. *Mol Pharm* 2007;4(3):360-72. doi: 10.1021/mp0700099
118. Jayasankar A, Somwangthanaroj A, Shao ZJ, Rodríguez-Hornedo N. Cocrystal formation during cogrinding and storage is mediated by amorphous phase. *Pharm Res* 2006;23(10):2381-92. doi: 10.1007/s11095-006-9110-6
119. Arora KK, Tayade NG, Suryanarayanan R. Unintended water mediated cocrystal formation in carbamazepine and aspirin tablets. *Mol Pharm* 2011;8(3):982-9. doi: 10.1021/mp200043u
120. Good D, Miranda C, Rodríguez-Hornedo N. Dependence of cocrystal formation and thermodynamic stability on moisture sorption by amorphous polymer. *CrystEngComm* 2011;13(4):1181-9. doi: 10.1039/c0ce00592d
121. Sanphui P, Kumar SS, Nangia A. Pharmaceutical cocrystals of niclosamide. *Cryst Growth Des* 2012;12(9):4588-99. doi: 10.1021/cg300784v
122. Yadav AV, Dabke AP, Shete AS. Crystal engineering to improve physicochemical properties of mefloquine hydrochloride. *Drug Dev Ind Pharm* 2010;36(9):1036-45. doi: 10.3109/03639041003642065
123. Forrest JO, George N, Burton RC, Parmar MM, Tandy MD, Buttar SM, Frampton CS, Brown AS, Chorlton AP, inventors; Syngenta Limited, assignee. Co-crystals. United States patent US 8,592,472, 2013.
124. Jayasankar A, Reddy LS, Bethune SJ, Rodríguez-Hornedo N. Role of cocrystal and solution chemistry on the formation and stability of cocrystals with different stoichiometry. *Cryst Growth Des* 2009;9(2):889-97. doi: 10.1021/cg800632r
125. Huang N, Rodríguez-Hornedo N. Effect of micellar solubilization on cocrystal solubility and stability. *Cryst Growth Des* 2010;10(5):2050-3. doi: 10.1021/cg1002176
126. Keramatnia F, Shayanfar A, Jouyban A. Thermodynamic Solubility Profile of Carbamazepine-Cinnamic Acid Cocrystal at Different pH. *J Pharm Sci* 2015;104(8):2559-65. doi: 10.1002/jps.24525
127. Shayanfar A, Velaga S, Jouyban A. Solubility of carbamazepine, nicotinamide and carbamazepine–nicotinamide cocrystal in ethanol–water mixtures. *Fluid Phase Equilib* 2014;363:97-105. doi: 10.1016/j.fluid.2013.11.024
128. Bansal IS, Sahu D, Bakshi G, Singh S. Evergreening-a controversial issue in pharma milieu. *J Intell Prop Right* 2009;14(7):299-306.
129. Brittain HG. Cocrystal Systems of Pharmaceutical Interest: 2007-2008. In: Brittain, HG, Editor. *Profiles of Drug Substances, Excipients, and Related Methodology, Vol 35.* Amsterdam: Elsevier Academic Press; 2010. P. 373-90.
130. Brittain HG. Cocrystal Systems of Pharmaceutical Interest: 2009. In: Brittain, HG, Editor. *Profiles of Drug Substances, Excipients, and Related Methodology, Vol 36.* Amsterdam: Elsevier Academic Press; 2010. P. 361-81.
131. Brittain HG. Cocrystal systems of pharmaceutical interest: 2011. *Cryst Growth Des* 2012;12(11):5823-32. doi: 10.1021/cg301114f
132. Trask AV. An overview of pharmaceutical cocrystals as intellectual property. *Mol Pharm* 2007;4(3):301-9. doi: 10.1021/mp070001z

133. Hoffman M, Lindeman JA. Co-crystals: Commercial opportunities and patent considerations. In: Wouters J, Quere L, Editors. Pharmaceutical Salts and Cocrystal. RSC Publishing; 2012. P. 318-28.
134. Letellier P, Lynch M, Pean JM, inventors; Les Laboratoires Servier, assignee. Co-crystals of agomelatine, a process for there preparation and pharmaceutical compositions containing them. United States patent US 8,710,101, 2014.
135. Holland J, Frampton C, Chorlton A, Gooding D, inventors; Nuformix Limited, assignee. Metaxalone cocrystals. United States patent US 8,871,793, 2014.
136. Hanna M, Shan N, Cheney ML, Weyna DR, inventors; Thar Pharmaceuticals, assignee. In vivo studies of crystalline forms of meloxicam. United States patent US 8,389,512, 2013.
137. Gadade DD, Pekamwar SS, Lahoti SR, Patni SD, Sarode MC. Cocrystallization of etodolac: prediction of cocrystallization, synthesis, solid state characterization and in vitro drug release. *Marmara Pharm J* 2017;21 (1).

Formulation and Optimization of Oral Mucoadhesive Patches of Myrtus Communis by Box Behnken Design

Mahbubeh Hashemi[1], Vahid Ramezani[1]*, Mohammad Seyedabadi[2], Ali Mohamad Ranjbar[3], Hossein Jafari[1], Mina Honarvar[1], Hamed Fanaei[4]

[1] *Department of Pharmaceutics, Faculty of Pharmacy, Shahid Sadoughi University of Medical Sciences, Yazd, Iran.*
[2] *Department of Pharmacology, School of Medicine, Bushehr University of Medical Sciences, Bushehr, Iran.*
[3] *Department of pharmacognosy, Faculty of Pharmacy, Shahid Sadoughi University of Medical Sciences, Yazd, Iran.*
[4] *Department of Physiology, School of Medicine, Zahedan University of Medical Sciences, Zahedan, Iran.*

Article info

Keywords:
- Myrtus communis
- Oral patch
- Methyl cellulose
- Gelatin
- Polyvinyl pyrrolidone
- Pectin

Abstract

Purpose: Recurrent aphthous stomatitis (RAS) is the most common painful ulcerative disease of oral mucosa happening in ~20% of people. Aimed to develop *Myrtus communis L. (Myrtle)* containing oral patches, we applied box-behnken design to evaluate the effect of polymers such as Polyvinyl pyrrolidone (PVP), Gelatin, Methylcellulose (MC) and Pectin.
Methods: The patches properties such as tensile strength, folding endurance, swelling index, thickness, mucoadhesive strength and the pattern of myrtle release were evaluated as dependent variables. Then, the model was adjusted according to the best fitted equation with box behnken design.
Results: The results indicated that preparation of myrtle patch with hydrophilic polymers showed the disintegration time up to 24h and more. Using of polyvinyl pyrrolidone as a water soluble polymer and a pore-former polymer led to faster release of soluble materials from the patch to 29 (min^{-1}). Also it decreases swelling index by increasing the patch disintegration. Gelatin and Pectin, with rigid matrix and water interaction properties, decreased the swelling ratio. Pectin increased the tensile strength, but gelatin produced an opposite effect. Thinner Myrtle patch (about 28μm) was obtained by formulation of methyl cellulose with equal ratio with polyvinyl pyrrolidone or gelatin.
Conclusion: Altogether, the analysis showed that the optimal formulation was achieved with of 35.04 mg of Gelatin, 7.22 mg of Pectin, 7.20 mg of polyvinyl pyrrolidone, 50.52 mg of methyl cellulose and 20 mg of Myrtle extract.

Introduction

Recurrent aphthous stomatitis (RAS) refers to recurring ovoid or round ulcers with yellow base and erythema in the surrounding tissue.[1] It is the most common painful ulcerative disease of oral mucosa happening in about 20% of people.[2,3] Even though the exact pathology is yet to be elucidated, several local, immunological and systemic factors play a role in RAS.[4-8] As such, RAS may be an adverse effect of some medications.[9] Clinically, RAS is classified to three classes of minor, major, and herpetiform ulcers. Having less than 5mm diameter, minor RAS is the most common type, and happens in 80% of people. Whereas, the major form usually has a diameter of more than 1cm.[10,11]Treatment protocol depends on RAS type and symptoms. In this regard, the minor ulcers will relieve after applying topical NSAIDs (Nonsteroidal anti-inflammatory drug), corticosteroids or local anesthetics.[12,13]

Myrtle is a perennial shrub widely distributed in the north of Iran. For many years, in Persian traditional medicine, Myrtle is known by its anti-hyperglycemic, antibacterial, anti-oxidant, anti-inflammatory and analgesic properties.[14-17] These properties suggest potential efficacy of Myrtle in RAS treatment.[18] Indeed, Myrtle paste is proven to be effective in decreasing size of ulcer, pain, severity and erythema.[19]

Mucoadhesive drug delivery systems are preferred dosage forms for treatment of RAS ulcers because; the drug is targeted to a specific region and maintained there for a long period of time. Oral patches, in particular, are more favorable because of their ability to localize the drug and its effects.[20,21] These formulations need to be resistant enough to maintain the integrity of drug delivery during jaw movement, and have to be flexible enough to avoid the interference with normal oral activity.[22,23]

Several factors ought to be optimized for an appropriate oral patch. In this regard, experimental design is a statistical method providing the possibility of evaluation of several independent variables on a specific response with minimum number of conducted experiments. In

***Corresponding author:** Vahid Ramezani, Email: vahidramezani@rocketmail.com particular, the effect of each independent variable is initially studied on a specific response. Subsequently, multiple regressions are performed to find the magnitude of effect (β) of each variable with respect to others. Finally, the interaction of independent variable was investigated to find possible synergy or antagonism. This method has been widely applied in numerous investigations to characterize and develop patch formulations.[24,25]

In the current study, we aimed to optimize a patch formulation for Myrtle drug delivery by applying box-behnken design.

Materials and Methods

Myrtle leaves were purchased from herbal medicine market, Yazd, Iran in January, 2015. The samples were authenticated at faculty of pharmacy, Shahid Sadoughi University of Medical Sciences, Yazd, Iran. Methyl cellulose (MC, M_W: 658.73 g/mole), Gelatin (M_W: 180.16 g/mole), Pectin (PE, M_W: 194.14 g/mole), Polyvinyl pyrrolidone (PVP, M_W: 112.89 g/mole), Propylene glycol (PG) and Folin-Ciocalteu reagent were purchased from Sigma (USA). All reagents were of analytical grade.

The leaves were powdered and then extraction was performed via percolation by Ethanol, 80% (v/v) at room temperature. Extraction was continued until no residual ingredient was observed in TLC (thin layer chromatography) followed by UV (ultra-violent) detection. Finally, the extracts were dried under vacuum evaporator and weighted to calculate the extractable material. Extraction efficiency was 12.5 percent.

Determination of total phenol

Total phenolic content of myrtle extract was determined in accordance with Folin–Ciocalteu method.[26] Briefly, 1.5 mL of Folin–Ciocalteu solution (diluted 10 times) was added to 200 μL of the diluted extract or gallic acid. They were mixed completely and placed at 22°C in water bath for 5 minutes. Then, 1.5 ml of sodium carbonate (60 $g.L^{-1}$) was added to test tubes, vortexed, and incubated at 22°C in water bath for 90 minutes. Subsequently, absorption at 725 nm was determined using a UV-visible spectrophotometer (UNICO, 4802 double beam, Dayton, NJ, USA). Finally, the total phenolic content of the extracts were determined using a calibration curve with different concentrations of gallic acid (25, 50, 75, 100, 125, 150 $\mu g.mL^{-1}$).

Preparation of muco-adhesive oral patches of Myrtle

Different formulation of myrtle oral patches were prepared by solvent casting method.[27] According to the Table 1, the proper amounts of each polymer was dispersed in deionized water and mixed for 24 h. Then, 20 mg of myrtle extract was diluted in 1ml of water, added to other ingredient, and mixed. Subsequently, proper amounts of PG, as plasticizer, were added to above mixture, and homogenized for 2 h. The total mixture was, then, degassed using a desiccator connected with vacuum pump for 6h. Finally, each formulation was casted in petri dish (diameter of 35 mm), and kept for 48h to dry.

Table 1. The high and low levels of independent variables

	Independent variables	-1 Level	+1 Level
A	Gelatin	1	25
B	Pectin	5	25
C	Polyvinyl pyrrolidone	5	25
D	Methylcellulose	25	75

Surface pH

Surface pH of the myrtle patches was determined with agar plate as described by Bottenberg *et al.*[28] Briefly, agar solution 2% (w/v) was prepared by mixing the required agar in water and then dispersed in simulated saliva (pH: 6.2). After solidification of agar and simulated salvia, the patches were placed on the surface of agar plate and allowed to swell for 2h. The surface pH finally determined by pH indicator strip. All measurements were carried out in triplicate.

Thickness, folding endurance and tensile strength

Screw gauge (model: 3D CAD) was employed to obtain the thickness of patches with a precision of 0.01 mm. The thickness was measured at different points and the average value was recorded.[10]

The folding endurance of patches was evaluated with continuous folding/re-folding episodes. According to the previous investigations, the suitable patch is defined as the one enduring more than 200 sequential folding/refolding challenges.[29]

The consistency of patches was evaluated using a tensilometer. In brief, a 2×1cm strip of patch was attached to two jaws; one of the jaws was fixed and the other was moving. The tensile strength was determined as resistance against breaking apart when the strip was pulled with increments of weight in moving jaw. The dial number was recorded as the tensile strength of the patch with unit of N/cm.

Swelling study

The swelling ratio was measured by placing the patches on the surface of 2% agar plates. Agar plates were, then, incubated at 37°C, and the patches were weighed at 5, 10, 60, and 120 min after incubation. Finally, the swelling index was calculated as: Swelling index (%) = $[(W_t - W_0) / W_0] \times 100$; Where, W_0 is the initial weight, and W_t is the weight of swelled patch after the incubation for time t.

Ex vivo mucoadhesive strength

The mucoadhesive strength of films were investigated using a modified physically balanced instrument described by Gupta.[30] In brief, the patch was placed between two parallel surfaces covered with buccal mucosa. The film was allowed for a while to stick to the buccal surfaces. While one of the surfaces remained constant, the other moved in response to increments of weight applied. Accordingly, the maximum required force to detach the buccal surfaces was measured by an accurate digital dynamometer. The buccal area was 2.4 cm^2 and muco-adhesive strength of the films was reported in N/cm^2scale.

In vitro release study

USP apparatus Type-2 rotating paddle (Erweka, Germany) was used to evaluate the release of myrtle extract from patches. Dissolution was performed in 500 mL of phosphate buffer (pH: 6.8) at 37±1°C and continuous stirring at 50 r/min.[31] The patches (3×3 cm) were floated in dissolution medium and 2ml of medium was extracted at different time intervals. Finally, Total phenol of each sample was analyzed and the rate of release was determined by modeling of the release pattern using regression with suitable R^2.

Statistical design

A box behnken method was applied to design, analyze, and optimize the myrtle patches. The concentration of gelatin, pectin, PVP, and methyl cellulose was selected as independent variables (Table 1). Accordingly, bioadhesion, patch thickness, the rate of polyphenol release, and swelling index were examined as dependent variables. Taken together, a total of 29 runs with 5 center points were designed and conducted (Table 2). The results were analyzed with model fitting based on ANOVA test, and P values< 0.05 were considered as significant.

Results and Discussion

Different parts of myrtle are rich in polyphenolic compounds such as phenolic acids, tannins, and flavonoids explaining its antiseptic effects.[32] Myrtle phenolic compounds are highly soluble in media resembling saliva. Therefore, the retention time of myrtle ingredients on aphthous ulcers is extremely low when is formulated in aqueous form.[33] Considering the chronic and recurrent nature of these ulcers, mucoadhesive patches seem appropriate to increase the drug exposure time and, hence, treatment efficiency.

In this investigation, a box behnken design was applied to develop an efficient mucoadhesive myrtle patch. As summarized in Table 2, the effect of several variables was studied in total of 29 formulations with different polymer combinations. At first, screening was performed to find the most critical factors. In this step, the concentration of myrtle, as active ingredient, and PG, as plasticizer, were considered as constant. The screening outcomes clarified methyl cellulose as the cornerstone polymer. Therefore, the ratio of other polymers was determined based on this polymer.

Thickness of the patch

the prepared films were uniform in thickness with smooth surface. The films thickness in different formulations was in the range of 27.60 to 38.30 μm (Table 3). Furthermore, a modified quadratic model with the following equation was fitted on the data (p: 0.0004); thickness of ptach =+28.58-0.56*A+0.73*B+0.11*C+1.07*D-3.07*A*D-1.30*C*D+1.58*A^2+1.11*C^2+1.84*D^2; where, A, B, C, and D are gela\
in, pectin, PVP, and MC, respectively. Indeed, MC (β: +1.07, p: 0.014) was the main determining factore for the patch thickness. That is, the more the ratio of MC, the thicker the final patch. Also, there were a significant interaction between MC and Gelatin (p: 0.0003). In this regard, the minimum thickness was obtained with combination of gelatin or PVP with the ratio of 1:1 (Figure 1). The thickness of film is essential factor in interaction of film with biological and patients compliance. As it was shown, the film thicness is affected by methyl cellullse as a film former agent. In parallel, Esmaeili A et al, showed that the thickness of methyl cellulose film is dependent on the ratio of film former and other additives.[34] Also it can be affected by the interaction of other polymers with MC in the film.[35]

Table 2. Design of experiment in case of 29 runs according to box-behnken design

Runs	Gelatin	Pectin	polyvinyl pyrrolidone	Methylcellulose
1	1	1	0	0
2	1	0	0	1
3	0	-1	1	0
4	0	0	0	0
5	1	0	0	-1
6	-1	0	0	1
7	0	0	0	0
8	1	0	-1	0
9	0	0	0	0
10	1	-1	0	0
11	0	0	-1	1
12	0	-1	0	1
13	-1	0	0	-1
14	1	0	1	0
15	0	-1	0	-1
16	0	1	-1	0
17	-1	1	0	0
18	0	0	0	0
19	0	1	0	-1
20	0	0	1	1
21	0	-1	-1	0
22	-1	-1	0	0
23	0	0	0	0
24	0	0	1	-1
25	-1	0	-1	0
26	-1	0	1	0
27	0	1	1	0
28	0	1	0	1
29	0	0	-1	-1

Table 3. The magnitude of various responses for all formulations

	Mucoadhesiveness (N/cm^2)	Release rate (min^{-1})	Swelling ratio (%)	Thickness (μm)	Tensile strength (N/cm)	Disintegration time
F1	125	37.87	222.8	30.3	295	10h
F2	75	39.04	256.8	31	225	9h
F3	200	35.8	209.9	29.3	400	11h
F4	140	37.26	189.3	29	355	10h
F5	130	38.07	276.6	33.3	215	4h
F6	160	35.33	136.4	38.3	695	>24h
F7	120	35.51	238	30.3	345	10h
F8	110	27.5	260.3	29.6	230	3h
F9	140	37.22	240.7	29.3	500	>24h
F10	140	33.44	272.6	28.6	345	10h
F11	100	33.57	259.7	35.3	550	>24h
F12	120	36.35	175	30	200	9h
F13	135	36.3	167.6	28.3	695	8h
F14	120	39.26	206.4	30.7	360	3h
F15	180	38.92	215	28.3	170	3h
F16	175	36	214.9	29	435	8h
F17	190	36.92	192.7	31.3	755	>24h
F18	130	38.37	205	28	355	10h
F19	125	37.96	198.4	30.3	445	9h
F20	135	39.38	195.5	30	460	6h
F21	210	35	195.6	29	335	6h
F22	165	41.17	131.9	29.6	705	11h
F23	180	38.16	220.8	27.6	610	6h
F24	150	39.88	316.9	30.6	660	6h
F25	180	36.45	192.4	30.7	605	12h
F26	210	38.84	208	32	560	10h
F27	155	37.37	229.4	33	715	9h
F28	90	39.52	241.3	29.7	1175	6h
F29	195	29.1	210.6	30.7	580	4h

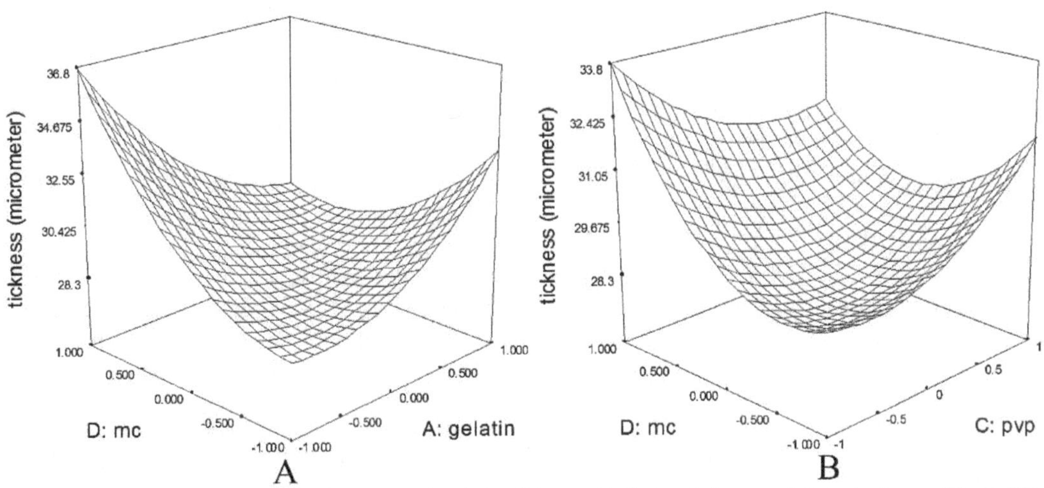

Figure 1. The interaction between Methyl cellulose and gelatin (A) and Methyl cellulose and Polyvinyl pyrrolidone (B) on thickness of patch. acording to figure, the minimum thickness can obtain with combination of gelatin or Polyvinyl pyrrolidone with the ratio of 1:1.

Tensile strength

As summarized in Table 3, the type of polymer played a crucial role in film resistance against breaking apart. A modified quadratic model with the following equation was fitted to the tensile strength data; tensile strenght =+424.57-195.42*A+93.58*B+35.00*C-0.17*D+53.75*BC+310.50 * BD-42.50 * CD+85.92 * B^2+97.79 * D^2; where, A, B, C, and D are gelatin, pectin, PVP, and MC, respectively. Indeed, gelatin with negative and pectin with positive coefficients significantly influenced the patch consistency. Furthermore, augmentation of MC with pectin resulted in dramatic increase in tensile strength (Figure 2). The data were in agreement with El Halal SL[36] and Dogan N[37] studies that showed the addition of cellulose resulted in increase in total strength of edible film. Also pectin is known as a rigid polymer[38] and need to modifications with different material to use in the films. This indicates that polysaccharides play a pivotal role in tensile endurance. In this regard, the hydroxyl groups in the structure of polysaccharides provide the possibility of hydrogen bond formation.[39] Accordingly, polymer chain cross linking as well as polymer interaction with myrtle ingredients results in a stronger matrix.[40] In addition, pectin, a complex polysaccharide, produces hydrogen and non-covalent bonds with cellulose, and acts as a binder. Therefore, pectin and cellulose synergistically increase the tensile strength. This explains why formulations containing these excipients exhibited maximal endurance against physical tension.[41]

Data analysis showed that there was no correlation between the tensile strength and thickness of patches. It showed that the containing polymer and polymer chain interactions determined the tensile strength of patch and polymer amount has minimal effect on this property.

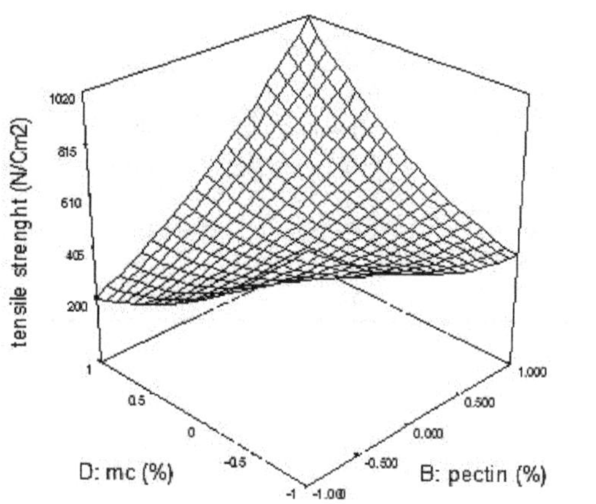

Figure 2. The interaction between Methyl cellulose and pectin on tensile of patch. according tothe Figure the interaction of Methyl cellulose and pectin content in formulation resulted in dramatic increase in patch tensile strength.

Swelling ratio and surface pH

Polymers with pK equal to that of extract helped develop films with narrow range of neutral surface pH (7-7.4) in all formulations that is suitable for oral ulcer which is sensitive to extreme acidic or basic condition and also it is suitable for oral application without mucosal irritation.[42]

Swelling behavior plays a pivotal role in the pattern of drug release as well as the mucoadhesiveness of patch.[43] It depends on several factors such as the physicochemical properties of the ingredients. Indeed, water solubility and wet ability of polymers determines the ability of water absorption. Accordingly, matrix integrity and disintegration rate defines the final extension of patch.[43] This indicates that the type and ratio of polymers determine the swelling index and, subsequently, the rate and pattern of drug release and bio-adhesiveness.

The swelling ratio in formulations varied from 131.90% to 316.90%.As such, different formulations exhibitted distinct patterns of swelling (Figure 3). Overal, a 2FI vs Linear model was fitted on the data (p: 0.0002); Swelling index =+216.57+38.88*A+8.29*B+2.72*C-10.03*D-27.65*A*B-42.63*C*D; where, A, B, C, and D are gelatin, pectin, PVP, and MC, respectively. This indicates that gelatin (β: +38.88) was the most crucial factor for swelling compared to other polymers. That is, the more the ratio of gelatin in formulation, the higher the swelling index of the resulted patch. Also, there was an interaction between glatin and pectin (p:0.0439). also there was an interaction between MC and PVP (p: 0.0033). In particular, maximum swelling index was observed in formulations containing maximum ratio of gelatin and minimum ratio of pectin. On the other hand, formulations containing equal amounts of PVP and MC exhibitted the lowest swelling index (Figure 4).

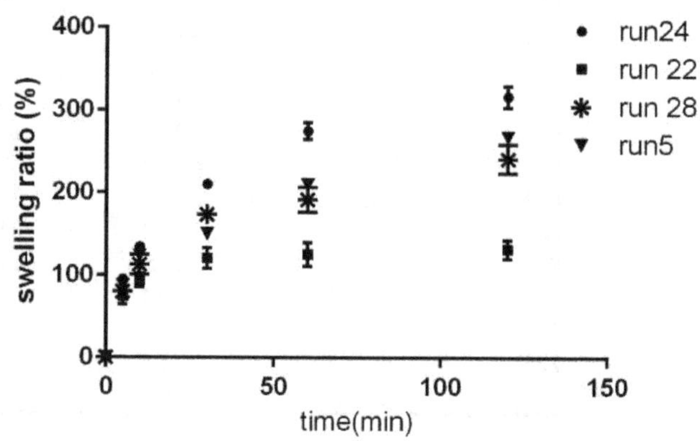

Figure 3. The swelling pattern of selected formulations (run 5 : 31.3% gelatin, 18.8 % pectin, 18.8% polyvinyl pyrrolidone, 31.3 % Methyl cellulose; run 22 : 1.4 % gelatin, 7 % pectin, 21.1 % polyvinyl pyrrolidone, 70.5 % Methyl cellulose; run 24 : 16.7 % gelatin, 19.2 % pectin, 32.1 % polyvinyl pyrrolidone, 32.1 % Methyl cellulose; run 28 10.2 % gelatin, 19.5 % pectin, 11.7 % polyvinyl pyrrolidone, 58.6 % Methyl cellulose).

Hydrophilic groups such as –OH, -COOH and –NH_2 in gelatin structure provides the possibility of hydrogen bond formation, and thereby high water absorption. This explains the positive impact of gelatin on swelling index. In this regard, the swelling index of gelatin depends on ionization of the functional groups. Therefore, the medium pH as well as electrolyte concentration and presence of other complexing agents influence the ionization state of gelatin.[44] This highlights the importance of other factors in gelatin-induced alteration of swelling index. In fact, formulations containing pectin and gelatin demonstrated lower swelling ratio compared to those containing only gelatin. This may be explained by the fact that pectin, with lots of -COOH group, interferes with –NH_2 groups in gelatin, thereby, decreases the capacity of gelatin for hydrogen bond formation and water absorption. In this regard, Mishara et al showed that increasing the ratio of gelatin in the pectin film enhanced the swelling index by improving the film porosity.[44]

PVP, by itself, didn't have any significant effect on swelling index. However, it did decrease the swelling ratio of patches containing MC (β: -42.63). This seems contrary to the high aqueous solubility of PVP which can enhance the wet ability and water absorption and disintegration rate of the hydrophilic matrix. In this regard, PVP enhanced the swelling of chitosan films, an insoluble polymer.[43] whereas no portion of highly soluble polymers such as HPMC lead to increasing the swelling of patch.[45]

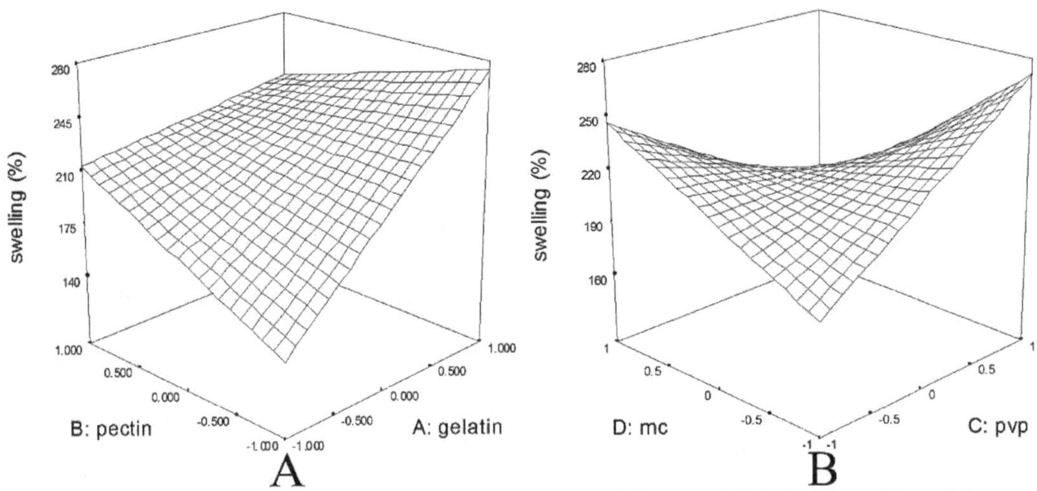

Figure 4. The interaction between pectin and gelatin (A) and Methyl cellulose and Polyvinyl pyrrolidone (B) on swelling of patch. According to figure, the maximum swelling index is approachable with maximum ratio of gelatin vs minimum ratio of pectin in formulation. On the other hand, there is the lowest swelling ratio when Polyvinyl pyrrolidone and Methyl cellulose are employed equally in the formuation.

Mucoadhesiveness test

We observed that gelatin (β: -25), MC (β: -19), and pectin (β: -12) were main factor influencing mucoadhesiveness of the patches. The result showed that the mucoadhesiveness of the myrtle patches was acceptable when polymers are used in low concentration. One of the most important factors affecting mucoadhesion is the concentration of polymers. Higher level of polymers is responsible for forming highly coiled structure of the polymers which can reduce the polymer chains flexibility and interaction with mucin. Subsequently, the mucoadhesion force will fall under acceptable value.[46] Namely, Malik and his coworkers indicated that increasing the concentration of chitosan in the ondansetron loaded beads will decrease the mucoadhesion force.[47] In this regard, the data best fitted to the following equation; mucoadhesiveness $=+138.24-25.00*A-12.92*B+3.33*C-19.58*D-20.00*A*D+20.00*C*D+17.18*B^2+20.30*C^2-17.82*D^2$; where, A, B, C, and D are gelatin, pectin, PVP, and MC, respectively. This indicates a synergistic effect between PVP and MC (β: +20).

Mucin in the structure of buccal surface is negatively charged. Therefore, positively charged excipients in formulation ought to enhance bioadhesion. In particular, high molecular weight polymers such as pectin as well as insoluble ones like chitosan produce stronger interactions with mucin.[48] However, we found that pectin had a negative impact on bioadhesion (β: -12). As such, positively charged PVP did not significantly alter this parameter (β: +3.33, $p > 0.05$). This observation is supported by Jiyeon and coworkers. They designed a bilayer mucoadhesive strip of lidocaine and showed that PVP was not able to enhance mucoadhesivity. However, they showed that addition of HPMC to the bilayer strips increased the mucoadhesion strength.[49] This indicates that bioadhesion is not determined only with surface charge density. In fact, several factors come to play including surface charge density, flexibility, polymer molecular weight, swelling rate, type of the biological surface to which the patch is adhered and the adherence time.[43] For instance, polymers enhancing the swelling index seem to reduce bioadhesion. In this regard, gelatin (β: +38.88) and MC (β: +10.03) significantly enhanced swelling index. In contrast, they had an inverse effect on bioadhesion (β: -25 and -19.58 for gelatin and MC, respectively). In this regard, patches produced with chitosan matrix having gelatin displayed less mucoadhesive strength compared to those having only chitosan.[50]

Myrtle release of patch

According to Table 3, almost the formulations composed the myrthys with long perod of disintegration time up to more than 24 houre in some formulations. Howevere polyphenolic compound was released of formulation between 3 to 6 houres.

Overal, the release rate best fitted to the following model; release rate $=+37.49-0.82*A+0.41*B+2.74*C+2.17*A*B+2.34*A*C-1.82*C^2$; where, A, B, C, and D are gelatin, pectin, PVP, and MC, respectively. This indicates PVP as the main factor determining polyphenol release from the patch. In fact, there was a positive correlation between the ratio of this cationic polymer and the rate of myrtle release from the patch (β: +2.74, F-value: 23.68).

Polyphenols are among water soluble materials. Therefore, their release from the matrix ought to have a direct relationship with the capacity of patch to absorb water. In this regard, water soluble polymers such as PVP enhance water absorption, promotes the drug release and patch dissolution. In addition, PVP as a pore-former polymer creates lots of water channels, and cause perturbation of the matrix consistency. Subsequently, these channels allow better water penetration, swelling and ultimately faster drug diffusion.[51] Similarly, PVP is shown to enhance the release of soluble drugs such as sumatriptan succinate and felodipine from polymeric matrix.[52,53]

In contrast, other polymers did not influence polyphenol release by themselves, although their effect was significant when used in combination. In this regard, co-formulation of gelatin and pectin (β: +2.17) as well as gelatin and PVP (β: +2.34) enhanced polyphenol release from the patch. Similarly, it was observed that gelatin concentration solely, does not play a crucial role in release of bupivacaine.[54] The failure of gelatin and MC, highly water soluble polymers, to influence drug release may seem contrary to the above mentioned direct relationship between the water solubility of polymer and drug release. This suggests a potential role for other factors. For instance, the composition of patch may influence the disintegration rate via mechanical properties of sol-gel interface with water.[55] In addition, total patch weight influenced the release rate (Figure 5). As such, solid content in the patch is another factor that can delay the extract release.[56] In fact, higher solid content diminishes matrix porosity, thereby inhibiting water penetration and outward movement of drug from matrix.[55] In this regard, increase in pectin and gelatin concentration delayed polyphenol release from the matrix (Figure 5A). Similarly, Ikram and coworkers showed that the release of drug from the matrix is dependent on the polymer properties and specially the viscosity of the polymeric matrix after water diffusion inside. Also the immobile water in the matrix by increasing the swelling index, create the new condition for drug release. All together the total tendency of polymer to water absorption and the ratio of patch swelling as well as polymer viscosity will identify the fate of drug release.[57] So the higher content of gelatin in combination with PVP or pectin in the myrtle patches, with high water absorption and swelling index, leads to increase the rate of drug release. However, optimization of the ingredients is necessary to obtain the patch with desire release rate.

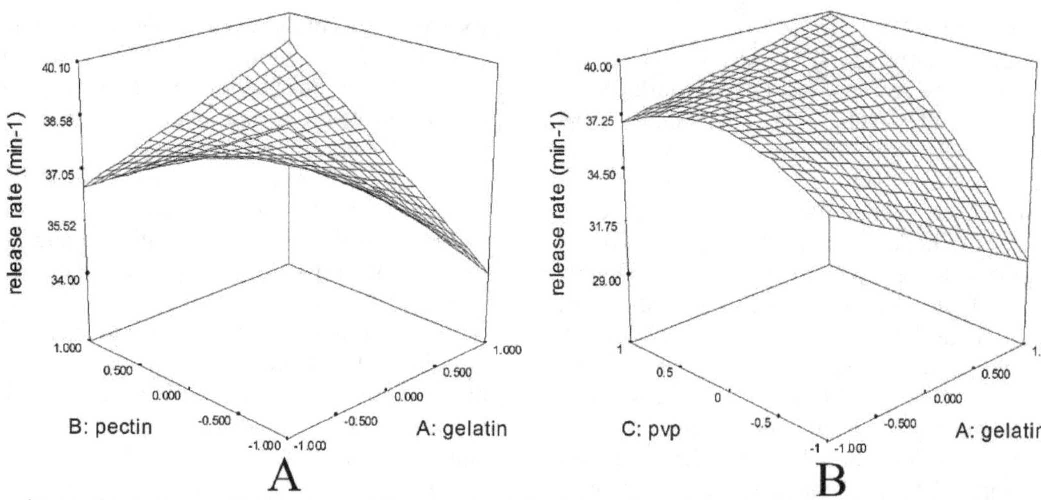

Figure 5. The interaction between Polyvinyl pyrrolidone and gelatin (A) and pectin and gelatin (B) on release myrtle from patch. According to the Figure, the correlation between the weight of patch and drug release. It shows that the amount of solid content in the patch is another factor that can delay the extract release.

Optimization

According to the optimal value for each response, the best formulation was predetermined. In fact, the ratio of each excipient was predicted to result in the desired response. Then, the final formulation was determined to get a patch with optimal values in all responses (Table 4). The calculated optimal formulation was composed of PVP, MC, pectin, gelatin and myrtle extract with ratios of 1:13:1:5:3, respectively.

Table 4. Predicted value of optimum formulation

	Gelatin	Pectin	Polyvinyl pyrrolidone	Methylcellulose	Release rate (min^{-1})	Swelling ratio (%)	Thickness (μm)	Desirability
Predicted value	25	5	5	65	27.5	291.9	30.0	0.92

The final patch was produced with the predicted ratios for optimal formulation. Then, dependent variables were studied once again for the final patch. The results demonstrated good agreement between the predicted and observed responses.

Conclusion

The suitable oral patch of *myrtus communis* L. can develop with the aid of soluble polymer including polyvinyl pyrrolidone, gelatin, pectin and methyl cellulose. Inclusion of gelatin in myrtus patches helps to higher swelling and hydration but with negative effect on mucuadhesive property. Pectin same as gelatin compose of oral patch with higher tensile strange. The release of myrtus extract is depended on water solubility of polymer. And, PVP as a low molecular water soluble polymer make the extract release faster. Altogether, optimization of the hydrophilic polymer in the patch, made it so flexible with degradation time more than 24 h and release rate of 27.5 (min^{-1}) and swelling ratio of about 300%.

Acknowledgments

This research was granted by research department of Shahid Sadoughi University of Medical Science and Health Services. This research was based on a thesis submitted for Pharm. D degree (No. 3602).

Conflict of Interest

The authors declare no conflict of interests.

References

1. Jurge S, Kuffer R, Scully C, Porter SR. Mucosal disease series. Number VI. Recurrent aphthous stomatitis. *Oral Dis* 2006;12(1):1-21. doi: 10.1111/j.1601-0825.2005.01143.x
2. Vincent SD, Lilly GE. Clinical, historic, and therapeutic features of aphthous stomatitis. Literature review and open clinical trial employing steroids. *Oral Surg Oral Med Oral Pathol* 1992;74(1):79-86.
3. Woo SB, Sonis ST. Recurrent aphthous ulcers: A review of diagnosis and treatment. *J Am Dent Assoc* 1996;127(8):1202-13. doi: 10.14219/jada.archive.1996.0412
4. Albanidou-Farmaki E, Poulopoulos AK, Epivatianos A, Farmakis K, Karamouzis M, Antoniades D. Increased anxiety level and high salivary and serum cortisol concentrations in patients with recurrent aphthous stomatitis. *Tohoku J Exp Med* 2008;214(4):291-6. doi: 10.1620/tjem.214.291
5. Arikan S, Durusoy C, Akalin N, Haberal A, Seckin D. Oxidant/antioxidant status in recurrent aphthous stomatitis. *Oral Dis* 2009;15(7):512-5. doi: 10.1111/j.1601-0825.2009.01580.x
6. Landesberg R, Fallon M, Insel R. Alterations of T helper/inducer and T suppressor/inducer cells in patients with recurrent aphthous ulcers. *Oral Surg Oral Med Oral Pathol* 1990;69(2):205-8. doi: 10.1016/0030-4220(90)90329-q
7. Savage NW, Mahanonda R, Seymour GJ, Bryson GJ, Collins RJ. The proportion of suppressor-inducer t-lymphocytes is reduced in recurrent aphthous stomatitis. *J Oral Pathol* 1988;17(6):293-7. doi: 10.1111/j.1600-0714.1988.tb01539.x
8. Berkenstadt M, Weisz B, Cuckle H, Di-Castro M, Guetta E, Barkai G. Chromosomal abnormalities and birth defects among couples with colchicine treated familial mediterranean fever. *Am J Obstet Gynecol* 2005;193(4):1513-6. doi: 10.1016/j.ajog.2005.03.043
9. Abdollahi M, Radfar M. A review of drug-induced oral reactions. *J Contemp Dent Pract* 2003;4(1):10-31.
10. Field EA, Brookes V, Tyldesley WR. Recurrent aphthous ulceration in children--a review. *Int J Paediatr Dent* 1992;2(1):1-10. doi: 10.1111/j.1365-263X.1992.tb00001.x
11. Scully C, Porter S. Recurrent aphthous stomatitis: Current concepts of etiology, pathogenesis and management. *J Oral Pathol Med* 1989;18(1):21-7. doi: 10.1111/j.1600-0714.1989.tb00727.x
12. Saxen MA, Ambrosius WT, Rehemtula al KF, Russell AL, Eckert GJ. Sustained relief of oral aphthous ulcer pain from topical diclofenac in hyaluronan: A randomized, double-blind clinical trial. *Oral Surg Oral Med Oral Pathol Oral Radiol Endod* 1997;84(4):356-61.
13. Khandwala A, Van Inwegen RG, Alfano MC. 5% amlexanox oral paste, a new treatment for recurrent minor aphthous ulcers: I. Clinical demonstration of acceleration of healing and resolution of pain. *Oral Surg Oral Med Oral Pathol Oral Radiol Endod* 1997;83(2):222-30. doi: 10.1016/s1079-2104(97)90009-3
14. Onal S, Timur S, Okutucu B, Zihnioglu F. Inhibition of alpha-glucosidase by aqueous extracts of some potent antidiabetic medicinal herbs. *Prep Biochem Biotechnol* 2005;35(1):29-36. doi: 10.1081/PB-200041438
15. Bonjar GH. Antibacterial screening of plants used in iranian folkloric medicine. *Fitoterapia* 2004;75(2):231-5. doi: 10.1016/j.fitote.2003.12.013
16. Yadegarinia D, Gachkar L, Rezaei MB, Taghizadeh M, Astaneh SA, Rasooli I. Biochemical activities of iranian mentha piperita l. And myrtus communis l. Essential oils. *Phytochemistry* 2006;67(12):1249-55. doi: 10.1016/j.phytochem.2006.04.025
17. Levesque H, Lafont O. Aspirin throughout the ages: A historical review. *Rev Med Interne* 2000;21(Suppl 1):8s-17s.
18. Feisst C, Franke L, Appendino G, Werz O. Identification of molecular targets of the oligomeric nonprenylated acylphloroglucinols from myrtus communis and their implication as anti-inflammatory compounds. *J Pharmacol Exp Ther* 2005;315(1):389-96. doi: 10.1124/jpet.105.090720
19. Babaee N, Mansourian A, Momen-Heravi F, Moghadamnia A, Momen-Beitollahi J. The efficacy of a paste containing Myrtus communis (Myrtle) in the management of recurrent aphthous stomatitis: A randomized controlled trial. *Clin Oral Investig* 2010;14(1):65-70. doi: 10.1007/s00784-009-0267-3

20. Parmar Viram J, Lumbhani AN, Vijayalakshmi P, Sajal Jha. Formulation development and evaluation of buccal films of carvedilol. *Int J Pharm Sci Res* 2010;1(8):149-56. doi: 10.13040/IJPSR.0975-8232.1(8-S).149-56
21. Guo JH. Investigating the surface properties and bioadhesion of buccal patches. *J Pharm Pharmacol* 1994;46(8):647-50. doi: 10.1111/j.2042-7158.1994.tb03875.x
22. Ebert CD, Heiber SJ, Dave SC, Kim SW, Mix D. Mucosal delivery of macromolecules. *J Control Release* 1994;28(1-3):37-44. doi: 10.1016/0168-3659(94)90151-1
23. Li C, Bhatt PP, Johnston TP. Transmucosal delivery of oxytocin to rabbits using a mucoadhesive buccal patch. *Pharm Dev Technol* 1997;2(3):265-74. doi: 10.3109/10837459709031446
24. Chawla A, Taylor KMG, Newton JM, Johnson MCR. Production of spray dried salbutamol sulphate for use in dry powder aerosol formulation. *Int J Pharm* 1994;108(3):233-40. doi: 10.1016/0378-5173(94)90132-5
25. Patel VM, Prajapati BG, Patel MM. Effect of hydrophilic polymers on buccoadhesive eudragit patches of propranolol hydrochloride using factorial design. *AAPS PharmSciTech* 2007;8(2):E119-26. doi: 10.1208/pt0802045
26. Singleton VL, Rossi JA. Colorimetry of total phenolics with phosphomolybdic-phosphotungstic acid reagents. *Am J Enol Vitic* 1965;16(3):144-58.
27. Khairnar A, Jain P, Baviskar D, Jain D. Developmement of mucoadhesive buccal patch containing aceclofenac: In vitro evaluations. *Int J PharmTech Res* 2009;1(4):978-81.
28. Bottenberg P, Cleymaet R, Muynck C, Remon JP, Coomans D, Michotte Y, et al. Development and testing of bioadhesive, fluoride-containing slow-release tablets for oral use. *J Pharm Pharmacol* 1991;43(7):457-64. doi: 10.1111/j.2042-7158.1991.tb03514.x
29. Surender V, Gupta N, Ashima. Formulation and evaluation of buccal patches of tramodol hydrochloride. *Eur J Pharm Med Res* 2016;3(8):339-46.
30. Gupta A, Garg S, Khre RK. Measurement of bioadhesive strength of mucoadhesive buccal tablet: Design of an in vitro assembly. *Indian Drugs* 1992;30:152–5.
31. Singh TP, Singh RK, Shah JN, Mehta TA. Mucoadhesive bilayer buccal patches of verapamil hydrochloride: Formulation development and characterization. *Int J Pharm Pharm Sci* 2014;6(4):234-41.
32. Amensour M, Sendra E, Abrini J, Perez-Alvarez J, Fernandez-Lopez J. Antioxidant activity and total phenolic compounds of myrtle extracts actividad antioxidante y contenido de compuestos fenólicos totales en extractos de myrtus. *CyTA-J Food* 2010;8(2):95-101. doi: 10.1080/19476330903161335
33. Shaikh R, Raj Singh TR, Garland MJ, Woolfson AD, Donnelly RF. Mucoadhesive drug delivery systems. *J Pharm Bioallied Sci* 2011;3(1):89-100. doi: 10.4103/0975-7406.76478
34. Esmaeili A, Ebrahimzadeh Fazel M. Optimization and preparation of methylcellulose edible film combined with of ferulago angulata essential oil (FEO) nanocapsules for food packaging applications. *Flavour Fragr J* 2016;31(5):341-9. doi: 10.1002/ffj.3321
35. Akhtar MJ, Jacquot M, Jasniewski J, Jacquot C, Imran M, Jamshidian M, et al. Antioxidant capacity and light-aging study of hpmc films functionalized with natural plant extract. *Carbohydr Polym* 2012;89(4):1150-8. doi: 10.1016/j.carbpol.2012.03.088
36. Dogan N, McHugh TH. Effects of microcrystalline cellulose on functional properties of hydroxy propyl methyl cellulose microcomposite films. *J Food Sci* 2007;72(1):E016-22. doi: 10.1111/j.1750-3841.2006.00237.x
37. El Halal SL, Colussi R, Biduski B, Evangelho JA, Bruni GP, Antunes MD, et al. Morphological, mechanical, barrier and properties of films based on acetylated starch and cellulose from barley. *J Sci Food Agric* 2017;97(2):411-9. doi: 10.1002/jsfa.7773
38. Mishra RK, Datt M, Banthia AK. Synthesis and characterization of pectin/pvp hydrogel membranes for drug delivery system. *AAPS PharmSciTech* 2008;9(2):395-403. doi: 10.1208/s12249-008-9048-6
39. Kondo T. The relationship between intramolecular hydrogen bonds and certain physical properties of regioselectively substituted cellulose derivatives. *J Polym Sci B Polym Phys* 1997;35(4):717-23.
40. Mistry P, Mohapatra S, Gopinath T, Vogt FG, Suryanarayanan R. Role of the strength of drug-polymer interactions on the molecular mobility and crystallization inhibition in ketoconazole solid dispersions. *Mol Pharm* 2015;12(9):3339-50. doi: 10.1021/acs.molpharmaceut.5b00333
41. Dufresne A, Cavaille JY, Vignon MR. Mechanical behavior of sheets prepared from sugar beet cellulose microfibrils. *J Appl Polym Sci* 1997;64(6):1185-94.
42. Krampe R, Visser JC, Frijlink HW, Breitkreutz J, Woerdenbag HJ, Preis M. Oromucosal film preparations: Points to consider for patient centricity and manufacturing processes. *Expert Opin Drug Deliv* 2016;13(4):493-506. doi: 10.1517/17425247.2016.1118048
43. Singh S, Jain S, Muthu MS, Tiwari S, Tilak R. Preparation and evaluation of buccal bioadhesive films containing clotrimazole. *AAPS PharmSciTech* 2008;9(2):660-7. doi: 10.1208/s12249-008-9083-3
44. Mishra RK, Majeed ABA, Banthia AK. Development and characterization of pectin/gelatin hydrogel membranes for wound dressing. *Int J Plast Technol* 2011;15(1):82-95. doi: 10.1007/s12588-011-9016-y

45. Deshmane SV, Channawar MA, Chandewar AV, Joshi UM, Biyani KR. Chitosan based sustained release mucoadhesive buccal patches containing verapamil HCL. *Int J Pharm Pharm Sci* 2009;1(1):216-29.
46. Roy S, Pal K, Anis A, Pramanik K, Prabhakar B. Polymers in mucoadhesive drug-delivery systems: A brief note. *Des Monomers Polym* 2009;12(6):483-95. doi: 10.1163/138577209X12478283327236
47. Malik RK, Malik P, Gulati N, Nagaich U. Fabrication and in vitro evaluation of mucoadhesive ondansetron hydrochloride beads for the management of emesis in chemotherapy. *Int J Pharm Investig* 2013;3(1):42-6. doi: 10.4103/2230-973x.108962
48. Lehr CM, Bouwstra JA, Schacht EH, Junginger HE. In vitro evaluation of mucoadhesive properties of chitosan and some other natural polymers. *Int J Pharm* 1992;78(1-3):43-8. doi: 10.1016/0378-5173(92)90353-4
49. Roh J, Han M, Kim KN, Kim KM. The in vitro and in vivo effects of a fast-dissolving mucoadhesive bi-layered strip as topical anesthetics. *Dent Mater J* 2016;35(4):601-5. doi: 10.4012/dmj.2015-369
50. Abruzzo A, Bigucci F, Cerchiara T, Cruciani F, Vitali B, Luppi B. Mucoadhesive chitosan/gelatin films for buccal delivery of propranolol hydrochloride. *Carbohydr Polym* 2012;87(1):581-8. doi: 10.1016/j.carbpol.2011.08.024
51. Charyulu NR, Jose J, Shetty V. Design and characterization of mucoadhesive buccal patch containing antifungal agent for oral candidiasis. *Int J Pharm Phytopharmacol Res* 2014;3(3):245-9.
52. Shidhaye SS, Saindane NS, Sutar S, Kadam V. Mucoadhesive bilayered patches for administration of sumatriptan succinate. *AAPS PharmSciTech* 2008;9(3):909-16. doi: 10.1208/s12249-008-9125-x
53. Karavas E, Georgarakis E, Bikiaris D. Application of PVP/HPMC miscible blends with enhanced mucoadhesive properties for adjusting drug release in predictable pulsatile chronotherapeutics. *Eur J Pharm Biopharm* 2006;64(1):115-26. doi: 10.1016/j.ejpb.2005.12.013
54. Foox M, Zilberman M. Drug delivery from gelatin-based systems. *Expert Opin Drug Deliv* 2015;12(9):1547-63. doi: 10.1517/17425247.2015.1037272
55. Kaur A, Kaur G. Mucoadhesive buccal patches based on interpolymer complexes of chitosan-pectin for delivery of carvedilol. *Saudi Pharm J* 2012;20(1):21-7. doi: 10.1016/j.jsps.2011.04.005
56. Rao NGR, Patel K. Formulation and evaluation of ropinirole buccal patches using different mucoadhesive polymers. *RGUHS J Pharm Sci* 2013;3(1):32-9.
57. Ikram M, Gilhotra N, Gilhotra RM. Formulation and optimization of mucoadhesive buccal patches of losartan potassium by using response surface methodology. *Adv Biomed Res* 2015;4:239. doi: 10.4103/2277-9175.168606

Novel Combination of Silver Nanoparticles and Carbon Nanotubes for Plasmonic Photo Thermal Therapy in Melanoma Cancer Model

Mohammad Ali Behnam[1], Farzin Emami[1], Zahra Sobhani[2]*, Omid Koohi-Hosseinabadi[3], Amir Reza Dehghanian[4], Seyed Mojtaba Zebarjad[5], Mohammad Hadi Moghim[5], Ahmad Oryan[6]

[1] *Nano Opto-Electronic Research Center, Electrical and Electronics Engineering Department, Shiraz University of Technology, Shiraz, Iran.*

[2] *Quality Control Department, Faculty of Pharmacy, Shiraz University of Medical Sciences, Shiraz, Iran.*

[3] *Center of Experimental and Comparative Medicine, Shiraz University of Medical Sciences, Shiraz, Iran.*

[4] *Pathology Department, Shiraz University of Medical Sciences, Shiraz, Iran.*

[5] *Materials Science and Engineering Department, Engineering School, Shiraz University, Shiraz, Iran.*

[6] *Pathology Department, School of Veterinary Medicine, Shiraz University, Shiraz, Iran.*

Article info

Keywords:
· Plasmonic photo thermal therapy
· Carbon nanotubes
· Silver nanorods
· Melanoma cancer
· Laser diode

Abstract
Purpose: Plasmonic photo thermal therapy (PPTT) is a therapeutic method in which the photon energy is rapidly transformed into heat via a series of radiative and non-radiative phenomena to ablate cancer. Plasmonic NPs, such as silver NPs (Ag NPs), have considerable properties in optical absorbance. Furthermore, good thermal conductivity and cell penetration ability of carbon nanotubes (CNTs) could improve the efficacy of Ag NPs for PPTT. Decoration of the multi-walled carbon nanotubes (MWCNTs) with silver has been developed to enhance thermal conductivity of the MWCNT particles.
Methods: The Ag NPs were decorated on the CNTs and the ability of these particles (CNT/Ag NPs) in reduction of melanoma tumor size after PTT was evaluated experimentally. For comparison, the PTT of silver nanorods (Ag NRs) and CNTs were investigated. The melanoma tumor was induced by injection of B16/F10 cell line to the inbred mice. Different NPs were injected into the tumors and then irradiated via laser diode (λ=670 nm, P=500 mW, and I= 3.5 W/cm^2) at scheduled time.
Results: Monitoring of tumor sizes showed that integration of CNTs with silver could enhance the optical absorption of CNTs and improve tumor destruction in PPTT technique.
Conclusion: The CNT/Ag NPs could act as a potent agent in PPTT method in curing solid tumors.

Introduction

Cancer is a disease defined by invasive and uncontrolled growth of abnormal cells. Current primary treatments for cancer are surgery, radiation, and chemotherapy. Surgical extirpation is efficacious in primary tumors, but limited to surgical detectable and accessible tumors. Chemotherapy is the other method but limited to the drug dosage forms and their side effects.[1] Radiation, a complementary method, is used to exterminate the remaining cancer cells after surgery, but it could be harmful to the healthy tissues in the vicinity of the tumor region or in the path of the radiation ray.[1,2] Recently, genesis of a novel class of photo thermally sensitized agents, nano-scale particles, called plasmonic photo thermal therapy (PPTT), made a revolution in photo thermal therapy (PTT). After entrance of nanoparticles (NPs) into the tumor sites, near infrared (NIR) or visible light excitation of NPs could induce a moderate temperature increment in vicinity of the NPs,[3] termed as hyperthermia, to destroy the cancer cells clinically.[4,5]

Hyperthermia is generally determined as heating tissues to a temperature in the range of 41-47°C for several minutes.[6] Tumors are selectively damaged due to their reduced heat tolerance in comparison to normal tissues. One of the specific characteristics of this method is to treat recurrent tumors conveniently while NPs are available in the tumor site. Hyperthermia makes irreversible cell damage by rupturing cell membranes, denaturing proteins, and cell cavitation and degeneration leading to cellular necrosis and apoptosis.[1,7] Thermal tumor therapies, based on hyperthermia phenomenon,[8] has been expanded by different kinds of nanomaterials, including gold NPs,[9,10] silver NPs,[11,12] and carbon nanotubes (CNTs).[13]

Metal NPs have ample applications in electronics, photonics,[14,15] chemical sensing, and imaging.[16] Lately, the plasmonic noble metal NPs have attracted a growing deal of interest to themselves. They have considerable impacts on the visible and invisible spectra, which could

***Corresponding author:** Zahra Sobhani, Email: sobhani@sums.ac.ir

improve their application in various approaches such as Raman scattering, radiative rate enhancement,[17] solar cell,[18] optical biosensor,[19] cancer treatment,[20,21] and biological and medical applications.[22,23] Plasmonic NPs have been distinguished from other nano-platforms such as semiconductor quantum dots, magnetic NPs,[24] and polymeric NPs by their distinctive surface plasmon resonance (SPR). This phenomenon is derived from photon confinement to a particle size which improves all the radiative and non-radiative properties of the NPs.[25] Plasmonic NPs, such as gold and silver, could be adjusted to absorb or scatter light at particular wavelengths in the visible and NIR spectra. Light absorption occurs when the energy of incident photons is dissipated via electron oscillation. Totally, optical absorption and scattering of NPs is related to their size, shape, and material nature.[26-28] In addition to the unique characteristics of metal NPs, the CNTs have specific physical and chemical characteristics like high aspect ratio, ultra-light weight, high mechanical strength, and high electrical and thermal conductivity[29-31] which are unique for nanotechnology, electronics, optics and biomedical engineering.[32] The ability of CNTs in heat energy induction after laser excitation in comparison to other materials is appreciable. CNTs have developed widely in drug delivery systems because they could internalize cells very simply[33] and operate as vehicles for drugs, antigens, genes, nucleic acids, and imaging agents.[31,34] Some pharmacokinetic studies have reported that CNTs dispersed by different procedures were free of nonspecific toxic effects in mice.[35,36] Combination of CNTs and noble metals could open up a new era to enhance the application of CNTs in both drug delivery systems and PTT technique.[37,38] Therefore, they could be an efficient choice to convert light energy into heat in cancer photothermal therapy.

In the present study, the efficacies of CNTs decorated with Ag NPs (CNT/Ag NP), CNTs and Ag nanorods (Ag NRs) as effective agents for PPTT were evaluated *in vivo*.

Materials and Methods

Synthesis procedure

Details of synthesis procedure of the CNT/Ag NPs can be found in our previous article.[39] Briefly, 100 mg of multi-walled carbon nanotubes (MWCNTs) (Plasmachem, Berlin, Germany) was dispersed in 40 ml deionized water by 30 min ultra-sonication. Number of walls, outer diameter and length of the MWCNTs were 3-15, 5-20 nm, and 1-10 μm, respectively. 40 ml aqueous solution of 0.1 M $AgNO_3$ was added drop wise to the prepared suspension. The pH of suspension was adjusted to 6 by adding 0.1 M NaOH solution, and it was again ultra-sonicated for 1 hour. Finally, the resultant CNT/Ag NPs were washed 5 times with deionized water and was centrifuged to be separated from the solution.

The Ag NRs and CNTs were used to be compared with CNT/Ag NPs as agents for PPTT. Ag NRs were a gift from Dr. Sabbaghi's laboratory, Shiraz University, Shiraz, Iran. To enhance the dispersability of CNT/Ag NPs, Ag NRs, and CNTs in aqueous solution, a layer of polyethylene glycol (PEG) (PEG_{1000}, Sigma-Aldrich, St Louis, MO, USA) was coated on them, which enhanced their hydrophilicity and dispersibility.[40,41] For this, 25 mg of nanoparticles was suspended in 25ml of deionized water containing 250 mg of PEG, separately. The suspensions were ultrasonicated for 3 min and were then stirred at room temperature overnight to allow for wrapping hydrophilic polymer around CNT/Ag NPs, Ag NRs, and CNTs. After stirring, the suspensions were centrifuged at 4000 rpm for 10 min to precipitate the unreacted reagents, and the supernatants were dialyzed and collected for further experiments.

Absorption spectra of light by CNT/Ag NPs, Ag NRs, and CNTs were measured by UV-Vis double beam spectrophotometer (PG instruments Ltd., T80+ UV–Vis spectrophotometer, Lutterworth, UK). The microscopic images were taken by transmission electron microscope (TEM) (Philips Electron Optics, The Netherlands).

Hyperthermia therapy of tumors

Cell culture

The murine melanoma cell line B16/F10 (NCBI C540), from the Cell Bank of Pasteur Institute of Iran, was cultured in RPMI 1640 medium (Shellmax, China) under 5% CO_2 at 37 °C. The culture medium was supplemented with 10% fetal bovine serum (Shellmax, China), 100 IU/mL of penicillin (Invitrogen, USA) and 100 μg/mL of streptomycin (Invitrogen, USA).

Tumor induction and hyperthermia therapy

All applicable international, national, and institutional guidelines for the care and use of animals were followed. This experiment was performed in the Center of Experimental and Comparative Medicine, Shiraz University of Medical Sciences.

25 female C57BL/6J inbred mice (age: 6-8 weeks and weight 25±5 g) were randomly allocated into five equal groups. The animals were housed in ordinary cages and maintained under conventional conditions with 14:10 hour light/dark cycle (lights on at 6:00 A.M), and ambient temperature of 22 ± 2 °C with 50% relative humidity. The animals received a balanced diet. They had access to water ad libitum.

200 μl of the B16/F10 melanoma cell suspension at 2.5×10^6 cells/ml in culture medium was injected to the mice subcutaneously. This highly metastatic cell line causes melanoma cancer in mice. Sixteen days after inoculation, melanoma tumors grew sufficiently (approximately 1cm^3) in order to begin treatment. At first, all mice were anesthetized by combination of Ketamine 10% (100-120 mg/kg) and Xylazine 2% (6-10 mg/kg). This injection was performed intramuscularly (IM). After shaving and rinsing, the tumors sizes were measured by a caliper and an ultrasound machine (Ultrasonix SonixOP; Burnaby, BC, Canada). They received treatment as follows:

In Group I (CNT/Ag group): CNT/Ag-PEG NPs (1 mg/ml) was injected into the tumor at a dose of 200 $\mu l/cm^3$ (tumor volume).
In Group II (Ag NR group): Ag NRs-PEG (1 mg/ml) was injected into the tumor at a dose of 200 $\mu l/cm^3$ (tumor volume).
In Group III (CNT group): CNT-PEG (1 mg/ml) was injected into the tumor at a dose of 200 $\mu l/cm^3$ (tumor volume).
Group IV (Laser therapy group) and group V (Control) did not receive any NPs.
The tumor area in groups I, II, III and IV were irradiated using a CW laser diode (λ= 670 nm, P=500 mW, and I=3.5 W/cm^2)[42] for 15 min daily for four days after the start of the treatment (at first, the mice were anesthetized and then their tumors were irradiated). The Control cases were not irradiated. The tumor sizes were measured daily during the period of the treatment. The tumor volume was calculated according to this formula: $[(L/2) * W^2]$[13,43] (L and W indicate the length and width of tumor). The laser wavelength was chosen according to the optical absorption peak of CNT/Ag NPs in visible-near IR range.

Histopathological examination

At the end of experiment, the animals were euthanized by chemical anesthetics overdosing, and the mass were excised for histopathological evaluations. The specimens were processed, and the formalin fixed paraffin embedded (FFPE) blocks were prepared and the slides were stained with Hematoxylin and Eosin (HE). The specimens were evaluated grossly and sampled for microscopic evaluation.

Statistical analysis

The results were presented as mean ± standard deviation (SD). Normality of the distribution was checked by One-Sample-Kolmogorov-Smirnov Test. Differences among the groups were determined using ANOVA and Duncan Post-Hoc Test. All the statistical analyses were done by SPSS® statistical software, version 20.0 (SPSS Inc., Chicago, IL, USA) for Windows®. Significance was regarded at *P-values< 0.05*.

Results and Discussion

Structural and optical characterization

Figure1 shows TEM images of different NPs. According to Figure1 (A), the Ag NPs with the average diameter of 20 nm which were attached to CNTs were synthesized. Also, it was observed that a continuous layer of PEG with the average thickness of a few nanometers was formed on the CNT/Ag NPs. TEM image of Ag NRs coated with PEG is shown in Figure 1(B). This image shows that a continuous layer of PEG with average thickness of 6 nm was formed on Ag NRs.
UV-Vis light absorption spectrum of CNT/Ag NPs is given in Figure 2. According to this spectrum curve, the maximum absorption wavelength of CNT/Ag NPs was in the range of 400-1100 nm which is in the visible-near IR range. The broad absorption in the visible-near IR range implies the suitability of the CNT/Ag NPs for PPTT application.

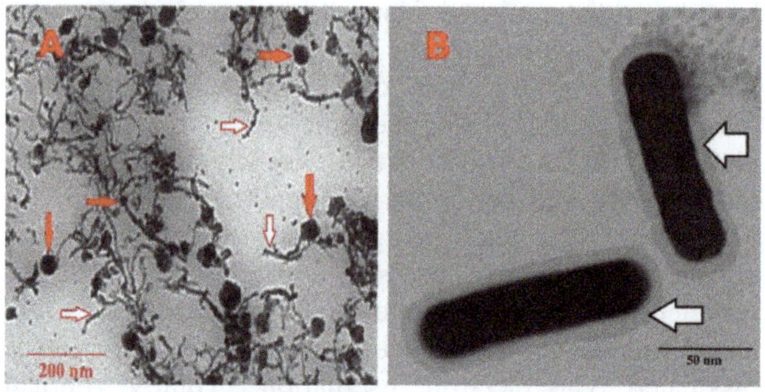

Figure 1. Ultramicrographs of different NPs. (**A**): Ultramicrograph of PEG coated CNT/Ag NPs. (**B**): Ultramicrograph of PEG coated Ag NRs; (open arrows indicate the PEG layer of different NPs and closed arrows indicate the Ag NPs on the surface of the CNTs)

The maximum absorption wavelength of CNT/Ag NPs occurred at 670 nm. These NIR wavelength ranges have considerable optical absorption which could penetrate skin and cells easily[1] and laser diode wavelength was overlapped with the SPR absorption of CNT/Ag NPs. According to Figure 2, CNT/Ag NPs absorb light in the range of 400-1100 nm significantly better than CNTs, which shows the unique effects of noble metal on enhancing optical absorption of CNTs.
The UV-Vis light absorption spectrum of Ag NRs was measured. Unlike CNT/Ag NPs, Ag NRs showed absorption at UV wavelength range and a weak peak between 360-600 nm. Lack of intense and broad absorption at UV-near IR range, in comparison to that of CNT/Ag NPs, implies unsuitability of Ag NRs for PPTT application. Moreover, UV-Vis light absorption spectrum of CNT is given in Figure 2. Based upon this figure, UV-Vis light absorption of CNT/Ag was improved in comparison to CNT and Ag NR.

Hyperthermia therapy of tumors

Tumor sizes were recorded during the experiment. Three prominent situations were reported: before the treatment, two days after the treatment, and four days after the treatment with PPTT technique. As shown in Figure 3, numerical analysis shows that the average tumor size in the Control group increased from 2785.60 mm^3 before the treatment to7243.93 mm^3 four days after the treatment, but it decreased significantly in the CNT/Ag group from 2205.12 mm^3 to1497.52 mm^3, respectively and in the CNT group from 2920.99 mm^3 to 2403.69 mm^3, respectively. The sizes of tumors in the Laser therapy group and in the Ag NR group were not significantly different but the growth of tumors was stopped in both groups. The rate of changes in the tumor size was calculated in different groups. The slopes of tumor size against time in the Control, Laser therapy, Ag NR, CNT, and CNT/Ag groups were approximately +1114.59 mm^3/days, +95.19 mm^3/days, –40.4

mm^3/days,–129.32 mm^3/days, and –176.90 mm^3/days, respectively (+ indicates increasing and – indicates decreasing of tumor size). The slope of tumor size reduction in the CNT/Ag group was remarkable.

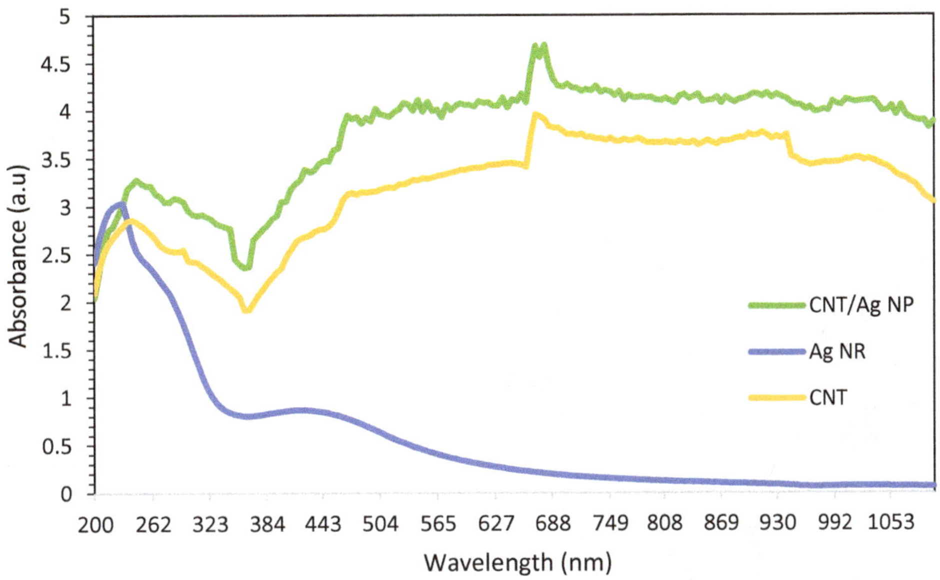

Figure 2. UV-Vis light absorption spectrum of CNT, Ag NR, and CNT/Ag NP

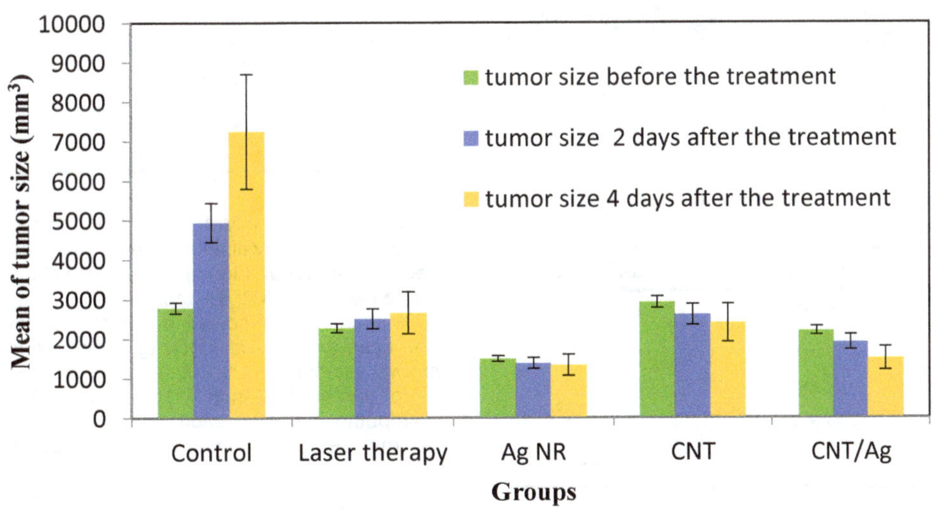

Figure 3. Tumor sizes in different groups at three conditions of measurement (before, two days after, and four days after the treatment with PPTT) (N= 5 in each group and data was shown as mean ± standard deviation).

In addition to these statistical analyses, the ultrasonography images and photographs of a cancerous mouse in the CNT/Ag group showed the healing effect of this technique on shrinking solid tumors, as shown in Figure 4. For more professional deliberation, histopathologic evaluation was done. Gross evaluation of the tumors showed severe necrosis in the CNT/Ag group. Histopathologic evaluation showed nodular subtype in all cases. Necrosis was the most important discriminator between the cases and its percentage was higher in the CNT/Ag group in comparison to the Control group, which is the result of therapy. Mitosis was higher in the Control cases when compared to other cases. There was no evidence of regressive fibrosis, lymphocytic infiltration, vascular invasion or neurotropism in the cases. The histopathologic results are shown in Table 1 and Figure 5.

Plasmonic NPs can absorb NIR light and convert its energy into heat. When NPs absorb light, electrons have to transit from the ground states to the excited states. The absorbed light is transformed into heat via a series of photo physical processes which contain electron-electron relaxation and electron-photon relaxation.[1,2,28] According to this phenomenon, the heat generated from plasmonic NPs after NIR irradiation can be used for treatment of solid tumors. The tumor cells are more sensitive to elevated temperature than normal cells.[13] In this study, we used CNTs decorated with Ag NPs (CNT/Ag) to evaluate their ability for tumor size reduction by PPTT technique. The efficacy of these NPs was compared to the effect of Ag NRs and CNTs. In the previous study we observed that irradiation of CNTs in the tumor region caused considerable damage to the melanoma *in vivo.*[13] Ag NRs have no significant absorption in the NIR range but the absorption of CNT/Ag NPs is very considerable even in comparison with CNTs.

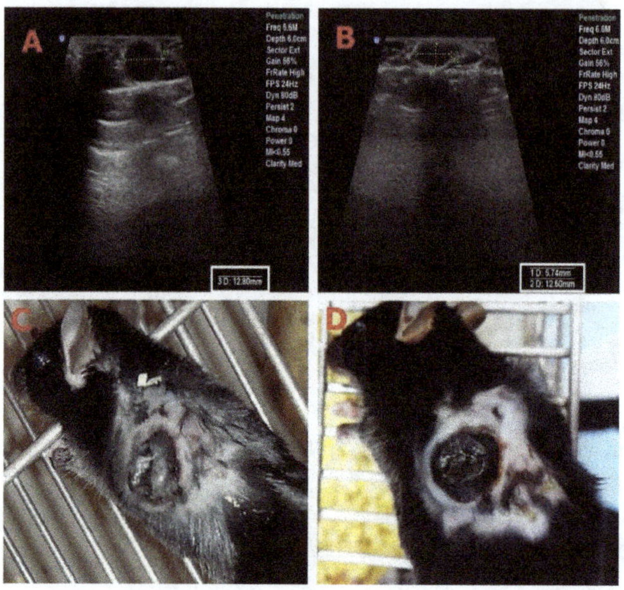

Figure 4. Ultrasonography images and photographs of a cancerous mouse in CNT/Ag group. (**A**, **C**): before the treatment with PPTT. (**B**, **D**): four days after the treatment with PPTT.

Table 1. Histopathologic results of tumor tissues after PTT in different groups of mice

Groups	*Necrosis (%)*	Mitotic rate
CNT/Ag	***~ 70%***	<1/mm^2
CNT	~ 60%	<1/mm^2
Ag NR	~ 45%	<1/mm^2
Laser therapy	~ 25%	<1/mm^2
Control	< 5%	>1/mm^2

At first, to improve the dispersibility of NPs in water, the hydrophilic polymer PEG was used to wrap the surface of NPs. Melanoma was induced in mice by injection of B16/F10 cell line. CNT/Ag NPs, Ag NRs, and CNTs were injected into the tumor. The tumor area was irradiated by a 670 nm CW laser diode after injection of NPs. Analyzing the results of this study showed that, in a definite period of irradiation, the CNT/Ag NPs resulted in tumor necrosis more effectively than the CNTs and Ag NRs in the melanoma cancer model. Based upon the attached UV-Vis light absorption spectra, this phenomenon was due to the enhanced optical absorbance of CNT/Ag NPs in comparison to CNTs and Ag NRs in the visible-near IR range. Laser excitation could increase hot electrons temperature rapidly in NPs and consequently resulted in elevated lattice temperature. Therefore, CNT/Ag NPs generated heat more efficiently than CNTs and Ag NRs. Monitoring the tumor size showed that in the groups receiving CNT/Ag NPs, Ag NRs, and CNTs, not only the tumor growth was stopped after irradiation but the tumor size also shrunk. However, in the group that underwent only laser therapy without any pretreatment, just the rate of tumor growth was slower than the Control group. Besides, histopathological examination showed 70% necrosis in the CNT/Ag group which demonstrated high efficiency of the CNT/Ag NPs as agents in PPTT method.

The results confirmed that combination of CNTs and silver could enhance the optical absorption of CNTs and, consequently, improve the tumor destruction in PPTT technique.

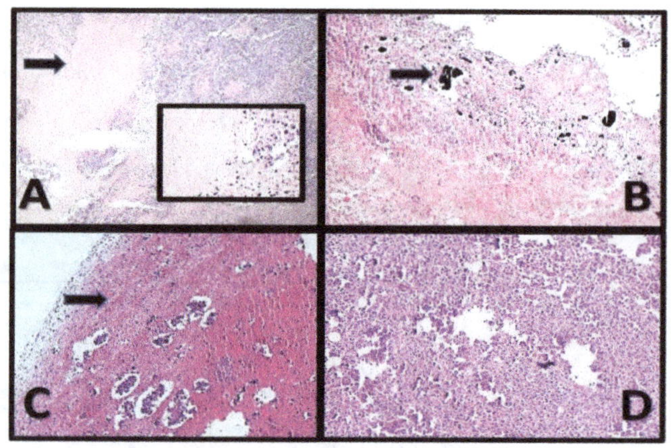

Figure 5. Malignant Melanoma. (**A**): The case treated with laser; Histopathologic evaluation shows the tumor with about 25% necrosis (arrow and inset) (×40-inset ×400) H&E. (**B**): The case treated with Ag NR; Histopathology of the case shows about 45% necrosis in association with NPs (arrow) (×100) H&E. (**C**): The case treated with CNT/Ag NPs; Histopathologic evaluation shows extensive necrosis (about 70% necrosis) with isolated tumor remnant islands (×100) H&E. (**D**): The Control case; Histopathologic evaluation shows sheets of tumor cells with minimal melanin pigments without necrosis (×100)

Conclusion

Integration of CNTs with silver increased the optical absorption of CNTs significantly. CNT/Ag NPs induced heat generation and resulted in considerable damage to melanoma cancer *in vivo*. Animal studies demonstrated high efficiency of this novel NPs in PPTT method with the specific parameters of excitation.

Acknowledgments

This work was financially supported by Shiraz University of Medical Sciences (grant No. 15986). We would like to thank Dr. Ali Mashreghi, a faculty member of Materials Science and Engineering Department, Shiraz University of Technology, Shiraz, Iran, for his helpful comments.

Conflict of Interest

The authors declare that they have no conflict of interests. Authors disclose all relationships or interests that could have direct or potential influence or impart bias on the work.

References

1. Huang X, El-Sayed MA. Plasmonic photo-thermal therapy (PPTT). *Alexandria J Med* 2011;47(1):1-9. doi: 10.1016/j.ajme.2011.01.001
2. Huang X, Jain PK, El-Sayed IH, El-Sayed MA. Plasmonic photothermal therapy (PPTT) using gold nanoparticles. *Lasers Med Sci* 2008;23(3):217-28. doi: 10.1007/s10103-007-0470-x
3. Yakunin AN, Avetisyan YA, Tuchin VV. Quantification of laser local hyperthermia induced by gold plasmonic nanoparticles. *J Biomed Opt* 2015;20(5):051030. doi: 10.1117/1.JBO.20.5.051030
4. Chatterjee DK, Diagaradjane P, Krishnan S. Nanoparticle-mediated hyperthermia in cancer therapy. *Ther Deliv* 2011;2(8):1001-14. doi: 10.4155/tde.11.72
5. Toraya-Brown S, Fiering S. Local tumour hyperthermia as immunotherapy for metastatic cancer. *Int J Hyperthermia* 2014;30(8):531-9. doi: 10.3109/02656736.2014.968640
6. Terentyuk GS, Maslyakova GN, Suleymanova LV, Khlebtsov NG, Khlebtsov BN, Akchurin GG, et al. Laser-induced tissue hyperthermia mediated by gold nanoparticles: Toward cancer phototherapy. *J Biomed Opt* 2009;14(2):021016. doi: 10.1117/1.3122371
7. Kang B, Austin LA, El-Sayed MA. Observing real-time molecular event dynamics of apoptosis in living cancer cells using nuclear-targeted plasmonically enhanced Raman nanoprobes. *ACS Nano* 2014;8(5):4883-92. doi: 10.1021/nn500840x
8. Banobre-Lopez M, Teijeiro A, Rivas J. Magnetic nanoparticle-based hyperthermia for cancer treatment. *Rep Pract Oncol Radiother* 2013;18(6):397-400. doi: 10.1016/j.rpor.2013.09.011
9. Jabeen F, Najam-ul-Haq M, Javeed R, Huck CW, Bonn GK. Au-Nanomaterials as a Superior Choice for Near-Infrared Photothermal Therapy. *Molecules* 2014;19(12):20580-93. doi: 10.3390/molecules191220580
10. Li JL, Gu M. Gold-nanoparticle-enhanced cancer photothermal therapy. *IEEE J Sel Top Quantum Electron* 2010;16(4):989-96. doi: 10.1109/JSTQE.2009.2030340
11. Patskovsky S, Bergeron E, Rioux D, Simard M, Meunier M. Hyperspectral reflected light microscopy of plasmonic Au/Ag alloy nanoparticles incubated as multiplex chromatic biomarkers with cancer cells. *Analyst* 2014;139(20):5247-53. doi: 10.1039/C4AN01063A
12. Thompson EA, Graham E, MacNeill CM, Young M, Donati G, Wailes EM, et al. Differential response of MCF7, MDA-MB-231, and MCF 10A cells to hyperthermia, silver nanoparticles and silver nanoparticle-induced photothermal therapy. *Int J Hyperthermia* 2014;30(5):312-23. doi: 10.3109/02656736.2014.936051
13. Sobhani Z, Behnam MA, Emami F, Dehghanian A, Jamhiri I. Photothermal therapy of melanoma tumor using multiwalled carbon nanotubes. *Int J Nanomedicine* 2017;12:4509-17. doi: 10.2147/IJN.S134661
14. Akhlaghi M, Emami F, Nozhat N. Binary TLBO algorithm assisted for designing plasmonic nano bi-pyramids-based absorption coefficient. *J Mod Opt* 2014;61(13):1092-6. doi: 10.1080/09500340.2014.920537
15. Akhlaghi M, Nozhat N, Emami F. Investigating the Optical Switch Using Dimer Plasmonic Nano-Rods. *IEEE Trans Nanotechnol* 2014;13(6):1172-5. doi: 10.1109/TNANO.2014.2349361
16. Katz E, Willner I. Integrated nanoparticle-biomolecule hybrid systems: Synthesis, properties, and applications. *Angew Chem Int Ed Engl* 2004;43(45):6042-108. doi: 10.1002/anie.200400651
17. Biteen JS, Pacifici D, Lewis NS, Atwater HA. Enhanced radiative emission rate and quantum efficiency in coupled silicon nanocrystal-nanostructured gold emitters. *Nano Lett* 2005;5(9):1768-73. doi: 10.1021/nl051207z
18. Catchpole KR, Polman A. Plasmonic solar cells. *Opt Express* 2008;16(26):21793-800. doi: 10.1364/OE.16.021793
19. Boriskina SV, Gopinath A, Dal Negro L. Optical gap formation and localization properties of optical modes in deterministic aperiodic photonic structures. *Opt Express* 2008;16(23):18813-26. doi: 10.1364/OE.16.018813
20. Kodiha M, Hutter E, Boridy S, Juhas M, Maysinger D, Stochaj U. Gold nanoparticles induce nuclear damage in breast cancer cells, which is further amplified by hyperthermia. *Cell Mol Life Sci* 2014;71(21):4259-73. doi: 10.1007/s00018-014-1622-3
21. Kossatz S, Grandke J, Couleaud P, Latorre A, Aires A, Crosbie-Staunton K, et al. Efficient treatment of breast cancer xenografts with multifunctionalized iron oxide nanoparticles combining magnetic hyperthermia and anti-cancer drug delivery. *Breast Cancer Res* 2015;17:66. doi: 10.1186/s13058-015-0576-1
22. Huang X, Jain PK, El-Sayed IH, El-Sayed MA. Gold nanoparticles: interesting optical properties and recent applications in cancer diagnostics and therapy. *Nanomedicine (Lond)* 2007;2(5):681-93. doi: 10.2217/17435889.2.5.681
23. Jain PK, Huang X, El-Sayed IH, El-Sayed MA. Noble metals on the nanoscale: Optical and photothermal properties and some applications in imaging, sensing, biology, and medicine. *Acc Chem Res* 2008;41(12):1578-86. doi: 10.1021/ar7002804
24. Bae S, Lee SW, Hirukawa A, Takemura Y, Jo YH, Lee SG. AC magnetic-field-induced heating and

physical properties of ferrite nanoparticles for a hyperthermia agent in medicine. *IEEE Trans Nanotechnol* 2009;8(1):86-94. doi: 10.1109/TNANO.2008.2007214
25. Link S, El-Sayed MA. Optical properties and ultrafast dynamics of metallic nanocrystals. *Annu Rev Phys Chem* 2003;54:331-66. doi: 10.1146/annurev.physchem.54.011002.103759
26. Sosa IO, Noguez C, Barrera RG. Optical Properties of Metal Nanoparticles with Arbitrary Shapes. *J Phys Chem B* 2003;107(26):6269-75. doi: 10.1021/jp0274076
27. Garcia MA. Surface plasmons in metallic nanoparticles: fundamentals and applications. *J Phys D Appl Phys* 2011;44(28):283001. doi: 10.1088/0022-3727/44/28/283001
28. Huang X, El-Sayed MA. Gold nanoparticles: Optical properties and implementations in cancer diagnosis and photothermal therapy. *J Adv Res* 2010;1(1):13-28. doi: 10.1016/j.jare.2010.02.002
29. Che J, Cagin T, Goddard WA. Thermal conductivity of carbon nanotubes. *Nanotechnology* 2000;11(2):65-9. doi: 10.1088/0957-4484/11/2/305
30. Park J, Bifano MFP, Prakash V. Sensitivity of thermal conductivity of carbon nanotubes to defect concentrations and heat-treatment. *J Appl Phys* 2013;113(3):034312. doi: 10.1063/1.4778477
31. Singh R, Torti SV. Carbon nanotubes in hyperthermia therapy. *Adv Drug Deliv Rev* 2013;65(15):2045-60. doi: 10.1016/j.addr.2013.08.001
32. Lin Y, Taylor S, Li H, Shiral Fernando KA, Qu L, Wang W, et al. Advances toward bioapplications of carbon nanotubes. *J Mater Chem* 2004;14(4):527-41. doi: 10.1039/b314481j
33. Lacerda L, Russier J, Pastorin G, Herrero MA, Venturelli E, Dumortier H, et al. Translocation mechanisms of chemically functionalised carbon nanotubes across plasma membranes. *Biomaterials* 2012;33(11):3334-43. doi: 10.1016/j.biomaterials.2012.01.024
34. Sahoo NG, Bao H, Pan Y, Pal M, Kakran M, Cheng HK, et al. Functionalized carbon nanomaterials as nanocarriers for loading and delivery of a poorly water-soluble anticancer drug: a comparative study. *Chem Commun (Camb)* 2011;47(18):5235-7. doi: 10.1039/c1cc00075f
35. Liu Z, Cai W, He L, Nakayama N, Chen K, Sun X, et al. In vivo biodistribution and highly efficient tumour targeting of carbon nanotubes in mice. *Nat Nanotechnol* 2007;2(1):47-52. doi: 10.1038/nnano.2006.170
36. Cherukuri P, Gannon CJ, Leeuw TK, Schmidt HK, Smalley RE, Curley SA, et al. Mammalian pharmacokinetics of carbon nanotubes using intrinsic near-infrared fluorescence. *Proc Natl Acad Sci U S A* 2006;103(50):18882-6. doi: 10.1073/pnas.0609265103
37. Amiri A, Shanbedi M, Eshghi H, Heris SZ, Baniadam M. Highly Dispersed Multiwalled Carbon Nanotubes Decorated with Ag Nanoparticles in Water andExperimental Investigation of the Thermophysical Properties. *J Phys Chem C* 2012;116(5):3369-75. doi: 10.1021/jp210484a
38. Moghim MH, Zebarjad SM. Fabrication and Structural Characterization of Multi-walled Carbon Nanotube/Fe3O4 Nanocomposite. *J Inorg Organomet Polym Mater* 2015;25(5):1260-6. doi: 10.1007/s10904-015-0235-0
39. Ahmadpoor F, Zebarjad SM, Janghorban K. Decoration of multi-walled carbon nanotubes with silver nanoparticles and investigation on its colloid stability. *Mater Chem Phys* 2013;139(1):113-7. doi: 10.1016/j.matchemphys.2012.12.071
40. Jahanbakhsh R, Atyabi F, Shanehsazzadeh S, Sobhani Z, Adeli M, Dinarvand R. Modified Gadonanotubes as a promising novel MRI contrasting agent. *Daru* 2013;21(1):53. doi: 10.1186/2008-2231-21-53
41. Foldvari M, Bagonluri M. Carbon nanotubes as functional excipients for nanomedicines: II. Drug delivery and biocompatibility issues. *Nanomedicine* 2008;4(3):183-200. doi: 10.1016/j.nano.2008.04.003
42. Zhang Z, Wang J, Nie X, Wen T, Ji Y, Wu X, et al. Near infrared laser-induced targeted cancer therapy using thermoresponsive polymer encapsulated gold nanorods. *J Am Chem Soc* 2014;136(20):7317-26. doi: 10.1021/ja412735p
43. Yan D, Teng Z, Sun S, Jiang S, Dong H, Gao Y, et al. Foot-and-mouth disease virus-like particles as integrin-based drug delivery system achieve targeting anti-tumor efficacy. *Nanomedicine* 2017;13(3):1061-70. doi: 10.1016/j.nano.2016.12.007

Anti Pneumococcal Activity of Azithromycin-Eudragit RS100 Nano-Formulations

Khosro Adibkia[1], Golrokh Khorasani[1], Shahriar Payab[1], Farzaneh Lotfipour[2]*

[1] *Drug Applied Research Center and Faculty of Pharmacy, Tabriz University of Medical Sciences, Tabriz, Iran.*
[2] *Food & Drug Safety Research Center and Faculty of Pharmacy, Tabriz University of Medical Sciences, Tabriz, Iran.*

Article info

Keywords:
· Azithromycin
· Anti Pneumococcal Activity
· Nano-Formulation
· Eudragit RS100

Abstract

Propose: Bacterial pneumonia is a common lung infection caused by different types of bacteria. Azithromycin (AZI), an azalide antibiotic, is widely used to manage pneumococcal infections. Studies have shown that antibiotics in nanocarriers may lead to increased antibacterial activity and reduced toxicity. The aim of this work was to valuate in vitro antibacterial performance azithromycin-Eudragit RS100 nano-formulations against *Streptococcus pneumoniae and Staphylococcus aureus.*

Methods: AZI-Eudragit RS100 nanoparticles were prepared via electrospinning technique and the *in* vitro antibacterial performance against *S. pneumoniae and S. aureus were assessed* using agar dilution method.

Results: Nanofibers in the sizes about 100-300 nm in diameter and micro scale in length and nanobeads in the range of 100-500 nm were achieved. The Minimum Inhibitory Concentrations (MIC) showed an enhancement in the antimicrobial effect of AZI-Eudragit RS100 nanofibers (40 µg/ml) compare to untreated AZI solution (>160 µg/ml) against *S. pneumonia*. The MIC value for AZI-Eudragit RS100 nanofibers against *S. aureus* was >128 µg/ml, same as that of the untreated AZI solution.

Conclusion: The enhanced efficiency of AZI in nanofibers could be related to the more adsorption opportunity of nanofibers to *S. pneumonia* capsulated cell wall which provides an antibiotic depot on the bacterial surface compared to *S. aureus*. AZI-Eudragit RS100 nanofibers with enhanced antimicrobial effect against S. *pneumonia* can be considered as a candidate for in vivo evaluations in antibiotic therapy of Pneumococcal infections.

Introduction

Azithromycin (AZI) is a semi-synthetic antibiotic from azalide class (14-membered ring macrolide) which was FDA approved for use in 1994. This antibiotic has been launched to pharmacy market as a result of notable limitations of former 14-membered ring macrolide i.e. erythromycin.[1] AZI achieves high tissue concentrations and reach the sites of infection by direct uptake via phagocytes.[2] Consequently the obtained high tissue concentrations are retained for extended periods resulted in once-daily dosing for 3 or 5 days. AZI like other macrolides inhibits bacterial protein synthesis by binding to the 50S ribosomal subunit of the bacterial 70S ribosome which inhibits peptidyl transferase activity and interferes with amino acid translocation during the translation process (Figure 1).[3] Remarkable microbiological features of make it a good candidate for the management of a wide range of bacterial infections especially those of bacterial pneumonia.[4]

Nevertheless, in line with the global antibiotic resistance trend, significant resistance among the formerly susceptible microorganisms like *Streptococcus pneumoniae* and *Staphylococcus aureus* has been detected. In fact the increasing numbers of reports on the failures of treatment of infections caused by macrolide resistant pneumococcal isolates in the last two decades has been a matter of concern.[4] Three prominent mechanisms for Pneumococcal macrolide resistance can be summarized as the alteration of the ribosomal target site, the production of inactivating enzymes, and the production and utilization of active efflux mechanisms. The first two approach are shown to be more important in the macrolide resistance development.[1]

Several approaches to overcome bacterial resistance issue were developed from which the use of drug carriers such as nanoparticles seems to be one of the promising strategies. Nanoparticles drug delivery vehicles are generally in dimensions of about 5 – 350 nm in diameter. These carriers for pharmaceutical purposes improve therapeutic efficacy of the drug by enhancing drug bioavailability, serum stability and pharmacokinetics.

Especially nanoparticle based antimicrobial vehicles could interact with microorganisms by fusing with their cell wall or membrane and releasing the load within them and/or adsorbing to cell wall and providing an antibiotic depot there to release drug molecules.[9-12]

***Corresponding author:** Farzaneh Lotfipour, Email: lotfipoor@tbzmed.ac.ir

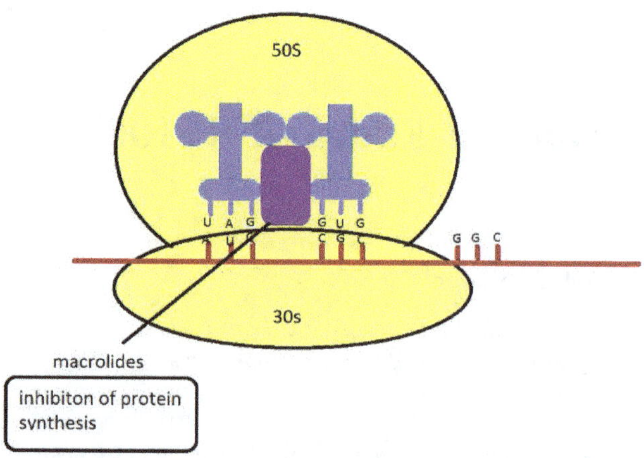

Figure 1. Schematic representation for antibacterial mechanism of macrolides.

Electrospinning is a promising method for nanoparticle production. A polymer-drug solution is injected into a capillary tube while applying electrical charge on the solution to create a liquid jet flying towards a grounded collector screen. By its movement to the collector, the solvent evaporates and a fine network of nanofibers or nanobeads would form on the collector.[13]

AZI loaded Eudragit RS100 nano-formulations were prepared using Electrospinning in our previous published work.[13] Here we aimed to evaluate the activity of the selected nano-formulations against AZI resistant *S. pneumonia* and *S. aureus* strains in comparison with the untreated drug.

Materials and Methods

Materials

AZI powder (Dr Reddy's Pharmaceutical Company, India) Eudragit RS100 (Degussa Darmstadt, Germany), HPLC grade methanol (Concord Technology (Tianjin) Co., Ltd.), Muller Hinton broth and agar media, blood base agar medium (DIFCO, U.K). *S. pneumonia* and *S. aureus* were previously isolated from clinical samples according to standard procedures and stored at -80°C.

Preparation and characterization of the nanobeads and nanofibers

The fabrication of AZI-Eudragit RS100 nanobeads and nanofibers was conducted according to our previously published paper.[13]

Nano-suspension preparation

The stock nano-suspension (containing equivalent AZI of 2.62 mg/ml) was prepared by dispersing 157.2 mg of the AZI-Eudragit RS100 nano-formulations, in 10 ml distilled water by vortexing. In the next step, the vortexed suspension was entered the process of serial dilution in order to obtain a bunch of distinct concentrations to use them within the ongoing agar dilution process. Furthermore, the stock of AZI solution in the same concentration (2.62 mg/ml) was prepared in 5% ethanol in distilled water as negative control.

Antibacterial activity of AZI-Eudragit RS100 nano-formulations

Antibacterial properties of the nano-formulations were investigated against AZI resistant *S. pneumonia* and *S. aureus* standard strains. After activating of the freezed bacteria, the culture was maintained in the blood base agar and nutrient agar media for *S. pneumonia* and *S. aureus* respectively at 4°C and used as stock cultures. A single colony from the stock plate was transferred into the relevant agar media and incubated over night at 37°C. After incubation time the cells were collected from the surface of agar medium, washed twice, and re-suspended in saline solution to provide an optical density equal to 0.5 McFarland or bacterial concentration around 10^8 CFU/ml.

Antibacterial performance against *S. pneumonia* was evaluated by agar dilution method. Firstly, a series of concentrations of antibiotics were prepared by 1:2 diluting trend in order to be added into the agar medium. Two millilitres from each concentration of AZI nano-formulation as well as untreated AZI solution (concentrations ranging from 0.625 to 160 μg/ml) was added to the plate containing 30 ml Haemophillus agar supplemented with 5% sheep blood (temperature=45°C). Therefore, for each concentration from each formulation two plates were obtained. After preparing the plates, they were inoculated with a swab from the adjusted *S. pneumoniae* inoculum suspension and incubated for 2 days at 37°C. The MICs were recorded after 48 h of incubation on the basis of the first concentration that inhibit the bacterial growth.

The antimicrobial activities of prepared nano-formulations against *S. aureus were assessed by* broth macrodilution method according to CLSI protocol. Briefly bacterial inoculum in Muller-Hinton Broth medium, added to serial diluted NPs suspension as well as drug solutions to reach the final concentration of 10^6 CFU/ml. After 24 h incubation at 37 °C , from the content of the tubes streak cultured onto Muller Hinton agar plates. MICs was designated as the first concentration of antibiotic with no sign of bacterial growth.[14]

Results and Discussion

Characteristics of prepared nano-formulations

Nanofibers in the sizes about 100-300 nm in diameter and micro scale in length as well as nanobeads in the range of 100-500 nm in diameter were achieved. As concluded from the SEM results depicted in Figure 2 (a and b), application of higher concentrations of solution resulted in production of nanofibers with smooth surfaces. On the other hand, lower solution concentration resulted in the production of nanobeads with concavities on their surfaces.[13,15-17]

Antibacterial activity of the nanosuspensions

S. pneumonia was cultured in Haemophilus agar containing 5% sheep blood used as an indicator to assess in vitro antibacterial activity of prepared nano-formulations compared to drug solution. According to the MIC test results, the tested *S. pneumonia* was shown to be *in vitro* resistant to AZI even at higher concentrations. In fact in all the tested concentrations (up to 160µg/ml) *S. pneumonia* colonies were observed on the surface of the cultured plates (Figure 3). While MIC values for sensitive strains were reported to be 0.5 to 2µg/ml in standard CLSI protocol that was significantly different from the MIC value obtained for our test strain. In spite of the obtained in vitro resistance pattern, it should be in vivo studies to extrapolate the data into clinical failures. In fact it has been shown that the host-defense responses lead macrolides and azalides after absorption to the infection site and release them at the infection site. Also, after phagocytosis of the pathogens, expose them to high intracellular drug concentrations.[1,18]

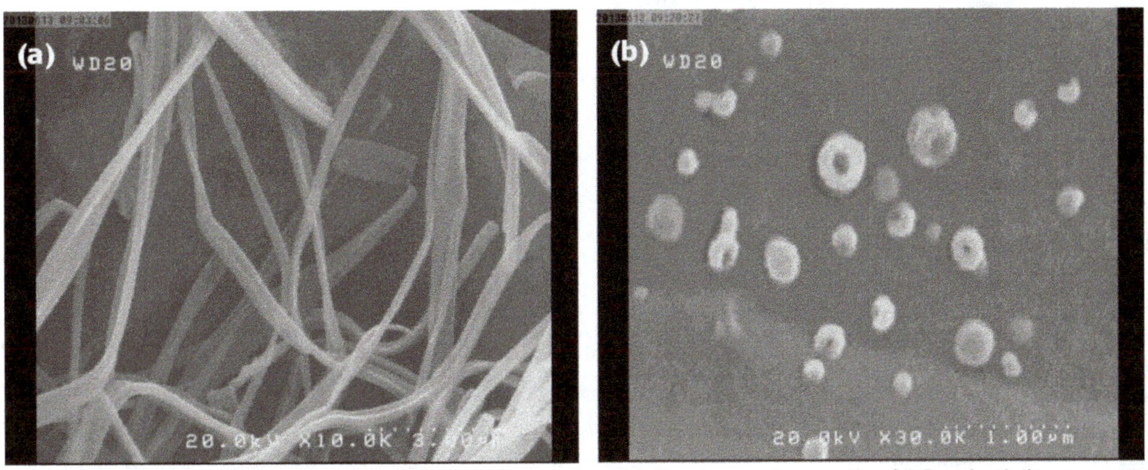

Figure 2. SEM images for AZI-Eudragit RS100 electrospuns. Samples with the drug: polymer ratio of 1:5 and solution concentrations of 20% (a) samples with the drug: polymer ratio of 1:5 and solution concentrations of 10% (b).

Sample ID	AZI Concentration (µg/ml)						
	160	80	40	20	10	5	Control
AZI-Eudragit RS100 NPs Suspention in water	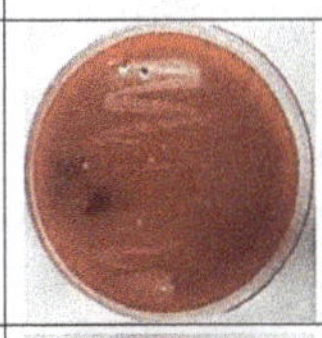	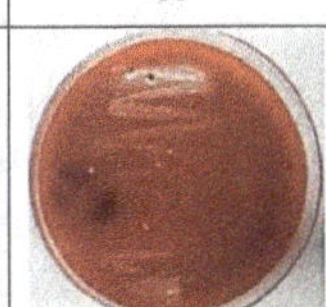	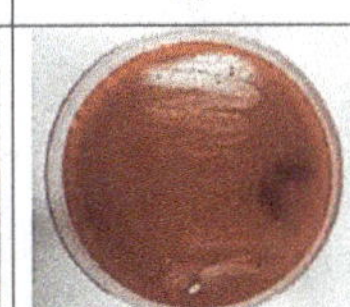	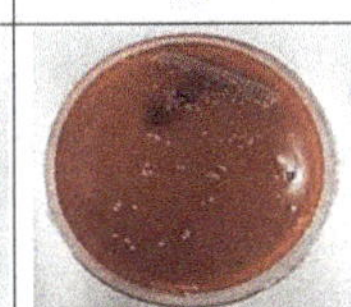	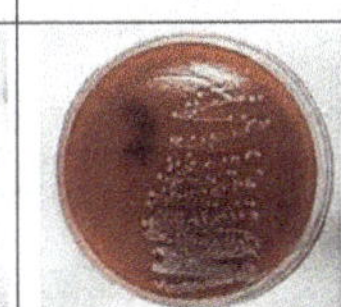	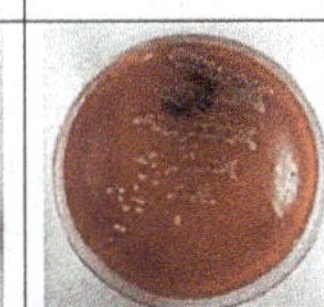	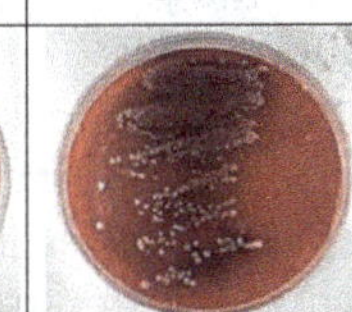
AZI solution in 5% v/v ethanol in water	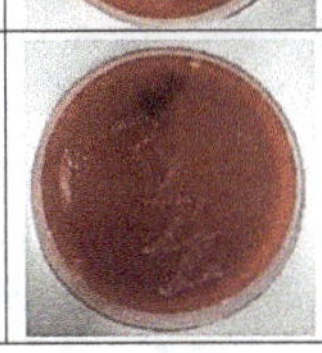	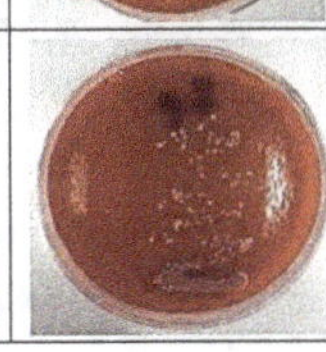	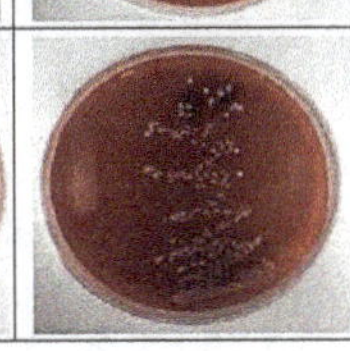	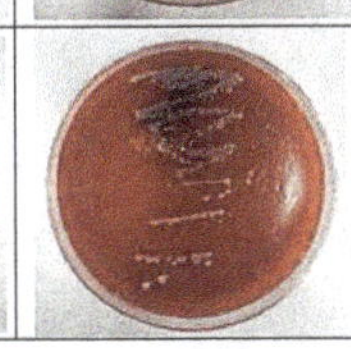	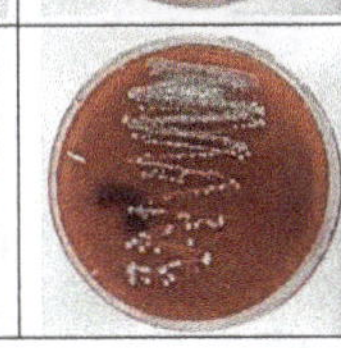	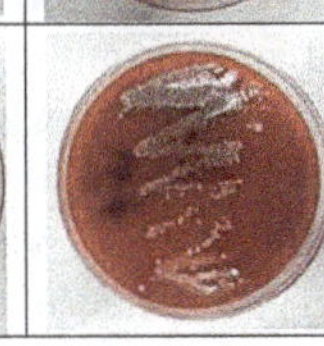	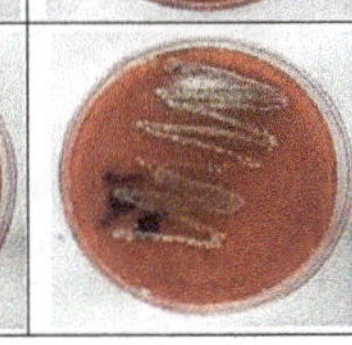

Figure 3. Haemophillus agar plates containing AZI-Eudragit RS100 nanofibers as well as untreated AZI solution with streak cultures of *S. pneumonia*.

On the other hand, the MIC values recorded for AZI-Eudragit RS100 nanofibers were 40 µg/ml, which was significantly lower than the MIC value of the untreated counterpart (Figure 4). This can be presumed as a remarkable improvement in the AZI performance. This improvement in the antibacterial performance of AZI in nano-form can be probably explained by some possible mechanisms. Overall, nanoparticle based antimicrobial delivery systems could interact with microorganisms via two mechanisms and consequently enhance the performance; by fusing with microbial cell wall or membrane and release the load within the cell wall or membrane; via adsorbing to cell wall and provide a antibiotic depot to continuously release drug molecules, which will diffuse into the interior of the microorganisms.[9] Furthermore, it has been reported that antibiotic-loaded NPs can enter host cells and tissues through endocytosis, followed by releasing the loaded drug to eradicate intracellular microorganisms.[19] In the case of AZI-Eudragit RS100 nanofiber the adsorption to the bacteria cell wall to provide an antibiotic depot on the bacterial surface seems to be more feasible due to the large surface area of the nanofibers with more interaction opportunity of the bacterial cell wall. Nevertheless, according to the fact that nano-fibres are nano size just in one dimension, they could not pass through absorption barriers and the fate of formulation in in vivo experiments could be different. Figure 4 shows the cellular structure of *S. pneumonia* which composed of cell wall and a rough polysaccharide capsule. Based on the capsule structure of *S. pneumonia*, it can be predictable that the adsorbing and trapping of the nanofibers within the complex capsule structure of the bacteria to provide an in situ antibiotic depot would not be farfetched.[20]

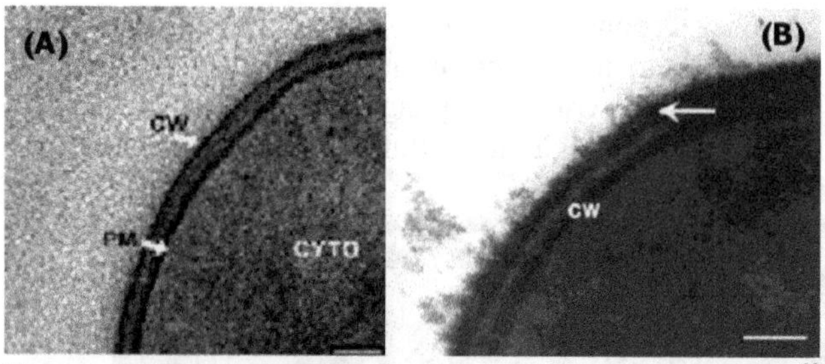

Figure 4. The cell wall structure of (A): *S. pneumonia*[20] with permission and (B): *S. aureus*[21] with permission. CW: cell wall, PM: plasma membrane, Bar = 100μm.

Nevertheless, based on the MIC value obtained for AZI-Eudragit RS100 nanobeads, the observed figures were >160 μg/ml, same as that of the untreated AZI solution indicating that the prepared nanobeads simply maintained the antibacterial efficiency of AZI. Still it would be valuable because of the potential benefits of prepared nanobeads which need to be evaluated in the upcoming in vivo or animal studies.

In vitro antibacterial activity of the prepared nano-suspensions *was* assessed against *S. aureus* by broth macrodilution method and compared to untreated drug solution.

According to the MIC test results, the experimented strain of *S. aureus* was shown to be *in vitro* resistant to AZI. In fact in all the tested concentrations (0.25 to 128μg/ml) *S. aureus* colonies were observed on the surface of the streak cultured plates (MIC >128μg/ml). According to standard CLSI protocol MIC values for susceptible strains were reported to be 2 to 8μg/ml. This finding is in good agreement with the various reports indicating growing in vitro resistance trends described about *S. aureus* against macrolides.

On the other hand, the MIC values recorded for both AZI-Eudragit RS100 nanofibers and nanobeads represented a resistant paradigm as well, with MIC values of >128μg/ml. Indeed, preparation of nano-formulation (nanofibers or nanobeads) could not improve the in vitro antibacterial activity of AZI in comparison with drug solution and just maintained the MIC values of AZI equal to untreated solution. Figure 5 (B) shows a schematic picture of a *S. aureus* cell wall structure. It seems that the adsorption and trapping opportunity of the nano-formulations to the capsule less cell wall structure of *S. aureus* would be lower than capsulated rough *S. pneumonia* cell wall.

Conclusion

In the current in vitro study we assessed the anti bacterial activity of formulated AZI- Eudragit RS100 nanobeads and nanofibers against S. *pneumonia* and *S. aureus;* two common cause of bacterial pneumonia. Herein, it was shown that AZI-Eudragit RS100 nanofibers with enhanced in vitro antimicrobial effect against S. *pneumonia* can be considered as a candidate for *in vivo* evaluations in antibiotic therapy of Pneumococcal infections.

Conflict of Interest

The Authors report no declaration of interest.

References

1. Amsden GW. Pneumococcal macrolide resistance--myth or reality? *J Antimicrob Chemother* 1999;44(1):1-6. doi: 10.1093/jac/44.1.1
2. Lode H, Borner K, Koeppe P, Schaberg T. Azithromycin--review of key chemical, pharmacokinetic and microbiological features. *J Antimicrob Chemother* 1996;37(Suppl C):1-8. doi: 10.1093/jac/37.suppl_c.1
3. Retsema J, Girard A, Schelkly W, Manousos M, Anderson M, Bright G, et al. Spectrum and mode of action of azithromycin (CP-62,993), a new 15-membered-ring macrolide with improved potency against gram-negative organisms. *Antimicrob Agents Chemother* 1987;31(12):1939-47. doi: 10.1128/AAC.31.12.1939
4. Reinert RR, Filimonova OY, Al-Lahham A, Grudinina SA, Ilina EN, Weigel LM, et al. Mechanisms of macrolide resistance among Streptococcus pneumoniae isolates from Russia. *Antimicrob Agents Chemother* 2008;52(6):2260-2. doi: 10.1128/AAC.01270-07
5. Samiei M, Farjami A, Dizaj SM, Lotfipour F. Nanoparticles for antimicrobial purposes in Endodontics: A systematic review of in vitro studies. *Mater Sci Eng C Mater Biol Appl* 2016;58:1269-78. doi: 10.1016/j.msec.2015.08.070
6. Hallaj-Nezhadi S, Dass CR, Lotfipour F. Intraperitoneal delivery of nanoparticles for cancer gene therapy. *Future Oncol* 2013;9(1):59-68. doi: 10.2217/fon.12.171
7. Nahaei M, Valizadeh H, Baradaran B, Nahaei MR, Asgari D, Hallaj-Nezhadi S, et al. Preparation and characterization of chitosan/β-cyclodextrin nanoparticles containing plasmid DNA encoding interleukin-12. *Drug Res (Stuttg)* 2013;63(1):7-12. doi: 10.1055/s-0032-1331165
8. Hallaj-Nezhadi S, Valizadeh H, Baradaran B, Dobakhti F, Lotfipour F. Preparation and characterization of gelatin nanoparticles containing pDNA encoding IL-12 and their expression in CT-26 carcinoma cells. *Future Oncol* 2013;9(8):1195-206. doi: 10.2217/fon.13.82
9. Zhang L, Pornpattananangku D, Hu CM, Huang CM. Development of nanoparticles for antimicrobial drug delivery. *Curr Med Chem* 2010;17(6):585-94. doi: 10.2174/092986710790416290
10. Lotfipour F, Valizadeh H, Milani M, Bahrami N, Ghotaslou R. Study of Antimicrobial Effects of

Clarithromycin Loaded PLGA Nanoparticles against Clinical Strains of Helicobacter pylori. *Drug Res (Stuttg)* 2016;66(1):41-5. doi: 10.1055/s-0035-1548910

11. Azhar SL, Lotfipour F. Magnetic nanoparticles for antimicrobial drug delivery. *Pharmazie* 2012;67(10):817-21.
12. Hallaj-Nezhadi S, Lotfipour F, Dass CR. Delivery of nanoparticulate drug delivery systems via the intravenous route for cancer gene therapy. *Pharmazie* 2010;65(12):855-9.
13. Payab S, Jafari-Aghdam N, Barzegar-Jalali M, Mohammadi G, Lotfipour F, Gholikhani T, et al. Preparation and physicochemical characterization of the azithromycin-Eudragit RS100 nanobeads and nanofibers using electrospinning method. *J Drug Deliv Sci Technol* 2014;24(6):585-90. doi: 10.1016/S1773-2247(14)50123-2
14. Wikler MA. Performance standards for antimicrobial susceptibility testing; 18th informational supplement. CLSI document M100-18 . Wayne PA: Clinical and Laboratory Standards Institute; 2008.
15. Liu H, Hsieh YL. Ultrafine fibrous cellulose membranes from electrospinning of cellulose acetate. *J Polym Sci Part B: Polym Phys* 2002;40(18):2119-29. doi: 10.1002/polb.10261
16. Frey MW, Li L. Electrospinning and porosity measurements of nylon-6/poly (ethylene oxide) blended non-wovens. *J Eng Fibers Fabrics* 2007;2(1):31-7.
17. Jafari-Aghdam N, Adibkia K, Payab S, Barzegar-Jalali M, Parvizpur A, Mohammadi G, et al. Methylprednisolone acetate-Eudragit® RS100 electrospuns: Preparation and physicochemical characterization. *Artif Cells Nanomed Biotechnol* 2016;44(2):497-503. doi: 10.3109/21691401.2014.965309
18. Ballow CH, Amsden GW, Highet VS, Forrest A. Pharmacokinetics of oral azithromycin in serum, urine, polymorphonuclear leucocytes and inflammatory vs non-inflammatory skin blisters in healthy volunteers. *Clin Drug Investig* 1998;15(2):159-67. doi: 10.2165/00044011-199815020-00009
19. Salouti M, Ahangari A. Nanoparticle based Drug Delivery Systems for Treatment of Infectious Diseases. In: Sezer AD, editor. Application of Nanotechnology in Drug Delivery. Vienna, Austria: InTech Publishing House: 2014. P. 155-92.
20. Chang YC, Jong A, Huang S, Zerfas P, Kwon-Chung KJ. CPS1, a homolog of the Streptococcus pneumoniae type 3 polysaccharide synthase gene, is important for the pathobiology of Cryptococcus neoformans. *Infect Immun* 2006;74(7):3930-8. doi: 10.1128/IAI.00089-06
21. Touhami A, Jericho MH, Beveridge TJ. Atomic force microscopy of cell growth and division in staphylococcus aureus. *J Bacteriol* 2004;186(11):3286-95. doi: 10.1128/JB.186.11.3286-3295.2004

Determining Abuse Deterrence Performance of Poly (ethylene oxide) Using a Factorial Design

Yogesh Joshi[1], Srinath Muppalaneni[2], Alborz Omidian[3], David Jude Mastropietro[4], Hamid Omidian[4]*

[1] Unipharma LLC., Tamarac, Florida, USA.
[2] Sancilio Pharmaceuticals Company, Inc., Riviera Beach, Florida, USA.
[3] The University of Chicago, Chicago, IL, USA.
[4] Department of Pharmaceutical Sciences, College of Pharmacy, Nova Southeastern University, Fort Lauderdale, Florida, USA.

Article info

Keywords:
- Abuse deterrent formulation
- Injecting drug use
- Crush resistance
- Opioid abuse
- Poly(ethylene oxide)

Abstract

Purpose: The purpose of this study was to determine the effects of thermal processing and antioxidant formulation variables on the abuse deterrence performance of a high molecular weight poly(ethylene oxide) (PEO) polymer.

Methods: A 2^4 factorial design with one categorical factor (antioxidant type) and three continuous factors (curing time, curing temperature, % antioxidant) was used. Abuse deterrence performance was evaluated using solution viscosity, surface melting temperature, and mechanical strength. Thermal degradation of PEO powders before compaction was also studied using DSC, FTIR spectroscopy, and viscosity analysis.

Results: Our results showed that curing temperature and type of antioxidant can significantly affect the deterrence performance of PEO. The main effect plot for viscosity shows the most prominent factors affecting viscosity are curing temperature and type of antioxidant. However, curvature in the linear model obtained was not sufficient to completely describe the behavior. For surface melting temperature, butylated hydroxytoluene was associated with higher surface melting temperatures compared to ascorbic acid. Additionally, higher percent of antioxidant resulted in higher melting temperature. Particle size distribution to indicate mechanical strength showed no significant effects of tested factors. This suggests that comminution method has more prominent effect on tablet fragment size than the formulation and processing factors studied.

Conclusion: While heat confers the mechanical strength to the polymer, it can diminish its physical stability and solution state viscosity. The experimental studies showed that prolonged exposure to high temperatures, even in the presence of antioxidants, can severely hamper polymer deterrence performance in both solid and solution states.

Introduction

The increasing use of prescription drugs in the United States suggests their major importance to clinical practice.[1] Along with their increased use, there has also been a rise in abuse of certain classes of medications, among which the prescription opioid pain relievers are perhaps the most widely-abused. For example, it has been reported that approximately 97.5 million people aged 12 or older were past year users of prescription pain relievers in 2015.[2] This represents more than one third (36.4 percent) of the United States population aged 12 and older. Additionally, misuse of prescription opioids as well as other classes has led to increased emergency room visits, overdose deaths, and treatment admissions for drug use disorders and addiction.[3] Furthermore, the rise in prescription drug abuse has also been associated with increased economic burden, particularly related to criminal and legal costs.[4] Therefore, methods and technologies aimed at decreasing such abuse are being actively researched and implemented.

One such technology uses unique dosage forms that are meant to decrease the abuse potential of certain medications such as opioids. Products equipped with these abuse deterrent features are commonly called abuse deterrent formulations (ADFs). It is believed that these formulations have the potential to decrease abuse without limiting access of opioid prescriptions to legitimate patients.[5] In general, ADFs lower the abuse desirability of a medication by preventing physical (e.g., crushing, chewing) and chemical (e.g., drug extraction) tampering, prevent drug metabolism or binding, or incorporate aversive materials (e.g., bittering agents, mucous membrane irritants) into the product.[6] Of these, those that physically and chemically hinder tampering have become most predominant in the market. Furthermore, within this category of commercialized ADFs, we see an extensive use of high molecular weight poly(ethylene oxide) (PEO).[7] Several formulations with approved ADF labeling use technologies that employ PEO as a primary

***Corresponding author:** Hossein Omidian, Email: omidian@nova.edu

means of providing abuse deterrence. These include opioid formulations such as Oxycontin, Targiniq ER, Hysingla ER, and Arymo ER.[8]

The popular use of PEO as a pharmaceutical excipient is based on several factors. PEO is associated with a high LD_{50} value, and therefore generally considered non-toxic for oral use.[9,10] Its non-ionic structure also provides a low tendency for drug interactions when used as a matrix for drug delivery. Additionally, it can easily be formulated into solid oral dosage forms (such as tablets) due to its good compressibility and lubricity characteristics. The low melting temperature of PEO (Tm, 65 – 70°C) allows extrusion, molding, and casting of solid dosage forms containing large amounts of the polymers.[11] PEO has several other desirable properties that can explain its prevalent use in ADFs. For example, PEO is a water-soluble polymer that is available in low (as low as 100,000 Da) to very high (7,000,000 Da) molecular weights. PEO hydrates rapidly in aqueous solvents and continues to swell to a large extent to form a thick gel-like solution,[12] that is believed to deter abuse by injection. Therefore, higher molecular weight PEOs are often used in ADFs to produce enhanced viscosities needed for abuse deterrence. PEO also shows pH-independent hydration, meaning it will provide viscosity in many different types of solvents that abusers may use for extraction processes. However, high molecular weight PEO solutions have been shown to exhibit some shear thinning behavior at high shear rates.[13] Since high shear stresses can occur when a PEO solution is aspirated into a syringe, abusers may still find it easy to abuse by injection despite a high viscous appearance. Furthermore, the ease of injecting a PEO solution is also evident by other studies showing parenteral drug delivery applications and injectable in-situ gel-forming systems based on PEO.[14,15] It is also known that the rheology of PEO solutions is largely influenced by hydrogen bonding in the solvent, as well as between the solvent and polymer.[16] Consequently, different solvents used during abuse may have variations in polarity or electrolyte concentrations that may significantly affect the rheological properties of aqueous PEO solutions. Even more, temperature can also influence the viscosity of PEO solutions. The effects of these solution variables are discussed further in the results section of this paper.

In terms of abuse deterrence, PEO has also been used to increase the mechanical strength of tablet dosage forms through thermal processing. For example, PEO-based matrix tablets can be exposed to a heat curing process after compression or manufactured directly using hot melt extrusion. Here, curing is a process where the temperature of the compressed tablets is brought up close to the melting temperature of the excipient polymer(s). Upon cooling, the polymer solidifies and imparts a plastic-like effect to the tablets with improved mechanical strength. Thermally processed PEO tablets are highly resistant to crushing, chewing, and grinding by common household instruments (e.g., blenders, coffee grinders, and hammer). The effectiveness of this thermal curing process is perhaps best highlighted by the prescription opioid OxyContin® ER. The reformulated version of this product currently has the widest market coverage, and its post-marketing data suggests a significant intervention to abuse.[17-19]

PEO used in hot melt extrusion is generally supplied with some required amounts of antioxidant (e.g., butylated hydroxytoluene) due to its susceptibility to thermo-oxidative degradation.[20,21] Temperature controlled manufacturing processes can be used to mitigate this process. However, in the realm of abuse, there will be no limit as to how long or at what high temperatures abusers may tamper with the medication. Abusers have been known to use microwares, stoves, and other heating devices to degrade the PEO polymer structure, and hence defeat its abuse deterrence properties.

Since most current ADFs are PEO-based and thermally manufactured, we aimed to investigate major factors during this process that may have the most significant effect on the final abuse deterrent properties of such a product. The objective of this study was therefore to analyze the effects of certain formulation and processing factors on the integrity of PEO-based compositions in terms of their abuse deterrence performance. This was done using a 2-level full factorial design with four chosen factors related to a curing process: 1) curing temperature, 2) curing time, 3) type of antioxidant, and 4) antioxidant percent. We measured abuse deterrence in terms of the effects of these parameters on solution viscosity (extraction potential), mechanical strength (crush resistance), and thermal behavior/stability (resistance to drug volatilization) of tablet compacts.

Materials and Methods

PEO (Sentry™ Polyox™ WSR-303) with a Mol. Wt. of 7,000,000 Da was obtained from Dow Chemical Inc. (Midland, MI, USA). Ascorbic acid and butylated hydroxytoluene were obtained from Amresco LLC. (Solon, OH, USA) and Sigma-Aldrich Inc. (St. Luis, MO, USA), respectively. Ultrapure water (≈ 18 MΩcm) from in-house Milli–Q® system (Bedford, MA, USA) was used for all aqueous solutions. All other chemicals were of analytical grade, and used as received.

Factorial design

In this study, a 2-level full factorial design with 4 factors was chosen. Three of the factors were continuous (*i.e.,* curing time, curing temperature, % antioxidant), and one was categorical (*i.e.,* antioxidant type). Therefore, a 2^4 full factorial experimental design where each factor was investigated at two levels (low and high) was generated. Each factor level and type were chosen based on preliminary experiments. Additionally, center points (one for each categorical factor) were also incorporated into the design to detect possible curvature in the fitted data. Three response variables (*i.e.,* viscosity, surface melting temperature, % particles >850 μm) were chosen to be measured for each run as a measure of abuse deterrence performance. Stepwise regression analysis of the factorial design was performed using Minitab 18.1 software to determine the main effects and possible interactions between factors. The stepwise regression procedure we selected systematically adds to the model the most significant variables and removes the least significant variables. Using no hierarchy restrictions, this process stops when all variables that are not in the model have *p*-values that are greater than that specified (i.e., $\alpha = 0.05$).

Preparation of Tablet Compacts

To eliminate the effects of several processing excipients, direct compression tablets were made of only PEO with or without an antioxidant to a total weight of 200 mg. Based on the amounts dictated in the experimental design, a physical mixture of either 0%, 1%, or 2% antioxidant (ascorbic acid (AA) or butylated hydroxytoluene (BHT) was combined with PEO. The powder mixtures were then compressed into tablets using a single station Carver press (Carver Inc., IN, USA) with a ½ inch diameter die and standard concave tooling at a compression force of 2000 lb. We refer to these compressed powder mixtures as tablet compacts in this paper. It should be noted that the PEO used in these experiments already contained 100-500 ppm BHT as claimed by the manufacturer.[22]

Thermal Curing

Each tablet compact was subjected to curing at various temperatures and time based on the factorial design. The curing step was performed inside an air recirculated oven with each tablet compact returned to room temperature before any experiments were conducted.

Evaluation and Characterization of Tablet Compacts

Viscosity Measurements

Tablet compacts were broken into fragments and dissolved in an appropriate amount of water to obtain a 1% w/v solution. Viscosities of the resultant solutions were measured using a cone and plate rheometer (Brookfield DV-III Ultra) at a shear rate of 300 sec^{-1} for 40 sec. We used viscosity values as an indicator of abuse deterrence via extraction for subsequent injection. The greater the viscosity, the greater resistance to syringeability was presumed.

Surface Melting Temperature

After curing, surface shavings from the tablet compacts were obtained for thermal analysis. Thermograms of the shavings were obtained using differential scanning calorimeter (DSC 4000, Perkin Elmer). Briefly, 10 mg of sample was weighed in a flat-bottomed aluminum pan and placed in the furnace. The sample was subjected to a gradual temperature increment and decrement cycle at the rate of 10°C/min from 25 to 250°C under a nitrogen gas purge (20 mL/min) to maintain an inert environment. The melting point was used as an indicator of solid state thermal stability and likelihood of drug volatilization. High thermal melting temperature was assumed to be associated with greater prevention of crushing and degradation of the product in the solid state.

Mechanical Strength

The resistance of cured tablet compacts to particle size reduction (mechanical strength) was determined using a high shear grinder (MicroMill® II, SP Scienceware Inc., NJ, USA). Each sample was placed alone in the mill and subjected to a steel blade revolving at full speed (≈10,000 rpm) for 60 seconds. Immediately following grinding, the contents were sieved to determine particle size distribution via sieve analysis. We considered the percent of fragments greater than 850 µm as an indication of crush resistance by commonly available household comminution practices.[23] We therefore used "% of fragments >850 µm" throughout the paper as an indicator of tablet compact mechanical strength. The higher the percentage of larger particles (>850 µm), the greater is the resistance to crushing, chewing, and grinding.

PEO Powder Thermal Degradation Properties

To further characterize the thermal properties of PEO, the following studies were performed on PEO powder.

FTIR Analysis

Infrared spectroscopy (FTIR Spectrum 100, Perkin Elmer) was used to observe any structural changes that may be occurring during the curing step. Spectra were obtained between wavelengths 650 and 4000 cm^{-1} on PEO powders that were exposed to different hot-air temperatures (80, 110, 150, and 180°C) for 1 hour.

DSC Analysis

DSC experiments were conducted using PEO powder to observe thermal behavior and degradation during heating in the presence of nitrogen and air using the same method as described previously.

Viscosity Analysis

Viscosities of 2% w/v aqueous solutions of non-heated and heat-treated PEO powder samples using the cone and plate rheometer procedure as previously described were obtained to observe any loss of viscosity caused by thermal degradation. Furthermore, the effect of solution temperature on the viscosity of PEO solutions was also performed using 0.5, 1, 2, 2.5, and 5% w/v PEO aqueous solutions at solution temperatures of 25, 50, and 90°C.

Results and Discussion

The influence of two formulation factors (antioxidant type and concentration) and two processing factors (curing temperature and curing time) on the final abuse deterrence performance of PEO-based tablets was evaluated using ANOVA and factorial plot graphs. The graphs included main effect, interaction, cube, and Pareto. Results for all runs are shown in Table 1.

Table 1. Full factorial design matrix and response parameter results

Run Order	Anti-oxidant Type	Anti-oxidant (%)	Curing Temp (°C)	Curing Time (min)	Viscosity (cP)	Surface melting temp (°C)	% of tablet fragments >850 μm
12	AA	2	25	180	2.4	76.89	64.25
2	AA	0	25	30	63	78.67	89.76
11	BHT	2	25	180	0	76.36	49.45
10	AA	0	25	180	2.18	74.45	58.28
1	BHT	0	25	30	58.64	80.89	83.77
4	AA	2	25	30	33.13	78.29	59.3
3	BHT	2	25	30	63	77.74	55.44
9	BHT	0	25	180	0.43	76.85	62.69
18	AA	1	87.5	105	8.5	69.82	34.67
17	BHT	1	87.5	105	2.83	71.55	68.84
7	BHT	2	150	30	2.18	71.22	62.88
8	AA	2	150	30	0.43	70.48	60.51
5	BHT	0	150	30	28.99	72.79	81.63
16	AA	2	150	180	83.71	76.65	86.36
6	AA	0	150	30	106.6	68.4	92.57
14	AA	0	150	180	33.13	62.42	77.49
15	BHT	2	150	180	2.83	74.41	86.15
13	BHT	0	150	180	54.5	65.58	76.24

Analysis of Factorial Design

For our 2^4 full factorial experiment, it would be possible for each response variable to have a model fit containing a mean term, four main effect terms, six two-factor interaction n terms, four three-factor interaction terms, and a four-factor interaction term (16 parameters). With this high number of terms, and the difficulty of interpreting higher order interaction terms existing at significant levels, a stepwise approach was chosen. The stepwise approach starts with a simple model having only the mean, and then adds or removes terms in a "stepwise" manner. Variables were deleted from the model if they had p-values greater than 0.05 or kept if their p-values was less than or equal to 0.05. This was done to keep only those factors in the model, which had the most significant main effects and interactions.

ANOVA results for each model showed not all factors and interaction terms were significant. Pareto charts showing only the significant terms and their relative importance for each model can be seen in Figure 1. The length of the horizontal lines in the charts are representative of the factors difference from zero. The vertical reference line indicates the critical value (p = 0.05), where a bar extending to the right indicates its significance.

The top graph in Figure 1 shows curing temperature and percent antioxidant were the most significant main effect factors influencing surface melting temperatures along with antioxidant type. Additionally, three 2-way interaction effects were also represented. For example, the surface melting temperature is also influenced by the relationship (interaction) between the type of antioxidant chosen and curing temperature, percent antioxidant and curing time, and percent antioxidant and curing temperature. These types of interactions would be expected since surface melting temperature might be affected, for example, not only by the percent of antioxidant but also the time or temperature of the curing process.

Similar to above, the middle graph in Figure 1 shows the response variables for viscosity. In this case, curing temperature and type of antioxidant were the only main effect variables shown to be significant. Furthermore, the type of antioxidant and percent antioxidant were the only 2-way interactions most influencing viscosity. In this case, the more ascorbic acid in the formula the lower the resultant viscosity compared to BHT. In the final graph of Figure 1, we see only a 4-way interaction for the model defining % of fragments >850 μm, which is challenging to interpret meaningfully.

Polynomial equations represented by the significant terms and interacts for all models are shown in Table 2. These functions represent how the independent variables and their interactions influence the response tested. The positive or negative value of each coefficient, along with its relative value, dictate how much of an increase or decrease will occur in the parameter being measured. The R^2 values representing the variations explained by the models were well fit for surface melting (91.13%) and less for viscosity (70.41%). The closeness of the values between R^2 and predicted R^2 for surface melting temperature shows how well the model predicts the response. However, the larger difference between these variables for viscosity indicates the likelihood the model is only predicting the observed data and not that of the true population. The ability of the model to fit the data from fragments >850 μm was very low (40.15%) and not relevant.

Additionally, the residual errors were partitioned into pure error, curvature, and/or lack of fit. The use of center points in the design allowed us to determine curvature in the fitted data. Curvature occurs when the mean response is greater or less than the corner points. While the lack of fit sum of squares, encompasses the effect of omitted interaction terms. We can see that for viscosity, curvature is suspected due to the low *p*-value and may explain why the model is not very predicative.

Table 2. Polynomial regression equations for response variables

Response	Equation	Model Summary			
		S	R-sq	R-sq (adj)	R-sq (pred)
Surface Melting Temp	= 73.539 - 1.028 ANTOXDT + 2.544 % ANTOXDT - 2.569 Curing temp - 1.994 ANTOXDT*Curing temp + 1.306 % ANTOXDT*Curing temp + 1.844 % ANTOXDT*Curing time	1.817	91.13%	86.30%	75.03%
Viscosity	= 25.68 - 14.40 ANTOXDT - 16.99 Curing temp- 11.35 ANTOXDT*% ANTOXDT + 42.1 Ct Pt	20.940	70.41%	61.31%	27.85%
% Fragments >850	=69.46- 10.28 ANTOXDT* % ANTOXDT*Curing temp*Curing time	12.553	40.15%	36.41%	23.85%

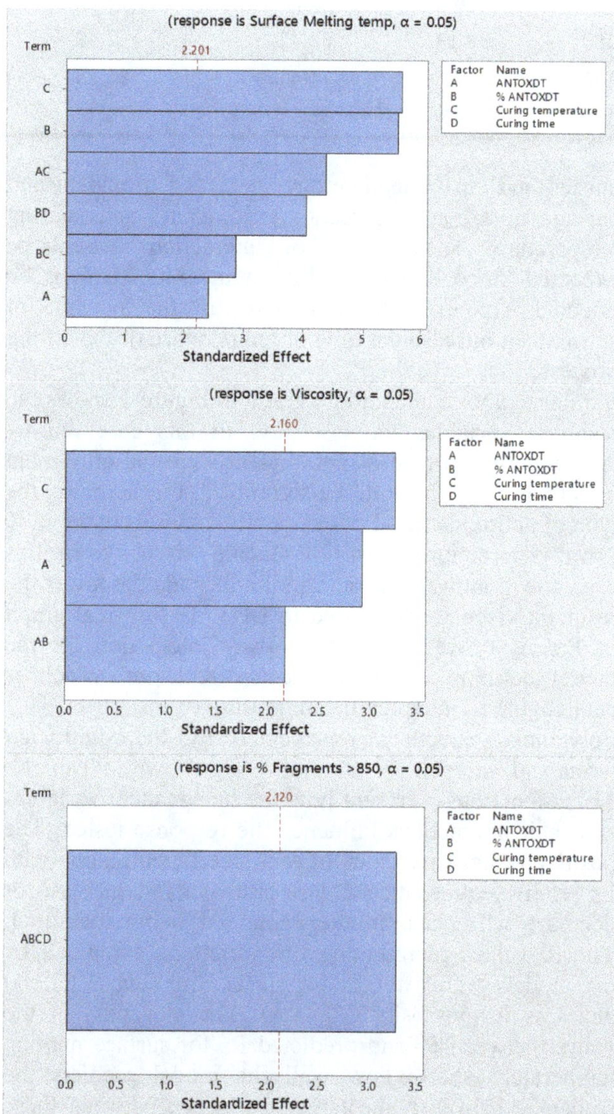

Figure 1. Pareto Charts of standardized effects

Surface melting Temperature

The temperature at which scrapings from the surface of the tablet compacts in the experimental design began to melt was used to assess thermal stability and as a way of measuring resistance to drug volatilization. For volatilization, we are assuming a soften or melted polymer would release drug easier when heated under abuse conditions used for this type of abuse. A plot of main factor effects for surface melting are shown in Figure 2. Main effect plots help in understanding how the response is affected by varying only one factor while keeping others constant. Main effect is indicated when average response changes across the levels of a factor. The main effect plot is created by plotting response against all levels of factors. If a line connecting the mean responses at factor levels is horizontal (parallel to X axis), it shows absence of main effect. However, if the line is not horizontal, and greater the slope of the line is, greater is the magnitude of the main effect.[24,25]

The significant main factors were antioxidant type, antioxidant percentage, and curing temperature. From Figure 2, we see that BHT is associated with higher surface melting temperatures compared to AA. Additionally, a higher percent of antioxidant will rise to a higher melting temperature. Since the antioxidant is used to prevent polymer degradation, a higher percent would likely result in a higher temperature of melting as the polymer molecular weight is better preserved. The beneficial effects of BHT on PEO stability over AA indicates that the primary source of oxidation reaction occurring on PEO at higher temperature are free radicals rather than oxygen. Curing temperature was also shown to be significant, meaning if PEO has been subjected to a thermal process, its melting temperature on re-heating (during abuse) would be less. This might suggest that ADFs may not need to be thermally treated to prevent melting, extraction, and drug volatilization. However, mechanical strength would likely be lower in such products. The Pareto chart for surface melting shows that 3 main effect terms (antioxidant type, antioxidant percent, and curing temperature) were significant, with curing temperature and percent antioxidant have greatest effects. However, the regression equation for surface melting shows that the impact of these to be minimal based on the low values of the coefficients. This may explain why the R^2 values are high. The highest interaction coefficient between antioxidant type and curing temperature (-1.994) may be explained based on the stability of the antioxidants at higher temperatures. The positive coefficients for the interaction of curing time and temperature with percent of antioxidant are also likely to be based on the lower degradation when lower temperatures and time are used along with the higher percent of antioxidant. When a response at one factor level depends on the levels of other factors, it shows an indication of an interaction. Interactions are critically important as they can reinforce or cancel out the main effects of factors. Thus, main effect cannot be interpreted without considering interaction effects.

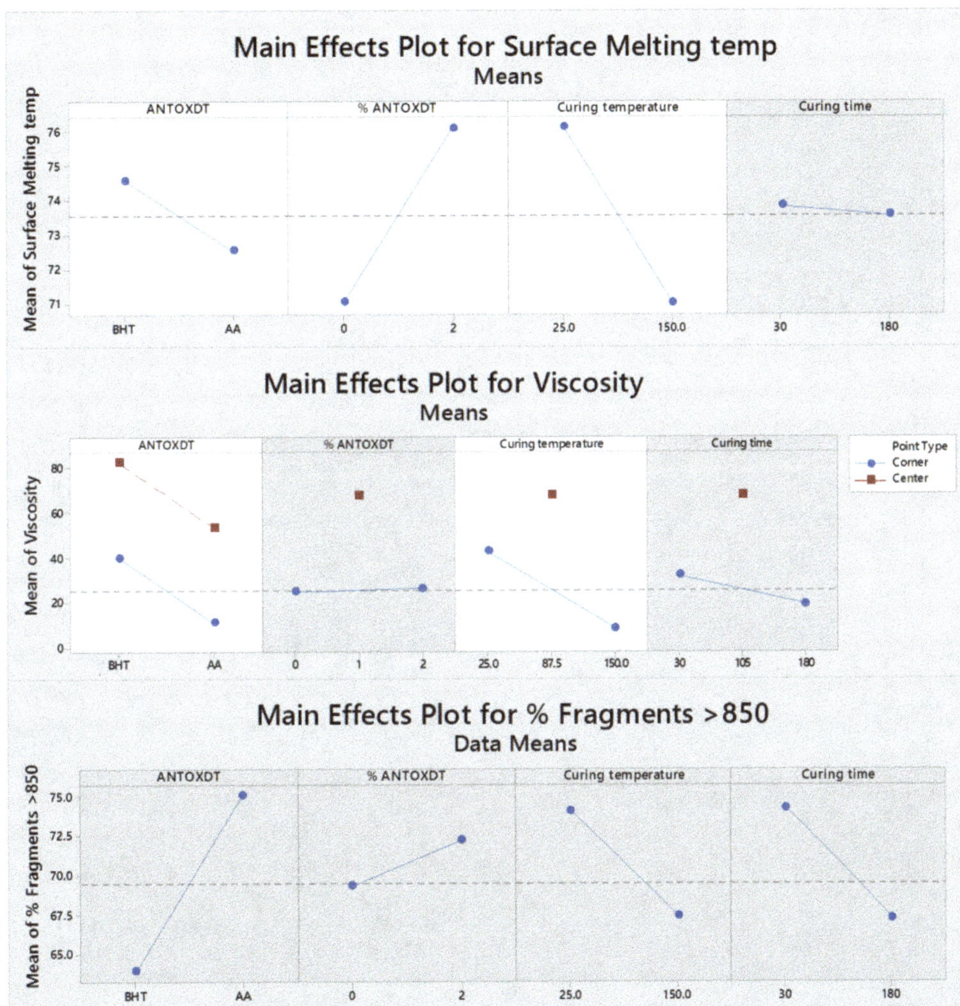

Figure 2. Main effect plots for response variables (a gray background represents a term not in the model)

The changes PEO experiences during a thermal event were also visually noticeable when exposed to heat curing having no additional antioxidant added. At high temperatures, the white polymer began to turn into a pale yellow starting at 150°C, indicating oxidative degradation. The pale yellow turned noticeably darker for samples exposed to 180°. Additionally, as the polymer began to soften and melt, the cohesive forces between powder particles were also increased and became more rigid on cooling. Furthermore, DSC analysis of PEO samples which were once heated (pre-heat treated) at different temperatures, showed gradual shifts in melting point peaks towards lower temperatures. The peak melting temperatures for these samples pretreated at 80°, 110°, 150°, and 180°C were 72.48°, 71.07°, 65.20°, and 54.65°C, respectively. Melting peak onset as well as heat of fusion were also decreased with an increase in temperature of the treatment. Therefore, it may be beneficial to manufacture an ADF composed of PEO at the lower temperatures to maintain greater resistance to thermal methods of tampering.

Further analysis via FTIR spectra of heat treated PEO samples showed appearance of a degradation peak at a wavelength of 1720 cm^{-1} for temperatures $\geq$ 150°C (Figure 3 (A)). This peak was absent in the spectrum at 110°C (Figure 3 (B)), whereas it shows prominent appearance at 150 and 180°C (Figures 3 (-C, -D, -E). Intensity of this peak was increased with increase in temperature as well as the duration of heat exposure (Figures 3 (-B, -C, -D). These observations provide significant evidence for PEO's oxidative degradation at high temperatures and correlate with the DSC results. Our experimental design used 180°C as a high range curing temperature and may explain why the results may not fit well to our models.

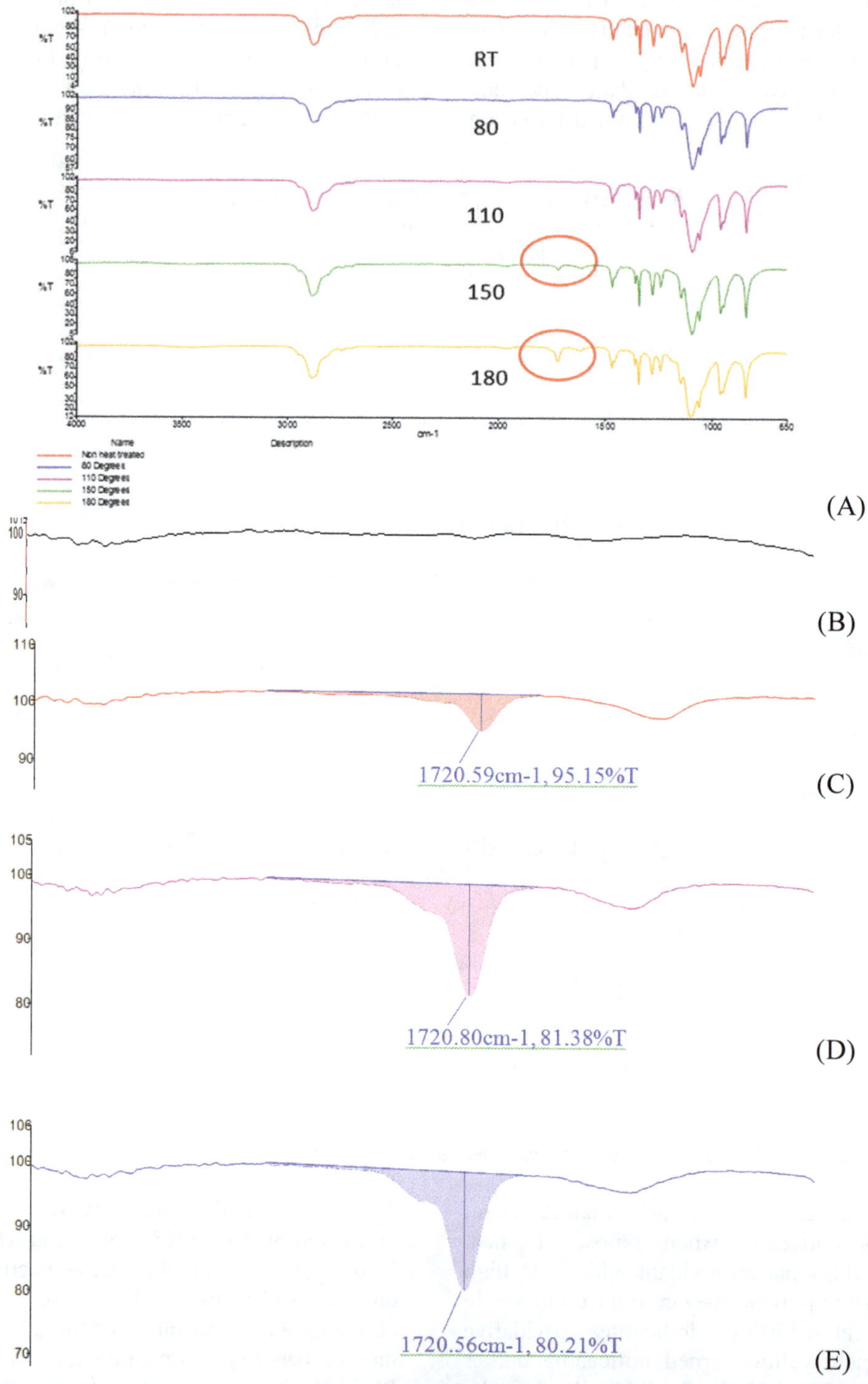

Figure 3. FTIR spectra of heat treated PEO (Polyox^{TM}, WSR coagulant) in solid state indicating oxidative degradation at higher temperatures (A), Magnification of degradation peak of PEO sample heat treated at (B) 110°C (B) 150°C, (C) 180°C for 1 hr and (D) 150°C for 3hrs at 1720 cm^{-1}

Viscosity

The main effect plot for viscosity (Figure 2) shows the most prominent factors (greatest slope) affecting viscosity are curing temperature and type of antioxidant. This would be expected as higher temperatures would lead to greater polymer degradation and shorter end-to-end distance for the polymer chains. Therefore, processing at a higher curing temperature (or abuse at higher temperatures) would lead to lower viscosity of the resultant aqueous extract. Additionally, the presence of BHT in the formula seems to impart higher viscosity compared to AA with the concentration effect not being significant. However, the curing time had less effect on viscosity compared to the temperature used during curing. The impact of these factors determined using stepwise regression show only curing temperature and antioxidant type along with one interaction factor to be significant. The interaction effect may occur since having more antioxidant would allow for greater stability of the polymer at higher temperatures as well as contribute to higher viscosity. The main effect plot also shows that curvature may exist for this model as was evidenced by the ANOVA table showing significance for curvature (p = 0.019). The significant p-value for curvature strongly suggests that a linear model would not be most appropriate, and more points would be needed in the model completely describe the equation curvature. The regression equation provided by the software with the design space, includes a center point. This indicates that a particular curing temperature and time may exist where the antioxidant would have the most significant effect on viscosity of solutions made from the crushed tablet compacts.

Other factors not considered in the model, which can still affect the viscosity experienced by an abuser, are the type of solution being used and the temperature of the solution being extracted. The effects of these variables can be seen in Figure 4. Figure 4 (A) shows a very viscous 5% w/v PEO aqueous solution at ambient room temperature and when heated to 95°C, Figure 4 (B). This mimics a common practice by abusers in which a tablet extract solution is heated (e.g., lighter, candle) in order to enhance drug solubility prior to intravenous abuse. Figure 4 (C) shows the same concentration of PEO but made using pure ethanol instead of water as the extraction solvent. This time we see complete loss of viscosity as the polymer precipitates out of solution, as can be seen on the bottom of the glass vial. In Figure 4 (D), even though the 5% w/v aqueous solution of PEO at room temperature appears viscous, it could still be drawn into a syringe with an attached needle. This provides evidence that high solution viscosity may not be an effective deterrent for parenteral abuse.

Temperature dependent viscosity was also further influenced by the concentration of PEO in solution. The viscosity of PEO solutions (made from non-heat treated PEO) was found to increase non-linearly with increasing concentrations (i.e., 0.5, 1, 2, 3, and 5%). Furthermore, for the same concentration, the viscosity was found to be lower as the temperature was increased. When a 2% (w/v) PEO solution was made using a heat-treated sample, we saw a gradual decrease in solution viscosity up to a solution temperature of 110°C (Figure 5). As the temperature was further increased from 110 to 150°C, a sharp drop of about 97.9% in viscosity was observed, which continued upon heating further to 180°C.

Results of these studies show that PEO undergoes oxidative degradation especially at elevated temperatures. The oxidative degradation presumably resulted in breaking up of long linear chains in the polymer structure into small fragments, which resulted in the loss of polymer viscosity. These findings corroborate various stability and degradation studies previously conducted on PEO.[20,21,26-28]

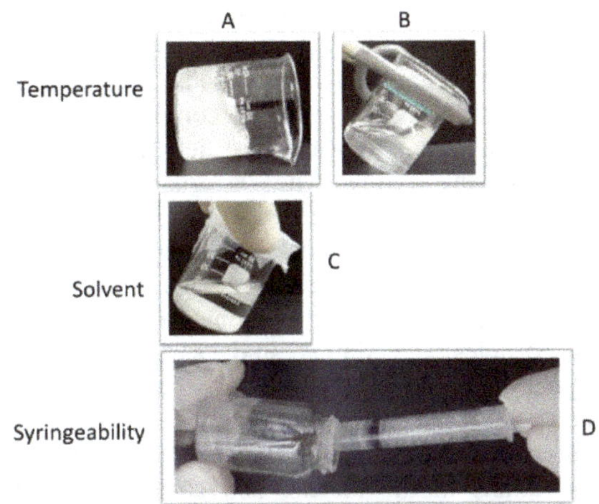

Figure 4. Susceptibility of a 2% w/v PEO solutions. Almost an 80% drop in viscosity was observed from at (A) ambient room temperature to (B) 95°C. (C) A complete precipitation was observed in ethanol. (D) The aqueous polymer (A) was easily syringeable at room temperature

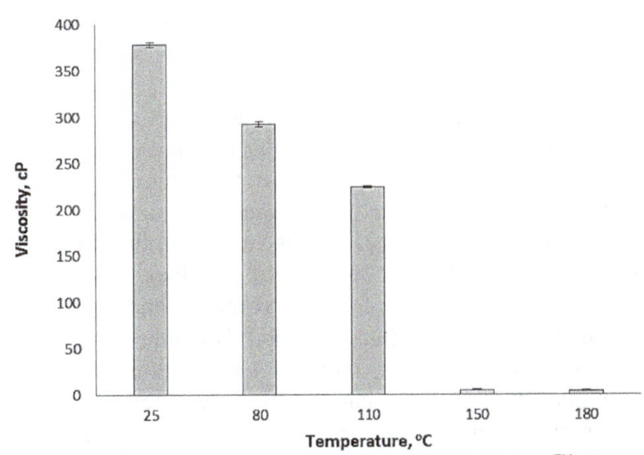

Figure 5. Drop in aqueous viscosity of PEO (Polyox™, WSR, coagulant) treated at different temperatures (n=3)

Mechanical Strength

Determining main factors that may influence mechanical strength (*i.e.,* % fragments >850μm) of a tablet compact showed no significant results of the factors we tested (Figure 2). Furthermore, the only interaction noted was a 4-way interaction that is hard to interpret at this high level (Figure 1). This resulted in a poor linear fit for the model at R^2 of 40.15%. It may be likely we have not chosen factors that would have great impact on the mechanical strength after curing. Since thermal processing is used to impart mechanical strength to the polymer upon cooling, other mechanisms may also be involved. Furthermore, the high amount of PEO in the cured tablets made them very resistant to our particle size reduction efforts. We therefore believe the testing method used may have such a large variability that the results were not conclusive. From our prior experience developing methods to test crush resistance, we have noticed the standard error in such measurements has been wide despite controlling several variables. A separate study also suggested that method of comminution used had the most prominent effect on tablet fragment size when powerful electric instruments such as high shear grinders are used.[23] Given this, we may conclude that grinding tablet compacts and further sieve analysis may not be the best determinant for such tamper resistant testing. The use of dynamic image analysis to assess the particle size of PEO based tablets crushed using a coffee grinder did show that the biggest factor affecting particle size was the curing temperature; higher curing temperatures and times resulted in more coarse particles.[29] A similar study assessing the abuse deterrence of cured PEO based formulations found that as the percent of PEO increased, so did the crush resistance.[30] However, the antioxidant type, antioxidant concentrations in the tablets, and curing temperatures were kept constant.

In summary, this study used a full factorial design of experiments to determine the impact of 4 different processing factors on the final abuse deterrent properties of a product having PEO as a matrix base. We looked at major factors and interactions of these effects on the crush resistance (mechanical strength), solution viscosity of the extracting medium, and final melting temperature of the polymer-based tablet compacts. The crush resistance testing was not adequate to report meaningful results. However, the other results can most easily be shown in 3D cube plots (Figure 6), which represent average responses of melting temperature, and viscosity at critical points. Critical points in cube plots are the points where all factors have limiting values.[25,31,32] Two cube plots were created for each response and represent two different curing times, 30 and 180 min. From the response cube plot of melting temperature, we can conclude that when curing is attempted at low temperatures, antioxidants do not impact the stability of the product. However, when the curing occurs at higher temperatures and for a longer period, the antioxidant BHT favors the surface melting at higher temperatures. The response cube plot for viscosity shows how the presence of BHT with or without heating also creates higher viscosity. Furthermore, the center points of this plot do not agree linearly as was previously discussed, making this model not ideal for full prediction. However, our results show that using BHT as an antioxidant and low curing temperature as well as shorter curing time would equip the solid dosage form with maximum resistance to abuse from tampering methods involving heat.

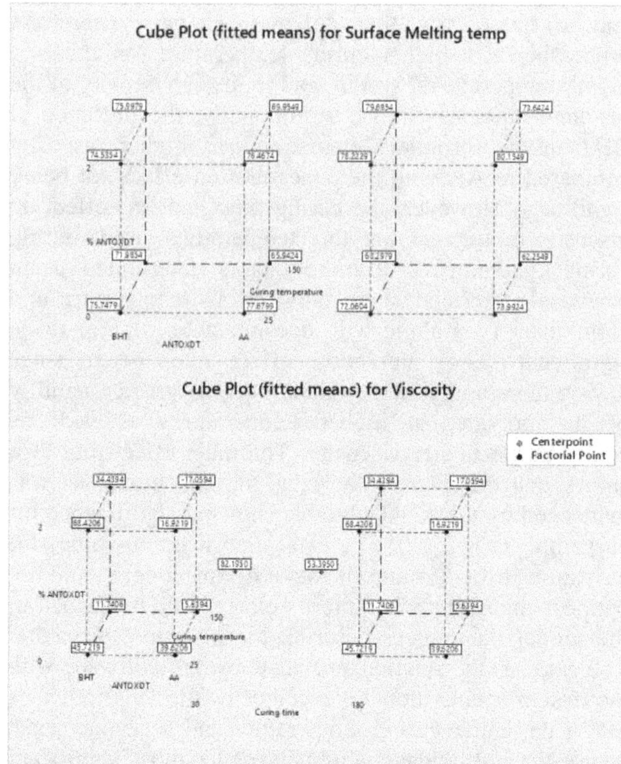

Figure 6. Cube plots for surface melting temperature (*top*) and viscosity (*bottom*)

Conclusion

Our data shows that high molecular weight PEO undergoes an oxidative degradation process at a rapid rate especially at high temperatures. This affects many aspects of polymer integrity particularly related to its deterrence performance. While heat confers the mechanical strength to the polymer, at the same time it diminishes its physical stability and solution state viscosity. The experimental studies showed that exposure to a high temperature for a long duration even in the presence of antioxidants can severely hamper polymer deterrence performance in solid and solution states.

Acknowledgments

This article is based on research performed as part of a Ph.D. thesis written by Yogesh Joshi.

Conflict of Interest

The authors declare that there is no conflict of interest regarding the publication of this article.

References

1. Kantor ED, Rehm CD, Haas JS, Chan AT, Giovannucci EL. Trends in prescription drug use among adults in the united states from 1999-2012. *JAMA* 2015;314(17):1818-31. doi: 10.1001/jama.2015.13766
2. Hughes A, Williams M R, Lipari R N, Bose J, Copello EAP, Kroutil LA. Prescription drug use and misuse in

the united states: Results from the 2015 national survey on drug use and health. NSDUH Data Review; 2016; Available from: https://www.samhsa.gov/data/sites/default/files/NSDUH-FFR2-2015/NSDUH-FFR2-2015.htm#appa.
3. National Institute on Drug Abuse. Misuse of prescription drugs. 2016 [2017 June 3]; Available from: https://www.drugabuse.gov/publications/research-reports/misuse-prescription-drugs.
4. Birnbaum HG, White AG, Schiller M, Waldman T, Cleveland JM, Roland CL. Societal costs of prescription opioid abuse, dependence, and misuse in the united states. *Pain Med* 2011;12(4):657-67. doi: 10.1111/j.1526-4637.2011.01075.x
5. Webster LR, Markman J, Cone EJ, Niebler G. Current and future development of extended-release, abuse-deterrent opioid formulations in the united states. *Postgrad Med* 2017;129(1):102-10. doi: 10.1080/00325481.2017.1268902
6. Mastropietro DJ, Omidian H. Abuse-deterrent formulations: Part 1 - development of a formulation-based classification system. *Expert Opin Drug Metab Toxicol* 2015;11(2):193-204. doi: 10.1517/17425255.2015.979786
7. Bulloch M. Abuse-deterrent opioids: A primer for pharmacists. 2015 [2017 June 3]; Available from: http://www.pharmacytimes.com/print.php?url=/contributor/marilyn-bulloch-pharmd-bcps/2015/10/abuse-deterrent-opioids-a-primer-for-pharmacists.
8. Litman RS, Pagán OH, Cicero TJ. Abuse-deterrent opioid formulations. *Anesthesiology* 2018;128(5):1015-26. doi: 10.1097/ALN.0000000000002031
9. Rowe RC, Sheskey PJ, Cook WG, Fenton ME. Handbook of pharmaceutical excipients. 7th ed. London: Pharmaceutical Press; 2006.
10. Safety data sheet polyox^{tm} wsr coagulant. The Dow Chemical Company; 2015 [2017 March 25]; Available from: http://www.dow.com/en-us/products/POLYOXNF.
11. Dow Chemicals. Msds polyox water-soluble resins. 2002 [2017 March 25]; Available from: http://msdssearch.dow.com/PublishedLiteratureDOWCOM/dh_0031/0901b8038003 1a4a.pdf?filepath=/326-00001.pdf&fromPage=GetDoc.
12. Palmer D, Levina M, Farrell T, Ali R. The influence of hydro-alcoholic media on drug release. *Pharm Technol* 2011;35(7):50-8.
13. Ebagninin KW, Benchabane A, Bekkour K. Rheological characterization of poly(ethylene oxide) solutions of different molecular weights. *J Colloid Interface Sci* 2009;336(1):360-7. doi: 10.1016/j.jcis.2009.03.014
14. Dhawan S, Dhawan K, Varma M, Sinha VR. Applications of poly(ethylene oxide) in drug delivery systems part ii. 2005 [2017 March 2017]; Available from: http://images.alfresco.advanstar.com/alfresco_images/pharma/2014/08/22/678845a2-b24c-4c47-bc3a-e711da795690/article-178636.pdf.
15. Gutowska A, Jeong B, Jasionowski M. Injectable gels for tissue engineering. *Anat Rec* 2001;263(4):342-9. doi: 10.1002/ar.1115
16. Briscope B, Luckham P, Zhu S. Rheological properties of poly(ethylene oxide) aqueous solutions. *J Appl Polym Sci* 1998;70(3):419-29.
17. Cicero TJ, Ellis MS, Surratt HL. Effect of abuse-deterrent formulation of oxycontin. *N Engl J Med* 2012;367(2):187-9. doi: 10.1056/NEJMc1204141
18. Coplan PM, Chilcoat HD, Butler SF, Sellers EM, Kadakia A, Harikrishnan V, et al. The effect of an abuse-deterrent opioid formulation (oxycontin) on opioid abuse-related outcomes in the postmarketing setting. *Clin Pharmacol Ther* 2016;100(3):275-86. doi: 10.1002/cpt.390
19. Dart RC, Surratt HL, Cicero TJ, Parrino MW, Severtson SG, Bucher-Bartelson B, et al. Trends in opioid analgesic abuse and mortality in the united states. *N Engl J Med* 2015;372(3):241-8. doi: 10.1056/NEJMsa1406143
20. Choukourov A, Grinevich A, Polonskyi O, Hanus J, Kousal J, Slavinska D, et al. Vacuum thermal degradation of poly(ethylene oxide). *J Phys Chem B* 2009;113(10):2984-9. doi: 10.1021/jp8107107
21. McGary CW Jr. Degradation of poly(ethylene oxide). *Int J Polym Sci* 1960;46(147):51-7. doi: 10.1002/pol.1960.1204614705
22. Dow Chemical Company. Technical data: Sentry polyox water-soluble resins. [2017 Jun 15]; Available from: https://dowac.custhelp.com/ci/fattach/get/57278/0/filename/SENTRY+POLYOX+WSR+Technical+Information+on+Stability.pdf.
23. Muppalaneni S, Mastropietro DJ, Omidian H. Crush resistance and insufflation potential of poly(ethylene oxide)-based abuse deterrent formulations. *Expert Opin Drug Deliv* 2016;13(10):1375-82. doi: 10.1080/17425247.2016.1211638
24. Halford GS, Baker R, McCredden JE, Bain JD. How many variables can humans process? *Psychol Sci* 2005;16(1):70-6. doi: 10.1111/j.0956-7976.2005.00782.x
25. Kukreja A, Chopra P, Aggarwal A, Khanna P. Application of full factorial design for optimization of feed rate of stationary hook hopper. *IJMO* 2011;1(3):205-9. doi: 10.7763/IJMO.2011.V1.36
26. Duval M, Gross E. Degradation of poly(ethylene oxide) in aqueous solutions by ultrasonic waves. *Macromolecules* 2013;46(12):4972-7. doi: 10.1021/ma400737g
27. Pielichowski K, Flejtuch K. Non-oxidative thermal degradation of poly(ethylene oxide): Kinetic and thermoanalytical study. *J Anal Appl Pyrolysis* 2005;73(1):131-8. doi: 10.1016/j.jaap.2005.01.003
28. Vijayalakshmi SP, Chakraborty J, Madras G. Thermal and microwave-assisted oxidative

degradation of poly(ethylene oxide). *J Appl Polym Sci* 2005;96(6):2090-6. doi: 10.1002/app.21676
29. Rahman Z, Yang Y, Korang-Yeboah M, Siddiqui A, Xu X, Ashraf M, et al. Assessing impact of formulation and process variables on in-vitro performance of directly compressed abuse deterrent formulations. *Int J Pharm* 2016;502(1-2):138-50. doi: 10.1016/j.ijpharm.2016.02.029
30. Rahman Z, Zidan AS, Korang-Yeboah M, Yang Y, Siddiqui A, Shakleya D, et al. Effects of excipients and curing process on the abuse deterrent properties of directly compressed tablets. *Int J Pharm* 2017;517(1-2):303-11. doi: 10.1016/j.ijpharm.2016.12.015
31. What is a cube plot? Minitab Inc; 2016 [2017 March 19]; Available from: http://support.minitab.com/en-us/minitab/17/topic-library/modeling-statistics/using-fitted-models/graphs/what-is-a-cube-plot.
32. Cube plot- factorial designs. Minitab Inc; 2007 [2017 March 20]; Available from: http://www.pinzhi.org/Minitab/help/Mtbsg/dofacdes/facp_030_cube_plot.htm.

23

Combined Activity of Colloid Nanosilver and *Zataria Multiflora Boiss* Essential Oil-Mechanism of Action and Biofilm Removal Activity

Maryam Shirdel[1], Hossein Tajik[1,2], Mehran Moradi[1]*

[1] *Department of Food Hygiene and Quality Control, Faculty of Veterinary Medicine, Urmia University, 1177, Urmia, West Azarbaijan, Iran.*

[2] *Department of Medicinal and Industrial Plant, Institute of Biotechnology, Urmia University, 1177 Urmia, Iran.*

Article info

Keywords:
- Antimicrobial
- Sanitizing
- Biofilm
- Essential oil
- Silver nanoparticle
- Combination

Abstract

Purpose: The aim of this study was to investigate antimicrobial and biofilm removal potential of *Zataria multiflora* essential oil (ZEO) and silver nanoparticle (SNP) alone and in combination on *Staphylococcus aureus* and *Salmonella* Typhimurium and evaluate the mechanism of action.

Methods: The minimum inhibitory concentration (MIC), and optimal inhibitory combination (OIC) of ZEO and SNP were determined according to fractional inhibitory concentration (FIC) method. Biofilm removal potential and leakage pattern of 260-nm absorbing material from the bacterial cell during exposure to the compounds were also investigated.

Results: MICs of SNP for both bacteria were the same as 25 µg/ mL. The MICs and MBCs values of ZEO were 2500 and 1250 µg/mL, respectively. The most effective OIC value for SNP and ZEO against *Salm.* Typhimurium and *Staph. aureus* were 12.5, 625 and 0.78, 1250 µg/ mL, respectively. ZEO and SNP at MIC and OIC concentrations represented a strong removal ability (>70%) on biofilm. Moreover, ZEO at MIC and OIC concentrations did a 6-log reduction of primary inoculated bacteria during 15 min contact time. The effect of ZEO on the loss of 260-nm material from the cell was faster than SNP during 15 and 60 min.

Conclusion: Combination of ZEO and SNP had significant sanitizing activity on examined bacteria which may be suitable for disinfecting the surfaces.

Introduction

Nanotechnology, the science of study and use of structures at nanoscale, is a promising tool for producing novel materials with biomedical applications. Silver nanoparticles (SNPs) has been extensively investigated in various scientific disciplines. Silver in the form of silver nitrate and silver sulfadiazine has been widely used to cure bacterial infections associated with burns. SNPs are considered as a potent antimicrobial, antifungal, antiviral and antiprotozoal compound and it is also reported to have anti-inflammatory activities.[1] Synthesis and use of SNPs as a new generation of antimicrobial agents would be a fascinating and economical tool to solve drug resistance. Microorganisms display different responses to nanoparticles which is related to differences in the bacterial structure and the composition of the cell wall.[1,2]

Essential oils (EOs), as a plant secondary metabolites, are volatile aromatic compounds extracted from different parts of plants. For centuries, EOs have been used in medicine, perfumery, cosmetics and food. They are primarily used in medicine, but in the nineteenth-century, EOs have found their importance to impart aroma and taste ingredients.[3] Lamiaceae is a family of plant with more than 230 genera, which distributed nearly worldwide. It contains many well- known species with fairly similar properties in botanical characteristics and applications, including *Thymus vulgaris*, *Thymus caramanicus*, *Zataria multiflora*, *Ziziphora clinopodioides* and *Ziziphora tenuior.*[3-5] *Zataria multiflora* Boiss is an important medicinal plant, distributed in Iran, Afghanistan, and Pakistan. The main antimicrobial compounds of *Zataria multiflora* Boiss essential oil (ZEO) are thymol, carvacrol, and p-cymene. The plant also contains tannins, flavonoids, saponins and some bitter substances.[6] Among the phenolic compounds, thymol is the most characteristic chemical substance of ZEO which founds in leaves, flowers, and roots at various amounts.[6,7] ZEO displays inhibitory activity on both gram-negative and gram-positive bacteria.[8]

The practical advantage of antimicrobial combinations has been comprehended for over 50 years. Combinations of two antimicrobial agents with a different mechanism of action, may enhance antimicrobial activity especially where resistance to a single agent develops by bacteria. Also, due to synergy or additive interaction, the combination of drugs allows utilizing lower antimicrobial concentration, reducing the harmful side effects and increasing treatment efficacy.[9] Tackling public health issues occur by the growing number of multidrug-resistant bacteria, proposes new antimicrobial formulation based on the combination of older antimicrobials with a rich source of new agents, such as natural products.[10] Simultaneous use of EOs and other antimicrobial compounds with great disinfectant properties has a high priority since using EOs in high concentrations make some unpleasant organoleptic changes in food and also on food contact surface when used as a sanitizing compound. Owing to the possible synergistic properties, combined use of EO with SNPs as a sanitizing mixture for food plant sanitation has been proposed.[11] The combined application of nanoparticles with EO has been reported.[2,12] To understand the combined antimicrobial and biofilm removal properties of SNP and ZEO, their effects on two important bacterial pathogens, *Staph aureus* and *Salm.* Typhimurium was investigated as a guideline for a possible application of formulated solution in sanitation schedule.

Materials and Methods

Silver nanoparticles solution (4000 µg/ mL with the particle size of 35 nm) was purchased from Pars Nano Nasb Co (Tehran, Iran) and sterilized by filtration through 0.22 µm filters before use. Peptone water, phosphate buffered saline (PBS), Luria-Bertani (LB) broth and agar, Agar-agar, and resazurin sodium were obtained from Sigma Chemical Co (St. Louis, MO., USA). All other chemicals were purchased from Merck (Darmstadt, Germany). The plant, *Zataria multiflora* Boiss, was purchased from local groceries. *Staph. aureus* ATCC 25923 and *Salm.* Typhimurium ATCC 14028 were obtained from the Department of Food Hygiene and Quality Control, Urmia University, Urmia, Iran.

Preparation of bacterial suspension

Staph. aureus and *Salm.* Typhimurium were grown at 37±1 °C for 18 h by transferring 10 microliters of frozen stocks (at -20 °C) into 10 mL of LB broth. Bacterial suspensions were adjusted to ~8 $\log_{10}$ CFU mL^{-1} using visible-ultraviolet spectrophotometer (Amersham Pharmacia Biotech Inc., Buckinghamshire, UK) at 600 nm (optical density: ~0.1) and confirmed by plating and counting on LB agar after 24 h incubation at 37±1 °C.

Essential oil extraction and quantification

The EO of *Zataria multiflora* Boiss (100 g) was extracted from dried aerial parts of plant using a Clevenger apparatus based on hydrodistillation procedure for 3 hours. The collected ZEO was dried over anhydrous Na_2SO_4, then filtrated and stored at 4 °C. The chemical composition of ZEOs was analyzed using a gas chromatograph (GC), as explained previously.[6]

Determination of Minimum inhibitory concentration (MIC) and minimum bactericidal concentrations (MBC)

The MICs and MBC of ZEO and SNP against both bacteria were determined in LB using broth microdilution assay in 96-wells polystyrene flat-bottomed microtitre plates based on CLSI guidelines.[13] Two-fold serial dilutions of ZEO were prepared in 0.1% peptone water containing 0.15% agar (to make a stable emulsion of EO in peptone water), whereas dilutions of SNP were made in 0.1% peptone water. The wells of a microplates with U-bottom were poured by 160 µL of LB and 20 µL of the bacterial suspension with OD_{600} = 0.1 to reach a suspension with 10^6 CFU/ mL in each well. Then, 20 µL either ZEO or SNP concentrations were added into the desired wells to achieve final concentrations of 312 to 5000 µg/ mL for ZEO and 62.5 to 2000 µg/mL for SNP. For every experiment, three controls, including LB alone, LB with bacteria and LB containing treatment agents without bacteria were used. The plate was mixed on a plate shaker at 250 rpm for 20 s and incubated at 37 ± 1 °C for 24 h. MICs were determined visually and by using 0.01% (w/v) resazurin sodium salt solution as explained previously. To determine MBCs, 10 µL from each well was inoculated into LB agar at 37 ± 1 °C for 24 h. The MBC was determined as the lowest concentration of antimicrobial agents that produces 99.99% inhibition in the initial population of microorganism. MBC: MIC ratio, which describes the relationship between the minimum *in vitro* bactericidal concentration and the MIC of antimicrobial agents, were also investigated.

Antimicrobial combination and interaction

Broth checkerboard micro-assay was carried out to evaluate the antagonistic, indifferent, additive and synergistic interactions of ZEO and SNP using the fractional inhibitory concentration (FIC) index method.[14] Eight different concentrations, 5 concentrations lower than MIC, two concentrations higher than MIC and one concentration as same as MIC of ZEO and SNP were used to design an 8 × 8 checkerboards of combinations. The microplates were prepared by dispensing 160 µL of LB and 20 µL of the logarithmic suspension of bacteria and 10 µL of different concentration of both antimicrobial agents into each well. Then, plates were kept in a plate shaker at 250 rpm for 20 s and incubated at 37 ± 1 °C for 24 h. MICs were determined visually and by resazurin reduction. MICs of the individual antimicrobials and all of the combinations were used to calculate Fractional inhibitory concentrations (FICs) of ZEO and SNP and FIC index using the following formula:

$$FIC\ of\ antibacterial \frac{MIC\ of\ antibacterial\ in\ combination}{MIC\ of\ antibacterial\ alone}$$

$$\text{FIC index (FICI)} = \text{FIC}_{\text{ZEO}} + \text{FIC}_{\text{SNP}}$$

If the FICI is < 0.5, the interaction is synergistic, if the FICI= 0.5-1, the interaction is additive, if the FICI= 1-4, the interaction is indifferent, and an FICI >4 is considered antagonistic. Optimal inhibitory combinations (OIC) is defined as the combinations producing an inhibitory effect by using the lowest concentration of one antimicrobial in combination with the other.[15]

Determination of the release of 260-nm absorbing material

260-nm absorbing material released into the supernatant was estimated according to the method described previously,[16] with some modifications. The bacterial suspension was prepared as described above. The procedure performed in 2 mL of harvested and washed cells (OD_{600nm} = 0.45) to which SNP and ZEO were added at final concentrations equivalent to their MICs and OIC and incubated in a shaker incubator (250 rpm at 37 °C). Two samples were taken at 15 and 60 min time points and centrifuged at 4000 *g* for 15 min and the absorbance was determined at 260 nm using PBS as blank. Controls containing bacterial supernatant without treatment agents and antibacterial compounds without bacteria were also prepared and analyzed.

Biofilm removal

Biofilm removal potential of both agents alone and in combination was assessed using 24-well flat-bottomed polystyrene microtiter plates according to the method explained previously with some modifications.[17] An aliquot of 200 µL of bacterial suspension with OD_{600} = 0.1 was dispensed into each well which was filled previously with 1800 µL of LB broth, using four repetitions per treatment to reach a suspension with 10^7 CFU/ mL per well. After incubation for 24 h at 37 ±1 °C, the planktonic cells in wells were then removed and the plates were washed three times with PBS and air-dried for 20 min at 23 ±2 °C. Then, 2000 µL of MIC, 2MIC and 4MIC concentrations of ZEO and SNP and their combinations (1/4 OIC, 1/2OIC, and OIC concentrations) were gently poured into the wells and incubated for 15 min at ambient temperature. The solutions were then removed and plates were washed three times with PBS and air-dried for 20 min at 23 ±2 °C. Following staining with 2 mL of 1% crystal violet (CV) (w/v) for 30 min, the contents of the wells were decanted and washed twice with tap water to remove the color excess and then allowed to air-dry for 30 min. The biomass of biofilms was quantified by solubilizing CV with 2 mL of acetic acid 33% and subsequent measuring optical absorbance (OD) at 540 nm. Wells containing LB broth and LB with bacteria without antibacterial were considered as negative and positive controls, respectively. Biofilm removal percentage was calculated as follow:

$$Reduction\ percentage = \frac{(C - B) - (T - B)}{(C - B)} \times 100$$

where C is OD_{540nm} of control wells, B is OD_{540nm} of negative controls and T is OD_{540nm} of treated wells.

Combined sanitizing activity

Sanitizing effects of ZEO and SNP combination were investigated by determining the growth of the microorganism in LB broth supplemented with different concentration of antimicrobials (1/4OIC, 1/2OIC, and OIC) to obtain optimal concentration for both compounds according to the method explained before with some modifications.[18] Bacterial cultures (1×10^7 CFU/ mL) (0.5 mL) were added to tubes containing 4.5 mL of antimicrobial agents in combination and then, tubes were incubated at 23± 2 °C for 15 min and bacterial growth was monitored by sampling (1mL) and counting the viable cells. After sampling, 1 mL aliquot were dispersed in a 9 mL neutralizing solution containing an equal volume of sodium thiosulphate 5% w/v and Tween-20 and remained for 10 min, to neutralize the subsequent activity of agents and then serial dilutions were prepared.

Statistical analysis

Each experiment was replicated in triplicate and carried out on three separate times and data were expressed as means ± S.E. Data were analyzed by analysis of variance (ANOVA, $P \leq 0.05$) using GraphPad Prism version 5.00 for Windows, GraphPad Software, San Diego California USA (www.graphpad.com).

Results

ZEO chemical analysis

As shown in Table 1, 26 different components were identified in ZEO, representing 97.23%, of total EO. General chemical profile of ZEO was characterized by an abundance concentration of thymol (44%). In addition to thymol, carvacrol (14.04%) and *p*-cymene (11.15%), as main constituents, and traces of linalool, ϒ-terpinene, and α-Pinene were also found in ZEO.

Antibacterial properties of ZEO and SNP

The inhibitory effects of ZEO and SNP alone and in combination against *Staph. aureus* and *Salm.* Typhimurium were investigated using microtiter plate assay. For *Staph. aureus*, the MIC values of ZEO and SNP were 1250 and 25 µg/mL and for *Salm.* Typhimurium the values were 2500 and 25 µg/mL, respectively. In all cases, MBC values were similar to MICs. The ZEO was found to be more effective on gram-positive than gram-negative bacteria whereas SNP displayed similar antibacterial activity on both bacteria. The MICs for SNP - ZEO combination were 0.78 and 12.5 µg/ mL against *Staph. aureus* and *Salm.* Typhimurium, respectively. ZEO-SNP combination inhibited *S. aureus* and *Salm.* Typhimurium at 625 µg/ mL. Based on the FICI scale (Table 2), the combination displayed a synergistic action on *Staph. aureus* (FICI=0.81) and *Salm.* Typhimurium (FICI= 0.75).

Loss of 260 nm absorbing material

Exposure of *Staph. aureus* and *Salm.* Typhimurium to ZEO at MIC concentrations over 15 min resulted in a significant increase in loss of 260 nm absorbing material from the bacterial cell compared with the control ($P<0.05$), indicating a stronger disruption of the cell membrane by ZEO (Figure 1, 2). Results also showed that the loss began before 15 min and continued up to 60 min. In general, loss of cytoplasmic materials by ZEO from both bacteria was faster than SNP. The leakage pattern of 260-nm absorbing material was directly linked to the sanitizing activity of both antimicrobial compounds. As shown in Figures 1 and 2, no significant release of 260 nm absorbing material with SNP- treated at MIC concentration over 15 min for both bacteria was found. Higher exposure time (60 min) significantly increased the cell leakage of *Salm.* Typhimurium, but not in case of *Staph. aureus.* Longer exposures (60 min) with OIC concentration of ZEO and SNP (Figures 1 and 2), caused 3 and 4-fold more gross membrane damage, in *Staph. aureus* and *Salm.* Typhimurium culture compared to the control sample, respectively.

Table 1. Chemical composition of ZEO.

Compounds	KI[a]	Area (%)	Compounds	KI	Area (%)
α-Thujene	931	0.15	linalool	1106	6.26
α-Pinene	639	3.66	Borneol	1163	0.19
Camphene	953	0.17	Terpinen-4-ol	1175	4.63
β-Pinene	980	1.55	Thymol methyl ether	1233	0.17
β-Mycrene	991	1.35	Bornyl acetate	1284	0.17
α-Phellandrene	1002	0.15	Thymol	1301	44
δ-3-Carene	1009	1	Carvacrol	1318	14.4
α-Terpinene	1016	1.74	Acetylthymol	1284	0.3
Cis-para-menth-2-en-1-o	1123	0.37	δ-Elemene	1340	0.24
p-Cymene	1028	11.15	Eugenol	1360	0.82
1,8-Cineole	1032	0.86	*Trans*-Caryophyllene	1423	2.78
Υ-Terpinene	1060	0.08	Caryophyllene oxide	1583	0.93
α-Terpinolene	1087	0.08			
Total					97.23%

[a]Kovats indices calculated against *n*-alkanes on HP-5 column.

Table 2. Survival population (log CFU/ mL) of *Staph. aureus* and *Salm.* Typhimurium treated with ZEO and SNP alone and in combination during 15 min contact time at room temperature.

Microorganism*	Alone at MIC concentration		In combination		
	ZEO	SNP	OIC	1/2OIC	1/4OIC
Staph. aureus	0	$3.11 \times 10^5 \pm 0.08^a$	0	$3.11 \times 10^5 \pm 0.67^a$	$4.74 \times 10^5 \pm 0.41^a$
Salm. Typhimurium	0	$4.69 \times 10^5 \pm 0.19^b$	0	$3.90 \times 10^5 \pm 0.21^b$	$5.30 \times 10^5 \pm 0.33^b$

*Initial bacterial counts: 10^6 CFU mL^{-1}. Different letters for each column of indicate a statistically significant difference ($P < 0.05$).

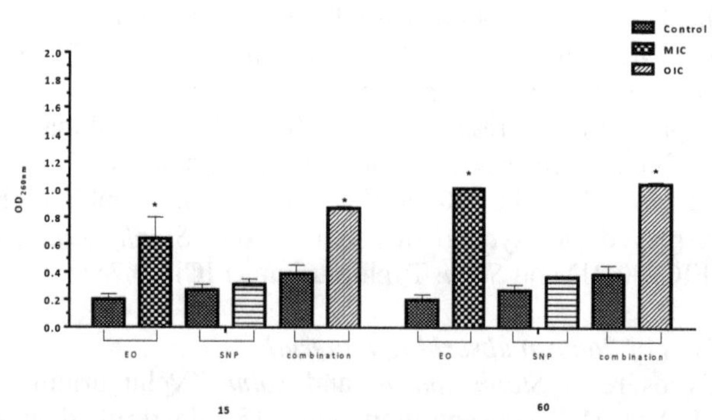

Figure 1. 260-nm absorbing material released from *Staph. aureus* cells after treatment with MIC concentration of silver nanoparticle (SNP), *Zataria multiflora* essential oil (EO) and their combination. Asterisks indicate significantly different values (P<0.05) when comparing optical density (OD) of control and each treatment at the same exposure time.

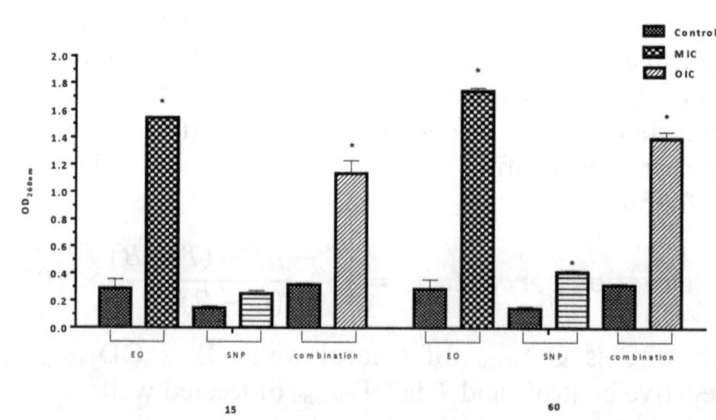

Figure 2. 260-nm absorbing material released from *Salm.* Typhimurium cells after treatment with MIC concentration of silver nanoparticle (SNP), *Zataria multiflora* essential oil (EO) and their combination. Asterisks indicate significantly different values (P<0.05) when comparing optical density (OD) of control and each treatment at the same exposure time.

Biofilm removal

As compared with *Salm.* Typhimurium (Figure 3b), higher removal of *Staph. aureus* biofilms were achieved at 15 min exposure time for SNP-ZEO (Figure 3a). Results demonstrated that biofilm of *Staph. aureus* is more sensitive to SNP - ZEO than *Salm.* Typhimurium. SNP at MIC, 2MIC, and 4MIC concentrations resulted in 93, 87 and 71.33% and 82, 79 and 58% removal of *Staph. aureus* and *Salm. Typhimurium* cells, respectively. For *Staph. aureus* and *Salm.* Typhimurium, 90.6%, and 89% bacteria were eliminated at a concentration of MIC for ZEO. Concerning the hydrophobicity property of ZEO, it can be observed in Figure 3, a reduction in the biofilm removal with increasing ZEO concentration supporting the use of surfactants could help in the disruption of such shortcoming.

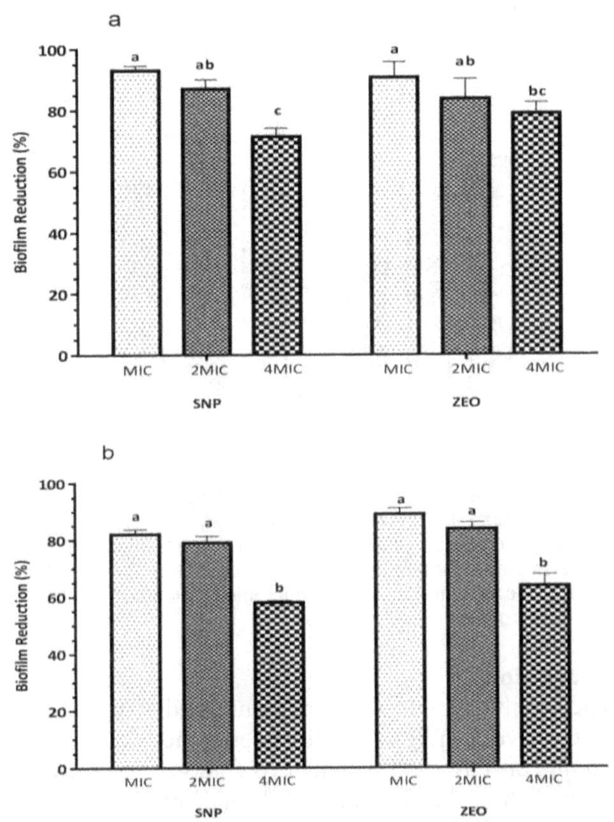

Figure 3. The effect of silver nanoparticle (SNP) and *Zataria multiflora* essential oil (ZEO) on removal one-day old biofilm of *Staph. aureus* (**a**) and *Salm.* Typhimurium (**b**) developed on polystyrene surface with 15 min contact time. Different letters for each concentration of antimicrobial indicate a statistically significant difference ($P < 0.05$).

Synergistic sanitizing activity

The purpose of this experiment was to achieve a best effective concentration of SNP and ZEO as a sanitizing solution. To assess the disinfectants efficiencies, MIC and OIC concentrations were determined. The reductions in the *Staph. aureus* and *Salm.* Typhimurium counts after 15 min exposure to MIC and various OIC concentrations were shown in Table 2. A reduction of 100% was achieved for both bacteria after 15 min exposure to ZEO. A similar reduction was also found for OIC concentration. Whereas, less than 0.4 $\log_{10}$ CFU/ mL reduction was observed for the samples treated with SNP in alone.

As shown by 260 nm absorbing material measurements, SNP displayed an antimicrobial activity after a long time of exposure (at least after 1 h) compared with ZEO. In comparison with *Staph. aureus*, *Salm.* Typhimurium had higher resistance to SNP. Additionally, no significant reduction ($P < 0.05$) was observed in the microbial counts of 1/2OIC and 1/4OIC with SNP treated samples.

Discussion

The components identified in ZEO (Table 1) in this study was similar to previous works. According to Saedi Dezaki et al. (2007),[19] the major components of ZEO were thymol (41.81%), carvacrol (28.85%), and *p*-cymene (5.63-13.16%). In the study of Saei-Dehkordi, et al. (2010),[7] a variation of the major components, thymol (27.5-64.87%), carvacrol (2.7-22.39), *p*-cymene (8.36%) and linalool (0-7.92%) of ZEO were observed, due to the collection of plant material from five main phytogeographic grown towns in Iran. Factors such as growth phase and geographic origin of plant, method of plant drying and processing affect EO content and chemical compositions.[7]

In our study, the antibacterial properties of ZEO was not different to the results reported from other studies, apart from some detected variable bacterial susceptibilities that may cause the differences in the chemical composition of ZEOs and the bacterial strains used by others. The hydrophobic property of most EOs could increase their permeability and accumulation in the bacterial cell membranes.[6,7]

Silver ions and silver-based compounds are widely known as highly toxic to 16 major species of bacteria due to their multiple mechanisms of action. Zarei et al. (2014) reported the MIC values of SNP against *Listeria monocytogenes*, *S.* Typhimurium, *Escherichia coli* O157:H7 and *Vibrio parahaemolyticus* in the range of 3.12- 6.25 μg mL^{-1} according to microdilution method in Tryptic soy broth.[20] The small size and high ratio of surface to volume in SNPs, allow them to more effectively contact with microorganisms and induce their antimicrobial activities.[21] It has been shown that antibacterial efficacy of SNP varies between different prepared SNPs. Given the fact that factors such as the type of bacteria, the media of inoculation, type and the size of nanoparticle and the method of preparation must be considered when comparing the antibacterial activity of different nanoparticles.[1]

The additive or partial synergy effect is a type of interaction in which the combined effect is equal to the sum of the effects of the individual agents. As shown previously,[22] SNP interaction with EO is a bacteria-dependent phenomenon. The synergistic properties of SNP with ZEO on *Staph. epidermidis* and *Staph. aureus* (FICI= 0.5-1) has been demonstrated, but no synergistic effects were found against Methicillin-resistant *Staph.*

aureus and *Ps. aeruginosa* (FICI value of 3 and 1.25, respectively).

The MBC: MIC ratio ≥ 8 is considered as an indicator of bacteriostatic activity.[23] In the current study, MIC/MBC of both SNP and ZEO were 1:1, suggesting a bactericidal effect on *Staph. aureus* and *Salm. Typhimurium*. It was demonstrated that oregano EO reveals a synergistic activity with common antibiotics such as gentamicin against some potential pathogens,[24] additive activity in combination with another antibiotic such as amoxicillin and polymyxin on Extended-Spectrum Beta-Lactamase (ESBL)-producing *E.coli,*[25] and synergistic with other EO obtained from *Thymus vulgare* and *Rosmarinus officinalis*.[26]

Measuring the loss of 260-nm absorbing material from the bacteria is an indicator of cell leakage which could be used to understand the mechanism of action of antimicrobial compounds. The presence of materials with an absorbance at 260 nm in the supernatant of bacterial solution indicates a loss of nucleic acids from the cell. Based on the results of this study (Figures 1 and 2), the higher values determined by the measurements at 260 nm are an indication for the leakage of bacterial contents which subsequently confirms the physical damages of bacterial cell walls by ZEO.[4] However, the reductions in the efficacy of SNP may be best explained by bacterial blocking caused by higher concentrations of SNP, which could reduce the contact surface of nanoparticles with bacteria and its antibacterial efficacy.

SNP can cause agglomeration after adding to the nutritious media such as LB and as shown previously,[2] treatment of *Staph. aureus* with a combination of EO and SNP, induced a reduction in cell density, exopolysaccharide, morphology changes, and cell destruction. However, membrane permeability created by EO might allow the small molecules of SNP to enter the cell.

Researchers are aware of the importance of biofilms in causing diseases and drug resistance, therefore finding a safe and effective method for biofilm removal is of great importance. Natural agents are considered as a safe way to remove biofilms. Although the research on SNP interaction with biofilm is still in its early phases, we currently know that removal of biofilm by SNP could occur in three steps: transportation to the vicinity of the biofilm, attachment, and penetration within the biofilm.[27] It has been shown that eradication of biofilms by SNP is not a concentration-dependent process, rather it occurs in a time-dependent manner.[28] The main compounds of ZEO are thymol, a monoterpene phenolic derivative, and its phenol isomer, carvacrol. Both of them contribute to antimicrobial and antioxidant properties of Lamiaceae family.[4] Additionally, hydrophobic characteristics of these ingredients allow the penetration of ZEO into outer exopolysaccharide and inner layers of biofilms.[29] In our study, by decreasing the OIC concentration from 1/2OIC to 1/4OIC (Figure 4), the biofilm removal properties were significantly decreased (P<0.05) from 64 % to 43.33 % for *Staph. aureus* (Figure 4) whereas OIC concentration, removed 76% of biofilm mass. For *Salm.* Typhimurium (Figure 4) the values were 96.46%, 81.50% and 68 % for OIC, 1/2OIC and 1/4OIC concentrations, respectively. It means that combined use of SNP and ZEO boosted biofilm removal potential of both antibacterial compounds against different pathogens. According to Gurunathan et al. (2014), the combined use of NPs and antibiotic such as ampicillin exhibit antibiofilm activity on Gram-positive and Gram-negative bacteria by 55 and 70%, whereas combining those NPs with vancomycin revealed a 75 and 55% reduction of biofilm of Gram-positive and Gram-negative bacteria.[1] It is worth mentioning that, differences in the method used to evaluate biofilm removal activity and differences in the sensitivity of different bacteria, the age of biofilm and type of surface which biofilm developed could cause different results in the biofilm removal percentage in previous studies.

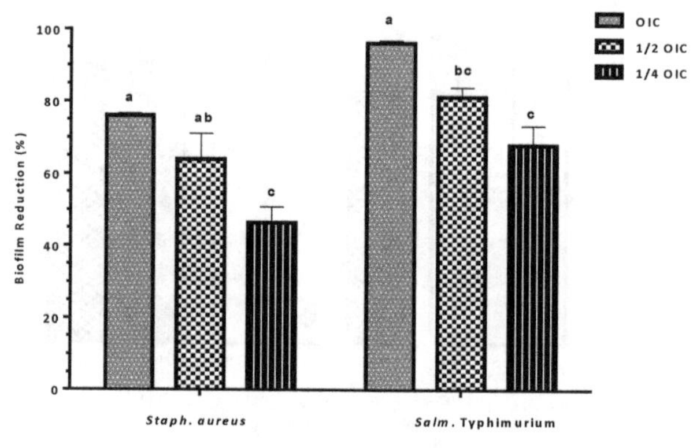

Figure 4. The effect of silver nanoparticle (SNP) and *Zataria multiflora* essential oil (ZEO) combination on removal one-day old biofilm of *Staph. aureus* and *Salm.* Typhimurium developed on polystyrene surface with 15 min contact time. Different letters for each concentration of antimicrobial indicate a statistically significant difference (P < 0.05).

Conclusion

The results of our study demonstrated that SNP and ZEO have synergistic antibacterial activities against *Staph. aureus,* and *Salm*. Typhimurium. It was also shown that the antimicrobial and biofilm removal properties of SNP and ZEO were affected by the type of microorganisms and concentrations of both compounds. ZEO displayed a fast antimicrobial activity. Both antimicrobials represented considerable biofilm removal activity on both bacteria. The combination of SNP and ZEO was additive, which means significant antibacterial and antibiofilm activity could achieve by use of agents at concentrations without compromising their antibacterial effects. The best concentrations for SNP- ZEO sanitizing solution were 12.5 µg/ mL for SNP and 625 µg/ mL for ZEO. Our results highlighted the powerful combination activity of SNP and ZEO which accelerated antibacterial activity, alleviated undesirable sensorial property of ZEO and reduced the concentration of both compounds.

Acknowledgments
This study was funded by a grant from Faculty of Veterinary Medicine and Institute of Biotechnology, Urmia University. The authors would like to thank Dr. Mahmoudian for his assistance.

Conflict of Interest
The authors declare no conflict of interest related to this work.

References
1. Gurunathan S, Han JW, Kwon DN, Kim JH. Enhanced antibacterial and anti-biofilm activities of silver nanoparticles against gram-negative and gram-positive bacteria. *Nanoscale Res Lett* 2014;9(1):373. doi: 10.1186/1556-276X-9-373
2. Scandorieiro S, de Camargo LC, Lancheros CA, Yamada-Ogatta SF, Nakamura CV, de Oliveira AG, et al. Synergistic and additive effect of oregano essential oil and biological silver nanoparticles against multidrug-resistant bacterial strains. *Front Microbiol* 2016;7:760. doi: 10.3389/fmicb.2016.00760
3. Hyldgaard M, Mygind T, Meyer RL. Essential oils in food preservation: Mode of action, synergies, and interactions with food matrix components. *Front Microbiol* 2012;3:12. doi: 10.3389/fmicb.2012.00012
4. Sajed H, Sahebkar A, Iranshahi M. Zataria multiflora boiss. (shirazi thyme)--an ancient condiment with modern pharmaceutical uses. *J Ethnopharmacol* 2013;145(3):686-98. doi: 10.1016/j.jep.2012.12.018
5. Shokri H, Sharifzadeh A. Zataria multiflora boiss.: A review study on chemical composition, anti-fungal and anti-mycotoxin activities, and ultrastructural changes. *J HerbMed Pharmacol* 2017;6(1):1-9.
6. Moradi M, Tajik H, Razavi Rohani SM, Mahmoudian A. Antioxidant and antimicrobial effects of zein edible film impregnated with Zataria multiflora Boiss. Essential oil and monolaurin. *LWT - Food Sci Technol* 2016;72:37-43. doi: 10.1016/j.lwt.2016.04.026
7. Saei-Dehkordi SS, Tajik H, Moradi M, Khalighi-Sigaroodi F. Chemical composition of essential oils in zataria multiflora boiss. From different parts of iran and their radical scavenging and antimicrobial activity. *Food Chem Toxicol* 2010;48(6):1562-7. doi: 10.1016/j.fct.2010.03.025
8. Sharififar F, Moshafi MH, Mansouri SH, Khodashenas M, Khoshnoodi M. In vitro evaluation of antibacterial and antioxidant activities of the essential oil and methanol extract of endemic Zataria multiflora Boiss. *Food Control* 2007;18(7):800-5. doi: 10.1016/j.foodcont.2006.04.002
9. Desbois AP, Lang S, Gemmell CG, Coote PJ. Surface disinfection properties of the combination of an antimicrobial peptide, ranalexin, with an endopeptidase, lysostaphin, against methicillin-resistant Staphylococcus aureus (MRSA). *J Appl Microbiol* 2010;108(2):723-30. doi: 10.1111/j.1365-2672.2009.04472.x
10. Bassetti M, Righi E. New antibiotics and antimicrobial combination therapy for the treatment of gram-negative bacterial infections. *Curr Opin Crit Care* 2015;21(5):402-11. doi: 10.1097/mcc.0000000000000235
11. Gutierrez J, Barry-Ryan C, Bourke P. The antimicrobial efficacy of plant essential oil combinations and interactions with food ingredients. *Int J Food Microbiol* 2008;124(1):91-7. doi: 10.1016/j.ijfoodmicro.2008.02.028
12. Taghizadeh M, Solgi M. The application of essential oils and silver nanoparticles for sterilization of bermudagrass explants in in vitro culture. *Int J Hort Sci Technol* 2014;1(2):131-40.
13. Clinical and laboratory standards institute. Performance standards for antimicrobial susceptibility testing; twentieth informational supplement. Document M100-S22. Wayne, Pa, USA: CLSI; 2012.
14. Moody JA. Synergism testing: Broth microdilution checkerboard and broth microdilution methods. In: Isenberg HD, editor. Clinical microbiology procedures handbook. Washington, DC: American Society for Microbiology; 2003. PP. 1-28.
15. Dong X, Chen F, Zhang Y, Liu H, Liu Y, Ma L. In vitro activities of rifampin, colistin, sulbactam and tigecycline tested alone and in combination against extensively drug-resistant acinetobacter baumannii. *J Antibiot (Tokyo)* 2014;67(9):677-80. doi: 10.1038/ja.2014.99
16. Rhayour K, Bouchikhi T, Tantaoui-Elaraki A, Sendide K, Remmal A. The mechanism of bactericidal action of oregano and clove essential oils and of their phenolic major components on escherichia coli and bacillus subtilis. *J Essent Oil Res* 2003;15(5):356-62. doi: 10.1080/10412905.2003.9698611
17. Mahdavi M, Jalali M, Kasra Kermanshahi R. The effect of nisin on biofilm forming foodborne bacteria using microtiter plate method. *Res Pharm Sci* 2007;2(2):113-8.
18. Phongphakdee K, Nitisinprasert S. Combination inhibition activity of nisin and ethanol on the growth inhibition of pathogenic gram negative bacteria and their application as disinfectant solution. *J Food Sci* 2015;80(10):M2241-6. doi: 10.1111/1750-3841.13015
19. Saedi Dezaki E, Mahmoudvand H, Sharififar F, Fallahi S, Monzote L, Ezatkhah F. Chemical composition along with anti-leishmanial and cytotoxic activity of *Zataria multiflora*. *Pharm Biol* 2016;54(5):752-8. doi: 10.3109/13880209.2015.1079223
20. Zarei M, Jamnejad A, Khajehali E. Antibacterial effect of silver nanoparticles against four foodborne

pathogens. *Jundishapur J Microbiol* 2014;7(1):e8720. doi: 10.5812/jjm.8720

21. Perez-Diaz M, Alvarado-Gomez E, Magana-Aquino M, Sanchez-Sanchez R, Velasquillo C, Gonzalez C, et al. Anti-biofilm activity of chitosan gels formulated with silver nanoparticles and their cytotoxic effect on human fibroblasts. *Mater Sci Eng C Mater Biol Appl* 2016;60:317-23. doi: 10.1016/j.msec.2015.11.036
22. Sheikholeslami S, Mousavi SE, Ahmadi Ashtiani HR, Hosseini Doust SR, Mahdi Rezayat S. Antibacterial activity of silver nanoparticles and their combination with zataria multiflora essential oil and methanol extract. *Jundishapur J Microbiol* 2016;9(10):e36070. doi: 10.5812/jjm.36070
23. Parhi AK, Zhang Y, Saionz KW, Pradhan P, Kaul M, Trivedi K, et al. Antibacterial activity of quinoxalines, quinazolines, and 1,5-naphthyridines. *Bioorg Med Chem Lett* 2013;23(17):4968-74. doi: 10.1016/j.bmcl.2013.06.048
24. Honorio VG, Bezerra J, Souza GT, Carvalho RJ, Gomes-Neto NJ, Figueiredo RC, et al. Inhibition of *Staphylococcus aureus* cocktail using the synergies of oregano and rosemary essential oils or carvacrol and 1,8-cineole. *Front Microbiol* 2015;6:1223. doi: 10.3389/fmicb.2015.01223
25. Rosato A, Piarulli M, Corbo F, Muraglia M, Carone A, Vitali ME, et al. *In vitro* synergistic antibacterial action of certain combinations of gentamicin and essential oils. *Curr Med Chem* 2010;17(28):3289-95.
26. Si H, Hu J, Liu Z, Zeng ZL. Antibacterial effect of oregano essential oil alone and in combination with antibiotics against extended-spectrum β-lactamase-producing *Escherichia coli*. *FEMS Immunol Med Microbiol* 2008;53(2):190-4. doi: 10.1111/j.1574-695X.2008.00414.x
27. Ikuma K, Decho AW, Lau BL. When nanoparticles meet biofilms-interactions guiding the environmental fate and accumulation of nanoparticles. *Front Microbiol* 2015;6:591. doi: 10.3389/fmicb.2015.00591
28. Khameneh B, Zarei H, Fazly Bazzaz BS. The effect of silver nanoparticles on staphylococcus epidermidis biofilm biomass and cell viability. *Nanomed J* 2014;1(5):302-7. doi: 10.7508/nmj.2015.05.003
29. Vazquez-Sanchez D, Cabo ML, Rodriguez-Herrera JJ. Antimicrobial activity of essential oils against staphylococcus aureus biofilms. *Food Sci Technol Int* 2015;21(8):559-70. doi: 10.1177/1082013214553996

24

Transdermal Evaporation Drug Delivery System: Concept to Commercial Products

Rabinarayan Parhi[1]*, **Suryakanta Swain**[2]

[1] *GITAM Institute of Pharmacy, GITAM (Deemed to be University), Gandhi Nagar Campus, Rushikonda, Visakhapatnam-530045, Andhra Pradesh, India.*

[2] *Southern Institute of Medical Sciences, College of Pharmacy, Department of Pharmaceutics, SIMS Group of Institutions, Mangaldas Nagar, Vijyawada Road, Guntur-522 001, Andhra Pradesh, India.*

Article info

Keywords:
· Transdermal
· Supersaturation
· Stratum corneum
· Crystallization
· Thermodynamic activity

Abstract

Since two decades or so transdermal route established itself as better alternative to traditional oral route. This is possible due to continuous innovations in transdermal drug delivery (TDD), which not only enables researchers from academia and industry to successfully develop and launch many new pharmaceuticals but also allow to include new classes of drugs that can be developed into transdermal formulations. These successes are achieved due to the use of novel techniques based on either physical or chemical approaches. However, both of these techniques suffer due to their own disadvantages. Comparatively, a simple method of supersaturation to enhance drug permeation across skin has created a new wave of interest. Even though the application supersaturated principle in topical and TDD has been used from 1960s, but proper control of drug release and formation of stable supersaturated states has been the core of intense research in the last decade. Out of various methods used to get supersaturated system, evaporation method is considered as most efficient and practically feasible for TDD. Therefore, in this review concept of supersaturation, selection of solvent system and the mechanism of inhibition of crystallization are discussed. Application of evaporation systems in the development of transdermal formulations such as solutions, semisolids and metered dose therapeutic systems (MDTS) and the commercial evaporative systems are also discussed in this review.

Introduction

Delivery of drug across the skin i.e., transdermal drug delivery (TDD) offer an alternative route to traditional oral and parenteral routes with many distinct advantages such as avoidance of first pass metabolism by liver and gastro-intestinal tract, improves patient compliance by reducing the frequency of drug administration, minimizes the side effect of drug caused due to temporary overdose, steadier drug plasma concentration, non-invasive drug delivery i.e., without any needle-phobia etc.[1-3] Common dosage forms applied topically to provide systemic effect are creams, ointments, gels and patches.[4] It is obviously difficult to sustain the effect of drugs present in creams and ointments for the considerable period of time after application because of every possibility of their removal from the skin surface as a result of movement, contact and wetting.[5]

Presently, patch and gel formulations are widely used in clinical settings owning to their increasing number of available formulations commercially such as Transderm Scop, Nitroderm, Nitrodisc etc. as patches and Androgels, Androderm etc. as gel. Contrary to creams and ointments, gels with bioadhesive polymer (s) provide optimum contact times for the drug absorption.[6,7] Gel formulation has the disadvantages such as to achieve desired plasma levels of drugs it has to apply over large surface area and there is always possibility of gel being transferred to female partners thereby further reducing the available drug amount for absorption. This particular problem can be avoided by using approved transdermal patches. However, local skin reactions such as redness, irritation, blistering and microbial proliferation caused by occlusion most often associated with patch formulation, which significantly reduces patient compliance as well as acceptance.[8-12] Not only that, manufacturing of multi-component systems such as patch has always been a challenge to formulation scientist. In addition, instability of patches especially drug crystallization on long storage is being a herculean task to be solved.

Skin is considered as largest organ of our body as it accounting for 10% of body mass. Despite of large surface area available for drug transport across the skin, penetration of drug into skin is limited by stratum corneum (SC), the uppermost layer of skin.[13] Manipulation of SC barrier can be carried out either by chemical[13,14] and several physical approaches[15-18] in order to improve drug permeation across the skin. Chemical approach using penetration enhancers (PEs) have definitive advantages such as they provide reversible damage to the skin, painless administration, give the flexibility to formulator to alter the formulation composition according to the need. Despite all this chemical PEs such as surfactants and organic solvents are resulting in different skin ailments such as stinging, burning, erythema and contact urticaria.[19] Furthermore, there is no report on the long-term effect of PEs on the SC.[20] No doubt that various physical techniques including iontophoresis, phonophoresis and more recently microneedle technique have tremendous potential in enhancing the drug permeation across the skin. But, the main concern with above techniques is the pain at the administration site. Furthermore, an additional step of microneedle sterilization increases the cost effectiveness of the system.[21] In this scenario, supersaturation technique seems to be one of the attractive alternatives.

Supersaturation

The concept of supersaturated systems originated from the crystallization theory, in which the formation of supersaturated solution is the first step of crystallization. A supersatuarated solution can be defined as the one which contains more amount of dissolved solute than it would normally contain in a saturated solution at a constant temperature. As supersaturated systems are considered as thermodynamically unstable (labile state), in most of the cases, there is spontaneous formation of crystals (Figure 1). Metastable is a state in which solute material remains in the supersaturated solution without crystallization. This state is maintained until any foreign solid particles are added intentionally/accidentally or the system is subjected to external forces (e.g., ultrasound). Thus, the line between labile and metastable states is mentioned as critical degree of saturation.[22]

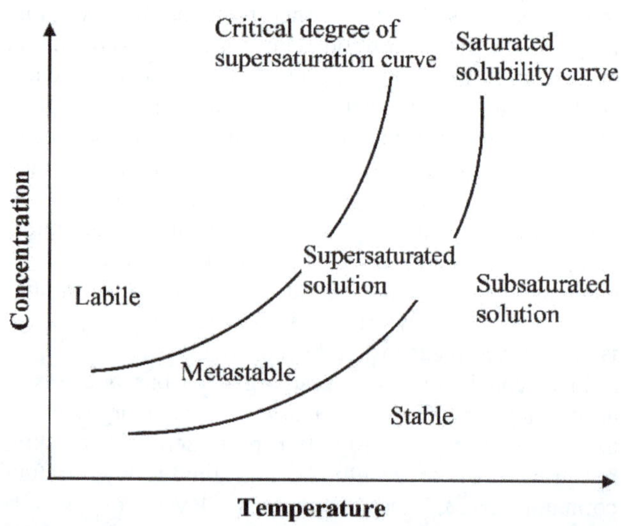

Figure 1. Diagram showing the critical degree of supersaturation and the different stability states of supersaturated systems.

Even though supersaturation concept is old concept, the benefits of it to transdermal/topical drug delivery were first recognized by Higuchi in 1960.[23] According to him the rate-controlling step to percutaneous absorption of drug from supersaturated system was resides in the outer layer of SC (Figure 2). Based on the definition of partition coefficient, when a vehicle is saturated with a drug applied on the skin surface, then it must lead to saturation of SC with the same drug. If excess than this saturation level of drug present in the vehicle, there will be increase in drug amount in the SC proportionately. Hence, it leads to penetration enhancement of drug in the same level of degree of supersaturation.[22] Later on, it was understood that above concept was also based on potential concentration gradient. Concentration gradient of a supersaturated system of drug is significantly higher than that of its saturated system across the skin surface. Therefore, a similar rise in concentration of the drug in the outer layer of SC in order to maintained equilibrium at least for a short period of time. This is only feasible if the lipids in the SC permit the drug to remain in higher concentration/activity level i.e., antinucleate agents.[22]

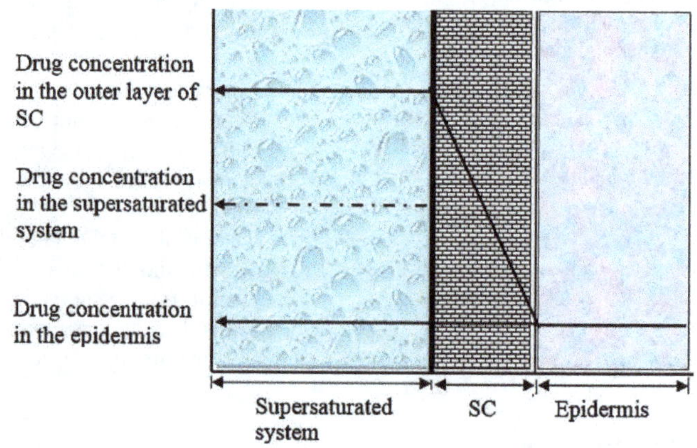

Figure 2. Schematic profile of steady-state diffusion across the skin (Modified from reference 22).

Broadly, there are five methods to obtain supersaturated systems:[24,25]

1. Heating and cooling
2. Evaporation of the solvent
3. By adiabatic evaporation i.e., cooling plus evaporation
4. Salting out i.e., addition of a substance to a solution that reduces the solubility of the primary solute
5. Formation of a new compound, due to the reaction between two or more solutes, which is poorly soluble compared to initial solute.

In addition, sometimes change in pH bring about change in solubility and resulted in supersaturated solution. Present review mainly focused on the formation of supersaturated system by evaporation method.

Advantages

1. Evaporative systems provide passive and nonocclusive delivery of drugs.[26] Therefore, this system is well tolerated and also demonstrates very low skin irritation rates.[27]
2. Compared to physical technologies they are having simple working mechanism and more importantly

they provide non-invasive drug delivery. Similarly these systems less likely to provoke skin irritation when compared with chemical PEs.[28]

3. These systems are inexpensive and provide penetration enhancement that is specific to the drug without disturbing the integrity of the SC.[22,29]
4. These formulations are fast drying products where the volatile component provides uniform distribution of drug on the skin surface with minimum vehicle deposition; thereby it reduces the uneasiness of patient.[30]
5. Manufacturing and scale-up of these systems are much less tedious than patch formulations.[27]
6. With single application of these systems, a sustained steady-state serum drug level can be maintained over 2-4 days.[31]
7. These systems offers ease of application, specifically when a metered dose transdermal system (MDTS) is used.
8. MDTS make sure that only pre-determined dose is administered which is aesthetically appealing and also able to eliminate concerns of residual drug associated with transdermal patches.[30]
9. In these systems, the patient have the flexibility to vary delivery dose according to the situation as it is packaged in a multi-dose container.[31]

Disadvantages

1. Like other transdermal dosage forms, these systems have relative low bioavailability compared to oral and parenteral dosage forms.[27]
2. Selection of solvent system is always posing a challenge to formulation scientist as the thermodynamic effect of drug depends on the solvent system selected.
3. Active ingredients for this technique would require a suitable drug-response profile.[31]
4. Supersaturated formulations are inheritently thermodynamically unstable and may lead to drug crystallization. In most of the case this problem can be overcome with antinucleate polymers which either inhibits nucleus formation or retard the crystallization.[20,28,29]

Selection of vehicle

The solvent in which a drug is present can increase the drug permeation through the skin by either ways: (i) by increasing the thermodynamic activity of the drug or (ii) altering the barrier property of the SC. Thermodynamic activity of a drug mainly depends on the solvent in which it is solubilized. Therefore, the selection of solvent is very crucial for enhanced permeation of drug across the skin. It has to keep in mind that maximization of thermodynamic activity is essential to achieve higher concentration of drug in the SC. The flux is related to thermodynamic activity as expressed in the following equation:

$$\frac{dm}{dt} = J\ (\text{flux}) = \frac{\alpha D}{\gamma h}$$

Where α is the thermodynamic activity of the drug in the donor formulation, γ is effective activity coefficient in the skin barrier, D is diffusivity and h is the thickness of the membrane. So, more the thermodynamic activity of a drug in a formulation higher will be the flux as the escaping tendency of the drug from the vehicle is at the peak.[32] Furthermore, thermodynamic activity of a drug in a solvent is proportional to the ratio of its concentration to solubility in that vehicle. Thus, more the solubility of drug in the vehicle less will be the thermodynamic activity. There are two approaches employed to study the effect of different vehicle/solvent on the permeation of a drug across the skin. In the first approach, a fixed concentration of a drug is prepared in different solvents. This method is helping in selecting appropriate solvent with higher thermodynamic activity for a drug whose concentration is already fixed. In second approach saturated solutions of a drug in different solvents are prepared (solute activity is considered as unity). This approach should give equal flux provided the solvents are not having skin barrier alteration potential.[33] Above equation also illustrates that different formulations of any particular drug at equal thermodynamic activity will provide equal penetration provided excipients in the formulation do not influence any property of drug. Implication of this is that by selecting appropriate formulation drug loading can be minimized by maintaining equal thermodynamic activity, thereby delivering equal amount of drug. For example; 0.1% hydrocortisone gel (Dioderm®) is clinically equivalent to 1% hydrocortisone cream, BP. Though both are having different concentrations of drug, but the thermodynamic activity is equal. Therefore in the successful development of transdermal/topical supersaturated systems it is essential to study the flux of various vehicles/solvents at fixed drug concentration as well as at saturation level.[34]

Mechanism of penetration enhancement by evaporation means of supersaturation

Any subsaturated or saturated solution can be converted to supersaturated one by evaporating the solvent as the same amount of solute will be present in gradually decreasing amount of solvent. This is more pronounced if any volatile component/solvent is present the solution. This principle is explored to develop transdermal and topical formulations in order to improve thermodynamic activity of active ingredient and thereby enhance its penetration into/across the skin.[35] For instance, an active ingredient not present in supersaturated level in any formulation, but when applied on the skin surface volatile solvent evaporates, thereby reducing solubility in the residual amount of solvent. The reduction of solvent amount lead to the formation of supersaturated state of the active ingredient. Certain topical formulations in the market (e.g., lotions) are forming supersaturated states, resulting in the penetration enhancement of active ingredients.

Basically, evaporation systems consisting of two components: drug and solvent mixture. The solvent mixture is composed of both volatile and nonvolatile solvents. Here the pre-requisite is that the selected drug must soluble in both the solvents. The volatile component ensures that the dose can be administered in a precise (volume per area and easy spreading of applied formulation) and reproducible manner. More importantly, it increases the concentration of drug in the formulation.[36] Non-volatile solvent prevents the precipitation of drug from the solution, when the volatile counterpart gets evaporated. Non-volatile solvent selected should have higher partitioning property. This physicochemical property not only helps in partitioning of solvent and drug into the SC, but also serving to disrupt the ordered intercellular lipids and enhance permeation.[31] Upon application of an evaporation delivery system on the skin surface, it creates a depot system in the SC from which the drug can be absorbed into systemic circulation for a longer period of time. Therefore, evaporation delivery systems ensure sustained plasma drug concentration for longer period of time.

Mechanism to inhibits or retard crystallization

It is mentioned in the earlier section that the instability is one of the major limitations for the supersaturated systems. The instability is due to rapid crystallization of drug when the volatile component is getting evaporated immediately after the application of these formulations. Formation of crystals not only reduces the initial high activity of the drug but also gives an irregular plasma drug concentration. Therefore, stabilization of thermodynamically unstable states is important step in the development of successful supersaturated systems with desired permeation enhancement across the skin. It is well known that the instability of supersaturated system lead to establish the foundation for crystallization i.e. formation of nucleus, which subsequently resulting in crystal growth. In addition, there are many external factors such as type of solvent, temperature variation (based on the heat of solution), impurities, pH and hydrodynamics. Furthermore, the nucleation time and the time needed to form critical sized nuclei, from where the crystal growth can take place, decreases with the increase in degree of saturation (DS). In order to stabilize the system, one or more of these factors are often used to control both the nucleus formation and its growth.[29,37]

When a supersaturated solution of a drug is applied on the skin surface, whether it contains PEs or not, the concentration of drug in the upper layer of SC is also supersaturated. This may lead to crystal formation in the upper layer of SC, which can reduce the rate of drug permeation into systemic circulation. In one study it was found that penetration enhancement of piroxicam was increased which may be due to antinucleating ability of the intercellular lipids of SC.[38] One of the very widely used methods is to selectively use antinucleant polymers to stabilize the unstable supersaturated systems.[20,39-41] Polymers such as hydroxypropyl methylcellulose (HPMC), methylcellulose (MC) and polyvinyl pyrrolidone (PVP) are already tested as antinucleate polymers.[29] Second method to prevent nucleus formation and crystal growth is to use tailor made additives (impurities). The inhibition of crystal growth of paracetamol was succefully performed by the addition of para-acetoxy acetanilide.[42] It was observed that by the addition of small quantities of fatty acid as additives was able alter the physiochemical properties of adipic acid tremendously by incorporating into crystal.[43,44] In addition to above techniques, a stable supersaturated solution is achievable with low DS compared to higher one. This is observed with ibuprofen; with higher DS the solution was converted to transulescent demonstrating the presence of ibuprofen micro-crystal whereas at lower DS the solution was found to be clear one.[41]

Mathematical modeling

Flux of a permeant across a membrane from a saturated solution is constant and independent of its concentration. Therefore, under normal conditions, the flux of a drug is limited by its saturated solubility. The flux of drugs across a membrane at the steady state is governed by Fick's first law of diffusion and expressed as:

$$J = \frac{DAK}{h\,(Cv - Cr)}$$

Where J is flux, D is the diffusion coefficient, K is partition coefficient between membrane and vehicle, h is the diffusional path length, and Cv and Cr are drug concentration in the solution/formulation and in receptor phase, respectively. Under sink condition ($Cv \geq 0.1Cr$), Cr is considered as negligible; therefore (Cv-Cr) term is usually approximated as Cv.[22,20]

Applications of evaporation based supersaturated principle

Supersaturated principle based on evaporation is mainly applied in transdermal/topical drug delivery and the formulations in which this concept is incorporated are topical solutions and semisolids and spray. The latter formulation is now being widely used in transporting drug across skin. In addition there are many commercial products available based on spray technique. A list of drugs, solvent systems, polymers with their references are presented in Table 1.

Solutions and semisolids

Poulsen *et al.* performed a series of experiments in order to find out the correct and optimum vehicle for the release of fluocinolone acetonide and its acetate derivatives from a gel comprising of propylene glycol (PG), water and isopropyl myristate (IPM) as vehicle. The solubility and concentration of the drug in the vehicle and partition coefficient between the vehicle and IPM were found to be determining factors for the release of drug from the prepared gel.[45]

Coldman *et al.* studied the potential of supersaturated systems of fluocinolone acetonide and its acetate esters and compared their penetration enhancement with that occluded formulations. The volatile component was isopropanol and non-volatile components were IPM and PG. After the application of above formulations, the volatile component gets evaporated leading to the formation of supersaturated state of the drug, thereby increased the penetration of drug. In the comparison between occluded and unoccluded systems, the unoccluded formulations were found to show higher penetration.[46]

Theeuwes *et al.* developed supersaturated solution of hydrocortisone using volatile/non-volatile co-solvent system. Acetone and water were volatile and non-volatile components, respectively. In the first step, mixture of acetone and water was prepared and then hydrocortisone was dissolved in it. After the application of above drug mixture on ethylene-vinyl acetate (EVA) membrane, acetone evaporates leaving supersaturated solution of hydrocortisone. This resulted in the 3.9 fold increase in saturation value, giving a proportional increase in flux.[47]

Kondo and Sugimoto investigated the diffusion of nifedipine across EVA copolymer membrane from different combinations of solvents such as IPM, PG and acetone. They observed that the initial flux was found to be higher than the steady-state fluxes. This was attributed to the initial evaporation of volatile solvent resulted in the formation of a saturated solution, thereafter the drug was crystallized out of the solution. The crystallization of drug was prevented by the incorporation of an antinucleate polymer into IPM:PG:acetone vehicle thereby enhancing the flux by 5-fold.[48]

In another study, the diffusion of nifedipine was studied across EVA copolymer membrane (*in-vitro*) and excised male Wistar rat skin (*in-vivo*) from vehicle consisting of ethanol (volatile component) and diethyl sabacate (nonvolatile component). With both *in-vitro* and *in-vivo* studies, highest diffusion was exhibited by ethanol:diethyl sebacate in the 75:25 ratio. Furthermore, the same combination showed 1.75 times of saturation after complete evaporation of the ethanol.[49] The same group of researchers investigated the *in-vivo* penetration of nifedipine from range of volatile (acetone)/ non-volatile solvent (PG and IPM) combinations across male Wister rat skin. The initial plasma concentrations of drug were higher from both binary mixture (PG:acetone and IPM: acetone) and ternary mixture (PG:IPM:acetone) due to the formation of supersaturated solution after the evaporation of acetone. The plasma concentrations of drug were decreased in the later stage due to precipitation of drug, but upon incorporation of an antinucleate polymer to the vehicles, higher plasma levels were observed. Furthermore, ternary systems exhibited greater degree of penetration compared to binary systems.[50]

Chiang *et al.* used ethanol as volatile component and PG and water as non-volatile components to enhance the flux of minoxidil through human cadaver skin. The evaporation of the volatile component mostly happened within 30 min of application at room temperature. The flux value was increased with increasing concentration up to a point where the crystallization of drug started. There were no statistically significant differences of minoxidil flux when PG content in the vehicle was varied at the expense of ethanol without changing drug concentration.[51]

McDaid and Deasy attempted to enhance the thermodynamic gradient of nifedipine across the hairless mouse skin by the use of evaporation system comprising of ethanol: butanone: water in the ratio of 18.75:37.5:43.75% v/v. The flux of nifedipine was enhanced using evaporation system compared to aqueous suspension by 1330, 2897 and 172-fold using three different types of membrane such as hairless mouse skin, Celgard 2400 and EVA 987192. They attributed the above results could be due to interaction between the solvent system and various membranes rather than the increased drug solubility in volatile/non-volatile vehicle.[52]

Pellett *et al.* prepared supersaturated solutions of piroxicam in a 40:60 (v/v) PG/water co-solvent mixture and studied the effect of different DS on the permeation of piroxicam across silicon membrane and full-thickness human skin. In general, there was a linear correlation between the flux and DS for the supersaturated systems, but flux values across human skin at 0.5 and 1 DS were found to be similar. This was partly due to difference in solubility of the drug at different donor phase temperatures. It was observed that solutions up to 4 DS were stable up to 16 h. It was also observed that addition of HPMC to the solution prevented the formation of hydrate form of piroxicam, which was less soluble than its anhydrous form in the mixture of aqueous solvent.[20]

Pellett *et al.* investigated the *in-vitro* permeation of piroxicam from supersaturated solutions up to 4 DS across human skin and the amount of permeant in SC was estimated by tape stripping method. It was observed that there was a linear relationship between the DS and the amount of piroxicam in the SC with R^2 value of 0.970. In addition, piroxicam amount in viable layers of the skin also increased with the increase in DS. Above result was attributed to the antinucleating ability of intercellular lipids of the SC that inhibits or retards the formation of drug crystals in SC.[38]

Cho and Choi tested various vehicles in order to evaluate their influence on the permeation rate of ketoprofen across mouse skin. Vehicles such as octanol, ethanol, and PG/Oleyl alcohol (OA) mixture exhibited the highest flux of 30 μg/cm^2/h from 5mg/ml solution. However, there was no correlation between the solubility of ketoprofen in those solvents and its permeation rate. This enhancement of ketoprofen was attributed to the change in barrier property of mouse skin and/or carrier mechanism of the vehicles used. When the effect of vehicles on the percutaneous absorption of ketoprofen from acrylic pressure sensitive adhesive (PSA), oleic acid exhibited marginally higher flux of 2 μg/cm^2/h compared to other solvents tested.[34]

Fang *et al.* developed aqueous ethanolic vehicle as evaporative system to enhance the delivery of sodium nonivamide acetate across rat skin. To stop the crystallization of drug as the volatile component evaporates on the skin surface, a range of potential antinucleant polymers were investigated. The delivery of drug was increased rapidly over the first 12 h thereafter a plateau up to 72 h. It was attributed to: (i) precipitation of drug on the skin surface and (ii) may be the crystallization within the skin membrane itself limited the continued increased in permeation. Among all, MC and hydroxypropyl cellulose (HPC) were found to be the best antinucleant polymers.[53]

Iervolino *et al.* developed supersaturated solutions of ibuprofen ranging from 0.5 to 5 DS in 40:60 (v/v) PG/water mixtures in the absence and presence of additives such as HPMC and 2-hydroxypropyl-β-cyclodextrin (CD) and investigated ibuprofen permeation across human epidermis from supersaturated solution. Supersatuarated solutions of drug showed significant flux enhancement compared saturated solutions of drug. In the absence of HPMC, the flux of ibuprofen was found to be below per expected for 4 and 5 DS. In the absence of additives, the flux was lower than expected for 4 and 5 DS whereas the addition of HPMC enhanced the flux in proportional to the DS because of stabilization of the supersaturated solutions. The stabilization is due to the formation of hydrogen bond between HPMC and ibuprofen which inhibit the growth of ibuprofen crystal. With CD at 2 and 3 DS, the flux of drug was found to be less compared not only to supersaturated solution with HPMC but also to saturated solutions due to the formation of ibuprofen/CD inclusion complex. But at 5 DS a higher enhancement of flux was observed indicating that CD might act as PE.[29]

Moser *et al.* prepared different supersaturated formulations of a lavendustin derivative (LAP) employing techniques such as (i) mixed co-solvent (e.g., PG-water, PEG-water, IPM-silicone oil), (ii) method of solvent evaporation such as ethanol-PG, and (iii) the method of dissolving the drug by heating. Formulations at 1 DS showed comparable permeation across the pig skin. Whereas formulations at 2 DS resulted in 2-fold increase in drug permeation and were independent of the type and composition of the vehicles, method of preparation and absolute concentration of the drug. Although supersatuarated solutions at 2 DS such as PG-water and ethanol-PG exhibited significant increase in LAP transport compared to 1 DS, but the later formulation showed highest increase (2.2-fold) in LAP transport.[54]

Santosh *et al.* prepared supersaturated solution of oxybutynin by solvent evaporation technique with solvent/vehicle such as ethanol, PG and octyl salicylate (OS) and studied the effect of different DS and solvents on the permeation of oxybutynin across human abdominal skin. There was an insignificant difference in oxybutynin permeation following the application of 25% PG containing formulations with 1, 2, and 5 DS. This result indicated that permeation enhancement could not be achieved employing supersaturated PG formulations. When 25% OS formulations with different DS were tested, 5 DS formulation showed lowest permeation (Q24h, 0.064±0.028 μm/cm^2) whereas with 50% OS formulations at 1 DS exhibited lowest permeation (Q24h, 0.052±0.008 μm/cm^2). Furthermore there were decrease in drug permeation with increase in DS of drug for OS containg formulations, which was attributed to decrease in both drug crystallization and solvent activity (OS uptake) with increase in DS.[35]

Wang *et al.* developed transdermal evaporation delivery system of praziquantel. They have used ethanol as volatile component and various non-volatile solvents such as ethylene glycol monophenyl ether (EGPE), tetrahydrofuran, 1, 4-dioxane, oleic acid and dimethyl sulfoxide (DMSO) and studied the solubility of drug in those solvents at different temperatures. Among all, EGPE was selected as non-volatile component as the drug solubility was found to be highest (more than 400 mg/mL) when it is mixed with ethanol (50% w/w) at 32°C. The serum drug concentration was found to be 35.93 mg/mL, which is 6.3 and 1.96 times higher than the oral administration and transdermal evaporation delivery system without ethanol, respectively, at the same dose.[55]

Santosh *et al.* studied the transport of fentanyl across silicone membranes from subsaturated, saturated and supersaturated residues prepared by employing co-solvent approach (PG:water, 60:40 % v/v) or by employing a volatile solvent (PG: ethanol, 60:40 % v/v). For both type of formulations (PG:water and PG:ethanol), there was a good correlation between the mean flux and theoretical DS. Furthermore, no significant differences were observed in the mean flux between PG:water and PG:ethanol finite dose studies except for the 2DS formulations. Higher permeation enhancement observed with ethanol-based formulations across the DS, which was clearly resulted from an enhanced thermodynamic activity of drug with ethanol evaporation. The only difference between finite and infinite dose studies is the donor reservoir capacity for the drug and solvent.[56]

Santosh *et al.* investigated the role of vehicles/PEs such as PG, OS and IPM on the permeation of fentanyl across human skin *in-vitro* and then a model spray formulations were prepared consisting of 10% (v/v) of individual PEs in ethanol. It was observed that increasing the DS did not promote drug permeation for formulation containing PG but increase of drug permeation observed with formulation containing IPM and OS. This was attributed to the faster permeation of PG from the skin surface compared to IPM and OS. PG and IPM were found to promote drug solubility in the membrane whereas OS acted as PE by increasing drug diffusion in the skin. Furthermore, OS containing formulation significantly improved drug permeation and reduces the lag time compared to IPM and PG.[57]

Intarakumhaeng and Li tried different solvents having different evaporation and penetration property such as ethanol, hexane, isopropanol, and butanol in order to explain their influence on skin deposition/absorption of corticosterone. There were no significant differences in solvent-induced deposition/permeation (i.e., skin permeation due to solvent convection) of corticosterone on/across the SC and also there was no correlation between the rate of absorption of the permeant and the rate of solvent evaporation/penetration was observed.

Conversely, for the slow evaporating solvents such as water, PG and PEG 400, there was relationship between permeant absorption and rate of solvent evaporation i.e., slower absorption of corticosterone was evident for the slow evaporating solvent which is due to the change in thermodynamic activity of the permeant during skin absorption.[58]

Spray systems (MDTS)

Until 2007, aerosols as topical spray were used to deliver the drug across the skin. It is known that aerosol system depends on the power of compressed or liquefied gas to expel the content from the container. Recently, these propellant based sprays have been substituted by propellant free and solvent and polymer based MDTS which can deliver metered amount of drug per actuation. The concept of MDTS was first developed by Victorian college of Pharmacy, Australia and the first commercial product was developed and marketed by Acrux limited.[59,60] MDTS represents evaporation topical aerosol product composed of drug, solvent systems (volatile:non-volatile), PEs and polymers.[61,62] Common drugs which are developed as MDTS are estradiol, testosterone, nestrone etc. Methanol, ethanol, dichloromethane, isopropanol are considered as volatile solvent whereas PG, water and diethyl sebacate are used as non-volatile component. In case of polymers, any natural or synthetic polymers can be used. Terpenes, pyrrolidone, azones, alcohol and surfactants are used as PEs.[59,61,63] In addition, Acrux company developed a lipid like and generally recognized as safe (GRAS) category of PE called as ACROSS® which is added to MDTS® to increase the drug permeation by forming depot system in skin.

This type of system has more advantages compared to solution and semisolid preparations: (i) as it is a spray system the volume per area of administration can be precisely defined with highly reproducible manner, and (ii) it also helps the formulation to be uniformly distributed on the skin over a defined area after application.[27,64,65] The major advantage of this system is that it can form drug reservoir/depot in the skin instead of over the skin as in case of patch.[64] These systems are forming drug reservoir/depot within the SC in step wise manner as illustrated in Figure 3. It is depicted in three steps: (a) actuation of MDTS released desired amount of formulation on to the skin surface, (b) the surface deposit of dosage form, which is shown as pyramid, gradually decreases in its size due to both rapid evaporation of volatile component of the solvent mixture and forced partitioning of drug and PEs into SC, and (C) this partitioning of drug and PEs resulting into formation of their reservoir within the SC and thereby releasing the drug into the systemic circulation in sustained manner. MDTS increases drug diffusivity by SC lipid fluidization or lipid phase.[61]

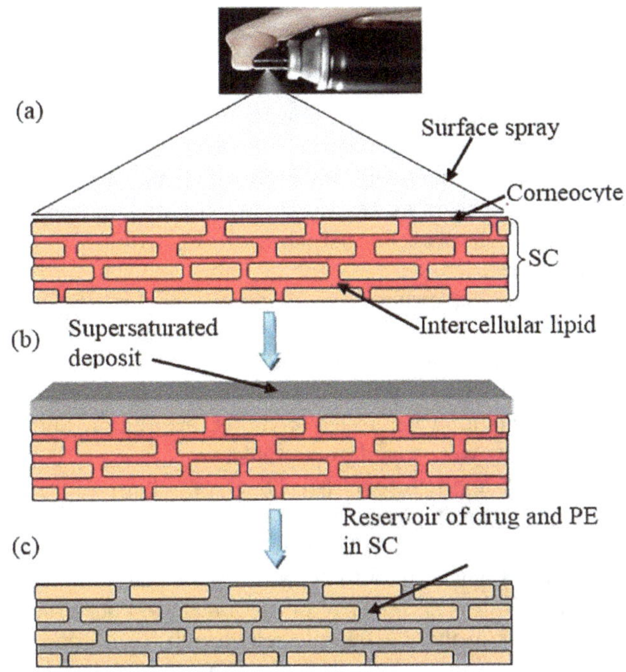

Figure 3. Schematic representation of mechanism of action of MDTS; (a) Surface spray applied to the SC, (b) forced partitioning concept where rapid evaporation of volatile vehicle followed by partitioning of drug and PE into SC, (c) drug and PE form a reservoir within the SC which is lipid in character and water resistant [Modified from Reference 31].

Leichtnam *et al.* evaluated testosterone permeation across hairless rat skin from a series of ethanol/PG/water formulations to obtain optimal composition followed by its incorporation with modification in to mechanical spray for feasible transdermal spray formulation. Among various combinations, saturated solution of testosterone in 1:1:1 ethanol/PG/water was exhibited highest flux of 1.7±0.2 mg/cm^2/h. Out of five formulation developed for mechanical spray only 1:1 ethanol/PG showed comparable flux and improved sprayability (due to absence of water). When propellant was added, only 3:1 ethanol/PG was found to be stable and all other formulations either showed phase separation or immediate crystallization. Furthermore, increasing the percentage of ethanol in the mixture increased evaporation rate without any alteration in testosterone permeation.[64]

Leichtnam *et al.* investigated various PEs in order find out suitable combination of PEs, solvent system and/or propellant for the delivery of testosterone from a spray/aerosol. Among the series of PEs used to pre-treat the skin before the application of spray, IPM was found to be most efficient as it increased the penetration enhancement of testosterone by more than 5 times from a solvent system containing 1:1 ethanol/water. The flux was further enhanced with solvent system of ethanol/PG (3:1), which is a more compatible vehicle for the spray. After incorporation of IPM in the range of 10-25% into aerosol system containing 50% v/v propellant, flux was found to be increased only 2.5-fold at highest level of IPM from both the spray and aerosol. The amount of pulverized drug finally contacted the skin surface represented only approximately 10% and 40 % from spray and aerosol, respectively, which was less than expected.[66]

Bakshi *et al.* developed oxybutynin containing metered dose spray formulation for transdermal delivery. A series of combinations of solvent system composed of ethanol/acetone/methylal were prepared and a ratio of 2:1:2 was selected as best combination based on various *in-vitro* parameters. Furthermore, different film forming agents were tried and carbopol and lutrol at 0.5 and 0.1%, respectively, have showed good clarity, spray pattern and evaporation rate. *In-vitro* diffusion study across semipermeable membrane demonstrated that the drug release was almost 59% over a period of 24 h. There was no skin irritation when tested on rabbit. In addition, above formulations were found to be stable.[67]

Terri *et al.* applied novel MDTS of estradiol (1.7%) to healthy postmenopausal women and investigated the steady state pharmacokinetics of estradiol and its metabolites such as estrone and estrone sulfate. The formulation was administered (1.53 mg/spray) once daily for 14 days in three different spray groups (1, 2, and 3) and samples were collected on day 1, before the first dose was administered, to 21 days including 7 days after the last dose administered). It was observed that the steady state was reached by day 7 or 8 for all the three groups and is maintained up to 21 day. The mean eastrdiol and estone concentrations at 14 days following 1, 2, 3-sprays were found to be 36 and 50, 57 and 54, and 54 and 71 pg/mL, respectively. Maximum concentration for estradiol was observed at 18-20 h (t_{max}). Finally, it was concluded that MDTS of estradiol produces low serum estron concentration.[68]

Davison *et al.* performed a pilot study on healthy postmenopausal women stabilized on estrogen in order to understand the effect of testosterone therapy on their cognitive performance such as visual and verbal as well as memory. Treatment group of women showed significant effect of testosterone on the cognitive performance in the domain of verbal and memory compared to untreated group.[69]

Lu *et al.* developed MDTS formulations of testosterone as topical solutions composed of volatile vehicle (ethanol) and non-volatile vehicle/PEs such as azone, IPM, PG, and NMP and film forming polymers (FFPs) such as Eudragit® E PO, Eudragit® RL PO, Plasdone® S630 and PVP K30 and evaluated their efficacy. Among the PEs and FFPs used in the permeation study, azone at 9% (v/v) and Plasdone® S630 exhibited highest flux for testosterone. Out of total 9 formulations prepared, formulation containing 10% (w/v) testosterone, 9% (v/v) azone and 91 % (v/v) ethanol showed good skin permeation and acceptable PE content and drug concentration. Furthermore, this optimized formulation was non-irritating in rat model and showed a different plasma-time profile from that of Testopatch® (commercially available product) with Testopatch® exhibited a more sustainable drug release.[27]

Lu *et al.* prepared different MDTS formulations containing dexketoprofen to screen different PEs such as azone, PG, IPM, lauryl lacetate (LA) and FFPs viz. Eudragit RL PO, Plasdone S-630, PVP K30 and Kollidone PF 12. There was no significant difference of drug permeation among all the FFPs. IPM among the PEs was found to be appropriate one and the optimized formulation was containing 7% (w/w) dexketoprofen, 7% (v/v) IPM and 93% (v/v) ethanol. Above formulation showed both anti-inflammatory and anti-nocieptive activities with no sign of skin irritation.[62]

Patel *et al.* developed an user friendly MDTS of Lopinavir to be used in combination of chemical and physical method (microneedle technique) to improve overall penetration enhancement across pig ear skin. Formulation having 5% w/v of Kollidon® showed best volatilization and spreadability property. *Ex-vivo* studies indicated a significantly higher penetration enhancement of 1.77 and steady state transdermal flux of 52.5 μg/cm^2/h across microporated pig ear skin. Furthermore, *in-vivo* investigation exhibited 3-fold increase in relative bioavailability of lopinavir through transdermal route compared to oral suspension of marketed tablet. In addition the system was found to be safe and stable as well as have potential to be used in clinical settings.[70]

Ranade *et al.* designed topical film-forming metered dose spray formulations of ropivacaine for the management of pain. Permeation study was performed on porcine skin and after the permeation study; skin sample was visualized under conofocal microscopy to ensure the potency of designed formulations. The results demonstrated a high level of drug concentration in the skin layers. The anti-nociceptive efficacy study showed that the formulation has comparable efficacy to the conventional lidocaine gel.[71]

Klose *et al.* prepared spray formulations of antiparkinson's agent such as ropinirole, pramipixole, sumanirole and cabergoline with aqueous ethanol as evaporating solvent and padimate O/OS as PEs. They observed that the formulations with PEs deliver more antiparkinson's agent through the shed skin of snake than the corresponding formulation.[72]

Morgan *et al.* successfully developed a topical spray system of oestradiol (1 and 1.7% w/v) and its derivative ethinyl oestradiol for its systemic delivery across the skin of animals and human. Other ingredients present in the system include OS/padimate O as PE and aqueous ethanol as evaporating solvent.[73]

Lulla *et al.* developed a topical spray system that can be sprayed onto the skin to form a stable breathable film or patch over a period of days. The system composed of estradiol and alendronate sodium as active ingredients, eudragit E 100 as a self-adhesive, plastoid B as a film former, PG as a humectant, sodium lauryl sulfate as a solubilizer for the drug, acetone as a volatile solvent for quick drying and non-occlusive vehicle and P11 as a propellant to expel the product out of the container. It was observed that the above composition was able to form stable thin film which was observed up to 24 h after formation and can deliver the drug in a sustained manner from 1 to 5 days.[74]

Lulla and Malhotra patented transdermal spray formulation for testosterone (16.66%). Vinyl pyrrolidone/vinyl acetate (VP/VA) copolymer was used as film forming polymer and ethanol and acetone combination was used as solvent system. The copolymer acted as antinucleating agent at a concentration 1-10%. Above formulation usually forms uniform thin film on the skin within 60 s when sprayed from metered dose spray container at a fixed distance from the skin surface. In addition the above concentration of testosterone in the formulation was able to penetrate the skin and reached to blood circulation in desired concentration.[75]

Watkinson *et al.* patented transdermal spray system for volatile active ingredients such as nicotine and selegiline and volatile solvents selected from ethanol, isopropanol or their mixture in a concentration ranging from 0.5 to 25% by weight to a area of human skin (20 cm^2). It was claimed to have better potential for the treatment or prophylaxis of Parkinson's disease and reduced craving for cigarettes in a smoker.[76]

Wan and Watkinson investigated transderrnal spray system of norethisterone acetate, nestorone, estradiol and testosterone containing PEG 200, 400 and OS as PE. They observed; (i) PEG 200 in combination with OS significantly enhance the permeation of norethisterone acetate and estradiol across the human epidermis in vitro, (ii) PEG 400 did not exhibit any significant effect on the permeation of Nestorone whereas it inhibit the permeation of ethylestradiol through human epidermis *in-vitro*, (iii) PEG 200 was significantly enhance the permeation of testosterone across human epidermis *in-vitro* which was not seen when PEG 400 was used as PE, (iv) PEG 200 showed significant increase in permeation enhancement of estradiol.[77]

Morgan *et al.* claimed that a transdermal spray formulation of testosterone comprising of 0.1 to 10% weight of testosterone, 0.1 to 10% weight of one or more PEs consisting of at least OS and padimate O, 85 to 99.8 % by weight of a volatile solvent selected from a group consisting of ethanol, isopropanol and their mixture and optionally a gelling agent. Upon application of the composition, evaporation of solvent at body temperature forms an amorphous deposits leading to enhanced delivery of testosterone across the skin. Similarly, buspirone exhibited maximum permeation across human epidermis when the formulation composed of 95% of ethanol and OS as volatile solvent and PE, respectively. This is because of the formation of amorphous form of the drug leading to both zero and first order kinetics.[78]

Table 1. List of evaporative drug delivery systems comprising of drugs, solvent systems and polymers

Types of formulation	Drug	Solvent systems (Non volatile/Volatile)	Polymer (s)	References
Solutions and semisolids	Fluocinolone acetonide and its acetate ester	PG, water and IPM	-	[45]
		PG and IPM/ Isopropanol	-	[46]
	Hydrocortisone	Water/Acetone	-	[47]
	Nifedipine	IPM and PG/ Acetone	-	[48]
		Diethyl sabacate/ Ethanol	-	[49
		PG and IPM/ Acetone	-	[50]
	Minoxidil	PG and water/ Ethanol	-	[51]
	Nifedipine	Butanone and water/ Ethanol	-	[52]
	Piroxicam	PG and water	HPMC	[20]
		-	-	[38]
	Ketoprofen	PG/ Octanol, ethanol and OA	-	[34]
	Sodium nonivamide acetate	Water/ Ethanol	-	[53]
	Ibuprofen	PG and water	MC and HPC	[29]
	Lavendustin derivative	PG, PEG, IPM and silicone oil/ Ethanol	HPMC and CD	[54]
	Oxybutynin	PG and OS/ ethanol	-	[35]
	Praziquantel	EGPE, tetrahydrofuran, 1, 4-dioxane, oleic acid and DMSO/ Ethanol	-	[55]
	Fentanyl	PG and water/ Ethanol	-	[56]
		PG, OS and IPM/ Ethanol	-	[57]
	Corticosterone	Water, PG and PEG 400/ Ethanol, hexane, isopropanol, and butanol	-	[58]
Sprays	Dexketoprofen	Azone, PG, IPM and LA/ Ethanol	Eudragit RL PO, Plasdone S-630, PVP K30 and Kollidone PF 12	[62]
	Testosterone	PG and water/ Ethanol	-	[64]
		IPM and water/ Ethanol	-	[66]
	Oxybutynin	-/ Ethanol, acetone, methylal	Carbopol and lutrol	[67]

Types of formulation	Drug	Solvent systems (Non volatile/Volatile)	Polymer (s)	References
	Estradiol	-	-	[68]
	Testosterone	-	-	[69]
		Azone, IPM, PG and NMP/ Ethanol	Eudragit® E PO, Eudragit® RL PO, Plasdone® S630 and PVP K30	[27]
	Lopinavir	-	Kollidon®	[70]
	Ropivacaine	-	-	[71]
	Ropinirole, pramipixole, sumanirole and cabergoline	Padimate O and OS/ Ethanol	-	[72]
	Oestradiol and ethinyl oestradiol	Padimate O and OS/ Ethanol	-	[73]
	Estradiol and alendronate sodium	PG/ Acetone	Eudragit E 100 a self adhesive, plastoid B	[74]
	Testosterone	-/ Ethanol and acetone	VA/VP	[75]
	Nicotine and selegiline	-/ Ethanol, isopropanol	-	[76]
	Norethisterone acetate, nestorone, estradiol and testosterone	PEG 200, 400 and OS/ -	-	[77]
	Testosterone and buspirone	OS and padimate O/ Ethanol, isopropanol	-	[78]

Commercial products

Acrux Pvt. Ltd. is the first company to commercialize MDTS with lunching number of products in market such as Evamist®, Lenzetto®, Ellavie®, Axiron®, Nestorone®. These products provide fast-drying, invisible sprays or liquids with outmost cosmetic acceptability. Moreover the other advantages of above system are attainment of steady state plasma concentration for four days after a single application and very low skin irritation rate because of non-occlusive delivery.[79,80] A list of commercial products based on evaporative principles with their brand name, marketing company, active ingredient, formulation type and use are presented in Table 2.

Table 2. List of commercial products based on evaporative principles

Product (Brand name)	Marketing company	Active ingredient	Formulation type	Purpose
Evamist®	Perrigo (From 2014) KV Pharmaceuticals (from 2007 to 2014)	Estradiol	Spray (MDTS)	Menopause symptoms related to vasomotor and hot flushes
Lenzetto®	Gedeon Richter			
Ellavie®	Aspen Pharmacare and Vifor pharma			
Axiron®	Eli Lilly	Testosterone	Solution	Hypogonadism or low/no testosterone
Nestorone (NES) MDTS®	Acrux Pvt. Ltd. (Phase-I trial completed) partnered with Population Council and Fempharm Pvt. Ltd	Nestorone	Spray (MDTS)	Contraception
Nicotine MDTS®	Acrux Pvt. Ltd. (Phase-I trial completed)	Nicotine	Spray (MDTS)	Smoking cessation
Recuvyra®	Elanco Pvt. Ltd.	Fentanyl	Spray (MDTS)	Postoperative pain (for veterinary use)

Evamist®, Lenzetto®, Ellavie® (Estradiol transdermal spray)

Estradiol spray system was the first MDTS developed by Acrux Pvt. Ltd. to treat menopause symptoms such as severe hot flushes and it was approved by FDA in three brand names such as Evamist, Lenzetto® and Ellavie®. These were licensed to different companies to market it all across the globe. In 2007, Evamist® licensed to KV Pharmaceuticals to market it in US, but latter on it was distributed by Perrigo from 2014 as the former company was acquired by the latter. Gedeon Richter received multiple marketing approvals for estradiol spray and in 2016 it was launched in Europe and Eurasia in the brand name of Lenzetto®. Ellavie® is a unique estradiol skin spray which is used to treat vasomotor symptoms associated with menopause. From 2009 Ellavie® was marketed and distributed in Australia by Aspen Pharmacare and in Switzerland by Vifor pharma.[81]

All the above products are small and hand-held spray (Figure 4), design to deliver a predetermined dose of estradiol in the systemic circulation on sustained basis over 24 h across the skin. They are placed gently against the skin following which an actuator button is pressed to release light spray containing estradiol. The spray is fast drying thereby leaving an invisible film after application.[31,82] When measured by radioimmunoassay after estradiol-MDTS post menopausal women have shown higher plasma level of estradiol than baseline value.[63]

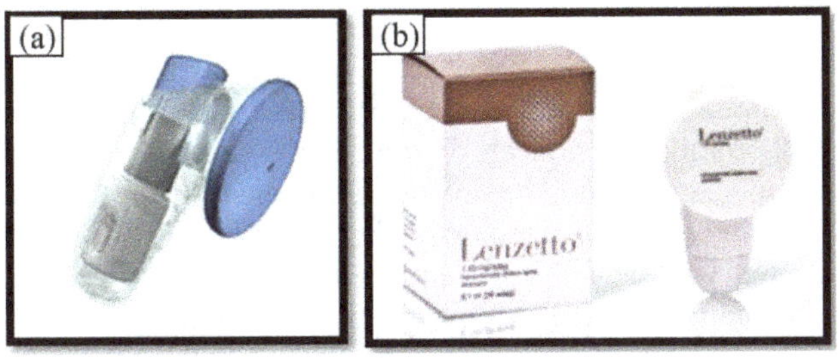

Figure 4. Commercial product of estradiol: (a) Evamist® and (b) Lenzetto®

Axiron® (Testosterone solution)

Testosterone topical solution was marketed in the brand name of Axiron®. It was licenced to Eli Lilly and was launched by the same company in the countries such as US, Canada, Australia Germany, Braziland South Korea. Axiron® is used to treat adult males who are suffering from hypogonadism or low/no testosterone. It is available in two forms; pump actuated (Figure 5a) and twist actuated (Figure 5b) metered dose pump and are approved for application with the help of an armpit (underarm) applicator.

Axiron® is consisting of three parts; pump, cap and applicator cup as soon as in Figure 5. Initially, the cap and the applicator cup are to be removed from the pump. Then, the nozzle of the pump is to positioned over the applicator and was pressed gently to release preset dose of testosterone (30, 60, 90, and 120 mg) on to the applicator. This is followed by the rubbing action (steady up and down movement) into the armpit application site. In case of twist actuated (Figure 5b), the applicator is fixed on the bottle. Therefore, it is directly rubbed on to the patient's armpit. The application site is to allow for drying for three minutes before wearing a dress.[83]

Acrux Pvt. Ltd. is also developing a fast drying testosterone MD-Lotion® which can be applied directly into the patient's armpit using an innovative "no-touch" applicator, in similar way as deodorant. In 2015, Elli Lily successfully completed phase III trial on the product in different countries over the world. The topical solution can only be applied by touching the applicator to the armpit. This necessitates an extra step of washing and drying of applicator prior to next use. In this context "no-touch" applicator is having a clear advantage.[84]

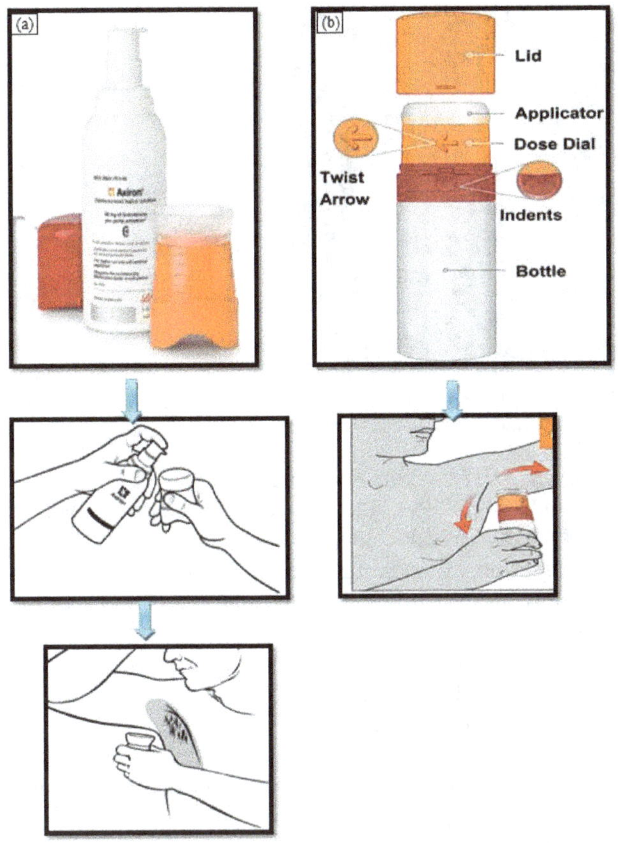

Figure 5. Commercial product of testosterone (Axiron®) and their way of application; (a) pump actuated, and (b) twist actuated

Nestorone (NES) MDTS® (Nestorone transdermal spray)

Nestorone is a non-androgenic novel progestin used for non-oral contraception. Acrux Pvt. Ltd. developed a progestin-only-spray-on-contraceptive MDTS for Nestorone (Figure 6 (a) and (b)). Nestorone spray is found to be highly active transdermally resulting in good systemic bioavailability.[85,86] Fraser *et al.* reported that serum levels of Nestorone was achieved within the range of 285-290 pmol/L and was able to block ovulation in case of 83% of the women taken the spray during the study. This result proven that the above serum concentration of the drug is sufficient enough to provide effective contraception.[87] Thereafter, Acrux Pvt. Ltd. partnered with Population Council and Fempharm Pvt. Ltd. to develop a MDTS spray system containing both Nestorone and an estrogen or 17-ethinylestradiol in order to explore the possibility of delivering once daily dose to illicit contraception. The product is under phase-1 trial and was found to be releasing the drug into blood circulation over a period of 72 h. The current status is that the company involved in the development process abandoned the project.[88]

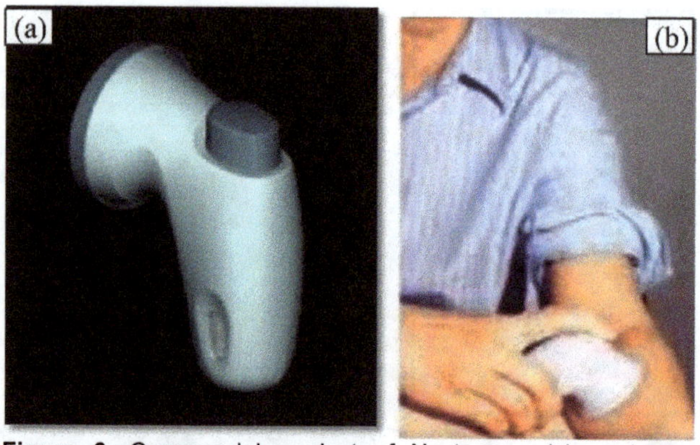

Figure 6. Commercial product of Nestorone; (a) nestorone MDTS®, and (b) its application

Nicotine MDTS® and Fentanyl MDTS®

In 2007, Acrux Pvt. Ltd. has announced that Nicotine MDTS®, a newly developed transdermal spray system for the cessation of smoking, is added to the pipeline. The company successfully completed phase I clinical trial of three different spray formulations of nicotine on sixteen subjects in Australia. Similarly, Acrux Pvt. Ltd. also developed fentanyl MDTS® to treat chronic pain and given distribution rights to CSL Ltd.

Apart from above MDTS® developed for human use, Acrux Pvt. Ltd. also developed transdermal fentanyl solution Recuvyra®, a veterinary product, used for the control of postoperative pain associated with major orthopaedic and soft tissue surgery (Figure 7). It is first of kind of innovative evaporative products (50mg/ml) lunched by Elanco Pvt. Ltd. to market it globally and has the ability to control pain for 4 days in a single dose.

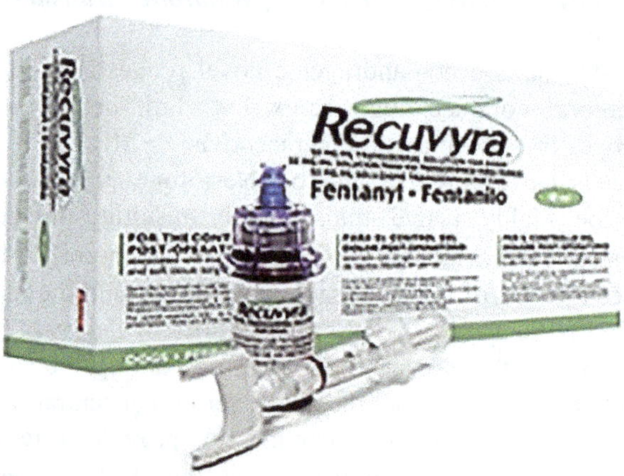

Figure 7. Commercial fentanyl transdermal solution for veterinary use (Recuvyra®).

Discussion

Drug delivery through transdermal route seems to be very attractive concept, but not all classes of drugs will be able to permeate the SC barrier in sufficient amount that can illicit the therapeutic action. The physico-chemical properties which are important for a drug to permeate the barrier layer of skin by passive diffusion includes small molecular size (less than 500Da), log partition coefficient preferentially within range of 1 to 3.5, aqueous solubility of greater than 100 μg/mL, low drug dose suitably less than 10mg/day and melting point less than 200°C.[21,89] The individual drugs suitable for TDD are those which undergoes first pass metabolism either in liver of GI tract, causing irritation in the stomach, elimination half life less than 3h and showing absorption window in oral route. At present, no such drug molecules are approved by USFDA which possess all above properties. However, it is possible only when the design and development of drug molecules with maximum number of desired properties to suit TDDD will be developed.

In these circumstances evaporation TDDS composed of only two component system can be explored to a maximum extent to include more drugs in to the fold of TDD route. The concept involved in evaporation system is supersaturation. The volatile component of the solvent mixture evaporates leaving behind supersaturated solution in non-volatile solvent component on the skin surface after application. The non-volatile component in which the drug is soluble thereby preventing the drug precipitation. This resulted in partitioning of drug across the skin in higher amount that can provide required drug concentration in systemic circulation.[31]

These systems can be formulated into various types of formulations such as solutions, semisolids, and sprays. The MDT spray systems have the added advantages of delivering the drug in metered manner that can provide precise dose. In addition these systems are able to deliver the dose at the site of action in case of topical drug delivery. There are many commercial products containing number of drugs such as Evamist®, Lenzetto®, Axiron®, Netorone MDTS®, Recuvyra®, and Nicotene MDTS® are already available and there are many drugs in the pipeline.

Conclusion

Despite of numerous constraints, drug delivery through transdermal route continues to grow and expand because of the development of new technologies such as the use of sonophoresis, electroporation, microneedle, chemical PEs and novel supersaturation concept. This technological advancement in TDD sector led to successful delivery of drugs ranging from potent (low dose) to moderately potent drug. Among all, supersaturation concept is standing tall as it has the flexibility of delivering the dose in solution, semisolid or in the spray form. In addition the drug dose can be precisely and accurately administered with MDTS which avoids the intra- and inter-patient dose variation. In this context, Aptar group taken a step ahead in developing metered dose spray pumps and dispenser for topical and transdermal products which can be combined with MDTS to achieve dial-a-dose of transdermal delivery with highest degree of accuracy and precision.[90]

Like other techniques, this concept is totally not free of disadvantages. The main issue remains is the stability of supersaturated formulations as with the increase in drug concentration there are more probability of drug crystallization. But to a large extent the problem is minimized by adding antinucleating excipients such as polymers. As of now the evaporative technique using supersaturated concept is restricted to drugs of fewer class e.g., hormones, anti-asthmatics, NSAIDs, central analgesics and drug addiction. But the positive outcome of this technique is that there are many formulations in the market and many are in the pipeline, particularly as MDTS. We anticipate more and more classes of drugs will be delivered using this technique and will be available in the market. We also hope that evaporative technique along with other TDD technique will improve health-related quality of life of patient globally by preventing, diagnosing and controlling the diseases.

Conflict of Interest

The author declares that this article content has no conflict of interest

References

1. Agrawal SS, Pruthi JK. Development and evaluation of matrix type transdermal patch of ethinylestradiol and medroxyprogesterone acetate for anti-implantation activity in female Wistar rats. *Contraception* 2011;84(5):533-38. doi: 10.1016/j.contraception.2011.03.005
2. Guo R, Du X, Zhang R, Deng L, Dong A, Zhang J. Bioadhesive film formed from a novel organic–inorganic hybrid gel for transdermal drug delivery system. *Eur J Pharm Biopharm* 2011;79(3):574-83. doi: 10.1016/j.ejpb.2011.06.006
3. Parhi R, Suresh P, Pattnaik S. Application of Response Surface Methodology for Design and Optimization of Reservoir-type Transdermal Patch of Simvastatin. *Curr Drug Deliv* 2016;13(5):742-53.
4. Gooren LJ, Bunck MC. Transdermal testosterone delivery: testosterone patch and gel. *World J Urol* 2003;21(5):316-19. doi: 10.1007/s00345-003-0368-6
5. Kang C, Shin SC. Preparation and evaluation of bioadhesive dibucaine gels for enhanced local anesthetic action. *Arch Pharm Res* 2010;33(8):1277-83. doi: 10.1007/s12272-010-0819-8
6. Shin SC, Kim JY, Oh IJ. Mucoadhesive and physicochemical characterization of carbopol-poloxamer gels containing triamcinolone acetonide. *Drug Dev Ind Pharm* 2000;26(3):307-12. doi: 10.1081/DDC-100100358
7. Parhi R, Suresh P, Pattnaik S. Transdermal Delivery of Diltiazem Hydrochloride from Poloxamer-HPMC Gel: in vitro, ex vivo, and in vivo Studies. *Drug Deliv Lett* 2015;5(3):163-72. doi: 10.2174/221030310503160401120711
8. Samsioe G. Transdermal hormone therapy: gels and patches. *Climacteric* 2004;7(4):347-56.
9. Valenzuela P, Simon JA. Nanoparticle delivery for transdermal HRT. *Nanomedicine* 2012; Suppl 1:S83-9. doi: 10.1016/j.nano.2012.05.008
10. Algın Yapar E, Inal O. Transdermal Spray in Hormone Delivery. *Trop J Pharm Res* 2014;13(3):469-74. doi: 10.4314/tjpr.v13i3.23
11. Lopez RF, Seto JE, Blankschtein D, Langer R. Enhancing the transdermal delivery of rigid nanoparticles using the simultaneous application of ultrasound and sodium lauryl sulfate. *Biomaterials* 2011;32(3):933-41. doi: 10.1016/j.biomaterials.2010.09.060
12. Taylor LJ, Lee RS, Long M, Rawlings AV, Tubek J, Whitehead L. Effect of occlusion on the percutaneous penetration of linoleic acid and glycerol. *Int J Pharm* 2002;249(1-2):157-64.
13. Parhi R, Suresh P, Mondal S, Kumar PM. Novel Penetration Enhancers for Skin Applications: A Review. *Curr Drug Deliv* 2012;9(2):219-30.
14. Asbill CS, El-Kattan AF, Michniak, B. Enhancement of transdermal drug delivery: chemical and physical approaches. *Crit Rev Ther Drug Carrier Syst* 2000;17(6):621-58.
15. Prausnitz MR. Microneedles for transdermal drug delivery. *Adv Drug Deliv Rev* 2004;56(5):581-87. doi: 10.1016/j.addr.2003.10.023
16. Wong TW, Chen CH, Huang CC, Lin CD, Hui SW. Painless electroporation with a new needle-free microelectrode array to enhance transdermal drug delivery. *J Control Release* 2006;110(3):557-65. doi: 10.1016/j.jconrel.2005.11.003
17. Batheja P, Thakur R, Michniak B. Transdermal iontophoresis. *Expert Opin Drug Deliv* 2006;3(1):127-38. doi: 10.1517/17425247.3.1.127
18. Kaushik D, Costach A, Michniak-Kohn B. Percutaneous penetration modifiers and formulation effects. *Int J Pharm* 2010;386(1-2):42-51. doi: 10.1016/j.ijpharm.2009.10.052
19. Choi WI, Lee JH, Kim JY, Kim JC, Kim YH, Tae G. Efficient skin permeation of soluble proteins via flexible and functional nano-carrier. *J Control Release* 2012;157(2):272-78. doi: 10.1016/j.jconrel.2011.08.013
20. Pellett MA, Castellano S, Hadgraft J, Davis AF. The penetration of supersaturated solutions of piroxicam across silicone membranes and human skin in vitro. *J Control Release* 1997;46:205-14. doi: 10.1016/S0168-3659(96)01595-7
21. Parhi R, Suresh P, Pattnaik S. Physical means of stratum corneum barrier manipulation to enhance transdermal drug delivery. *Curr Drug Deliv* 2015;12(2):122-38.
22. Pellett M, Raghavan SL, Hadgraft J, Davis A. The Application of Supersaturated Systems to Percutaneous Drug Delivery. In: Guy RH, Hadgraft J, editors. Transdermal Drug Delivery. New York and Basel: Marcel Dekker, Inc; 2003.
23. Higuchi T. Physical chemical analysis of percutaneous absorption process from creams and ointments. *J Soc Cosmet Chem* 1960;11:85-97.
24. Khamskii EV, Crystallisation from Solutions. New York: Consultants Bureau, 1969.

25. Davis AF, Hadgraft J. Supersaturated solutions as topical drug delivery systems. In: Walters KA, Hadgraft J, editors. *Pharmaceutical Skin Penetration Enhancement*. New York: Marcel Dekker Inc;1993.
26. Morgan TM, Reed BL, Finnin BC. Enhanced skin permeation of sex hormones with novel topical spray vehicles. *J Pharm Sci* 1998;87(10):1213-8. doi: 10.1021/js980025k.
27. Lu W, Luo H, Wu Y, Zhu Z, Wang H. Preparation and characterization of a metered dose transdermal spray for testosterone. *Acta Pharm Sinica* B 2013;3:392-9.
28. Moser K, Kriwet K, Kalia YN, Guy RH. Stabilization of supersaturated solutions of a lipophilic drug for dermal deliver. *Int J Pharm* 2001;224(1-2):169-76.
29. Iervolino M, Cappello B, Raghavan SL, Hadgraft J. Penetration enhancement of ibuprofen from supersaturated solutions through human skin. *Int J Pharm* 2001;212(1):131-41.
30. Ibrahim SA. Spray-on transdermal drug delivery systems. *Expert Opin Drug Deliv* 2015:12(2):195-205. doi: 10.1517/17425247.2015.961419
31. Thomas BJ, Finnin BC. The transdermal revolution. *Drug Discov Today* 2004;9(16):697-703. doi: 10.1016/s1359-6446(04)03180-0
32. Barry BW. Transdermal drug delivery. In: Aulton ME, Taylor KMG, editors. Aulton's Pharmaceutics: The design and Manufacture of Medicines. London: Churchill Livingstone, Elsevier; 2007.
33. Twist JN, Zatz JL. The effect of solvents on solute penetration through fuzzy rat skin in vitro. *J Soc Cosmet Chem* 1989;40(4):231-42
34. Cho YJ, Choi HK. Enhancement of percutaneous absorption of ketoprofen: effect of vehicles and adhesive matrix. *Int J Pharmaceut* 1998;169:95-104. doi:10.1016/S0378-5173(98)00115-X
35. Santos P, Watkinson AC, Hadgraft J, Lane ME. Oxybutynin permeation in skin: The influence of drug and solvent activity. *Int J Pharm* 2010;384(1-2):67-72. doi: 10.1016/j.ijpharm.2009.09.043
36. Morgan TM, Reed BL, Finnin BC. Metered-dose transdermal spray (MDTS). New York: Marcel Dekker: 2003.
37. Mullin JW. Crystallization.uk:Butterworth-Heinemann: 2001.
38. Pellett MA, Roberts MS. Hadgraft J. Supersaturated solutions evaluated with an in vitro stratum corneum tape stripping technique. *Int J Pharmaceut* 1997;151:91-98. doi: 10.1016/S0378-5173(97)04897-7
39. Pellett MA, Davis AF, Hadgraft J. Effect of supersaturation on membrane transport: 2. Piroxicam. *Int J Pharmaceut* 1994;111:1-6. doi: 10.1016/0378-5173(94)90395-6
40. Schwarb FP, Imanidis G, Smith EW, Haigh JM, Surber C. Effect of concentration and saturation of topical Fluocinonide formulations on in vitro membrane transport and In vivo availability on human skin. *Pharm Res* 1999;16(6):909-15.
41. Iervolino M, Raghavan SL, Hadgraft J. Membrane penetration enhancement of ibuprofen using supersaturation. *Int J Pharm* 2000;198(2):229-38.
42. Chow AH-L, Chow PKK, Zhongshan W, Grant DJW. Modification of acetaminophen crystals: influence of growth in aqueous solutions containing p acetoxyacetanilide on crystal properties. *Int J Pharm* 1985;24:239-58. doi: 10.1016/0378-5173(85)90024-9
43. Fairbrother JE, Grant DJ. Crystal engineering studies with an excipient material (adipic acid). *J Pharm Pharmacol* 1979;31(Suppl.):27.
44. Chow KY, Go J, Mehdizadeh M, Grant DJW. Modification of adipic acid crystals: influence of growth in the presence of fatty acid additives on crystal properties. *Int J Pharm* 1984;20:3-24. doi:org/10.1016/0378-5173(84)90214-X
45. Poulsen BJ, Young E, Coquilla V, Katz M. Effect of topical vehicle composition on the in vitro release of fluocinolone acetonide and its acetate ester. *J Pharm Sci* 1968;57(6):928-33.
46. Coldman MF, Poulsen BJ, Higuchi T. Enhancement of percutaneous absorption by the use of volatile: nonvolatile systems as vehicles. *J Pharm Sci* 1969;58(9):1098-102.
47. Theeuwes F, Gale RM, Baker RW. Transference: a comprehensive parameter governing permeation of solutes through membranes. *J Membrane Sci*1976;1:3-16. doi: 10.1016/S0376-7388(00)82254-1
48. Kondo S, Sugimoto I. Enhancement of transdermal delivery by superfluous thermodynamic potential. I. Thermodynamic analysis of nifedipine transport across the lipoidal barrier. *J Pharmacobiodyn* 1987;10(10):587-94.
49. Kondo S, Yamasaki-Konishi H, Sugimoto I. Enhancement of transdermal delivery by superfluous thermodynamic potential. II. In vitro-in vivo correlation of percutaneous nifedipine transport. *J Pharmacobiodyn* 1987a;10(11):662-68.
50. Kondo S, Yamanaka C, Sugimoto I. Enhancement of transdermal delivery by superfluous thermodynamic potential. III. Percutaneous absorption of nifedipine in rats. *J Pharmacobiodyn* 1987b;10(12):743-49.
51. Ming CC, Flynn GL, Weiner N, Szpunar GJ. Bioavailability assessment of topical delivery systems: effect of vehicle evaporation upon in vitro delivery of minoxidil from solution formulations. *Int J Pharmaceut* 1989;55(s 2-3):229-36. doi: 10.1016/0378-5173(89)90046-X
52. McDaid DM, Deasy PB. An investigation into the transdermal delivery of nifedipine. *Pharm Acta Helv* 1996;71(4):253-58.
53. Fang JY, Kuo CT, Huang YB, Wu PC, Tsai YH. Transdermal delivery of sodium nonivamide acetate from volatile vehicles: Effects of polymers. *Int J Pharmaceut* 1999;176(2):156-67. doi: 10.1016/S0378-5173(98)00301-9

54. Moser K, Kriwet K, Kalia YN, Guy RH. Enhanced skin permeation of a lipophilic drug using supersaturated formulations. *J Control Release* 2001;73(2-3):245-53.
55. Wang L, Zheng X, Fang Y, Wang Y, Duan C, Yao B. Transdermal evaporation delivery system of praziquantel for Schistosomiasis Japonicum chemotherapy. *J Pharm Sci* 2011;100(7):2769-777. doi: 10.1002/jps.22508
56. Santos P, Watkinson AC, Hadgraft J, Lane ME. Enhanced permeation of fentanyl from supersaturated solutions in a model membrane. *Int J Pharm* 2011;407(1-2):72-77. doi: 10.1016/j.ijpharm.2011.01.025
57. Santos P, Watkinson AC, Hadgraft J, Lane ME. Influence of penetration enhancer on drug permeation from volatile formulations. *Int J Pharm* 2012;439(1-2):260-68. doi: 10.1016/j.ijpharm.2012.09.031
58. Intarakumhaeng R, Li SK. Effects of solvent on percutaneous absorption of nonvolatile lipophilic solute. *Int J Pharm* 2014;476(1-2):266-76. doi: 10.1016/j.ijpharm.2014.09.034
59. Kumar R, Philip A. Modified Transdermal Technologies: Breaking the barriers of drug permeation via the skin. *Trop J Pharm Res* 2007; 6(1): 633-44. doi: 10.4314/tjpr.v6i1.14641
60. Humberstone AJ, Evans AM, Nation RL, MacLennan AH. Comparison of pharmacokinetics and tolerability following application of an Estraderm® 50 patch or anovel Estradiol Metered-Dose Transdermal Spray (MDTS®). Paper presented at North American Menopause Society 13th Annual Meeting: Chicago, IL, US; 2002.
61. Morgan TM. Metered dose transdermal spray (MDTS). In: Hagraft J, editor. Modified release drug delivery technology. New York: Marcel Dekker; 2003.
62. Lu W, Luo H, Zhu Z, Wu Y, Luo J, Wang H. Preparation and the biopharmaceutical evaluation for the metered dose transdermal spray of dexketoprofen. *J Drug Deliv* 2014;2014:697434 doi: 10.1155/2014/697434
63. Finnin BC, Morgan TM. Transdermal penetration enhancers: applications, limitations and potential. *J Pharm Sci* 1999;88(10):955-58.
64. Leichtnam ML, Rolland H, Wuthrich P, Guy RH. Formulation and evaluation of a testosterone transdermal spray. *J Pharm Sci* 2006;95(8):1693-1702. doi: 10.1002/jps.20641
65. Reid ML, Benaouda F, Khengar R, Jones SA, Brown MB. Topical corticosteroid delivery into human skin using hydrofluoroalkane metered dose aerosol sprays. *Int J Pharm* 2013;452(1-2):157-65. doi:10.1016/j.ijpharm.2013.04.083
66. Leichtnam ML, Rolland H, Wüthrich P, Guy RH. Identification of penetration enhancers for testosterone transdermal delivery from spray formulations. *J Control Release* 2006;113(1):57-62. doi:10.1016/j.jconrel.2006.03.008
67. Bakshi A, Bajaj A, Malhotra G, Madan M, Amrutiya N. A novel metered dose transdermal spray formulation for oxybutynin. *Indian J Pharm Sci* 2008;70(6):733-39. doi: 10.4103/0250-474X.49094
68. Morton TL, Gattermeir DJ, Petersen CA, Day WW, Schumacher RJ. Steady-state pharmacokinetics following application of a novel transdermal estradiol spray in healthy postmenopausal women. *J Clin Pharmacol* 2009;49(9):1037-46. doi: 10.1177/0091270009339187
69. Davison SL, Bell RJ, Gavrilescu M, Searle K, Maruff P, Gogos A, et al. Testosterone improves verbal learning and memory in postmenopausal women: Results from a pilot study. *Maturitas* 2011;70(3):307-11. doi: 10.1016/j.maturitas.2011.08.006
70. Patel D, Kumar P, Thakkar HP. Lopinavir metered-dose transdermal spray through microporated skin: Permeation enhancement to achieve therapeutic needs. *J Drug Deliv Sci Tec* 2015;29:173-80. doi:10.1016/j.jddst.2015.07.004
71. Ranade S, Bajaj A, Londhe V, Babul N, Kao D. Fabrication of topical metered dose film forming sprays for pain management. *Eur J Pharm Sci* 2017;100:132-41. doi: 10.1016/j.ejps.2017.01.004
72. Klose KT-J, Tran NTK, Morgon TM, Finnin BC, Reed BL. inventors; Monash University, assignee. Transdermal delivery of antiparkinson agents. United States patent US 20040013620A1. 2004 Jan 22.
73. Morgan T, Bakalova M, Klose K, Finnin B, Reed B. inventors; Monash University, assignee. Transdermal delivery of hormones. United States patent US20040028725 A1. 2004 Feb 12.
74. Lulla A, Malhotra G, Raut P. inventors. U & I Pharmaceuticals Ltd., assignee. Topical spray compositions. United States patent US6962691 B1. 2005 Nov 5.
75. Lulla A, Malhotra G. inventors; Cipla Pvt. Ltd., assignee. Transdermal pharmaceutical spray formulations comprising a vp/va copolymer and a non-aqueous vehicle. US2005041943A1. 2005 May 12
76. Watkinson A, Finnin BC, Wilkins NF, inventors; AcruX DDS Pty Ltd., assignee. Method and system for transdermal administration of volatile active. United States patent US2008128280A1. 2008 Oct 30.
77. Wan KS, Watkinson A. inventors; AcruX DDS Pty Ltd., assignee. Transdermal delivery system for hormones and steroids. United States patent US 20100279988A1. 2010 Nov 4.
78. Morgan TM, Wilkins NF, Klose KT-J, Finnin BC, Reed BL, inventors; AcruX DDS Pty Ltd., assignee. Transdermal delivery rate control using amorphous pharmaceutical compositions. United States patent US 008784878B2. 2014 Jul 22.
79. Khafagy ELS, Morishita M, Onuki Y, Takayama K. Current challenges in non-invasive insulin delivery systems: A comparative review. *Adv Drug Deliv Rev* 2007;59(15):1521-46. doi:10.1016/j.addr.2007.08.019

80. http://www.acrux.com.au. Accessed 21 November 2017.
81. http://www.acrux.com.au/product/ellavie-evamist]. Accessed 21 November 2017.
82. Yoo JW, Lee CH. Drug delivery systems for hormone therapy. *J Control Release* 2006;112(1):1-14. doi: 10.1016/j.jconrel.2006.01.021
83. http://www.acrux.com.au/product/axiron/. Accessed 21 November 2017.
84. https://www.eurekalert.org/pub_releases/2007-07/ra-ado071607.php. Accessed 26 November 2017.
85. Sitruk-Ware R. Routes of delivery for progesterone and progestins. *Maturitas* 2007;57(1):77-80. doi: 10.1016/j.maturitas.2007.02.015
86. Sitruk-Ware R, Small M, Kumar N, Tsong YY, Sundaram K, Jackanicz T. Nestorone: clinical applications for contraception and HRT. *Steroids* 2003;68(10-13):907-13.
87. Fraser IS, Weisberg E, Kumar N, Kumar S, Humberstone AJ, McCrossin L, et al. An initial pharmacokinetic study with metered dose transdermal systemfor delivery of the progestogen Nestorone as a possible future contraceptive. *Contraception* 2007;76(6):432-38. doi: 10.1016/j.contraception.2007.08.006
88. https://pipeline.ctiexchange.org/products/nes-transdermal-spray. Accessed 21 December 2017.
89. Coulman S, Allender C, Birchall J. Microneedles and other physical methods for overcoming the stratum corneum barrier for cutaneous gene therapy. *Crit Rev Ther Drug Carrier Syst* 2006;23(3):205-58.
90. https://pharma.aptar.com/en-us/delivery-routes/dermal-transdermal.html. Accessed 22 December 2017.

Preparation and Characterization of *Pistacia khinjuk* Gum Nanoparticles Using Response Surface Method: Evaluation of Its Anti-Bacterial Performance and Cytotoxicity

Ali Fattahi[1,2,3], Tahereh Sakvand[4], Marziyeh Hajialyani[3], Behzad Shahbazi[2], Mohammad Shakiba[5], Ahmad Tajehmiri[1], Ebrahim Shakiba[6]*

[1] *Medical Biology Research Center, Kermanshah University of Medical Sciences, Kermanshah, Iran.*
[2] *Nano Drug Delivery Research Center, Faculty of Pharmacy, Kermanshah University of Medical Sciences, Kermanshah, Iran.*
[3] *Pharmaceutical Sciences Research Center, Faculty of Pharmacy, Kermanshah University of Medical Sciences, Kermanshah, Iran.*
[4] *Department of Medicinal plants, Kermanshah Jahade-Daneshgahi, Institute of Higher Education, Kermanshah, Iran.*
[5] *Student Research Committee, Kermanshah University of Medical Sciences, Kermanshah, Iran.*
[6] *Department of Biochemistry, Medical School, Kermanshah University of Medical Sciences, Kermanshah, Iran.*

Article info

Keywords:
· Antibacterial activity
· Cytotoxicity
· Nanoparticle
· *Pistacia Khinjuk*
· Response Surface Model

Abstract
Purpose: This study aims to prepare a novel, natural nanoparticle (NP) as a drug carrier, which also has inherent therapeutic effects.
Methods: *Pistacia khinjuk* gum NPs were prepared and Response surface methodology (RSM) was used for statistical analysis of data and optimizing the size of NPs.
Results: NPs were in the range of 75.85–241.3 nm. The optimization study was carried out, and an optimized size (70.86nm) was obtained using DMSO as a solvent. The volume of the organic phase was 111.25µl, and the concentration of gum was 1% w/v. The cell viability assay was performed on the pure gum and NPs toward β-TC_3, MCF7, and HT29 cell lines. It was observed that NPs have higher cytotoxic activity in comparison with pure gum, and that the IC_{50}value was achieved at 1% of NPs in β-TC_3 cells. The obtained NPs demonstrated antibacterial activity against two bacterial strains (*Pseudomonas aeruginosa* and *Staphylococcus aureus*).
Conclusion: Altogether, according to the obtained results, these NPs with inherent cytotoxicity and antibacterial activity are an attractive carrier for drug delivery.

Introduction

Pistacia khinjuk is one of the major Pistacia species that grows in some of Mediterranean countries (they have especially been widely distributed in the *Zagrossian* region of Iran) and classified into the *Anacardiaceae* family. Different parts of the plant, including resin, leaf, bark, fruit, and aerial parts, can be used as traditional medicine.[1] They have been used for a long time as useful remedies for the treatment and prevention of different kinds of diseases such as asthma and stomach discomfort, throat infections, burns, nausea, eczema, vomiting, and toothaches;[2-5] specifically, the gum resin has exhibited wound healing activity that could be used for the treatment of brain and gastrointestinal disturbances.[2] Due to the literature reports, *p. khinjuk* has exhibited inherent anti-inflammatory, antileishmanial, antipyretic, antioxidant, antitumor, antiviral, antiasthmatic, and antimicrobial properties.[2,6,7] In addition to these common medical applications *p.khinjuk* gum could be a candidate as a new natural biopolymer for drug delivery systems.

According to the literature review, the fabrication of p.khinjukgum NPs and using them as a novel delivery vehicle has not been previously investigated. Due to the numerous desirable characteristics and advantages of *p.khinjuk* gum in therapeutic objectives, the fabrication of *p.khinjuk* gum NPs as drug carriers was investigated in this study. The obtained data was statistically analyzed using RSM, which combines statistical and mathematical techniques to fit experimental data to the model for optimization processes.[8]

Materials and Methods

Materials

P.khinjuk gum was collected from the exudates of the trunk of *p.khinjuk* tree (from Oshtoran-Kooh Mountain, in Azna, Lorestan province, Iran) in July 2014. The organic solvents (acetone, ethanol and DMSO) were purchased from Merck (Germany). Trypsin-ethylenediamine tetra acetic acid (EDTA) was supplied from Ben Yakhte, Iran. DMEM (Dulbecco's Modified Eagle's Medium) and Roswell Park Memorial Institute

***Corresponding author:** Ebrahim Shakiba, Email: eshakiba@kums.ac.ir medium (RPMI) were procured from Gibco, Scotland. Thiazolyl blue (MTT) was purchased from Merck, Germany.All of the other compounds were of analytical grade from Merck.

Preparation of NPs

The organic solutions were prepared using three organic solvents (ethanol, acetone, and DMSO). *P.khinjuk* gum with three different amounts of 0.1, 0.55, and 1g, was dissolved in 100 ml of each organic solvent to prepare three different concentrations of *p.khinjuk* gum (0.1%, 0.55%, and 1%w/v).Then 100, 500, and 1000 µl of each stock solution was added dropwise to 10 ml of distilled water under stirring. The resulting solutions were stirred for 1 h at 2500 rpm and at room temperature.

Experimental design

In this study, optimization of the size of NPs was carried out according to the Central Composite Face-Centered Design (CCFD) and using Design-Expert software (Version 8.0.7.1, statEase, Inc., USA).

Characterization of NPs

The size of fabricated particles was assessed and analyzed by Zetasizer (Nano-ZS, Malvern, UK) using dynamic light scattering (DLS).
The morphology and structure of NPs were observed by a transmission election microscope (TEM, Zeiss-EM10C, 80 KV, Germany).

Cell viability assay

In this study, β-TC_3 (a mouse beta pancreatic cell line), was purchased from Iran genetic resources center. MCF7 (a human breast cancer cell line) and HT29 (a human colon adenocarcinoma cell line) were purchased from Pasteur Institute of Iran. The thiazolyl blue assay has been used in experiments for the assessment of cell viability. Briefly, cells were seeded at density of 5×10^4 cells/ml in 96-well tissue culture. After 24 h, cells were incubated with increasing concentrations of pure gum and NPs (1%, 0.5%, 0.25%, and 0.125% w/v) for 48 h separately. Then the MTT assay was performed to measure the cell viability according to previous study.[9]

Antibacterial test

Pseudomonas aeruginosa (ATCC27853), as a standard strain, and *Staphylococcus aureus*, as a clinicallyisolated strain, in the Microbiology Laboratory of Imam Khomeini Hospital (Kermanshah, Iran) were used in this study.
Serial dilutions (1.5%, 1.3%, 1.1%, 0.9%, and 0.7%) of the NPs were made in Mueller-Hinton Broth containing 5% DMSO for bacteria, in 96-well micro titer plates. 20 µl of fresh microbial suspensions was prepared from overnight grown cultures containing 1.5×10^8 organisms/ml and were added to each well. The final volume of culture was 200 µl per each well.
Ampicillin and water were used as positive and negative controls, respectively. The MTT assay was performed to assess the (MIC) and MBC of the extract of NPs using MTT solution with concentration of 5.0 mg/ml.

Results and Discussion

Response Surface Model

Table 1 shows the actual form of factors and the experimental size of NPs, as the response. Based on the data, the range of responses was found from 75.85–241.3 nm. The response function was fitted by a quadratic polynomial model.

Table 1. Factors in actual form, and experimental size data

Organic phase volume (µl)	Concentration of gum (w/v%)	Solvent type	Size(nm)
1000	0.55	Ethanol	159
1000	0.55	Acetone	195.6
1000	0.55	DMSO	118.2
550	0.55	Acetone	189.66
550	0.55	DMSO	114.6
550	0.55	Acetone	183.3
550	0.55	Ethanol	117.1
550	0.55	Ethanol	116.5
550	0.55	Ethanol	113.5
550	0.55	Acetone	149.66
550	0.55	DMSO	105.9
550	0.55	Acetone	164.1
550	0.55	DMSO	100.9
550	0.55	DMSO	98.02
550	0.55	Ethanol	138
550	0.55	DMSO	107.3
550	0.55	Ethanol	134.1
550	0.55	Acetone	168.4
100	0.55	DMSO	78.86
100	0.55	Acetone	135.6
100	0.55	Ethanol	107.1
1000	1	DMSO	102
1000	1	Ethanol	186.6
1000	1	Acetone	241.3
550	1	DMSO	87.52
550	1	Acetone	202.3
550	1	Ethanol	164.5
100	1	Acetone	186.6
100	1	DMSO	97.2
100	0.1	Ethanol	144.8
1000	0.1	DMSO	155.2
1000	0.1	Acetone	140
1000	0.1	Ethanol	118
550	0.1	DMSO	114.5
550	0.1	Ethanol	82.96
550	0.1	Acetone	106.9
100	0.1	Acetone	96.32
100	0.1	DMSO	104.5
100	0.1	Ethanol	75.853

To find the best model correlating the response to process variables the analysis of variance (ANOVA) by calculating F-value was employed. It is important to note that the p-values< 0.05 indicate a better significance of model terms. The lack of fit F-value of 0.7007 revealed that the lack of fit is not significant in response, which indicates low error and accuracy of the model (Table 2). According to the experimental results and using RSM, the response function was fitted by a quadratic polynomial equation. This equation is given as follows in terms of coded factors:

$$\text{Z average} = +50.85+0.05828A+89.116B-0.0145\ AB\ \text{(ethanol)} \quad (1)$$

$$\text{Z average} = +71.027+0.0666A+114.2620B-0.0145\ AB\ \text{(acetone)} \quad (2)$$

$$\text{Z average} = +100.63+0.0431A-24.427B-0.0145\ AB\ \text{(DMSO)} \quad (3)$$

Where Z average is the average of size, A is the volume of the organic phase, and B is the percentage of gum in the solution.

The regression analysis shows that all the linear coefficients of the independent variables, and also the interaction of the volume of the organic phase and the percentage of gum in the solution, are significant (where $p<0.05$).

The coefficient of determination (R^2), adjusted R^2, and predicted R^2 of the model were found 0.93, 0.92, and 0.90, respectively.

Table 2. Analysis of Variance

Source	Sum of Squares	D_f	Mean Square	F-Value	p-value	Prob> F
Model	55183.41	6.00	9197.24	76.88	< 0.0001	Significant
A-Organic solvent volume	8409.62	1.00	8409.62	70.30	< 0.0001	
B-Concentration of gum	9734.17	1.00	9734.17	81.37	< 0.0001	
C-Type of solvent	23772.23	2.00	11886.12	99.36	< 0.0001	
BC	13267.39	2.00	6633.70	55.45	< 0.0001	
Residual	3827.95	32.00	119.62			
Lack of Fit	2143.51	20.00	107.18	0.76	0.7132	not significant
Pure Error	1684.44	12.00	140.37			
Cor Total	59011.36	38.00				

Figure 1 shows the distributed plot of the predicted amounts versus the actual amounts for the size of NPs. The closer the points are to the 45 degree line, the better the estimations of the RSM model. Based on this plot, the model could appropriately fit the data.

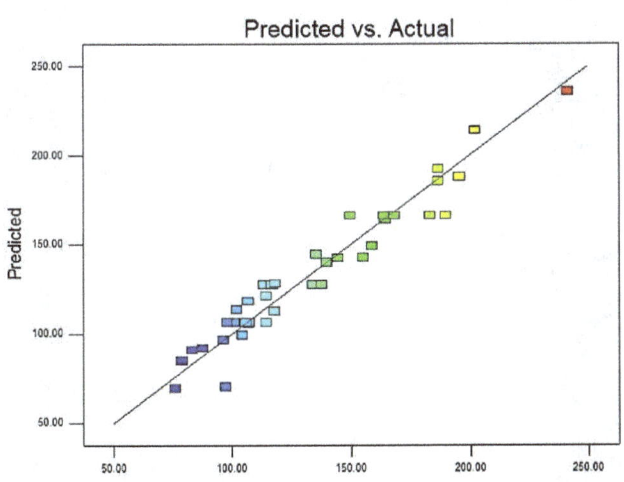

Figure 1. Predicted versus actual values of Zaverage for RSM mode

Figure 2 shows the response surface 3D plots exhibiting the effects of interactions between the volume of the organic phase and the concentration of gum in the organic phase.

Effect of process parameters on the size of NPs

The size of the fabricated NPs was measured and the results are tabulated in Table 1. In the presence of ethanol and acetone, increasing the gum concentration causes fabrication of larger NPs. But in the presence of DMSO, the results were the inverse, and increasing the concentration of gum resulted in the reduction in the size of NPs. As the concentration of gum in the organic phase increases, the size of fabricated NPs increases due to an increase in the viscosity of organic solution and the hindering of the diffusion of solvents to water. Diminution in viscosity leads to the facilitation of solvent diffusion to the outer aqueous solution and consequently, production of smaller particles.[10] This trend was conversely when DMSO was used as the organic solvent. This incongruity may arise from possible interactions between *p.khinjuk* gum and DMSO molecules.

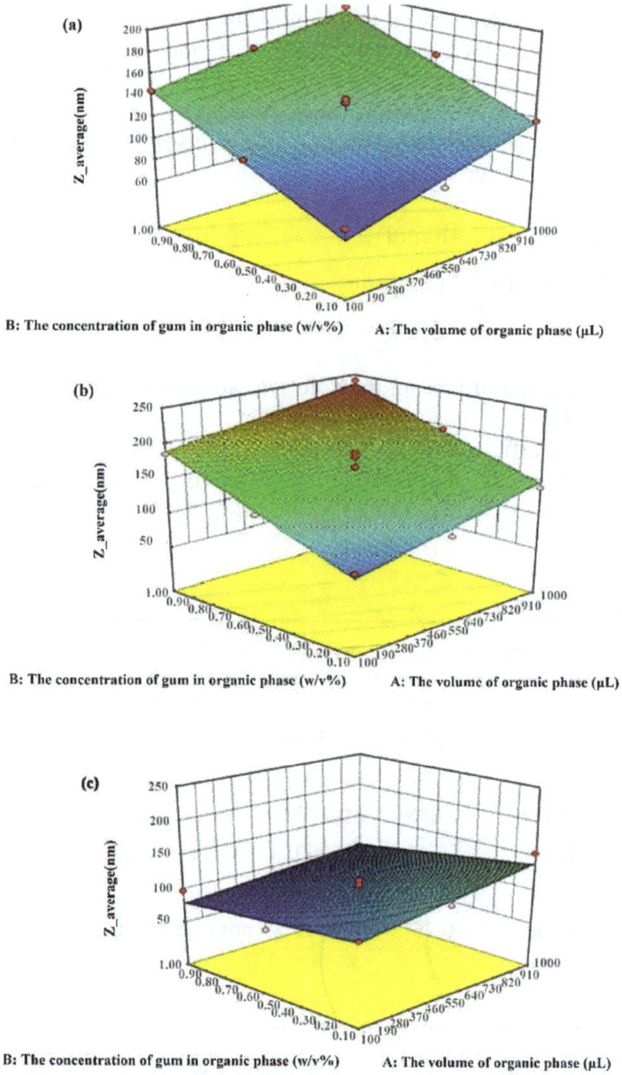

Figure 2. The effect of volume of organic phase and the concentration of gum in organic solution on Z average of NPs obtained by a) ethanol; b) acetone; and c) DMSO as organic solvent.

The results also revealed that, at constant volume of aqueous solution, increasing the volume of the organic phase (increasing the volume ratio of the organic to aqueous solutions) results in an increase in the size of fabricated NPs. Decreasing the ratio of organic to aqueous solutions can improve the diffusion of organic solvent, and it increases the distribution efficiency of the organic phase into the external phase, leading to formation of smaller NPs. This reason has been evoked in the similar studies.[11]

The size of NPs using different solvents is exhibited in Table 1. The comparison revealed that using DMSO as the solvent, results in smaller NPs at the highest concentration of gum. DMSO was chosen as the most suitable solvent due to the production of smaller particles. It is worthmentioning that the selection of organic solvent could be directly affected by individual key parameters, such as a solvent dielectric constant and the affinity of the solvent for water. The miscibility of solvents in water is an important parameter that should be considered. The higher miscibility of the solvent in water causes the higher rate of diffusion into the aqueous phase, and consequently, the production of smaller NPs. The miscibility of solvents in water could be evaluated regarding the mutual solubility parameter ($\Delta\delta$), The smaller $\Delta\delta$ indicates the higher affinity.The $\Delta\delta$ has been evaluated 27, 28.7, and 34.4 MPa$^{1/2}$ for ethanol, DMSO, and acetone, respectively.[12]

Optimization and model validation

To determine the optimum condition for the lowest Z average, some solutions would be suggested by the software. Based on these results, the optimum size of NPs was obtained using DMSO as the organic solvent (using 111.25 μl of organic phase and 1% of gum). For model validation, experiments were performed by using the aforementioned optimum conditions. The experimental response for optimized NP size was 73.18 nm, and the prediction error was found 0.0327 (<0.05), which confirms the validity of model in optimizing the size of NPs.

Morphology of NPs

The TEM result of the suspension of NPs (at the concentration of 1% w/v using DMSO as organic phase) is visualized in Figure 3. The polydispersity index of these NPs was measured using Zetasizer. According to the TEM observation, particles were found to be relatively spherical, and the size of the obtained NPs was less than 100 nm. The obtained NPs were monodisperse, and the polydispersity of NPs was found 0.07, which confirms the narrow size distribution of NPs. The measured values resulted from TEM was comparable with the DLS results.

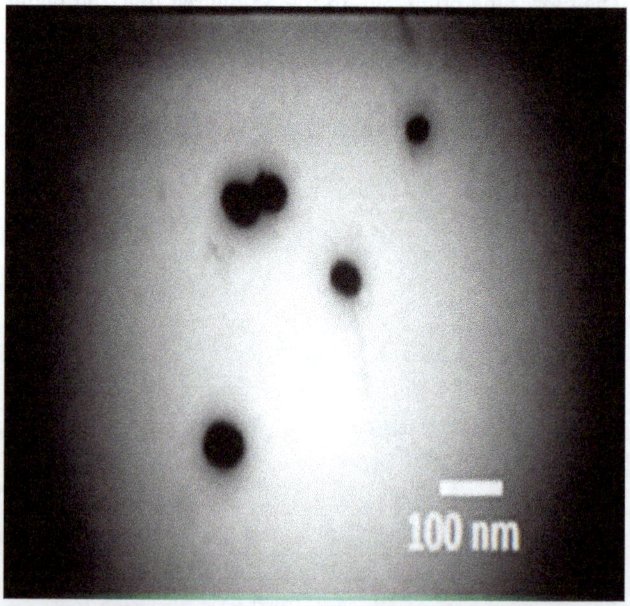

Figure 3. TEM of the suspension of NPs in DMSO with the concentration of 1% w/v.

The cytotoxicity test

The MTT results indicated that NPs have higher cytotoxic activity compare to pure gum in all three cell lines (β-TC_3, MCF7, and HT29), while NPs and gum exhibited the relatively highest cytotoxic activity towards β-TC_3 (Figure 4). The IC_{50}value was achieved at 1% of NPs in β-TC_3. The results revealed that the cytotoxicity of pure gum and NPs does not reach IC_{50} in HT29 and MCF7 cell line. The cytotoxic activity of NPs and pure gum can be attributed to the high content of terpenes in *p.khinjuk* gum structure.[13] The Hedgehog (Hh) signaling pathway is a critical element regulating cellular growth and organizing differentiation during embryonic development, which plays a significant role in different types of cancer.[14,15] Terpenes possess the ability to affect and target the Hh pathways and have been used for treating cancer. This pathway has been frequently discussed in the treatment of pancreatic cancer and has a significant effect on the treatment of this cancer, but it has no significant effect on HT29; the effect of this pathway on colon cancer is not clear. The Hh pathway also affects breast cancer, but there have some inconsistent reports on the effect of Hh on the MCF7 cell line. While this pathway has been found effective on the MCF7 cell line, its growth could not be inhibited by cyclopamine.[15,16] There is no clear report for the mechanism of Hh activation in breast cancer, and the mechanism of Hh effect on MCF7 is not clear yet.

The higher cytotoxic activity of NPs could be due to the small size of the particles and advantageous for nano-sized particles. Furthermore, it could be noted that pure gum is insoluble in water, while NPs could disperse homogenously in water and are able to transport more into cells, thus achieving lower cell viability and showing greater cytotoxicity compared to gum.

Measurement of antibacterial activity

Table 3 shows the results of antibacterial activity of NPs towards both performed bacterial strains.The inhibition activity of the samples can be attributed to the fact that the major constituent of gum is α-pinene. The antimicrobial activity of α-pinene has been reported in the literature.[17]

Conclusion

In the current study, *p.khinjuk* gum NPs, were prepared as novel drug carriers and the size of particles could be altered with different affecting parameters. The optimization was performed, and the optimum size was achieved using 111.25μl of DMSO, and 1% (w/v) of gum, with the NP size of 70.86 nm (obtained by model). The effect of experimental parameters on the size of NPs was obtained by fitting experimental data with a quadratic equation with a prediction error less than 0.05. The obtained NPs were found monodisperse and spherical, according to the DLS and TEM results. The obtained NPs had higher cytotoxic activity in comparison with pure gum and its IC_{50} value was achieved at 1% of NPs in β-TC_3. These NPs also possess inherent antibacterial activity and could be good candidates for treatment and as carriers in drug delivery systems.

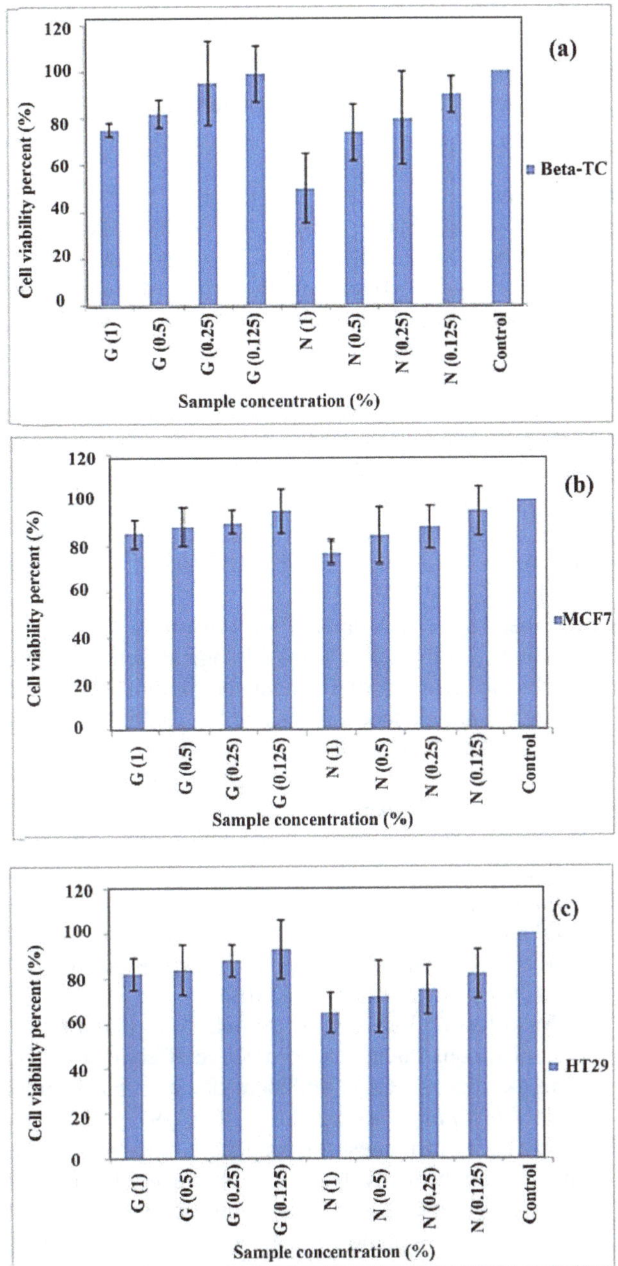

Figure 4. Cell viability of pure gum and NP on a) β-TC_3; b) MCF7; and c) HT29 cell lines (*G refers to Gum and N refers to NP).

Table 3. The antibacterial activity of NPs.

Bacterial Strains	Concentration				
	0.7%	0.9%	1.1%	1.3%	1.5%
Pseudomonas aeruginosa	+	+	MIC	+	MBC
staphylococcus aureus	+	+	MIC	MBC	_

Acknowledgments
The authors would like to acknowledge the Research Council of Kermanshah University of Medical Sciences for supporting this work (Research grant No.94219).

Conflict of Interest
The authors declare no conflict of interests.

References
1. Ezatpour B, Saedi Dezaki E, Mahmoudvand H, Azadpour M, Ezzatkhah F. In vitro and in vivo antileishmanial effects of Pistacia khinjuk against leishmania tropica and leishmania major. *Evid Based Complement Alternat Med* 2015;2015:149707. doi: 10.1155/2015/149707
2. Bozorgi M, Memariani Z, Mobli M, Salehi Surmaghi MH, Shams-Ardekani MR, Rahimi R. Five Pistacia species (P. vera, P. atlantica, P. terebinthus, P. khinjuk, and P. lentiscus): a review of their traditional uses, phytochemistry, and pharmacology. *Scientific World J* 2013;2013:219815. doi: 10.1155/2013/219815
3. Hacibekiroglu I, Yilmaz PK, Hasimi N, Kilinc E, Tolan V, Kolak U. In vitro biological activities and fatty acid profiles of Pistacia terebinthus fruits and Pistacia khinjuk seeds. *Nat Prod Res* 2015;29(5):444-6. doi: 10.1080/14786419.2014.947492
4. Ghasemi Pirbalouti A, Aghaee K. Chemical composition of essential oil of Pistacia khinjuk stocks grown in bakhtiari zagross mountains, iran. *Electron J Biol* 2011;7(4):67-9.
5. Tohidi M, Khayami M, Nejati V, Meftahizade H. Evaluation of antibacterial activity and wound healing of Pistacia atlantica and Pistacia khinjuk. *J Med Plant Res* 2011;5(17):4310-4.
6. Moussa AY, Labib RM, Ayoub NA. Isolation of chemical constituents and protective effect of Pistacia khinjuk against CCl4–induced damage on HepG2 cells. *Phytopharmacology* 2013;4(4):1-9.
7. Nazari H, Yavarmanesh M, Haddad Khodaparast MH. In vitro study to evaluate the antibacterial effect of Pistacia khinjuk stocks oil as compared with olive oil on food borne pathogenic bacteria (staphylococcus aureus, escherichia coli, listeria monocytogenes). *J Essent Oil Bear Plants* 2016;19(1):125-33. doi: 10.1080/0972060X.2014.971067
8. Bezerra MA, Santelli RE, Oliveira EP, Villar LS, Escaleira LA. Response surface methodology (RSM) as a tool for optimization in analytical chemistry. *Talanta* 2008;76(5):965-77. doi: 10.1016/j.talanta.2008.05.019
9. Shahbazi B, Taghipour M, Rahmani H, Sadrjavadi K, Fattahi A. Preparation and characterization of silk fibroin/oligochitosan nanoparticles for sirna delivery. *Colloids Surf B Biointerfaces* 2015;136:867-77. doi: 10.1016/j.colsurfb.2015.10.044
10. Chorny M, Fishbein I, Danenberg HD, Golomb G. Lipophilic drug loaded nanospheres prepared by nanoprecipitation: Effect of formulation variables on size, drug recovery and release kinetics. *J Control Release* 2002;83(3):389-400. doi: 10.1016/S0168-3659(02)00211-0
11. Budhian A, Siegel SJ, Winey KI. Haloperidol-loaded plga nanoparticles: Systematic study of particle size and drug content. *Int J Pharm* 2007;336(2):367-75. doi: 10.1016/j.ijpharm.2006.11.061
12. Galindo-Rodriguez S, Allemann E, Fessi H, Doelker E. Physicochemical parameters associated with nanoparticle formation in the salting-out, emulsification-diffusion, and nanoprecipitation methods. *Pharm Res* 2004;21(8):1428-39. doi: 10.1023/B:PHAM.0000036917.75634.be
13. Mirian M, Behrooeian M, Ghanadian M, Dana N, Sadeghi-Aliabadi H. Cytotoxicity and antiangiogenic effects of Rhus coriaria, Pistacia vera and Pistacia khinjuk oleoresin methanol extracts. *Res Pharm Sci* 2015;10(3):233-40.
14. Kubo M, Nakamura M, Tasaki A, Yamanaka N, Nakashima H, Nomura M, et al. Hedgehog signaling pathway is a new therapeutic target for patients with breast cancer. *Cancer Res* 2004;64(17):6071-4. doi: 10.1158/0008-5472.CAN-04-0416
15. Rifai Y, Arai MA, Koyano T, Kowithayakorn T, Ishibashi M. Terpenoids and a flavonoid glycoside from Acacia pennata leaves as hedgehog/GLI-mediated transcriptional inhibitors. *J Nat Prod* 2010;73(5):995-7. doi: 10.1021/np1000818
16. Zardawi SJ, O'Toole SA, Sutherland RL, Musgrove EA. Dysregulation of hedgehog, wnt and notch signalling pathways in breast cancer. *Histol Histopathol* 2009;24(3):385-98. doi: 10.14670/HH-24.385
17. Habibi Najafi MB, Hajimohamadi Farimani R, Tavakoli J, Madayeni S. GC-MS Analysis and Antimicrobial Activity of the Essential Oil of Trunk Exudates of Pistacia atlantica var. mutica. *Chem Nat Compd* 2014;50(2):376-8. doi: 10.1007/s10600-014-0959-z

Improvement of Meloxicam Solubility Using a β-Cyclodextrin Complex Prepared via the Kneading Method and Incorporated into an Orally Disintegrating Tablet

Ahmad Ainurofiq[1,2], Syaiful Choiri[1,2]*, Muhamad Ali Azhari[1], Chaterin Romauli Siagian[1], Bambang Budi Suryadi[1], Fea Prihapsara[1], Sholichah Rohmani[1]

[1] *Department of Pharmacy, Sebelas Maret University, Ir. Sutami 36A, Surakarta, 57126, Indonesia.*
[2] *School of Pharmacy, Institut Teknologi Bandung, Ganesha 10, Bandung, 40132, Indonesia.*

Article info

Keywords:
· Meloxicam
· β-cyclodextrin
· Kneading
· Orally disintegrating tablet
· Quality by design

Abstract
Purpose: The aim of this research was to formulate and develop an orally disintegrating tablet (ODT) that incorporated a MEL/β-CD complex, using a quality by design (QbD) approach to enhance solubility and drug release.
Methods: Multiple regression linear analysis was conducted to develop the kneading process and ODT formulation. Mixing time and amount of solvent were used as independent variables in kneading process optimisation, while the superdisintegrants were used to obtain the desired formulation. Fourier transform infrared spectroscopy and differential scanning calorimetry were performed for complex characterization.
Results: MEL/β-CD complexation was successful in enhancing MEL solubility. The results suggest that increasing the amount of solvent and mixing time enhances drug loading and drug release. However, increased solvent amounts present the problem of removing the solvent. Primojel and Polyplasdone had a significant effect on the water wicking and tablet disintegration process ($p<0.05$), although Polyplasdone negatively affected tablet hardness. Both an optimized KN process and ODT formulation were obtained using a QbD approach.
Conclusion: Incorporation of the MEL/β-CD complex during ODT formulation using the QbD approach serves as a model for ODT product development, with optimal product performance based on the specification of quality target product profiles. To understand more specific phenomena, one point in the middle of the design for each factor should be added to more powerfully estimate this effect and avoid the lack of estimate due to an inadequate equation.

Introduction

Drugs with poor water solubility present the challenge of low bioavailability. Furthermore, the rate limiting step in the absorption of a poorly water-soluble drug depends on its solubility.[1] Several methods have been developed to enhance the solubility of poorly water-soluble drugs, e.g. addition of solubilizing agents, dispersion of amorphous solids,[2] cyclodextrin complexation,[3] co-crystal formulation,[4] nano crystal formulation,[5] lipid formulation,[6] etc.

Cyclodextrin (CD) complexation is feasible method that has been used in the pharmaceutical industry to enhance solubility, drug release, and drug stability. Depending on the glucopyranose units, CD is divided into three types, i.e. α, β, and γ-CD, and to enhance their water solubility, modification of functional groups and substitution have been used.[7,8] In CD complexation, many preparation methods have been utilized, e.g. grinding, kneading, co-precipitation, spray drying, freeze drying, microwave radiation, etc.[3,9,10] These methods give different results in terms of yield, complexation efficiency, and input energy required.

The kneading (KN) method is a feasible, economic, less time consuming, and simple preparation method, obtains higher complexation yields, and is easier and more reproducible than the other methods.[10,11] Studies on the kneading process have been reported that interaction between guest molecules and CD occur during solidification of the paste.[9,10] Enhancement of dissolution using kneading was also observed for diclofenac sodium and CD with better results than their physical mixtures.[12] Some process parameters of kneading using carvedilol and β-CD, i.e. mixing time, amount added and frequency of solvent addition, affected the complex.[13] The result of complex formation is related to the level of interaction between drug and β-CD in aqueous solution and in solid state; therefore, it depends on the kneading process.[10]

Quality by design (QbD) is a development approach that uses statistical and multivariate analyses to assess and investigate the influence of each factor/critical process

***Corresponding author:** Syaiful Choiri, Emails: syaiful.apt@student.uns.ac.id; s.choiri@yahoo.co.id

parameter (CCP) on critical quality attributes (CQAs) based on a quality target product profile (QTPP). Design experimentation (DoE) based on the QbD approach can minimize the number of runs and help obtain product knowledge.[14] The purpose of this study was to formulate and develop an orally disintegrating tablet (ODT) that incorporated meloxicam (MEL)/β-cyclodextrin (β-CD) to enhance its solubility and drug release, using the QbD approach to assess the factors studied.

Materials and Methods

Materials

Meloxicam (MEL, Lot No. 400240798) was obtained from Dexa Medica (Palembang, Indonesia), Avicel PH 102 was obtained from FMC Biopolymer (NJ, USA), Polyplasdone was obtained from ISP Pharmaceuticals (NJ, USA), and β-Cyclodextrin (β-CD, Kleptose) was obtained from Roquette (France). Sodium starch glycolate (Primojel), mannitol (Pearlitol 400DC) and sodium stearyl fumarate (Pruv) were obtained from DFE Pharma (Foxhol, the Netherlands), Roquette (Lestrem, France) and JRS Pharma (Rosenberg, Germany), respectively. All of the APIs and excipients were used as received.

Methods

MEL/β-CD complex preparation

Preparation of the MEL/β-CD complex was performed by the kneading method. Optimization of the kneading method was conducted to obtain an optimized complex that would be incorporated into the ODT formulations. A 2^2 factorial design was applied to optimize the KN process. Mixing time and the amount of solvent were used as independent variables, while the dependent variables were drug release (dissolution efficiency over 30 min; DE_{30min}) and entrapment efficiency (%EE) of the complex. The experimental design of the KN process is presented in Table 1 (in the KN Process section).

The drug release of the complex was determined via a dissolution test using the USP apparatus II model. A 500 ml of deionized water was used as a dissolution medium at a stirring rate of 100 rpm, and temperature was kept constant at 37±0.5°C. A MEL/β-CD complex equivalent to 5 mg MEL was used as the sample. 5 ml aliquots were withdrawn at 10, 15, 30, 45, and 60 min, with replacement of fresh medium at the same temperature. All the samples were analysed spectrophotometrically at λ_{max} 361 nm. Dissolution efficiency (DE) was calculated using following equation:

$$\mathrm{DE} = \frac{\int_0^{30} y\delta t}{100T} \times 100\% \qquad (1)$$

Where y is the amount of drug released over time t and T is total time. DE was calculated for drug release over 30 min (DE_{30min}).

Entrapment efficiency (%EE)/drug loading was calculated based on the free amount of MEL in the MEL/β-CD complex. 100 mg of complex was washed with a small amount of 0.1 mol/L sodium hydroxide in methanol followed by methanol, and the amount of MEL in treated complex was determined spectrophotometrically at 361 nm. %EE was calculated using following equation:

$$\%\mathrm{EE} = \frac{A-B}{A} \times 100\% \qquad (2)$$

Where A is the theoretical amount of MEL in the MEL/β-CD complex and B is the amount of MEL after washing.

The optimized complex was obtained based on the desirability function of DE_{30min} and %EE using factorial design as an experimental design.

Table 1. Design of experiments of KN process and ODT formulation

Run	Coded level			
	KN Process		ODT formulation*	
	A	B	C	D
1	-1	-1	-1	-1
2	+1	-1	+1	-1
3	-1	+1	-1	+1
4	+1	+1	+1	+1
Coded level			-1	+1
A : Mixing time (min)			20	40
B ; Amount of solvent (ml)			4	12
C; Primojel (mg)			2	18
D ; Polyplasdone (mg)			2	18

*center point was added triplicates to estimate the curvature

Characterization of optimized complex

The optimized complex was characterized using spectroscopic analysis, thermal analysis, and solubility.

Solubility characterization for MEL and the MEL/β-CD complex was performed. Briefly, 50 mg of MEL or optimized complex was added to 5 ml double distilled water and sonicated for 15 min, followed by stirring for 48 h at ambient temperature. The saturated solubility of MEL in pure MEL and in complex was measured spectrophotometrically using UV spectroscopy at 361 nm.

In spectroscopic analysis, Fourier transform infrared spectroscopy Shimadzu 8400S (Kyoto, Japan) was utilized to identify the interaction between MEL and β-CD using potassium bromide pellets. 1% of the sample was dispersed on potassium bromide and compressed with 6 kN of compression force for 5 min. The pellet was scanned at wavenumber of 4000 – 400 cm^{-1} with resolution of 2 cm^{-1} and 10 iterations.

In thermal analysis, LINSEIS PT1600 (NJ, USA) differential scanning calorimetry was performed using 10 mg samples at 20°C/min under nitrogen atmosphere.

Tablet preparation

The direct compression method was used for tablet preparation. The optimized complex equivalent to 7.5 mg MEL was used in tablet formulation. The weight of the tablet for all formulations was kept constant at 200 mg and contained 30 mg Avicel PH102, 2 mg Pruv, and variable mounts of Pearlitol 400DC depending on

Primojel and Polyplasdone concentrations. The proportions of Primojel and Polyplasdone as independent variables in tablet formulation are presented in Table 1 (in the ODT Formulation section). All of the components in the formulation, except for lubricant, were passed through a 60 mesh sieve and blended in a cube mixer for 15 min at 25 rpm. Pruv was passed through a 100 mesh sieve, added to the blend and mixed for 2 min at 25 rpm. The final blends were compressed using a Korsch XP-1 single punch tablet (flat-face punch, diameter 8 mm).

Post-compression evaluation

Post-compression evaluation of the tablets looked at weight variation (n = 20 tablets), friability testing (n = 20 tablets) using a Gouming friability tester, and tablet hardness (n = 10 tablets) using a Gouming YD-1 hardness tester.

Water wicking was assessed based on tablet wetting time. The wetting time evaluation was performed using a petri dish and filter paper. Briefly, two pieces of paper filter were placed in the petri dish (diameter 10 cm) and 5 ml of 0.1% (w/v) dye solution was used. Wetting time was reported as the time required for the dye to reach the entire surface of the tablet.

The disintegration test was carried out using a USP model disintegration tester, with 900 ml of distilled water as the medium. Six tablets were used as samples and the disintegration time was measured semi-automatically until the tablet passed through the sieve.

In vitro drug release

Drug release was determined using an Electrolab TDT 08L dissolution tester type apparatus II (paddle method), with 900 ml of phosphate buffer (pH 7.5) as the dissolution medium, temperature maintained at 37±0.5°C, and a stirring rate of 50 rpm. 5 ml aliquots were withdrawn at 0.5, 1, 2, 3, 5, 7, and 10 min, with replacement of 5 ml of the fresh medium. All samples were analysed spectrophotometrically at λ_{max} 361 nm. The amount of drug released at 1 minute (Q_{1min}) and DE_{30min} (calculated based on Equation 1) were used as drug release parameters to determine the optimized formulation.

Statistical analysis and optimization

The data obtained were analysed using Design Expert® software version 7.1.5 (Stat-Ease Inc., Minneapolis, MN, USA). Factorial models, including the intercept, main effect, and interactions, were generated for all the response variables using multiple linear regression analysis (MLRA). The models were evaluated based on several statistical parameters, including the determination coefficient (R^2), adjusted determination coefficient (Adj. R^2), predicted determination coefficient (Pred. R^2) and adequate precision (adeq. precision).

The significance of a factor's effect on the response was determined by F test or p-value of analysis of variance (ANOVA), with a confidence interval of 95% (p=0.05). These were calculated using the Design Expert® software. Contour plots were constructed based on the equations of the responses; such plots are useful for elucidating the interaction effects of factors on the response. The optimal formulation, was obtained by superimposing the contour plots for each parameter.[15]

Results and Discussion

Complex preparation and optimization

Enhancing the solubility of poorly water soluble drugs can be achieved via β-CD complexation.[7,8] The greater the solubility, the faster the drug release. The drug release profiles of MEL from the MEL/β-CD complex are presented in Figure 1. Almost all of the drug was released by 60 min, indicating that the complexation of MEL and β-CD enhanced drug release compared to MEL alone (about 40% of MEL was released at 60 min; data not shown). Differences in process parameters, i.e. the amount of solvent and mixing time, lead to different amounts of drug released. Therefore, to estimate the effects of the amount of solvent and mixing time on drug release and drug loading, and to obtain the optimized process parameters for kneading, the QbD paradigm using factorial design was employed.

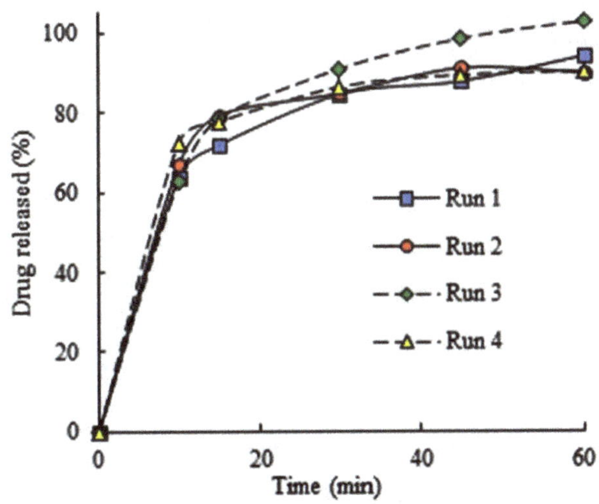

Figure 1. MEL released from MEL/β-CD complexes using kneading method

Since the DE_{30min} shows the drug release profiles from point to point,[15] the DE_{30min} was used to assess drug release. Based on a factorial design approach for DE_{30min}, the mathematical function for MLRA of DE_{30min} is presented in Table 2. In the equation for DE_{30min}, the intercept was 63.93, and is obtained in the centre point combination of each level. The amount of solvent (regression coefficient of 1.54) significantly affected DE_{30min} ($p < 0.05$) while mixing time did not (regression coefficient of 0.79; $p > 0.05$). An increase in solvent increased the dissolved β-CD and thus increased the possibility interaction between MEL and β-CD more so than β-CD in solid state, where interaction occurs only on the surface of the solid[9]. Interaction between the amount of solvent and mixing time (regression coefficient of -0.54) did not significantly decrease

DE_{30min} ($p > 0.05$). Figure 2a shows the influence of the amount of solvent and mixing time on DE_{30min}. At low mixing times, an increase in solvent increased the DE_{30min} higher than at high mixing times. The lowest DE_{30min} values were obtained with low mixing time and amount of solvent, while the highest DE_{30min} values were obtained with high mixing time and amount of solvent. Thus, increasing the mixing time and amount of solvent increased the drug release.

Table 2. Statistical parameter and regression coefficient of equation of DE_{30min} and %EE in KN process optimization

Parameters	β_0	A	B	AB	Model (p-value)	R^2	Adj.R^2	Pred R^2	AP
DE_{30min} (p-value)	63.93	0.79** (0.073)	1.54* (0.009)	-0.58** (0.150)	0.0235*	0.886	0.800	0.543	7.11
%EE (p-value)	83.39	1.64* (0.027)	3.41* (0.002)	-0.27** (0.598)	0.0066*	0.940	0.895	0.761	10.55

β_0 = intercept; A,B, and AB = regression coefficient of (A), (B), and (A) (B); AP = adequate precision; * = significant term ($p < 0.05$); ** = not significant term ($p > 0.05$)

Efficiency of complexation can be assessed using drug loading/MEL trapped on β-CD (%EE). This function is based on free MEL after the KN process. Based on the factorial design approach for %EE, the mathematical function of the MRLA of %EE is presented in Table 2. From this equation, an intercept of 83.39 was obtained. While the amount of solvent (regression coefficient of 3.41) was a more dominant factor in terms of increasing the %EE than mixing time (regression coefficient of 1.64), both of factors were statistically significant ($p < 0.05$). However, the interaction of both was not statistically significant ($p > 0.05$). An increase in the amount of solvent enhanced MEL and β-CD dissolution, therefore increasing the interaction between MEL and β-CD, and MEL was incorporated into the β-CD cavity, but not completely. The contour plot of %EE is presented in Figure 2b, and shows a similar pattern to the DE_{30min} contour plot. To obtain the optimal process conditions for both DE_{30min} and %EE, the contour plots were combined to create desirability function and are presented in Figure 2c. A high mixing time (40 min) and amount of solvent (12 ml) were chosen as the optimized KN process and incorporated into the ODT formulations based on their giving the highest desirability value.

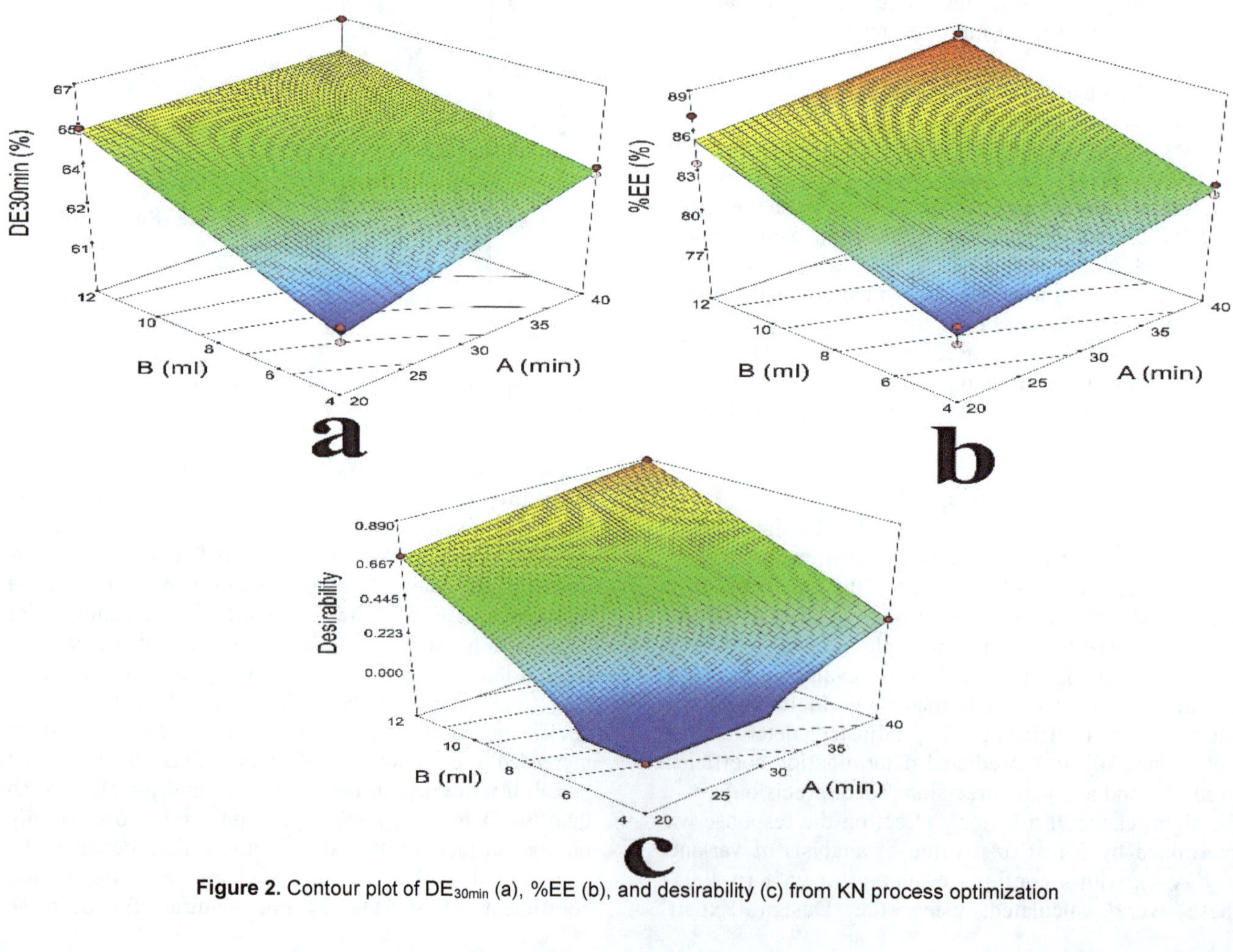

Figure 2. Contour plot of DE_{30min} (a), %EE (b), and desirability (c) from KN process optimization

Complex characterization

Characterization of the optimized KN MEL/β-CD complex was conducted, including evaluation of solubility enhancement, spectroscopic analysis using FTIR and thermal analysis using DSC. The solubility study showed that the MEL solubility and optimized KN in water (pH 6.7) were 10.57±1.11 and 58.68±4.00 μg/ml (measured at 27±1°C; ambient temperature), respectively. Therefore, complexation of MEL and β-CD increased the solubility of MEL 5.55-fold. The FTIR study was done to characterize the interaction between MEL and β-CD, and the results are presented in Figure 3. The MEL spectrum showed the vibration of N-H stretching at wavenumber 3300 cm^{-1}. The peaks at wavenumbers 1600 and 1150 cm^{-1} are due to C=N and S=O stretching vibrations, respectively. The spectrum FTIR of β-CD was assigned with peaks at wavenumbers 3300 (OH stretching vibration; broad peak) and 1000 cm^{-1} (OH bending vibration). Moreover, the FTIR spectrum of the physical mixture was the combination of both peaks of MEL and β-CD. Overall, in the KN complex, all of the MEL peaks appeared, and the KN and MEL spectra showed decreased intensity, especially at wavenumber 1200 to 1600 cm^{-1}. Therefore, the FTIR spectra confirmed that MEL was not completely loaded into the β-CD. The DSC thermogram (Figure 4) of MEL showed an endothermic peak with an onset at 259°C due to melting point. The β-CD and optimized KN thermograms showed a broad spectrum from 90–150°C (onset around 140°C) due to loss of water crystals from the structure lattice. An endothermic peak at around 259°C was not observed in the KN complex, although a small endothermic peak with low intensity was observed at 257°C due to peak shifting. The shifting to a lower melting point corresponded to an increase in solubility, and a decrease in intensity corresponded to the amount of unloaded MEL.

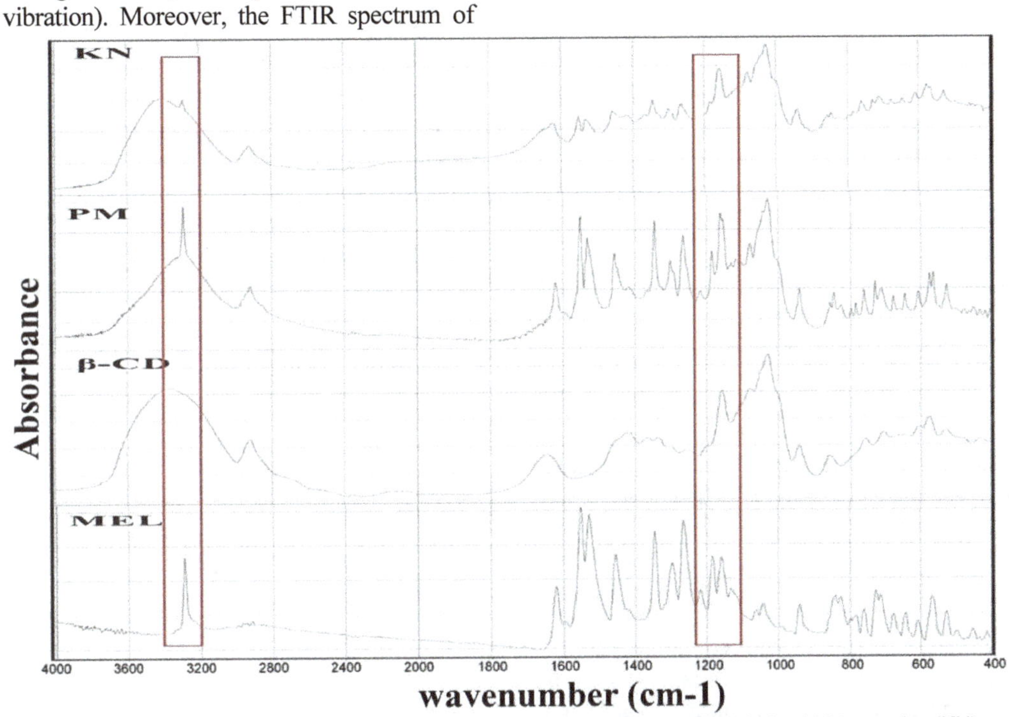

Figure 3. FTIR spectra of MEL, β-CD, their physical mixture (PM), and optimized KN complex (KN)

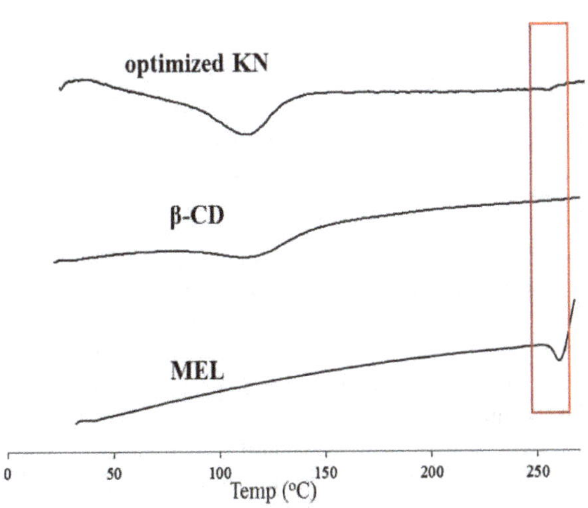

Figure 4. DSC thermogram of MEL, β-CD, and optimized KN complex

Tablet formulation and optimization

The optimal KN process to obtain an optimized complex with the highest DE_{30min} and %EE was incorporated into ODT formulations. Development of ODT formulations was conducted via the QbD approach, using factorial design. A preliminary study found a unique effect of the combination of crospovidone (Polyplasdone) and sodium starch glycolate (Primojel) on water wicking and disintegration process (data not shown). Thus, the effect of these factors on tablet physical properties (hardness, friability, wetting time (WT), disintegration time (DT) and drug release) was determined using the QbD approach to obtain the preferred design space or control strategy. Based on a factorial design approach, a mathematical model that describes the influence of Primojel and Polyplasdone was developed and is presented in Table 3.

Table 3. Statistical parameter and regression coefficient of ODT optimization

Statistic		Hardness	Friability	WT	DT	DE_{20min}
Regression coefficient	Intercept	31.13	0.55	26.21	18.99	73.06
	C	0.025**	-0.049*	-4.51*	-0.88*	-0.28**
	(p-value)	(0.9383)	(0.0176)	(<0.0001)	(0.0424)	(0.5549)
	D	-3.93*	-0.087*	-6.79*	-3.47*	1.39*
	(p-value)	(<0.0001)	(0.0005)	(<0.0001)	(<0.0001)	(0.0123)
	CD	3.78*	-0.033**	6.77*	4.51*	2.05*
	(p-value)	(<0.0001)	(0.0818)	(<0.0001)	(<0.0001)	(0.0012)
p-value	Curvature	0.3493**	0.6048**	0.1313**	0.2205**	0.0168*
	Model	<0.0001*	0.0010*	<0.0001*	<0.0001*	0.0024*
Fitting equation	R^2	0.9676	0.7883	0.9789	0.9590	0.7489
	Adj. R^2	0.9579	0.7248	0.9725	0.9467	0.6736
	Pred. R^2	0.9272	0.5237	0.9524	0.9078	0.4351
	AP	24.45	7.88	27.53	21.20	7.54

* = significant term ($p < 0.05$); ** = not significant term ($p > 0.05$); AP = adequate precision

ODT formulations must have sufficient strength to maintain their physical properties;[16] thus, hardness and friability as CQAs were used to determine the tablet strength. Hardness of all ODT formulations ranged from 22.9 to 39.4 N, with similar compression pressures and friability varying from 0.366 to 0.701%. The factorial design approach was applied to assess the effects of Primojel and Polyplasdone on the hardness and friability of ODT formulations, and the results are presented in Table 3.

Based on the hardness equation, the model was significant, with an intercept of 31.13 for the centre point of design and no significant difference with the curvature ($p > 0.05$). Polyplasdone (regression coefficient of -3.93) significantly decreased hardness ($p < 0.05$), while Primojel (regression coefficient of 0.025) had no significant affect on ODT hardness ($p > 0.05$). This indicates that Primojel is more compactible than Polyplasdone. Sodium starch glycolate is a more plastic, deformable material than crospovidone, and this characteristic therefore significantly affected hardness.[17,18] The interaction of Primojel and Polyplasdone significantly increased hardness due to recovery by Primojel's plastic deformation characteristic ($p < 0.05$). The friability equation was significant ($p < 0.05$), while the curvature was not ($p > 0.05$), and the intercept was 0.55. Polyplasdone (regression coefficient of -0.087) had a preferable effect on the friability, reducing it to a greater extent than Primojel (regression coefficient of -0.049) and was statistically significant ($p < 0.05$). Although Primojel did not reduce the hardness of the ODT formulation, lower interparticle bonding of Primojel increased friability; a similar result was reported in which an increased concentration of Primojel increased tablet friability.[17] The contour plots of tablet hardness and friability were used to elucidate the effects of Primojel and Polyplasdone on hardness and friability in the range of the design space. The lowest and highest hardness values were obtained at a low level of Primojel/high level of Polyplasdone and a low level of each factor, respectively. This indicates that increased superdisintegrant concentration reduces the hardness. With Primojel at a low concentration, an increase in Polyplasdone reduced the hardness to a greater extent than with Primojel at a high concentration. The greatest hardness value does not necessarily mean the lowest friability, as the lowest friability was obtained at a high level of each factor, and friability proportionally decreased with an increase in concentration of both superdisintegrants.

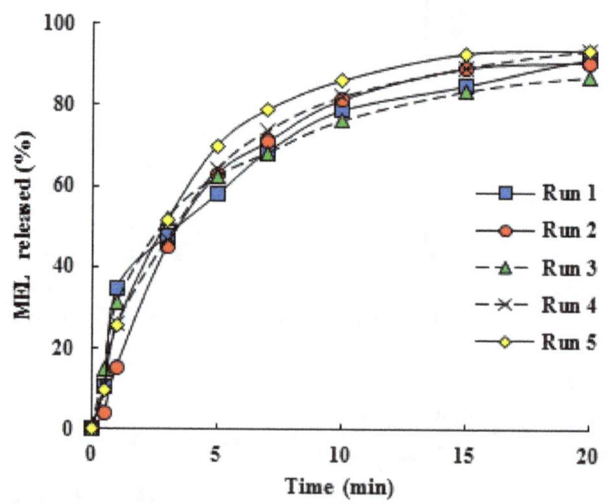

Figure 5. MEL released profiles from ODT MEL/β-CD complex

Rapid disintegration time was the desirable characteristic for the ODT formulations. In this phenomenon, the water wicking process and swelling mechanism is followed by interparticular breaking. The water wicking process was evaluated by WT. The WT and DT varied from 17.34 to 46.79 s and 10.63 to 28.88 s, respectively. Factorial design was applied to assess and elucidate the effects of Primojel and Polyplasdone on WT and DT, and the results are presented in Table 3. The WT and DT equations were significant ($p < 0.05$ for both) and the curvatures did not have a significant difference from intercept ($p > 0.05$ for both). The intercepts for WT and DT were 26.21 and 18.99, respectively. Primojel, Polyplasdone, and the interaction of both had significant effects on WT and DT ($p < 0.05$ for all). Polyplasdone (WT and DT regression coefficients of -6.79 and -3.47, respectively) reduced WT and DT to a greater extent than Primojel (WT and DT regression coefficients of -4.51 and -0.88, respectively). This effect was induced by the disintegration mechanism of the superdisintegrant. Polyplasdone is dominant in water wicking through water capillary action, although Primojel has a swelling mechanism.[16,17,19] The combination of both had an undesirable effect, increasing the WT and DT based on the factorial design approach. This phenomenon involved an increase in the distance of water wicking due to the swelling action of Primojel and Primojel's gelling characteristic at high concentrations.

Drug release was depicted by the drug release profiles of the ODT formulations, which are presented in Figure 5. The drug release profiles for all runs showed a similar drug release pattern; for all drug runs, almost all of the MEL was released by 20 min. Therefore, DE_{20min} was used to compare the drug release profiles, and factorial design was applied to assess the drug release. The DE_{20min} equation was significant, but undesirable fitting of the curvature was found to be statistically significant ($p < 0.05$). This indicated that the fit of model was not appropriate to fit the model at the centre point of design space. Primojel (regression coefficient of -0.28) had not statistically significant effect on DE_{20min} ($p > 0.05$), but Polyplasdone and the interaction of both (regression coefficient of 1.39 and 2.05, respectively) significantly increased DE_{20min}. Although Primojel did not significantly affect drug release, the coefficient of regression had a negative sign, indicating the gelling properties of Primojel at high concentrations.

The desired model required a significant model term to indicate that the model could be used to describe the CQAs and that curvature was not significant. Therefore, the factorial model is adequate for estimating the pure error. The fitting model was used to characterize an appropriate and adequate equation for describing the CPPs on CQAs, i.e. the R^2 should be sufficiently high (more than 0.7), the difference between Adj. R^2 and Pred. R^2 should not more than 0.2, and AP should be more than 4. The inability to obtain an estimate occurs due to an inadequate or inappropriate equation.

The design space for an optimal formulations could be determined by the QTPP of the ODT formulations, such as sufficient tablet strength (hardness greater than 25 N and friability less than 0.5%; in pharmaceutical development, friability less than 0.8 is preferable[20]), rapid water wicking (WT less than 30 s), rapid disintegration (DT less than 20 s) and high drug release (DE_{20min} greater than 75%). Based on these criteria, the non-linear optimal design space of the ODT formulation was achieved and is presented in Figure 6f. The non-linear combination is yellow in colour, and from it, the linear combination to obtain the optimum design space is shown to be Primojel 8.5-9% and Polyplasdone 8-9%, and the optimized ODT formulation was obtained at Primojel 8.5% and Polyplasdone 9%.

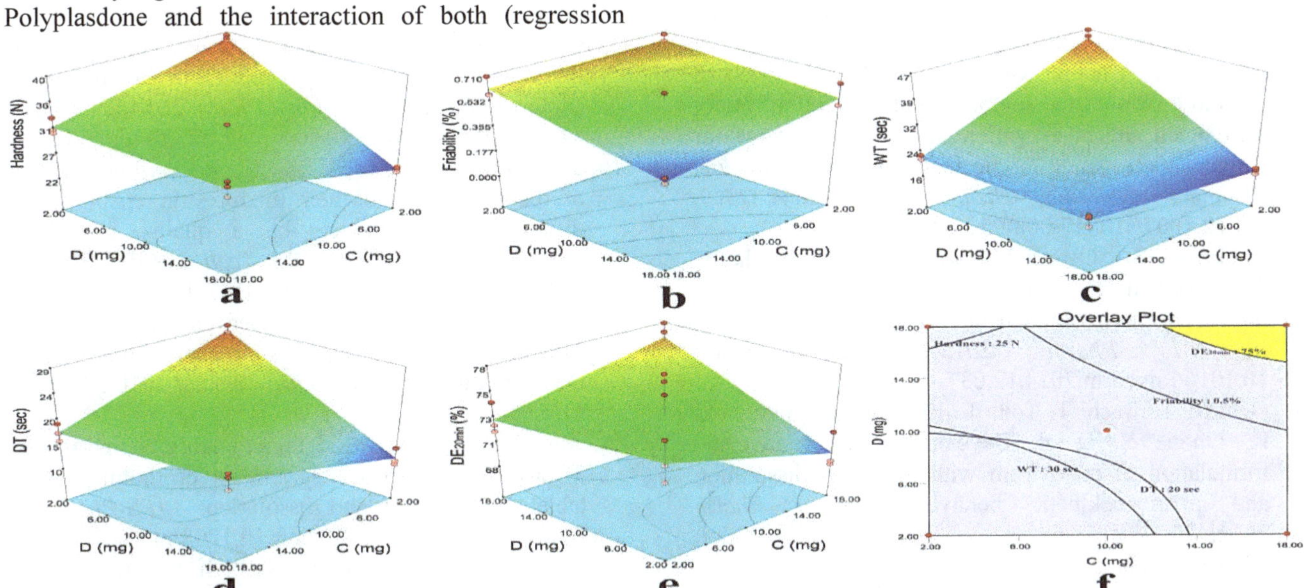

Figure 6. Contour plot of hardness (a), friability (b), WT (c), DT (d), DE_{20min} (e), and superimposed contour plot (f)

Conclusion

The QbD approach was successful for assessing and investigating the effect of mixing time and amount of solvent in the KN process and obtaining the optimized KN process conditions to be incorporated into ODT formulations. The results suggest that increasing the amount of solvent and mixing time enhances drug loading and drug release, although increasing the amount of solvent appears to have the problem of solvent removal. In the ODT formulation, Primojel and Polyplasdone had a significant effect on wicking properties, the disintegration process, and hardness. Incorporation of the MEL/β-CD complex into the ODT formulation using the QbD approach serves as a model for ODT product development with optimal product performance based on the specifications of the QTPP. To understand more specific phenomena, one point in the middle of the design space for each factor called as curvature should be added into the 2^2 factorial design, providing a powerful equation to estimate the effects on drug release and drug loading, and to avoid the inability to obtain an estimate due to an inadequate equation.

Acknowledgments
Muhammad Ali Azhari, Chaterin R. Siagian, and Bambang R. Suryadi would like to thank the DIPA UNS for financial support. Syaiful Choiri also would like to thanks Dexa Medica (Palembang, Indonesia), Roquette (Lestrem, France), DFE Pharma (Foxhol, the Netherlands), JRS pharma (Rosenberg, Germany) for providing API and excipients. All authors declare that they have no conflict on interest.

Conflict of Interest
The authors report no conflicts of interest in this work.

References
1. Loftsson T, Muellertz A, Siepmann J. For the special ijp issue "poorly soluble drugs". *Int J Pharm* 2013;453(1):1-2. doi: 10.1016/j.ijpharm.2013.05.056
2. Rahman Z, Zidan AS, Khan MA. Risperidone solid dispersion for orally disintegrating tablet: Its formulation design and non-destructive methods of evaluation. *Int J Pharm* 2010;400(1-2):49-58. doi: 10.1016/j.ijpharm.2010.08.025
3. Obaidat AA, Khanfar RA, Khawam MN. The effect of β-cyclodextrin on the solubility and dissolution rate of meloxicam and investigation of the driving force for complexation using molecular modeling. *J Incl Phenom Macro Chem* 2009;63(3-4):273–9. doi:10.1007/s10847-008-9517-2
4. El-Gizawy SA, Osman MA, Arafa MF, El Maghraby GM. Aerosil as a novel co-crystal co-former for improving the dissolution rate of hydrochlorothiazide. *Int J Pharm* 2015;478(2):773-8. doi: 10.1016/j.ijpharm.2014.12.037
5. Ochi M, Kawachi T, Toita E, Hashimoto I, Yuminoki K, Onoue S, et al. Development of nanocrystal formulation of meloxicam with improved dissolution and pharmacokinetic behaviors. *Int J Pharm* 2014;474(1-2):151-6. doi: 10.1016/j.ijpharm.2014.08.022
6. Prabhu S, Ortega M, Ma C. Novel lipid-based formulations enhancing the in vitro dissolution and permeability characteristics of a poorly water-soluble model drug, piroxicam. *Int J Pharm* 2005;301(1-2):209-16. doi: 10.1016/j.ijpharm.2005.05.032
7. Brewster ME, Loftsson T. Cyclodextrins as pharmaceutical solubilizers. *Adv Drug Deliv Rev* 2007;59(7):645–66. doi:10.1016/j.addr.2007.05.012
8. Kurkov SV, Loftsson T. Cyclodextrins. *Int J Pharm* 2013;453(1):167–80. doi:10.1016/j.ijpharm.2012.06.055
9. Gil A, Chamayou A, Leverd E, Bougaret J, Baron M, Couarraze G. Evolution of the interaction of a new chemical entity, eflucimibe, with gamma-cyclodextrin during kneading process. *Eur J Pharm Sci* 2004;23(2):123-9. doi: 10.1016/j.ejps.2004.06.002
10. Salustio PJ, Feio G, Figueirinhas JL, Pinto JF, Cabral Marques HM. The influence of the preparation methods on the inclusion of model drugs in a beta-cyclodextrin cavity. *Eur J Pharm Biopharm* 2009;71(2):377-86. doi: 10.1016/j.ejpb.2008.09.027
11. Torricelli C, Martini A, Muggetti L, Eli M, De Ponti R. Stability studies on steroidal drug/β-cyclodextrin kneaded systems. *Int J Pharm* 1991;75(2):147–53. doi:10.1016/0378-5173(91)90188-T
12. Das S, Subuddhi U. Studies on the complexation of diclofenac sodium with β–cyclodextrin: Influence of method of preparation. *J Mol Struct* 2015;1099:482–9. doi:10.1016/j.molstruc.2015.07.001
13. Pamudji JS, Mauludin R, Lestari VA. Improvement of carvedilol dissolution rate through formation of inclusion complex with B-cyclodextrin. *Int J Pharm Pharm Sci* 2014;6(4):228–33.
14. International Conference on Harmonisation. Guidance for Industry Q8 (R2) Pharmaceutical Development. 2009. http://www.fda.gov/downloads/Drugs/.../Guidances/ucm073507.pdf. Accessed 22 August 2015
15. Choiri S, Sulaiman TNS, Kuncahyo I. Optimization and acessing the influence of xanthan gum, effervescent components and hardness on floatation behavior and drug release of gastro-floating captopril tablet. *Indonesian J Pharm* 2014;25(4):255–64. doi:10.14499/indonesianjpharm25iss4pp255
16. Desai PM, Er PX, Liew CV, Heng PW. Functionality of disintegrants and their mixtures in enabling fast disintegration of tablets by a quality by design approach. *AAPS Pharm Sci Tech* 2014;15(5):1093-104. doi: 10.1208/s12249-014-0137-4
17. Zhang Y, Wrzesinski A, Bertran H, Moses M. Comparison of Superdisintegrants in Orally Disintegrating Tablets. *Pharm Technol* 2010;34(7):54–61.
18. Zhao N, Augsburger LL. Functionality comparison of 3 classes of superdisintegrants in promoting aspirin tablet disintegration and dissolution. *AAPS Pharm Sci Tech* 2005;6(4):E634-40. doi: 10.1208/pt060479
19. Rahman Z, Siddiqui A, Khan MA. Orally disintegrating tablet of novel salt of antiepileptic drug: Formulation strategy and evaluation. *Eur J Pharm Biopharm* 2013;85(3 Pt B):1300-9. doi: 10.1016/j.ejpb.2013.06.006
20. United States Pharmacopeial Convention. Tablet Friability. In: United Stated Pharmacopoeia 35-National Formulary 30. Rockville, Maryland, USA: The United States Pharmacopeial Convention; 2012.

Permissions

 Every chapter published in this book has been scrutinized by our experts. Their significance has been extensively debated. The topics covered herein carry significant findings which will fuel the growth of the discipline. They may even be implemented as practical applications or may be referred to as a beginning point for another development.

The contributors of this book come from diverse backgrounds, making this book a truly international effort. This book will bring forth new frontiers with its revolutionizing research information and detailed analysis of the nascent developments around the world.

We would like to thank all the contributing authors for lending their expertise to make the book truly unique. They have played a crucial role in the development of this book. Without their invaluable contributions this book wouldn't have been possible. They have made vital efforts to compile up to date information on the varied aspects of this subject to make this book a valuable addition to the collection of many professionals and students.

This book was conceptualized with the vision of imparting up-to-date information and advanced data in this field. To ensure the same, a matchless editorial board was set up. Every individual on the board went through rigorous rounds of assessment to prove their worth. After which they invested a large part of their time researching and compiling the most relevant data for our readers.

The editorial board has been involved in producing this book since its inception. They have spent rigorous hours researching and exploring the diverse topics which have resulted in the successful publishing of this book. They have passed on their knowledge of decades through this book. To expedite this challenging task, the publisher supported the team at every step. A small team of assistant editors was also appointed to further simplify the editing procedure and attain best results for the readers.

Apart from the editorial board, the designing team has also invested a significant amount of their time in understanding the subject and creating the most relevant covers. They scrutinized every image to scout for the most suitable representation of the subject and create an appropriate cover for the book.

The publishing team has been an ardent support to the editorial, designing and production team. Their endless efforts to recruit the best for this project, has resulted in the accomplishment of this book. They are a veteran in the field of academics and their pool of knowledge is as vast as their experience in printing. Their expertise and guidance has proved useful at every step. Their uncompromising quality standards have made this book an exceptional effort. Their encouragement from time to time has been an inspiration for everyone.

The publisher and the editorial board hope that this book will prove to be a valuable piece of knowledge for researchers, students, practitioners and scholars across the globe.

List of Contributors

Mathrusri Annapurna Mukthinuthalapati, Venkatesh Bukkapatnam and Sai Pavan Kumar Bandaru
Department of Pharmaceutical Analysis & Quality Assurance, GITAM Institute of Pharmacy, GITAM University, Visakhapatnam-530045, India

Elham Ghasemian, Parisa Motaghian and Alireza Vatanara
Pharmaceutics Department, Faculty of Pharmacy, Tehran University of Medical Sciences, Tehran, Iran

Tadiboyina Sirisha and Bannimath Gurupadayya
Department of Pharmaceutical Chemistry, JSS College of Pharmacy, JSS University, Mysore, India

Sridhar Siddiraju
Department of Pharmaceutical Chemistry, Malla Reddy College of Pharmacy, Osmania University, Secunderabad, India

Hamed Hamishehkar
Drug Applied Research Center, Tabriz University of Medical Sciences, Tabriz, Iran

Ali Nokhodchi
Medway School of Pharmacy, Universities of Kent and Greenwich, Central Ave., Chatham Maritime, Kent ME4 4TB, United Kingdom

Saeed Ghanbarzadeh
Biotechnology Research Center, Tabriz University of Medical Sciences, Tabriz, Iran

Maryam Kouhsoltani
Dental and Periodontal Research Center and Faculty of Dentistry, Tabriz University of Medical Sciences, Tabriz, Iran

Sunethra Kalvakuntla, Zenab Attari and Koteshwara Kunnatur B
Department of Pharmaceutics, Manipal College of Pharmaceutical Sciences, Manipal University, Manipal

Mangesh Deshpande
Dr. Reddy's Laboratories Ltd., Hyderabad, India

Mohammad Reza Siahi-Shadbad and Mohammad Barzegar-Jalali
Drug Applied Research Center, Tabriz University of Medical Science, Tabriz, Iran
Faculty of Pharmacy, Tabriz University of Medical Science, Tabriz, Iran

Khosro Adibkia
Drug Applied Research Center, Tabriz University of Medical Science, Tabriz, Iran
Faculty of Pharmacy, Tabriz University of Medical Science, Tabriz, Iran
Research Center for Pharmaceutical Nanotechnology, Tabriz University of Medical Sciences, Tabriz, Iran

Hadi Valizadeh and Alireza Taherpoor
Faculty of Pharmacy, Tabriz University of Medical Science, Tabriz, Iran

Saeed Ghanbarzadeh
Faculty of Pharmacy, Tabriz University of Medical Science, Tabriz, Iran
Student Research Committee, Tabriz University of Medical Sciences, Tabriz, Iran
Research Center for Pharmaceutical Nanotechnology, Tabriz University of Medical Sciences, Tabriz, Iran

Ghobad Mohammadi
School of Pharmacy, Kermanshah University of Medical Science, Kermanshah, Iran

Azim Barzegar-Jalali
Faculty of Medicine, Islamic Azad University, Ardabil Branch, Ardabil, Iran

Abbas Akhgari
Targeted Drug Delivery Research Center, School of Pharmacy, Mashhad University of Medical Sciences, Mashhad, Iran

Ali Tavakol
Nanotechnology Research Center and School of Pharmacy, Ahvaz Jundishapur University of Medical Sciences, Ahvaz, Iran

Mehdi Hassanpour Aghdam
Research Center for Pharmaceutical Nanotechnology, and Students' Research Committee, Tabriz University of Medical Sciences, Tabriz, Iran

Saeed Ghanbarzadeh
Zanjan Pharmaceutical Nanotechnology Research Center, and Department of Pharmaceutics, Faculty of Pharmacy, Zanjan University of Medical Sciences, Zanjan, Iran
Drug Applied Research Center, Tabriz University of Medical Sciences, Tabriz, Iran

Hamed Hamishehkar
Drug Applied Research Center, Tabriz University of Medical Sciences, Tabriz, Iran

Yousef Javadzadeh
Biotechnology Research Center and Department of Pharmaceutics, Faculty of Pharmacy, Tabriz University of Medical Sciences, Tabriz, Iran

Elham Nazemiyeh and Hossein Sheikhloie
Department of Food Engineering, Maragheh Branch, Islamic Azad University, Maragheh, Iran

Morteza Eskandani
Research Center for Pharmaceutical Nanotechnology, Tabriz University of Medical Sciences, Tabriz, Iran

Hossein Nazemiyeh
Faculty of Pharmacy, Tabriz University of Medical Sciences, Tabriz, Iran

Ali Shirani, Samaneh Mohammadi and Samad Mussa Farkhani
Research Center for Pharmaceutical Nanotechnology and Department of Medical Nanotechnology, Faculty of Advanced Medical Sciences, Tabriz University of Medical Sciences, Tabriz, Iran

Ahmad Yari Khosroshahi and Javid Shahbazi Mojarrad
Biotechnology Research Center and Faculty of Pharmacy, Tabriz University of Medical Sciences, Tabriz, Iran

Parvin Zakeri- Milani
Liver and Gastrointestinal Diseases Research Center and Faculty of Pharmacy, Tabriz University of Medical Sciences, Tabriz, Iran

Naser Samadi
Faculty of Advanced Medical Sciences, Tabriz University of Medical Sciences, Tabriz, Iran

Simin Sharifi and Hadi Valizadeh
Drug Applied Research Center and Faculty of Pharmacy, Tabriz University of Medical Sciences, Tabriz, Iran

Jafar Akbari, Majid Saeedi and Maryam Lashkari
Department of Pharmaceutics, Faculty of Pharmacy, Mazandaran University of Medical Sciences, Sari, Iran

Katayoun Morteza-Semnani
Department of Medicinal Chemistry, Faculty of Pharmacy, Mazandaran University of Medical Sciences, Sari, Iran

Hamidreza Kelidari
Pharmaceutical Sciences Research Center, Mazandaran University of Medical Sciences, Sari, Iran

Shringika Soni, Rakesh Kumar Ruhela and Bikash Medhi
Department of Pharmacology, Postgraduate Institute of Medical Education & Research, Chandigarh, 160012, India

Mitra Jelvehgari and Hadi Valizadeh
Drug Applied Research Center, Tabriz University of Medical Sciences, Tabriz, Iran
Faculty of Pharmacy, Tabriz University of Medical Sciences, Tabriz, Iran

Seyed Hassan Montazam
Islamic Azad University of Bonab Unit, Bonab, Iran

Sanam Abbaszadeh
Biotechnology Research Center, Tabriz University of Medical Sciences, Tabriz, Iran
Student Research Committee, Tabriz University of Medical Sciences, Tabriz, Iran

Md. Lutful Amin, Tajnin Ahmed and Md. Abdul Mannan
Department of Pharmacy, Stamford University Bangladesh

Somayeh Sadighian and Hassan Hosseini-Monfared
Faculty of Science, Department of Chemistry, University of Zanjan, Zanjan, Iran

Kobra Rostamizadeh
Zanjan Pharmaceutical Nanotechnology Research Center, Zanjan University of Medical Sciences, Zanjan, Iran
Department of Medicinal Chemistry, School of Pharmacy, Zanjan University of Medical Sciences, Zanjan, Iran

Mehrdad Hamidi
Zanjan Pharmaceutical Nanotechnology Research Center, Zanjan University of Medical Sciences, Zanjan, Iran
Department of Pharmaceutics, School of Pharmacy, Zanjan University of Medical Sciences, Zanjan, Iran

Saieede Soltani
Drug Applied Research Center, Tabriz University of Medical Sciences, Tabriz, Iran
Student Research Committee, Tabriz University of Medical Sciences, Tabriz, Iran

Mitra Jelvehgari
Drug Applied Research Center, Tabriz University of Medical Sciences, Tabriz, Iran
Department of Pharmaceutics, Faculty of Pharmacy, Tabriz University of Medical Sciences, Tabriz, Iran

Parvin Zakeri-Milani
Liver and Gastrointestinal Diseases Research Center, Tabriz University of Medical Sciences, Tabriz, Iran
Department of Pharmaceutics, Faculty of Pharmacy, Tabriz University of Medical Sciences, Tabriz, Iran

Mohammad Barzegar-Jalali
Department of Pharmaceutics, Faculty of Pharmacy, Tabriz University of Medical Sciences, Tabriz, Iran

Vnira Rakhimovna Akhmetova, Nail Salavatovich Akhmadiev and Galiya Maratovna Nurtdinova
Institute of Petrochemistry and Catalysis, Russian Academy of Sciences, 141 Prospekt Oktyabrya, 450075 Ufa, Russia

Rozalia Akramovna Galimova, Albina Midkhatovna Galimova, Eduard Feliksovich, Agletdinov and Valery Alekseevich Kataev
Bashkir State Medical University, 3 Lenin Str., 450008 Ufa, Russia

Ravil Akhmetzyanovich Khisamutdinov
Ufa Institute of Chemistry, Russian Academy of Sciences, 71 Prospekt Oktyabrya, 450054 Ufa, Russia

Dipak Dilip Gadade and Sanjay Sudhakar Pekamwar
School of Pharmacy, S.R.T.M. University, Vishnupuri, Nanded - 431606, India

Mahbubeh Hashemi, Vahid Ramezani, Hossein Jafari and Mina Honarvar
Department of Pharmaceutics, Faculty of Pharmacy, Shahid Sadoughi University of Medical Sciences, Yazd, Iran

Mohammad Seyedabadi
Department of Pharmacology, School of Medicine, Bushehr University of Medical Sciences, Bushehr, Iran

Ali Mohamad Ranjbar
Department of pharmacognosy, Faculty of Pharmacy, Shahid Sadoughi University of Medical Sciences, Yazd, Iran

Hamed Fanaei
Department of Physiology, School of Medicine, Zahedan University of Medical Sciences, Zahedan, Iran

Mohammad Ali Behnam and Farzin Emami
Nano Opto-Electronic Research Center, Electrical and Electronics Engineering Department, Shiraz University of Technology, Shiraz, Iran

Zahra Sobhani
Quality Control Department, Faculty of Pharmacy, Shiraz University of Medical Sciences, Shiraz, Iran

Omid Koohi-Hosseinabadi
Center of Experimental and Comparative Medicine, Shiraz University of Medical Sciences, Shiraz, Iran

Amir Reza Dehghanian
Pathology Department, Shiraz University of Medical Sciences, Shiraz, Iran

Seyed Mojtaba Zebarjad and Mohammad Hadi Moghim
Materials Science and Engineering Department, Engineering School, Shiraz University, Shiraz, Iran

Ahmad Oryan
Pathology Department, School of Veterinary Medicine, Shiraz University, Shiraz, Iran

Khosro Adibkia, Golrokh Khorasani and Shahriar Payab
Drug Applied Research Center and Faculty of Pharmacy, Tabriz University of Medical Sciences, Tabriz, Iran

Farzaneh Lotfipour
Food & Drug Safety Research Center and Faculty of Pharmacy, Tabriz University of Medical Sciences, Tabriz, Iran

Yogesh Joshi
Unipharma LLC., Tamarac, Florida, USA

Srinath Muppalaneni
Sancilio Pharmaceuticals Company, Inc., Riviera Beach, Florida, USA

Alborz Omidian
The University of Chicago, Chicago, IL, USA

David Jude Mastropietro and Hamid Omidian
Department of Pharmaceutical Sciences, College of Pharmacy, Nova Southeastern University, Fort Lauderdale, Florida, USA

Maryam Shirdel and Mehran Moradi
Department of Food Hygiene and Quality Control, Faculty of Veterinary Medicine, Urmia University, 1177, Urmia, West Azarbaijan, Iran

Hossein Tajik
Department of Food Hygiene and Quality Control, Faculty of Veterinary Medicine, Urmia University, 1177, Urmia, West Azarbaijan, Iran
Department of Medicinal and Industrial Plant, Institute of Biotechnology, Urmia University, 1177 Urmia, Iran

Rabinarayan Parhi
GITAM Institute of Pharmacy, GITAM (Deemed to be University), Gandhi Nagar Campus, Rushikonda, Visakhapatnam-530045, Andhra Pradesh, India

Suryakanta Swain
Southern Institute of Medical Sciences, College of Pharmacy, Department of Pharmaceutics, SIMS Group of Institutions, Mangaldas Nagar, Vijyawada Road, Guntur-522 001, Andhra Pradesh, India

Ahmad Tajehmiri
Medical Biology Research Center, Kermanshah University of Medical Sciences, Kermanshah, Iran

Ali Fattahi
Medical Biology Research Center, Kermanshah University of Medical Sciences, Kermanshah, Iran
Nano Drug Delivery Research Center, Faculty of Pharmacy, Kermanshah University of Medical Sciences, Kermanshah, Iran
Pharmaceutical Sciences Research Center, Faculty of Pharmacy, Kermanshah University of Medical Sciences, Kermanshah, Iran

Behzad Shahbazi
Nano Drug Delivery Research Center, Faculty of Pharmacy, Kermanshah University of Medical Sciences, Kermanshah, Iran

Marziyeh Hajialyani
Pharmaceutical Sciences Research Center, Faculty of Pharmacy, Kermanshah University of Medical Sciences, Kermanshah, Iran

Tahereh Sakvand
Department of Medicinal plants, Kermanshah Jahade-Daneshgahi, Institute of Higher Education, Kermanshah, Iran

Mohammad Shakib
Student Research Committee, Kermanshah University of Medical Sciences, Kermanshah, Iran

Ebrahim Shakiba
Department of Biochemistry, Medical School, Kermanshah University of Medical Sciences, Kermanshah, Iran

Muhamad Ali Azhari, Chaterin Romauli Siagian, Bambang Budi Suryadi, Fea Prihapsara and Sholichah Rohmani
Department of Pharmacy, Sebelas Maret University, Ir. Sutami 36A, Surakarta, 57126, Indonesia

Ahmad Ainurofiq and Syaiful Choiri
Department of Pharmacy, Sebelas Maret University, Ir. Sutami 36A, Surakarta, 57126, Indonesia
School of Pharmacy, Institut Teknologi Bandung, Ganesha 10, Bandung, 40132, Indonesia

Index

www.ingramcontent.com/pod-product-compliance
Lightning Source LLC
LaVergne TN
LVHW060554210926
848485LV00005B/1313